Clinical Organ Transplantation

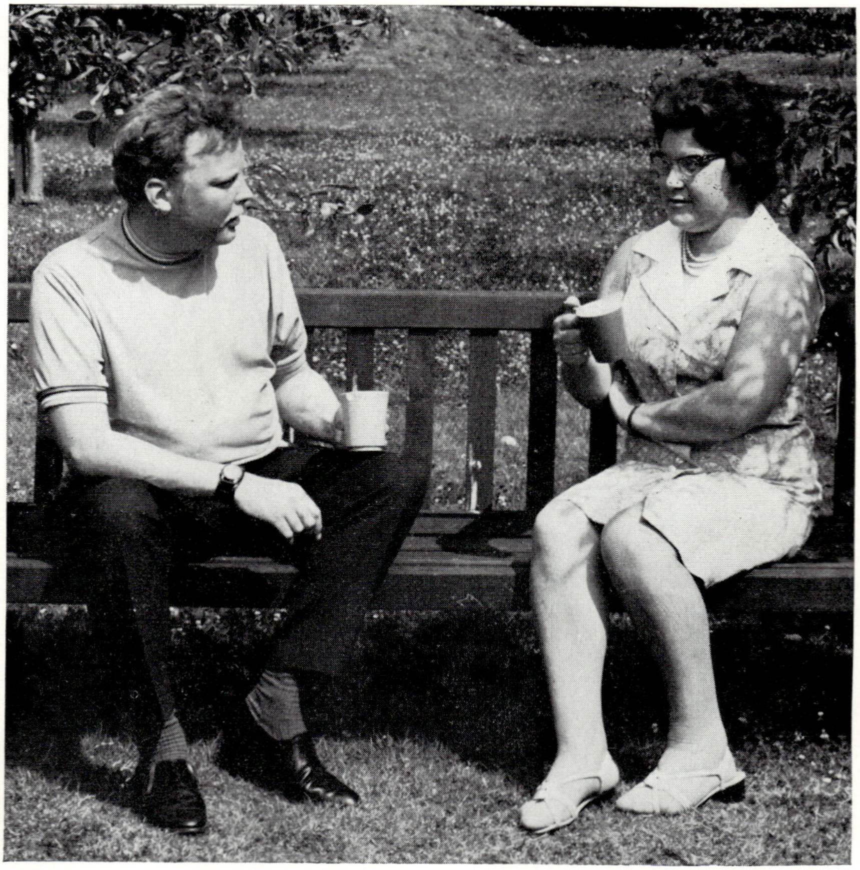

Left: Mr J. L. 5 years after cadaveric renal transplantation; right: Mrs W. S. 2 years after orthoptic liver transplantation.

Clinical Organ Transplantation

edited by R. Y. Calne

M.A. M.S. F.R.C.S.
Professor of Surgery, University of Cambridge
and Fellow of Trinity Hall, Cambridge

Blackwell Scientific Publications
Oxford and Edinburgh

5 Alfred Street, Oxford, England and
9 Forrest Road, Edinburgh, Scotland

ISBN 0 632 07890 1

First published 1971

Distributed in the U.S.A. by
F. A. Davis Company, 1915 Arch Street,
Philadelphia, Pennsylvania

Printed in Great Britain by
Adlard & Son Ltd, Bartholomew Press,
Dorking, Surrey
and bound by
The Kemp Hall Bindery
Osney Mead, Oxford

Contents

PART 2 · KIDNEY TRANSPLANTATION

PART 3 · LIVER TRANSPLANTATION

Acknowledgements

I am extremely grateful to all the contributors in this book for their collaboration in providing their sections on time and to Mr D.C. Dunn, Mr A. Robson and Dr S. Tomlinson for help with proof reading. I am indebted to my secretary, Miss P. Hagan, for her untiring efforts in getting this volume to press. Last, but not least, I thank the Publishers for their help and encouragement.

The authors of chapters 20, 25, 26 and 27 are grateful to the research fellows and clinical staff of the Liver Unit at King's College Hospital, as well as Mr John Winch and Mr John Dawson of the Department of Surgery, who have helped at one time or another in the care of these patients. Members of the Department of Chemical Pathology have also been of invaluable assistance in the post-operative management. We are also indebted to Dr M.G.M. Smith for his considerable assistance with the immunological studies and to Dr M.O. Rake for his work on the haematological changes. Various aspects of the research have been generously supported by grants from the Wellcome Trust and the Wates Foundation.

Introduction

R.Y. Calne

There are now many texts and a huge literature on tissue transplantation. The scientific background is exceptionally wide, stretching from protein chemistry and serology to surgical technique and including most of the disciplines of medicine and pathology. Theory and laboratory speculations have often been out of phase with clinical practice. The objective of organ transplantation differs in no way in principle from that of established medical therapy, it is to restore to a happy and useful life, patients doomed to premature deaths from fatal disease of a vital organ. The cardinal feature of organ transplantation is that the function of the diseased organ is replaced by a biologically active graft. The large numbers of young people dying from renal disease has been a powerful stimulus to progress in organ transplantation. The surgical technique was developed 60 years ago, so to the clinician, graft rejection has been a frustrating humiliation; a poorly understood biological nuisance acting as a barrier against potential therapy. Drs Murray, Merrill and their colleagues at the Peter Bent Brigham Hospital in Boston chose the one situation where the barrier was defective for their early studies of kidney transplantation. They demonstrated more than 15 years ago that excellent treatment could result from [illegible] kidney grafted between identical twins. Since most people dying of fatal [illegible]disease do not have the luxury of a perfect twin donor, the early [illegible] in Boston served to increase efforts directed towards an understanding and overcoming of graft rejection. Unfortunately the body has no discriminatory powers in its natural mechanisms for eliminating foreign invaders. Potentially lethal bacteria and viruses are dealt with in the same way as life-saving tissue grafts. Although to the transplanter this may be infuriating, it is perhaps not surprising. A highly efficient and effective apparatus designed to overcome infection is of obvious survival advantage in evolutionary selection. It happens that this basic biological attribute operates by an exquisitely sensitive recognition ability that mounts a continuous surveillance of all the body constituents, admitting without protest all products belonging to the individual, but immediately recognizing and reacting against any foreign material. The immunity apparatus can detect differences in the biochemical constitution of the cell membrane, that are beyond the capabilities of analytical chemists. Thus the histocompatibility differences between individuals of the same species are recognized and behave as sensitizing antigens.

Efforts to overcome rejection have been crude and empirical. Moreover most work devoted to the subject has been on skin grafts in rodents and it was subsequently found that skin is the most difficult tissue to protect from rejection and immunosuppressive agents effective in rodents did not necessarily have similar actions in man and vice versa. Despite prognostications of gloom and allegations of irresponsibility from some transplantation immunologists, surgeons proceeded to transplant kidneys in man, basing their immunosuppressive regimen on results obtained in the dog. The results have been in excess of the most optimistic hopes of the transplanters. Since every patient surviving with a functioning graft would otherwise be dead or blocking a dialysis space and thereby preventing others from receiving treatment, a survival rate of around 50% at 2 years for grafts from cadavers and approaching 80% when the donor was a close relative, must be considered even by the most bitterly prejudiced opponents of transplantation as worthwhile treatment. Certainly it compares favourably with the results of much effort devoted to the treatment of many forms of cancer. Techniques are now available to transplant every organ, but for a variety of reasons the results of kidney transplantation are at present much the best.

There are only three possible donor sources for clinical organ transplantation, namely live animals, live humans and dead humans. It is most unlikely that organ transplantation across species will be a practical possibility until there is almost full control of the rejction process within a species. This is unfortunate, since the concept of breeding germ free animals to varying required sizes for organ grafting into man is attractive. Entirely normal organs could be grafted with minimal ischaemic damage and many of the present ethical difficulties would be eliminated.

Live humans can only be donors of one of a pair of vital organs, for example the kidney. There are many reasons for preferring not to interfere with a healthy normal individual in order to provide a donor kidney, nevertheless there are situations where grafting a kidney between relatives offers the best chances of success and if certain rather rigorous requirements are fulfilled, the procedure is justified. Grafting from the dead cannot hurt the donor and would seem to be the most suitable donor source at present. There are many difficulties in utilizing organs from cadavers, yet most of these could be solved if there was sufficient understanding within the medical profession and goodwill in the community.

In this book an attempt has been made to present organ transplantation from the point of view of the Clinician. The practical features of transplanting the major parenchymatous organs are discussed. There are preliminary chapters summarizing present knowledge on rejection, immunosuppression, organ storage, prevention of infection and tissue typing, which are problems common to all types of organ transplants. There are individual sections on kidney, liver, heart and lung transplantation and a brief discussion of the possibilities of transplanting other organs and a final chapter concerned with ethics and the law relating to organ grafting. No attempt has been made to provide an exhaustive bibliography, only key references are given, intended as a guide for further reading.

It is hoped that this book may be of use to those embarking on clinical organ grafting, that their patients may profit from the mistakes and experience of others.

Part 1
General

CHAPTER **I**

The Allograft Reaction

B.M. Herbertson

I. INTRODUCTION

Of the numerous factors now known to determine the fate of transplanted living tissue the most significant features in the context of human organ transplantation are the genetic relationship and the consequent antigenic similarities and differences between the donor and the recipient. The impressive clinical study of skin grafting in man by Gibson & Medawar (1943) and the associated investigations in the rabbit by Medawar (1944, 1945) demonstrated beyond reasonable doubt that destruction of allografts ('homografts') is a specific immune phenomenon provoked by antigenic components in the grafted foreign tissue. Various discoveries, including the adoptive transfer of transplantation immunity (Mitchison 1953, 1954; Billingham *et al* 1954), soon provided overwhelming experimental support for this concept. Although an immune mechanism for allograft rejection had been previously proposed on a number of occasions, the investigations of Medawar and his colleagues and of other workers at this time undoubtedly provided the vital evidence. With hindsight it seems strange that uncertainty about the nature of the response should have persisted for so many years. As Medawar (1958) puts it: 'Yet no one now doubts that the homograft reaction is immunological in character. The difficulty nowadays is to put oneself in the position of those who at one time believed that it was not.'

During the last 25 years there have been dramatic advances in transplantation biology and in its application to the treatment of human disease. However, despite fundamental discoveries in general immunology and related sciences, practical methods of preventing rejection of human organ allografts are often either inadequate or dangerously non-specific.

II. NOMENCLATURE

With the growth of interest in tissue transplantation numerous terms were introduced to describe the various kinds of graft and, as frequently happens, terminology became confusing. In transplantation biology the special problem has been to find appropriate words to indicate the genetic relationship between the donor and recipient of a graft. Lack of uniform practice in biological terminology, especially in the use of the prefixes iso- and homo-, has not made this task any simpler. However, Gorer *et al* (1961) and, later, Snell (1964) proposed improved nomenclature. Snell's suggestions in particular have received wide acceptance and are used in this volume.

Other terms commonly employed in transplantation include words which indicate the position in which the graft is placed, the method of grafting, and the frequency with which grafts have been made between two individuals.

A Relationship between donor and recipient

Relationship between donor and recipient	*Name given to graft*	*Synonyms*
Same individual	Autograft	Autogenous graft Autogeneic graft
Individuals of same species and identical genotype	Isograft	Isogeneic graft Syngeneic graft
Individuals of same species but different genotype	Allograft	Homograft Allogeneic graft
Different species	Xenograft	Heterograft Xenogeneic graft

B Anatomical position of graft

Orthotopic graft	The transplanted tissue is placed in a site anatomically normal for the particular tissue. Example: skin transplanted to graft bed prepared on skin surface.

Heterotopic graft — The transplanted tissue is placed in an anatomically unnatural position for the particular tissue. Example: skin transplanted to peritoneal cavity or inserted into brain.
A heterotopic graft may be called accessory, or auxiliary, if it is additional to the recipient's own tissues. Example: an extra liver grafted in the abdomen.

C Method of grafting

Free graft — The transplanted tissue is completely detached from the donor and no vascular anastomoses are created by the surgeon between the graft and the recipient's circulatory system at the time of transplantation. Example: conventional skin grafting.

Graft employing vascular anastomoses — A graft in which vascular anastomoses are created by the surgeon at the time of transplantation. Example: renal and hepatic transplantation.

Pedicle graft — The graft at first remains partially attached to its site of origin by a pedicle containing blood vessels. The pedicle may later be severed when the graft has developed vascular connections with the new graft bed.

D Frequency of grafting between two individuals

First-set grafts
Second-set grafts — These terms are used to denote the first, second and subsequent grafts of living tissue from the same donor, or genetically identical donor, to a particular recipient. The significance of these terms is that after rejecting a first-set allograft from a particular donor, the recipient will be immune (i.e. 'sensitized' or 'allergic') and will probably reject a second-set graft more quickly. If on a first occasion several pieces of tissue are transplanted to a recipient from the same donor, the grafts as a group would be designated first-set grafts.

III. GENERAL DESCRIPTION

Provided their physiological needs are met and infection is prevented, autografts and isografts of tissues and organs survive and function indefinitely. For example, if a skin autograft is placed on a suitable graft bed and kept firmly in place during the healing phase the transplanted skin is accepted and survives for the lifetime of the recipient. Similarly, renal and hepatic autografts and isografts are permanently accepted and function normally if their nutritional and secretory requirements are fulfilled. Obviously grafts of this kind must be provided with an adequate blood supply and appropriate outlets for the secretions they produce. This involves immediate surgical anastomosis of large blood vessels and the creation of suitable excretory channels.

On the other hand, if allografts are transplanted in a similar fashion to immunologically competent recipients, the transplanted tissue or organ will usually be destroyed. On a first occasion such allografts initially behave as if they were autografts but after a variable number of days the transplant undergoes necrosis. The response causing this destruction is known as the allograft reaction ('homograft reaction'). If an animal has already rejected an allograft, second and subsequent grafts from the same recipient are more rapidly destroyed. Among his initial skin-grafting experiments with rabbits, for example, Medawar (1944) found that second-set allografts of skin survived for only about 6 days in comparison with a survival time of about 10 days for large first-set grafts. At that time this accelerated rejection of second-set allografts was one of the major features supporting the concept that allograft rejection is an immune process.

A Skin allografts (Figs 1–4)

When full thickness allografts of skin are transplanted on a first occasion, they often survive for between 8 and 16 days, the survival time depending, among other factors, on the species of animal, the antigenic disparity between donor and recipient, and the amount of skin transplanted. Initially, for a period of 5 days or more, such allografts are usually indistinguishable from autografts similarly transplanted. They become vascularized in the same fashion by end-to-end anastomoses between the vessels in the graft and graft bed and become firmly bound to the recipient's tissues. However, towards the end of the 1st week the dermis of the graft becomes infiltrated by mononuclear cells (compare Figs. 1 and 2). These cells are blood borne and, after adhering to the endothelium of capillaries and venules in the graft, many migrate into the connective tissue of the dermis. During this process the walls of the vessels may be injured and disintegrate (Fig. 3). Dilatation of capillaries and venules and diminished blood flow are other notable features. At this stage the macroscopic appearance often changes dramatically. For example, the graft may become a livid blue colour (Fig. 4) and in certain species oedema is a prominent feature. Substantial numbers of mononuclear cells with platelets and fibrin

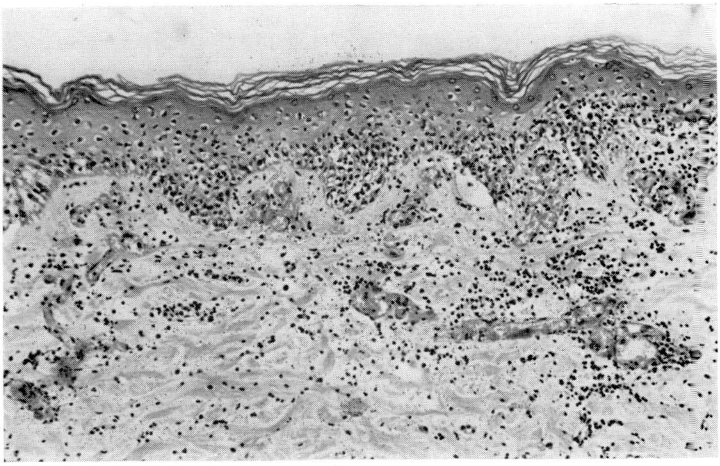

FIG. 1. Pig skin allograft (first-set) 5 days after transplantation. Mononuclear cell infiltration of dermis and epidermis with disintegration of some epithelial cells. Conspicuous dilatation and congestion of dermal blood vessels. The junction between the graft and graft bed is not included in the photograph. H.E. ×110.

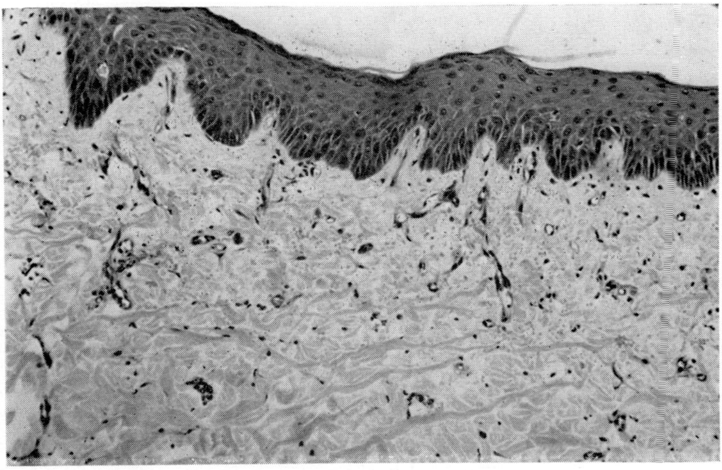

FIG. 2. Pig skin autograft 5 days after transplantation. The epidermis and dermis are essentially normal. The junction between the graft and graft bed is not included in the photograph. H.E. ×110.

may also accumulate in small arteries and veins and contribute to the vascular stasis. Necrosis of the epidermal cells of the graft then rapidly occurs, followed later by necrosis of the graft dermis. The necrotic graft may become detached from the graft bed leaving a gaping wound which is gradually covered by host epithelium. Alternatively the dead tissue may remain firmly attached until it is separated from the graft by ingrowing epithelium.

The mononuclear cells infiltrating the graft vary in their morphology but with light microscopy their type is difficult to distinguish. Employing

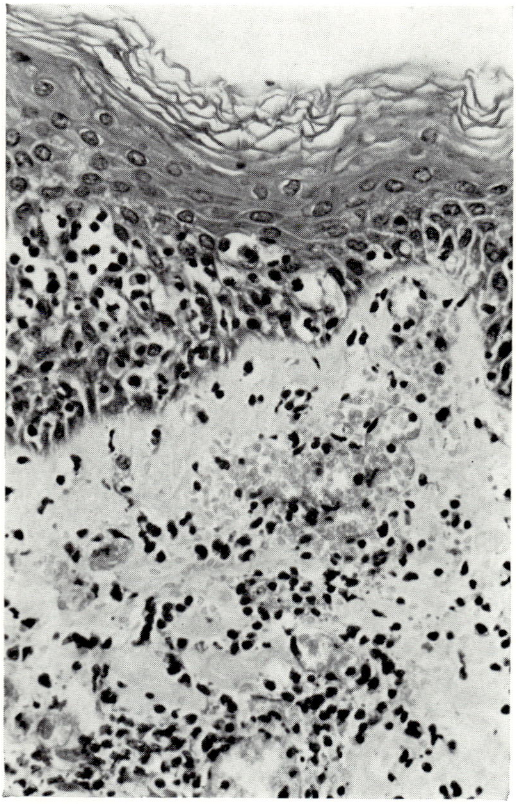

FIG. 3. Pig skin allograft (first-set) 5 days after transplantation. Higher power photograph of another part of allograft illustrated in Fig. 1. Conspicuous dilatation and congestion of blood vessels with partial disintegration of their walls and haemorrhage into the surrounding tissue. Mononuclear cell infiltration of dermis and deeper part of epidermis with disintegration of related epidermal cells. A few polymorphs are also present. H.E. ×300.

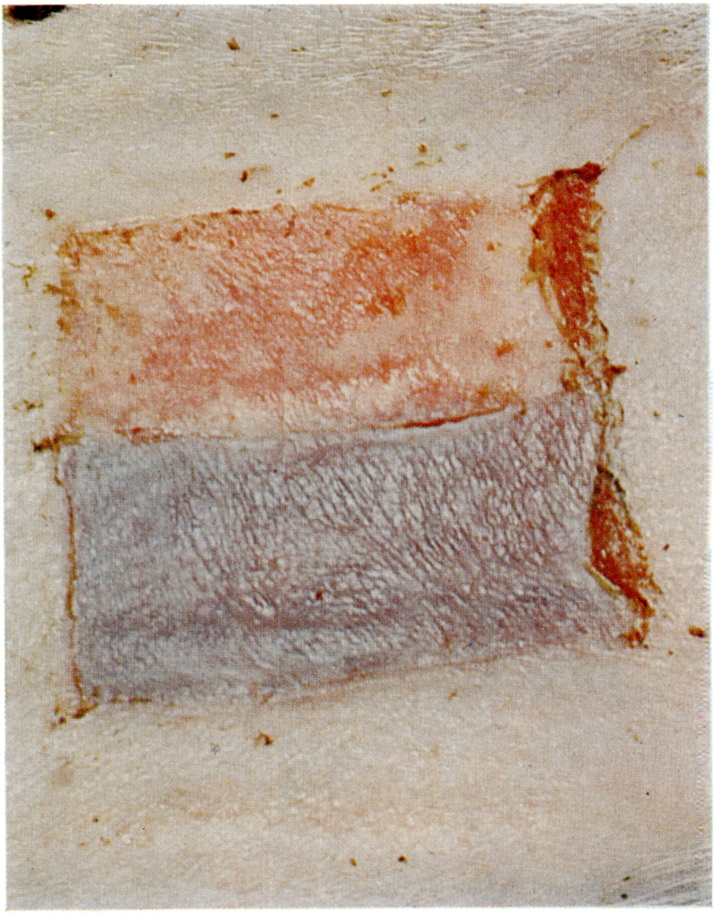

FIG. 4. Pig skin autograft and allograft (first-set) 6 days after transplantation. Apart from slight excoriation near its centre, the autograft (above) appears healthy and has a normal whitish-pink colour. The allograft (below) is wrinkled and livid blue; it became totally necrotic a few days later.

paraffin sections the most that can usually be claimed is that some appear to be small lymphocytes and that a proportion of the larger mononuclear cells possess pyroninophilic cytoplasm. In the later stages some typical plasma cells also appear. However, fine structure studies with the electron microscope have added considerable information. Many of the infiltrating cells possess a relatively large nucleus with prominent nucleoli and their cytoplasm contains several mitochondria, a well developed Golgi apparatus and numerous polyribosomes but little or no rough-surfaced endoplasmic reticulum. In the literature these cells have been given various names, such as 'graft rejection cells' (Wiener *et al* 1964) and 'immunocytes', but they are generally thought to belong to the family of lymphocytes. Typical small lymphocytes and macrophages are also present and, later, immature and mature plasma cells with increasing amounts of endoplasmic reticulum may be found.

Although the morphological changes associated with skin allograft rejection appear to be fundamentally similar in different species, there are considerable differences of detail. For example, mononuclear cell infiltration is prominent in rabbits and cattle but is much slighter in mice, rats and guinea-pigs. Similarly, oedema is a conspicuous feature in skin allografts in rabbits and cattle but is comparatively trivial in most other common laboratory animals. An interesting aspect of human skin allografts is that considerable infiltrations of eosinophil leucocytes are occasionally observed (Rogers *et al* 1953).

Survival of second-set skin allografts is considerably shorter than similar first-set grafts and the morphological features also differ. Sometimes the graft never becomes vascularized and perishes within 2 or 3 days of transplantation. This form of response has been called the 'white graft reaction' (Rapaport & Converse 1958). On other occasions, vascularization of the graft begins but blood flow soon ceases with disruption of blood vessels, haemorrhage and thrombosis. In such accelerated allograft reactions the cellular infiltration is often much less pronounced than in first-set grafts and is concentrated in the graft bed and immediately adjacent portions of the allograft dermis rather than in the interior of the graft. In other words, the reaction tends to be centred on the interface between the recipient's tissue and the graft. The morphological appearances suggest that ischaemia is a major cause of graft destruction.

B **Renal allografts** (Figs. 5–8)

When a renal allograft is transplanted to a normal recipient it functions for the first few days in virtually the same fashion as a similarly transplanted renal autograft. However, after a variable period, frequently towards the end of the 1st week, secretion of urine rapidly ceases. At this time the kidney is much enlarged, often being two to three times its normal weight. The macroscopic appearances of the kidney tissue vary considerably. Frequently the broadened cortex is much paler than usual, while the medulla is somewhat congested. On other occasions the kidney is a blotchy deep reddish-purple with numerous haemorrhages scattered throughout its substance (Fig. 5).

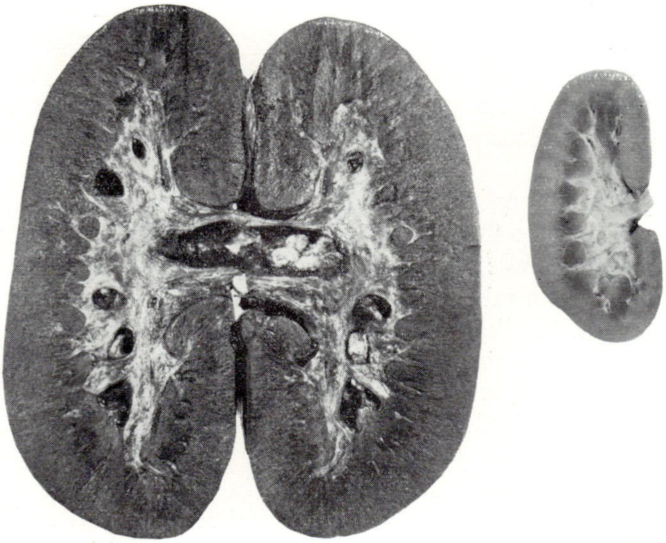

FIG. 5. Pig renal allograft (first-set) 7 days after transplantation with a comparable normal pig kidney. The allograft (left) is greatly enlarged, deeply congested and the boundary between cortex and medulla poorly defined. The main renal blood vessels were patent. Necrotic debris fills renal pelvis. The normal kidney (right) was from a pig of similar weight to the donor of the allograft. Two-fifths natural size.

During the first few hours after transplantation some small lymphocytes may be seen in contact with the endothelium of intertubular capillaries and venules within the allograft. During the 3rd or 4th day mononuclear cells of large lymphoid type with pyroninophilic cytoplasm, seemingly identical with those seen in skin allografts, begin to collect in the intertubular capillaries and venules. These cells appear closely adherent to the endothelial cells. Although the cell membranes of the mononuclear and endothelial cells are usually distinct, adjoining portions of the cell membranes sometimes disappear at particular places and continuity between the cytoplasm of the two cells seems to be established (Kountz *et al* 1963).

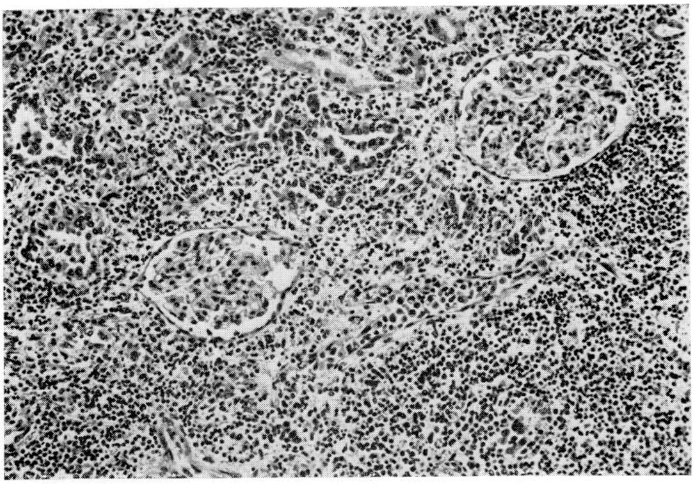

FIG. 6. Rhesus monkey renal allograft (first-set) 25 days after transplantation. Extensive mononuclear cell infiltration in oedematous interstitial tissue. The glomeruli have survived but many tubules have been destroyed. H.E. × 110.

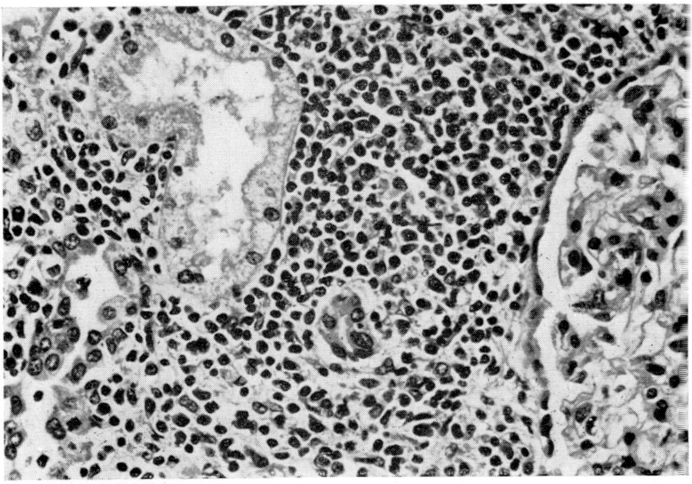

FIG. 7. Rhesus monkey renal allograft (first-set) 25 days after transplantation. Higher power photograph of another part of allograft illustrated in Fig. 6. Epithelial cells lining surviving tubules are abnormal and some are undergoing necrosis. H.E. × 300.

These lymphoid cells, accompanied by a considerable number of macrophages and small lymphocytes, migrate into the interstitial tissue of the kidney (Figs. 6 and 7). They are particularly prominent in the cortex and at the corticomedullary boundary and are often aggregated around veins. Among the infiltrating cells mitoses are fairly frequently seen. Later, mononuclear cells with increasing amounts of rough-surfaced endoplasmic reticulum (i.e. immature and mature plasma cells) also appear in the interstitial tissue. As the cellular infiltration develops the interstitial tissue usually becomes oedematous, and, if capillary and venular walls are disrupted, haemorrhage also occurs. In addition, mural and occluding

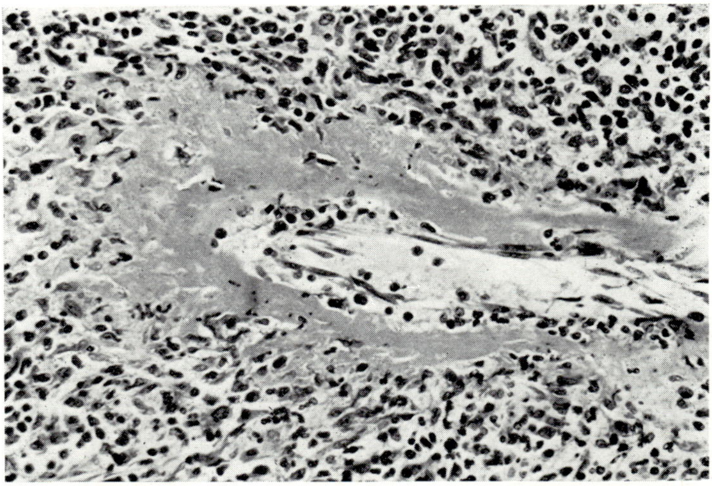

FIG. 8. Dog renal allograft (first-set) 11 days after transplantation. Fibrinoid necrosis of an interlobular artery with a few mononuclear cells beneath surviving endothelium. Substantial mononuclear cell infiltration in oedematous perivascular tissue. H.E. ×300.

thrombi may develop in small and larger veins and massive aggregations of platelets may be seen in glomerular capillaries. In the later stages there is extensive tubular necrosis and the dead and dying tissue is infiltrated by neutrophil polymorphs. In some species fibrinoid necrosis of interlobular arteries and glomerular arterioles with or without thrombosis may develop before the allograft is totally destroyed (Fig. 8).

A renal allograft transplanted into an animal previously sensitized by a graft of living cells from the same donor is rapidly rejected and, if it functions at all, does so for only a day or two. The major morphological features in such a kidney are dilatation and engorgement of glomerular and intertubular capillaries, thrombosis of small and large vessels, fibrinoid necrosis of interlobular arteries and glomerular arterioles, extensive haemorrhage, tubular necrosis and neutrophil polymorph infiltration. Any mononuclear cell infiltration is slight.

For a more extensive description the authoritative reviews by Porter (1966a, b) should be consulted.

C **Hepatic allografts** (Figs. 9–13)

Experimental liver transplantation in immunologically normal recipients has been studied in various species including the dog (Moore *et al* 1960; McBride *et al* 1962; Groth *et al* 1968), the pig (Cordier *et al* 1966; Hunt 1967; Calne *et al* 1967), the rat (Lee & Edgington 1968), and the rhesus monkey (Calne *et al* 1970). In all these species livers are rejected more slowly than renal allografts.

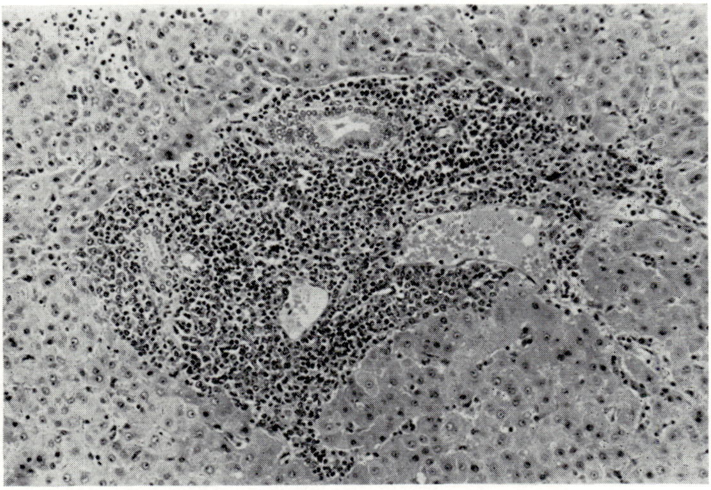

FIG. 9. Rhesus monkey hepatic allograft (first-set) 15 days after transplantation. Substantial mononuclear cell infiltration in enlarged portal tract with a few similar cells in sinusoids in periphery of surrounding liver lobules. H.E. ×110.

Liver allografts in dogs, rats and rhesus monkeys are usually destroyed by the recipient and the process of rejection appears to follow a pattern essentially similar to the changes observed in renal allografts. On the 3rd or 4th day after transplantation mononuclear cells begin to adhere to the endothelium of the portal veins and venules and to infiltrate the connective tissue of the portal tracts. There is a similar accumulation in and around

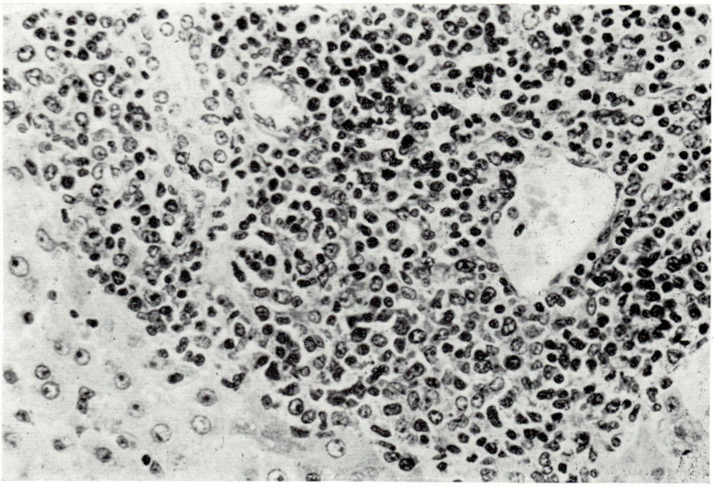

FIG. 10. Rhesus monkey hepatic allograft (first-set) 15 days after transplantation. Higher power photograph of part of Fig. 9. Considerable variation in morphology of mononuclear cells. H.E. × 300.

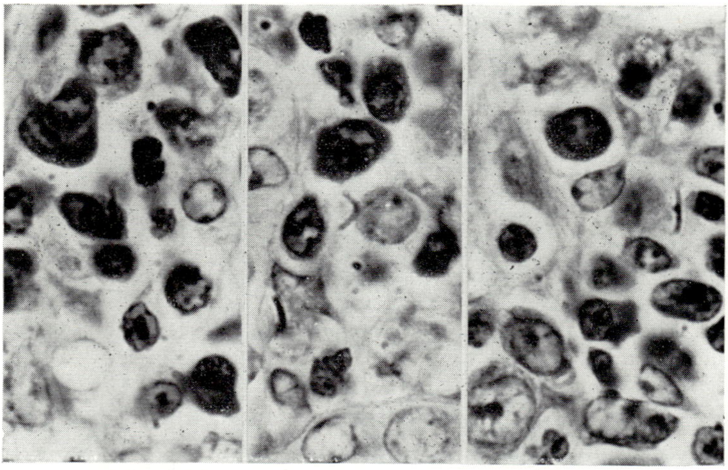

FIG. 11. Rhesus monkey hepatic allograft (first-set) 15 days after transplantation. Higher power photographs of mononuclear cells in a portal tract of allograft illustrated in Figs. 9 and 10. The pyroninophilic cells have dark cytoplasm. Pyronin—Methyl green. × 1050.

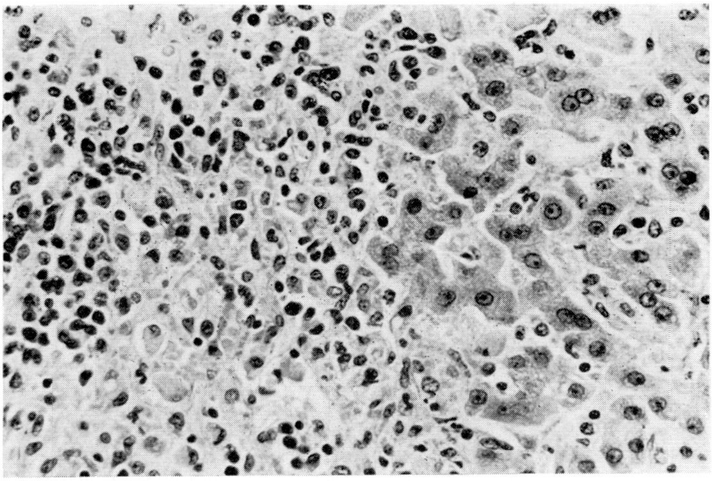

FIG. 12. Rhesus monkey hepatic allograft (first-set) 15 days after transplantation. Another part of the allograft illustrated in Figs. 9, 10 and 11. Mononuclear cell infiltration in liver lobule with necrosis of liver cells in the left half of the field. The mononuclear cells are much more numerous in the necrotic portion. H.E. × 300.

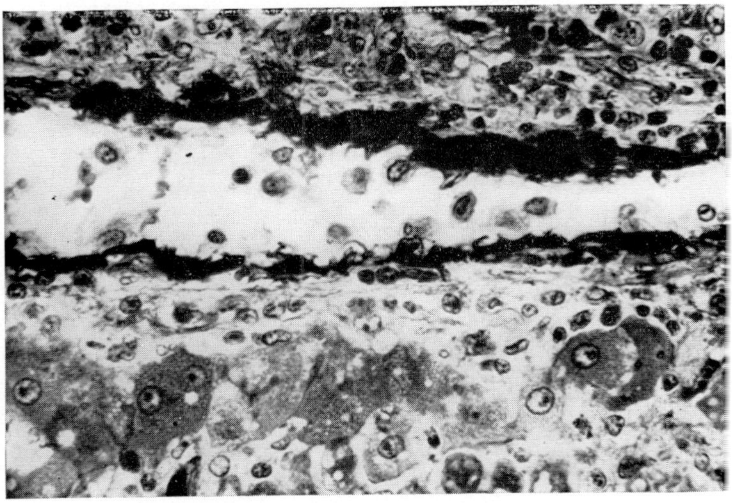

Fig. 13. Rhesus monkey hepatic allograft (first-set) 7 days after transplantation. Darkly-stained fibrin-like material in wall of vein in portal tract with almost complete loss of endothelium. P.T.A.H. × 360.

the central veins. During subsequent days this infiltration increases substantially (Figs. 9 and 10) and mononuclear cells also adhere to Kupffer cells and endothelial cells lining the sinusoids. These cells migrate into the space of Disse and may penetrate between the liver cells. A considerable proportion of the mononuclear cells possess pyroninophilic cytoplasm (Fig. 11) and from their fine structure appear to be essentially the same as the large lymphoid cells seen in skin and renal allografts. At this time many liver cells, particularly in the central and middle zones of the lobules begin to degenerate and undergo necrosis (Fig. 12). The reticular framework in the necrotic areas then tends to collapse and bile pigment accumulates in bile canaliculi and in Kupffer cells. In a small proportion of animals fibrinoid necrosis of small intrahepatic arteries occurs and fibrin-like material may accumulate beneath the endothelium of veins in the portal tracts (Fig. 13).

Rejection of hepatic allografts in the rat and the rhesus monkey seems to follow a fundamentally similar pattern. On the other hand, although rejection has been reported in the pig, most porcine liver allografts are accepted. Pigs, however, reject skin and renal allografts rapidly.

D **Cardiac allografts** (Fig. 14)

There have been numerous experimental studies of the functional behaviour of cardiac allografts and of the morphological changes developing in them. Until the recent introduction of satisfactory techniques for orthotopic cardiac transplantation, most were grafted heterotopically, often in the neck or abdomen, but the process of allograft rejection appears essentially the same wherever the transplanted heart is placed. The species studied have included the dog (Lower & Shumway 1960; Chiba *et al* 1962; Lower *et al* 1965), the rat (Abbott *et al* 1965) and the calf (Hardy *et al* 1964).

In many experiments the rejection of cardiac allografts in immunologically unmodified recipients seems to follow a fundamentally similar pattern to the changes observed in allografts of other organs and tissues. For example, in their study of rat cardiac allografts Abbott *et al* (1965) found increasing infiltrations of mononuclear cells, oedema, vascular changes including loss of endothelium, and extensive myocardial necrosis. In first-set allografts the mononuclear cell infiltration began to appear beneath the endocardium and adjoining heart muscle 3 days after transplantation. The cellular infiltrate rapidly became much more extensive and at 5 days some myocardial fibres had undergone necrosis. Nine to 13 days after transplantation much of the myocardium had been destroyed and there was conspicuous interstitial haemorrhage and fibroblastic proliferation. With second-set allografts the changes were similar but rejection occurred more quickly.

In first-set canine cardiac allografts the process of rejection takes a generally similar form but Chiba *et al* (1962) found in serial biopsies that various cellular changes began to occur shortly after transplantation. At 3 h there was a slight perivascular infiltration of lymphocytes and soon a few macrophages and plasma cells were also present. At 19 h some cells resembling Anitschkow and Aschoff cells appeared. During subsequent days the mononuclear cell infiltration gradually increased throughout

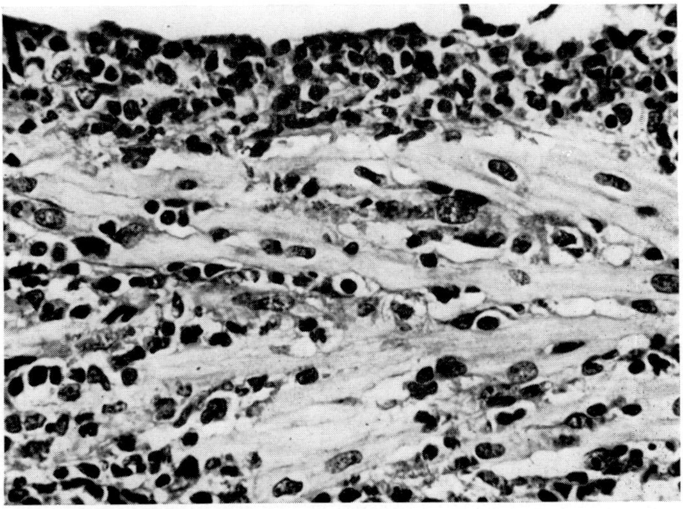

Fig. 14. Auxiliary pig cardiac allograft (first-set) 7 days after transplantation. Substantial mononuclear cell infiltration in between muscle fibres of ventricle and in endocardium. Some muscle fibres are degenerating. H.E. ×340.

the myocardium and after 8 days there was conspicuous swelling of vascular endothelium and necrosis of myocardial fibres. In dogs previously sensitized with donor spleen cells an accelerated reaction developed, myocardial necrosis sometimes occurring within 4 h of transplantation.

In their study of orthotopic canine cardiac allografts Lower *et al* (1965) found that of 20 dogs the survival time varied from 4 to 21 days, the mean being 7 days. Again the main features of rejection were dense infiltrations of mononuclear cells, particularly in the subendocardial, subpericardial and perivascular regions, and myocardial necrosis. A notable feature was calcification of necrotic muscle fibres which sometimes occurred within 6 days of transplantation.

Preliminary studies with heterotopic cardiac allografts in the pig suggest that rejection is basically similar to the changes described in other species (Fig. 14).

IV. MECHANISM OF ALLOGRAFT REJECTION

Much experimental work on tissue transplantation has been directed towards an understanding of the mechanism of allograft rejection. Despite many uncertainties there is general agreement that allograft destruction is a specific immune phenomenon and in elementary terms takes the following pattern. First, immunologically competent cells are somehow made aware of histocompatibility antigens possessed by the allograft but not by the recipient. Second, appropriate competent cells respond and produce immune lymphocytes and immunoglobulins. Third, these products of the immune response then react with components in the graft and in some fashion cause its destruction. On theoretical grounds it is conceivable that uncommitted immunologically competent cells are brought to the graft by the blood stream and that all the other events occur within the substance of the transplant. However, with most forms of allograft there is very strong evidence that host lymphatic tissue (including regional lymph nodes and/or more distant lymph nodes and the spleen) is directly involved in the process. Indeed, it seems virtually certain that antigenic components derived from the grafted cells, or information about such antigens, are transferred to host lymphatic tissue where certain immunologically competent cells enlarge, multiply and produce (1) immune lymphocytes and (2) plasma cells which form and secrete immunoglobulins. These products then enter the bloodstream, probably directly and via the thoracic duct, and react with the grafted cells. The immune lymphocytes are generally regarded as the principal agent responsible for destroying the transplanted tissue but in certain circumstances immunoglobulins may also affect the allograft. Although present uncertainties about various aspects of allograft rejection prevent precise analysis, it is convenient for descriptive purposes to distinguish three phases in the process. These are: (1) the afferent pathway to lymphatic tissue, (2) the cellular response in lymphatic tissue, and (3) the efferent pathway from lymphatic tissue and immune interaction within the graft causing its destruction.

A First-phase: afferent pathway to lymphatic tissue

With orthotopic skin allografts most experimental investigation strongly favours the concept that histocompatibility antigens, or information about them, pass via the lymphatic vessels to the regional lymph nodes. The evidence for this view is provided by the prolonged survival of heterotopic skin allografts placed in sites where lymphatic vessels are absent, such as the brain (Medawar 1948) and the hamster cheek pouch (Billingham & Silvers 1964). It is also supported by the discovery that orthotopic skin allografts with a blood vascular supply but deprived of lymphatic drainage also survive for considerable periods (Barker & Billingham 1967). Moreover, with conventional orthotopic skin allografts the major morphological response in lymphatic tissue usually occurs in the regional lymph nodes (Scothorne & McGregor 1955). On the other hand, there is very little reliable information about the form in which the antigens reach the lymph nodes. Such antigens may be carried freely in the lymph in molecular form or as fragments of discarded cell membrane or endoplasmic reticulum. Alternatively, small lymphocytes reaching the graft via the blood stream may be 'induced' within the graft and then drain to and settle in the regional lymph nodes. Clearly, more information is needed about the composition of lymph draining from sites of skin allografts during the first hours and days after transplantation.

With renal allografts experimental evidence suggests that the blood stream is the major route but there is conflicting opinion about the way in which sensitization occurs. From their experiments with dogs May *et al* (1965) believed that transplantation antigens were liberated into and transported by the blood plasma. On the other hand, Strober & Gowans (1965), using inbred strains of rats, provided substantial evidence that during the first few hours after transplantation host lymphocytes in the circulating blood make contact with the vascular endothelium of the graft and after leaving the kidney in the blood enter and settle in the spleen and lymph nodes.

B Second-phase: cellular response in lymphatic tissue

Within a few days of applying a skin allograft the regional lymph node or nodes become considerably enlarged and a substantial number of large lymphoid cells with strongly pyroninophilic cytoplasm appear in what have been referred to as the 'tertiary cortical nodules' (Scothorne & McGregor 1955), or 'paracortical areas' (Oort & Turk 1965). Various names have been given to such cells, including 'activated lymphoid cells', 'blast cells', 'lymphoblasts' and 'immunoblasts', but, like the pyroninophilic cells which infiltrate allografts, they are generally considered to be members of the lymphocyte family. The germinal centres in the cortex usually remain normal.

These large lymphoid cells in the lymph nodes initially proliferate but when the graft is destroyed they gradually disappear. Similar cells are not seen in the regional lymph nodes after applying autografts and much other evidence suggests that these cells have an important and specific role in graft rejection. Investigations of graft-versus-host reactions, for example by Gowans *et al* (1962) and Porter & Cooper (1962), support the view that following the application of allografts, small lymphocytes exposed to histocompatibility antigens become transformed into large lymphoid cells within lymphatic tissue. A fresh population of small lymphocytes and cells transitional between small lymphocytes and the large lymphoid cells appear to be produced and are probably the source of at least some of the mononuclear cells infiltrating allografts.

C Third-phase: efferent pathway from lymphatic tissue and immune interaction within graft causing its destruction

Although allograft destruction is accepted to be an immune phenomenon there continues to be considerable controversy about the respective roles of immune lymphoid cells and of humoral immunoglobulins. Many features suggest that the process of allograft destruction is predominantly cell-mediated and is essentially similar to delayed-hypersensitivity reactions like the tuberculin response. The evidence was primarily provided by the discovery that transplantation immunity can usually be transmitted from sensitized to normal animals by transferring lymphoid cells (Mitchison 1953, 1954; Billingham *et al* 1954) but not by serum (Billingham *et al* 1954; Billingham & Brent 1956). In other words, activated or immune lymphoid cells are thought to be released from lymphatic tissue, to migrate into the graft and then destroy the foreign cells. Most investigators interested in transplantation immunity agree that a cell-mediated mechanism of this kind plays a vital role in allograft rejection. On the other hand, some workers, for example Stetson (1963), have steadfastly continued to hold that humoral mechanisms, involving immunoglobulins and complement, are important. The relative significance of these two views will doubtless emerge but it appears that much of the dispute is rather artificial and that depending upon the circumstances either or both mechanisms may be involved. For example, it seems probable that a cell-mediated mechanism is the major factor destroying many first-set allografts. On the other hand, humoral factors may be much more significant, for instance, in the immediate rejection of a renal allograft in a person previously sensitized by multiple pregnancies or blood transfusion.

There has also been much uncertainty about the role of ischaemia in destroying transplanted tissue. Some believe that direct immune destruction of the allogeneic cells is all important and that ischaemia is incidental.

Others, however, hold that immune injury to blood vessels of the graft is the primary event and that much of the necrosis of parenchymal cells in organ allografts is due to subsequent ischaemia.

Despite these different views there is at the present time a fairly well based working concept of the likely events leading to destruction of first-set allografts. First, it has been established that the vast majority of mononuclear cells appearing in allografts during rejection are of host origin (i.e. belong to the recipient). In his initial account of rejection of rabbit skin allografts Medawar (1944) regarded the mononuclear cells as being derived from the recipient; but in their studies of renal allografts Dempster (1953) and Simonsen (1953) raised the possibility that many are of donor origin and are responding to recipient antigens. More recently, however, various investigations, including the autoradiographic studies in the dog by Porter & Calne (1960), have convincingly demonstrated that the majority of the infiltrating mononuclear cells are derived from the recipient. Second, during experiments with rat skin allografts Gowans *et al* (1962) showed that many of the mononuclear cells are newly formed and from other work it seems likely that they are derived from the large pyroninophilic lymphoid cells which appear in host lymphatic tissue. The pyroninophilic cells infiltrating allografts are usually smaller than the large lymphoid cells in the lymph nodes draining such grafts but in other respects their structure is very similar (Porter 1969). Third, contrary to what might be expected but in keeping with observations on the tuberculin reaction, it appears that many of the infiltrating cells are not specifically activated against the particular graft. In elegantly designed skin-grafting experiments in the rabbit Prendergast (1964) found that in the invasion of grafts there is either little or no specific selection of lymphoid cells in the sense that mononuclear cells derived from a regional lymph node draining an allograft from a particular donor equally invade identical and unrelated allografts transplanted at the same time. These surprising results are in accord with the observations of various workers including Turk (1962) and Turk & Oort (1963) on the non-selective character of the mononuclear response in delayed-hypersensitivity reactions.

The mononuclear cells which infiltrate allografts arrive via the blood stream and initially adhere to the foreign endothelium lining the blood vessels within the graft. At present the factors determining this adherence are obscure but this is manifestly a most important feature. If the graft were invaded only by immune lymphocytes (i.e. lymphocytes specifically active against histocompatibility antigens in the particular graft), specific immune attachment might well be the vital factor, but, as mentioned, present evidence suggests that there is little or no selection of this kind. As many of the invading cells seem to be newly formed, there may be some particular quality about their cell surface which makes them specially prone to adhere to the endothelium but there is no well based evidence for this at present. After emigrating from the blood vessels the mononuclear cells appear to wander through the interstitial tissue of the graft and some at least may then react specifically with the allogeneic cells and destroy them. In morphological studies numerous workers, including Wiener *et al* (1964) and Lee & Edgington (1968), have observed close contact between the infiltrating and the allograft cells and believe that this association is of vital significance.

There is abundant evidence that immune lymphocytes can cause destruction of foreign cells ('target cells'), such as those present in allografts, but the mechanism by which such target cells are destroyed remains uncertain. In *in vitro* studies Govaerts (1960), Rosenau & Moon (1964) and Wilson (1965a, b), among others, have shown that sensitized lymphocytes can destroy a wide range of foreign cells. This cytotoxic action of immune lymphoid cells occurs in the absence of complement but is immunologically specific and only takes place when there is contact between the lymphoid and target cells. However, the properties which enable sensitized lymphocytes to destroy allogeneic cells are still unknown. The most widely held belief is that immune lymphocytes have themselves synthesized and retained a specific antibody-like moiety (i.e. 'cell-bound antibody') which is active at the cell surface. Various workers, including Coombs & Franks (1969), believe that there may be two stages in the process of target cell destruction. First, the immune lymphocytes become specifically attached to the target cells to which they are sensitized. This specific attachment could be due to an interaction between specific receptors on the surface of the lymphocytes and the related antigens on the cell membrane of the target cells. Knowledge about the second phase in which the target cells are destroyed is even less certain but it is thought that it may be immunologically non-specific.

Most allografts appear to elicit a humoral response in addition to cell-mediated immunity. The immunoglobulins formed after applying an allograft can be detected by various procedures. These include agglutination and haemolysis of red cells and the cytotoxic effects of such antibodies on certain kinds of somatic cells. Nevertheless, evidence about the role of humoral immunoglobulins in the allograft reaction is particularly confusing. On the one hand, certain alloantibodies in the presence of complement can unquestionably destroy various types of cell. In other circumstances, however, antibodies may reduce the response to an allograft so that it survives much longer than expected ('enhancement'). The factors determining the effects of such alloantibodies are still poorly understood but presumably include the differing activities of the various classes of immunoglobulins and the properties of the cell types involved. In the present context the destructive capacity of alloantibodies is the major concern. Experimental work with mouse cell lines suggests that the sensitivity of different types of target cell varies greatly. For example, lymphocytes and some neoplastic cells tend to be readily destroyed but many other cell types seem to be much more resistant. In certain instances the sensitivity or resistance of target cells to the cytotoxic activity of antibody and complement appears to be related to the concentration of alloantigens on the cell surface. These differences may well be responsible for the variable and apparently contradictory results of certain experimental work and the conflicting views about the significance of immunoglobulins in graft rejection.

Direct evidence of the role of humoral immunoglobulins in allograft destruction has been difficult to achieve. However, IgG and IgM have often been demonstrated in the cytoplasm of a proportion of infiltrating mononuclear cells in experimental and human renal and hepatic allografts and it is conceivable that release of immunoglobulins from antibody-forming cells within the graft itself may sometimes be more effective in causing allograft rejection than is usually considered. The detection of IgG and IgM and complement components in the walls of glomerular arterioles and interlobular arteries undergoing fibrinoid necrosis in human renal allografts provides some evidence that humoral antibodies are significant in allograft destruction. Similarly, the immediate rejection of renal allografts in previously sensitized recipients possessing cytotoxic antibodies seems much more likely to be due to serum immunoglobulins than a cell-mediated mechanism. This view is supported by the investigations of Cochrum *et al* (1969) who showed that goat renal autografts could apparently be rejected by immune serum in circumstances which excluded any possibility of a cell-mediated component. Similarly, in technically rather complicated experiments involving the temporary transfer of renal allografts to specifically sensitized dogs, rendered leucopenic by X-irradiation, and with subsequent return of the kidneys to the original donors, Clark *et al* (1968) also believed that specific humoral factors were responsible for destruction of the grafts. Although these various observations do not perhaps provide conclusive evidence, at present it would seem both unwise and unscientific to disregard the possibility of a humoral mechanism.

Apart from immunoglobulins freely suspended in blood and tissue fluids, it is conceivable that cytophilic antibodies carried on the surface of macrophages may be significant in graft rejection. For example, Granger & Weiser (1964, 1966) and Weiser *et al* (1965) found that allogeneic cells may be destroyed both *in vitro* and *in vivo* by a seemingly pure suspension of macrophages from immunized mice. This reaction appears to be immunologically specific and is thought to depend on the presence of cytophilic antibody attached to the cell membrane of the macrophages. From a theoretical viewpoint macrophage–cytophilic antibodies may also determine other aspects of macrophage behaviour during graft rejection. For instance, cytophilic antibody might cause 'immune macrophages' (macrophages to which cytophilic antibody has become attached) to adhere specifically to the vascular endothelium in the graft. Such a mechanism might be responsible for the substantial aggregation of macrophages which occurs. However, the role of cytophilic antibodies in graft rejection remains uncertain and deserves further investigation.

Although there can be no doubt about the immune nature of allograft rejection, whatever the precise mechanism may be, there is considerable variation of view about the possible role of ischaemia. As suggested earlier, some tend to regard destruction of all or most of the grafted tissue as being directly due to immune mechanisms. Others, however, while agreeing about the nature of the primary injury, believe that ischaemia resulting from immune vascular injury is often responsible for much of the parenchymal cell necrosis in allografts, especially of organs such as the kidney and liver. Diminished blood flow through organ allografts has been amply demonstrated but as with other forms of injury it is often difficult to determine whether ischaemia is causing tissue damage or is a consequence of it. Most morphologists, however, regard ischaemia as an important feature in graft rejection.

For more extensive treatment of the mechanisms of allograft rejection the reader should consult the authoritative reviews by Brent (1958), Lawrence (1959), Billingham & Silvers (1963), Stetson (1963), Gowans (1965) and Brent & Medawar (1967).

V. XENOGRAFTS (Figs. 15 and 16)

Skin, kidney, liver, heart and other tissues and organs have frequently been transplanted on an experimental basis from one species to another. For example, skin has been grafted from ducks to chickens, from rats to mice and from guinea-pigs to rabbits. Similarly, kidneys have been grafted from cats to dogs and from goats to sheep, and livers from pigs to primates and between different primate species. Recently, in attempts to treat human disease, kidney, liver and heart xenografts have also been transplanted to man from rhesus monkey, baboon and chimpanzee.

The fate of skin xenografts varies considerably. Frequently the transplanted tissue never becomes vascularized and perishes within 2 or 3 days. Sometimes, however, a skin xenograft heals in place, gains a blood supply

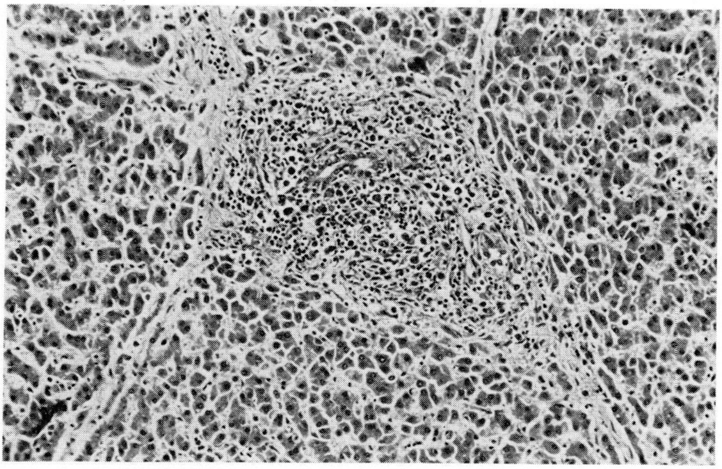

FIG. 15. Pig-to-baboon hepatic xenograft (first-set) $3\frac{1}{2}$ days after transplantation. Considerable mononuclear cell infiltration in oedematous portal tract. Few mononuclear cells in sinusoids in adjoining liver lobules. The recipient had been given steroid hormones. H.E. × 110.

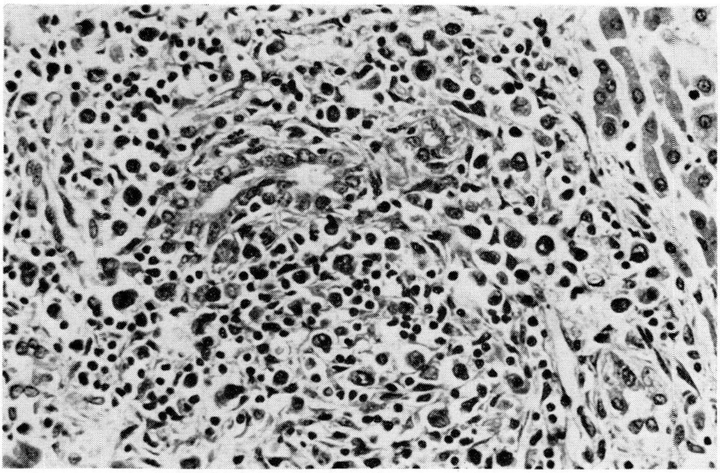

FIG. 16. Pig-to-baboon hepatic xenograft (first-set) $3\frac{1}{2}$ days after transplantation. Higher power photograph of part of Fig. 15. Conspicuous pleomorphism of mononuclear cells. H.E. × 300.

and survives for a longer period. For example, when skin from Wistar rats is transplanted to A/Jax mice the graft is initially accepted and may appear relatively healthy for up to about a week before being rejected (Monaco *et al* 1966).

With organ xenografts, in which vascular anastomoses have to be created at the time of transplantation, these two patterns of xenograft reaction are seen more clearly. Frequently such grafts are rapidly destroyed, the first changes developing within minutes of revascularization. For example, Calne (1961) found that a goat's kidney transplanted to a dog became pale within 5 min of satisfactory revascularization and soon became deeply cyanosed. Microscopically, the kidney showed oedema, congestion, disruption of fine blood vessels and extensive haemorrhage. Perper & Najarian (1966a) also observed similar immediate reactions when kidneys were transplanted from dog to pig and vice versa. In these experiments the serum of both donor and recipient animals contained natural antibodies reactive against the cells of the other species. The behaviour of such grafts closely resembles the immediate rejection of human renal allografts which may occur when the ABO blood group of the donor is incompatible with the recipient or when the recipient has been previously sensitized. It seems likely that natural antibodies are responsible for the rapid and violent rejection of such renal xenografts but the detailed mechanism has still to be determined. On the other hand, particularly if the donor and recipient belong to closely related species, renal xenografts may survive and function for at least several days in unmodified recipients before being rejected. For instance, Perper & Najarian (1966b) transplanted kidneys between non-sensitized sheep and goats and found that the xenografts secreted urine for about 10 days, the animals dying 1 or 2 days later. Microscopically, the xenografts were extensively infiltrated by mononuclear cells, many of which possessed pyroninophilic cytoplasm. The changes were virtually identical with those found in renal allografts in these two species and it appears that the process of rejection was essentially similar.

Experiments with hepatic xenografts are often complicated by disturbances of blood coagulation and at the present time interpretation of the results tends to be less clear than with renal xenografts. Nevertheless, similar patterns appear to be emerging. In other words, hepatic xenografts between certain species rapidly fail but between others the xenograft may function for some days and when rejection takes place the process is similar to allograft rejection (Figs. 15 and 16) (Calne *et al* 1968, 1970).

Although much more information is needed about the factors controlling the fate of xenografts, experimental and clinical studies support the concept that there are two major forms of xenograft rejection. First, if the donor and recipient belong to widely disparate species, the graft is often rejected immediately. In such circumstances it appears that pre-existing natural antibodies are usually the cause of graft failure. However, biological incompatibility of other kinds may sometimes be responsible and this possibility needs more thorough investigation. Second, if the donor and recipient are members of closely related species, the xenograft may at first be accepted and when rejection occurs the mechanism is similar to that which destroys allografts. Moreover, this second form of xenograft rejection may be modified by certain procedures which prolong or reduce the survival time of allografts (Monaco *et al* 1966; Perper & Najarian 1966b; Lance & Medawar 1968). The effect of immunosuppressive treatment is well illustrated by the prolonged survival of some baboon and chimpanzee renal xenografts transplanted therapeutically to man (Starzl *et al* 1964; Reemtsma *et al* 1964).

Calne (1970) has recently suggested that the adjectives 'discordant' and 'concordant' might be used to describe these two forms of xenograft. If first-set grafts between two particular species were immediately rejected, they would be said to be 'discordant'. On the other hand, if the reaction were essentially similar to the response to a first-set allograft, the xenografts would be described as being 'concordant'.

REFERENCES

Abbott C.P., De Witt C.W. & Creech O. (1965) The transplanted rat heart: histologic and electrocardiographic changes. *Transplantation*, **3**, 432.

Barker C.F. & Billingham R.E. (1967) The role of regional lymphatics in the skin homograft response. *Transplantation*, **5**, 962.

Billingham R.E. & Brent L. (1956) Further attempts to transfer transplantation immunity by means of serum. *Br. J. exp. Path.* **37**, 566.

Billingham R.E., Brent L. & Medawar P.B. (1953) 'Actively acquired tolerance' of foreign cells. *Nature, Lond.* **172**, 603.

Billingham R.E., Brent L. & Medawar P.B. (1954) Quantitative studies of tissue transplantation immunity. II. The origin, strength and duration of actively and adoptively acquired immunity. *Proc. R. Soc.* B **143**, 58.

Billingham R.E. & Silvers W.K. (1963) Sensitivity to homografts of normal tissues and cells. *Ann. Rev. Microbiol.* **17**, 531

Billingham R.E. & Silvers W.K. (1964) Syrian hamsters and transplantation immunity. *Plast. reconst. Surg.* **34**, 329.

Brent L. (1958) Tissue transplantation immunity. *Progr. Allergy* **5**, 271.

Brent L. & Medawar P.B. (1967) Cellular immunity and the homograft reaction. *Br. med. Bull.* **23**, 55.

Calne R.Y. (1961) Observations on renal homotransplantation. *Br. J. Surg.* **48**, 384.

Calne R.Y. (1970) Organ transplantation between widely disparate species. *Transplantation Proc.* (in press).

CALNE R.Y., DAVIS D.R., PENA J.R., BALNER H., DE VRIES M., HERBERTSON B.M., MILLARD P.R., JOYSEY V.C., SEAMAN M.J., SAMUEL J.R., STIBBE J. & WESTBROEK D.L. (1970) Hepatic allografts and xenografts in primates. *Lancet* i, 103.

CALNE R.Y., WHITE H.J.O., HERBERTSON B.M., MILLARD P.R., DAVIS D.R., SALAMAN J.R. & SAMUEL J.R. (1968) Pig-to-baboon liver xenografts. *Lancet* i, 1176.

CALNE R.Y., WHITE H.J.O., YOFFA D.E., BINNS R. M., MAGINN R.R., HERBERTSON B.M., MILLARD P.R., MOLINA V.P. & DAVIS D.R. (1967) Prolonged survival of liver transplants in the pig. *Br. med. J.* iv, 645.

CHIBA C., WOLF P.L., GUDBJARNASON S., CHRYSOHOU A., RAMOS H., PEARSON B. & BING R.J. (1962) Studies on the transplanted heart: its metabolism and histology. *J. exp. Med.* **115,** 853.

CLARK D.S., FOKER J.E., GOOD R.A. & VARCO R.L. (1968) Humoral factors in canine renal allograft rejection. *Lancet* i, 8.

COCHRUM K.C., DAVIES W.C., KOUNTZ S.L. & FUDENBERG H.H. (1969) Renal autograft rejection initiated by passive transfer of immune plasma. *Transplantation Proc.* **1,** 301.

COOMBS R.R.A. & FRANKS D. (1969) Immunological reactions involving two cell types. *Prog. Allergy* **13,** 175.

CORDIER G., GARNIER H., CLOT J.P., CAMPLEZ P., GORIN J.P., CLOT P., RASSINIER J.P., NIZZA M. & LEVY R. (1966) La greffe de foie orthotopique chez le porc: premiers résultats. *Mém. Acad. Chir.* **92,** 799.

DEMPSTER W.J. (1953) Kidney homotransplantation. *Br. J. Surg.* **40,** 447.

GIBSON T. & MEDAWAR P.B. (1943) The fate of skin homografts in man. *J. Anat., Lond.* **77,** 299.

GORER P.A., LOUTIT J.F. & MIEKLEM H.S. (1961) Proposed revisions of 'transplantese'. *Nature, Lond.* **189,** 1024.

GOVAERTS A. (1960) Cellular antibodies in kidney homotransplantation. *J. Immunol.* **85,** 516.

GOWANS J.L. (1965) The role of lymphocytes in the destruction of homografts. *Br. med. Bull.* **21,** 106.

GOWANS J.L., MCGREGOR D.D., COWEN D.M. & FORD C.E. (1962) Initiation of immune responses by small lymphocytes. *Nature, Lond.* **196,** 651.

GRANGER G.A. & WEISER R.S (1964) Homograft target cells: specific destruction *in vitro* by contact interaction with immune macrophages. *Science, N.Y.* **145,** 1427.

GRANGER G.A. & WEISER R.S. (1966) Homograft target cells: contact destruction *in vitro* by immune macrophages. *Science, N.Y.* **151,** 97.

GROTH C.G., PORTER K.A., OTTE J.B., DALOZE P.M., MARCHIORO T.L., BRETTSCHNEIDER L. & STARZL T.E. (1968) Studies of blood flow and ultrastructural changes in rejecting and nonrejecting canine orthotopic liver homografts. *Surgery* **63,** 658.

HARDY J.D., KURRUS F.D., CHAVEZ C.M. & WEBB W.R. (1964) Heart transplantation in infant calves: evaluation of coronary perfusion to preserve organ during transfer. *Ann. N.Y. Acad. Sci.* **120,** 766.

HUNT A.C. (1967) Pathology of Liver Transplantation in the Pig. In *The Liver*, ed. READ A.E., pp. 337-349. London: Butterworth.

KOUNTZ S.L., WILLIAMS M.A., WILLIAMS P.L., KAPROS C. & DEMPSTER W.J. (1963) Mechanism of rejection in homotransplanted kidneys. *Nature, Lond.* **199,** 257.

LANCE E.M. & MEDAWAR P.B. (1968) Survival of skin heterografts under treatment with antilymphocyte serum. *Lancet* i, 1174.

LAWRENCE H.S. (1959) Homograft sensitivity. *Physiol. Rev.* **39**, 811.

LEE S. & EDGINGTON T.S. (1968) Heterotopic liver transplantation utilising inbred rat strains. I. Characterization of allogeneic graft rejection and the effects of biliary obstruction and portal vein circulation on liver regeneration. *Amer. J. Path.* **52**, 649.

LOWER R.R., DONG E. & SHUMWAY N.E. (1965) Long-term survival of cardiac homografts. *Surgery* **58**, 110.

LOWER R.R. & SHUMWAY N.E. (1960) Studies on orthotopic homotransplantation of the canine heart. *Surg. Forum* **11**, 18.

MAY J., MAY L.W. & NAJARIAN J.S. (1965) Onset, duration, and mechanism of antigen release from the homotransplanted kidney. *Surg. Forum* **16**, 250.

MCBRIDE R.A., WHEELER H.B., SMITH L.L., MOORE F.D. & STARZL T.E. (1962) Homotransplantation of the canine liver as an orthotopic vascularized graft. Histologic and functional correlations during residence in new host. *Amer. J. Path.* **41**, 501.

MEDAWAR P.B. (1944) The behaviour and fate of skin autografts and skin homografts in rabbits. *J. Anat., Lond.* **78**, 176.

MEDAWAR P.B. (1945) A second study of the behaviour and fate of skin homografts in rabbits. *J. Anat., Lond.* **79**, 157.

MEDAWAR P.B. (1948) Immunity to homologous grafted skin. III. The fate of skin homografts transplanted to the brain, to subcutaneous tissue, and to the anterior chamber of the eye. *Br. J. exp. Path.* **29**, 58.

MEDAWAR P.B. (1958) The homograft reaction. *Proc. R. Soc.* B **149**, 145.

MITCHISON N.A. (1953) Passive transfer of transplantation immunity. *Nature, Lond.* **171**, 267.

MITCHISON N.A. (1954) Passive transfer of transplantation immunity. *Proc. R. Soc.* B **142**, 72.

MONACO A.P., WOOD M.L., GRAY J.G. & RUSSELL P.S. (1966) Studies on heterologous anti-lymphocyte serum in mice. II. Effect on the immune response. *J. Immunol.* **96**, 229.

MOORE F.D., WHEELER H.B., BEMISSIANOS H.V., SMITH L.L., BALANKURA O., ABEL K., GREENBERG J.B. & DAMMIN G.J. (1960) Experimental whole-organ transplantation of the liver and of the spleen. *Ann. Surg.* **152**, 374.

OORT J. & TURK J.L. (1965) A histological and autoradiographic study of lymph nodes during the development of contact sensitivity in the guinea-pig. *Br. J. exp. Path.* **46**, 147.

PERPER R.J. & NAJARIAN J.S. (1966a) Experimental renal transplantation. I. In widely divergent species. *Transplantation* **4**, 377.

PERPER R.J. & NAJARIAN J.S. (1966b) Experimental renal heterotransplantation. II. Closely related species. *Transplantation* **4**, 700.

PORTER K.A. (1966a) Tissue Transplantation. In *Recent Advances in Pathology.* Eighth Ed., ed. HARRISON C.V., pp. 242–319. London: Churchill.

PORTER K.A. (1966b) Renal Transplantation. In *Pathology of the Kidney*, by HEPTINSTALL R.H., pp. 601–643. London: Churchill.

PORTER K.A. (1969) Pathology of liver transplantation. *Transplant. Rev.* **2**, 129.

PORTER K.A. & CALNE R.Y. (1960) Origin of the infiltrating cells in skin and kidney homografts. *Transplant. Bull.* **26**, 458.

PORTER K.A. & COOPER E.H. (1962) Transformation of adult allogeneic small lymphocytes after transfusion into newborn rats. *J. exp. Med.* **115,** 997.

PRENDERGAST R.A. (1964) Cellular specificity in the homograft reaction. *J. exp. Med.* **119,** 377.

RAPAPORT F.T. & CONVERSE J.M. (1958) The immune response to multiple-set skin homografts: an experimental study in man. *Ann. Surg.* **147,** 273.

REEMTSMA K., MCCRACKEN B.H., SCHLEGEL J.V., PEARL M.A., PEARCE C.W., DEWITT C.W., SMITH P.E., HEWITT R.L., FLINNER R.L. & CREECH O. (1964) Renal heterotransplantation in man. *Ann. Surg.* **160,** 384.

ROGERS B.O., CONVERSE J.M., TAYLOR A.C. & CAMPBELL R.M. (1953) Eosinophile in human skin homografting. *Proc. Soc. exp. Biol. Med.* **82,** 523.

ROSENAU W. & MOON H.D. (1964) The specificity of the cytolytic effect of sensitised lymphoid cells *in vitro*. *J. Immunol.* **93,** 910.

SCOTHORNE R.J. & MCGREGOR I.A. (1955) Cellular changes in lymph nodes and spleen following skin homografting in the rabbit. *J. Anat., Lond.* **89,** 283.

SIMONSEN M. (1953) Biological incompatibility in kidney transplantation in dogs. II. Serological investigations. *Acta path. microbiol. scand.* **32,** 36.

SNELL G.D. (1964) The terminology of tissue transplantation. *Transplantation* **2,** 655.

STARZL T.E., MARCHIORO T.L., PETERS G.N., KIRKPATRICK C.H., WILSON W.E.C., PORTER K.A., RIFKIND D., OGDEN D.A., HITCHCOCK C.R. & WADDELL W.R. (1964) Renal heterotransplantation from baboon to man: experience with six cases. *Transplantation* **2,** 752.

STETSON C.A. (1963) The role of humoral antibody in the homograft reaction. *Advances in Immunology* **3,** 97.

STROBER S. & GOWANS J.L. (1965) The role of lymphocytes in the sensitization of rats to renal homografts. *J. exp. Med.* **122,** 347.

TURK J.L. (1962) The passive transfer of delayed hypersensitivity in guinea-pigs by the transfusion of isotopically-labelled lymphoid cells. *Immunology*, **5,** 478.

TURK J.L. & OORT J. (1963) A histological study of the early stages of the development of the tuberculin reaction after passive transfer of cells labelled with [^{3}H]thymidine. *Immunology* **6,** 140.

WEISER R.S., GRANGER G.A., BROWN W., BAKER P., JUTILA J. & HOLMES B. (1965) Production of acute allogeneic disease in mice. *Transplantation* **3,** 10.

WIENER J., SPIRO D. & RUSSELL P.S. (1964) An electron microscopic study of the homograft reaction. *Amer. J. Path.* **44,** 319.

WILSON D.B. (1965a) Quantitative studies on the behaviour of sensitized lymphocytes *in vitro*. I. Relationship of the degree of destruction of homologous target cells to the number of lymphocytes and to the time of contact in culture and consideration of the effects of isoimmune serum. *J. exp. Med.* **122,** 143.

WILSON D.B. (1965b) Quantitative studies on the behaviour of sensitised lymphocytes *in vitro*. II. Inhibitory influence of the immune suppressor, Imuran, on the destructive reaction of sensitised lymphoid cells against homologous target cells. *J. exp. Med.* **122,** 167.

ACKNOWLEDGEMENTS

I wish to thank Dr R.M. Binns for Fig. 4 and Mr L. Beard, Miss J. Fendick and Mr S.W. Patman for their help with the preparation of the illustrations.

CHAPTER 2

Biological Aspects of Allograft Rejection and Immunosuppression

D.B. Evans
R.A. Sells

INTRODUCTION

From the foregoing account it will be apparent that morphologically the principal cell type involved in rejection is the small lymphocyte. This chapter describes the properties of the small lymphocyte with respect to the allograft reaction, followed by a description of theoretical and practical aspects of immunosuppression.

HISTOCOMPATIBILITY ANTIGENS

The stimulus to rejection is the presence of substances (antigens) on donor cells which are absent in the recipient. As these substances elicit an immune response when they encounter an antigenically disparate recipient, they are termed histocompatibility antigens. They are present on nucleated mammalian cells and their distribution is genetically polymorphic and their genetic transmission is Mendelian. The significance of their existence is a matter for speculation at present. Thomas (1959) has suggested a useful function for this antigen system in terms of autogenous tumour suppression: normal nonmutant cells replicate to form identical progeny with identical histocompatibility antigens; mutation, such as may occur at the genesis of a potential neoplasm, may be accompanied by minute alteration in surface antigen which would lead to a suppressive immune reaction from the host. It is probable that such mutation does occur in mammalian cells very frequently and that a minority of such cellular changes results in a growth developing, which suggests that some host reactivity does exist to early genetic neoplastic change. It is also known that tumour specific antigens may be detected on artificially induced tumours and an immune response may be naturally or artificially stimulated by transplantation within an isogeneic strain. However, until the genetic and chemical characteristics of neoplasia are known in more detail, interpretation of histocompatibility antigen function must remain speculative.

If rejection depends on the genetic disparity of donor and recipient then one would expect to find a correlation between disparity and immune reactivity. Confirmation of this prediction is found in three groups of grafts:

a Isografts between identical twins or members of a genetically pure inbred strain of experimental animal will survive indefinitely without showing any signs of rejection.

b Allografts produce a wide range of rejection response, ranging from minimal cellular infiltration with little evidence of graft damage on the one hand, to massive infiltration, arterial damage, thrombosis and graft necrosis on the other. Evidence is accumulating that the vigour of rejection response (as measured by graft function, e.g. creatinine clearance in human renal transplants) shows a correlation with histocompatibility antigen disparity (as measured by donor and recipient tissue typing).

c Grafts between members of different species (xenografts or heterografts) are usually immediately rejected within minutes, the characteristic lesion being cell disruption, vascular thrombosis, and haemorrhage. This is probably due to gross biological incompatibility involving naturally occurring species specific antibody and antigen.

THE IMMUNE COMPETENT CELL

A Developmental aspects

The role of the lymphocyte in rejection has recently been closely studied and a clearer picture of the properties and distribution of lymphocytes has emerged, although the mode of their activation is still obscure. A short account follows of the properties of lymphocytes in immune cellular response.

1 *The thymus*

The development of a normal cellular reactive mechanism appears to be governed by the thymus. Thymectomy in neonatal mice (Miller 1962; Martinez *et al* 1962) and other mammals, produced deficient maturation of lymph nodes with diminished lymphoid reactivity and inability to reject homografts and to produce antibody. Examination of the thoracic duct lymph and peripheral blood revealed a deficiency of circulating lymphocytes (Metcalf 1960) and typical histological changes in the lymph nodes showed lymphocyte depletion in the paracortical region of the node.

Grafting syngeneic thymic tissue to thymectomized animals restored immune capability to normal. It is thought that the thymus performs an inductive function in the development of the lymphoreticular system rather than providing a source of immune competent cells. The thymocytes are derived originally from foetal bone marrow cells, and in early life the gland is the centre of differentiation of 'immunocytes', which eventually colonize the peripheral lymphoid tissue. In addition, there is evidence that the thymus exerts a humoral effect on the development of peripheral lymphoid tissue in that grafting thymectomized mice with thymus enclosed in a millipore chamber (Osaba & Miller 1963) or injecting the animals with extract of thymus (Hardy *et al* 1969) restores a degree of cellular immune responsiveness, and results in a return of the proliferation reaction to skin grafting in the paracortical regions of the draining lymph node.

The role of the paracortical or 'thymus dependent' region of the node is still variously interpreted by researchers. In that the cells of this region remain inactive in the absence of a normal thymic gland during the neonatal period and that paracortical proliferation is seen in regional nodes draining an area of chemical hypersensitivity reaction in skin or skin homograft (Oort & Turk 1965) the indirect dependence of cellular immune response on thymic induction is evident. Some workers feel, however, that the paracortical area, being endowed with a profuse post-capillary venous plexus, simply provides a large surface area for the interaction of incoming informant cells (afferent phase) with the intermediary immune cells (cf. efferent phase). Recent work suggests strongly that in the mouse at least thymus derived cells form a substantial proportion of the small lymphocyte population resident in the lymph nodes. (Schlesinger & Yron 1969). An antigen ('theta') has been detected in high concentrations in mouse brain and thymus cells and is not part of the mouse H-2 antigen system. Antibody to mouse thymus cells (ATS) raised in the rabbit and administered intraperitoneally to mice of the donor strain caused a diminution in sensitivity of lymph node cells to anti-theta antibodies *in vitro*; 3 days after the last dose of ATS, sensitivity to anti-theta antibody was nil, but 7 days afterwards the lymph node cells were found to have recovered their sensitivity. It seems that the loss of sensitivity after ATS administration represents the disappearance of a population of thymus dependent cells from the lymph nodes, an observation which is in accord with the theory of lymphoreticular thymic dependence and is substantiated by the recent observation that thymectomy results in the permanent loss of theta-positive cells from the lymph nodes (Schlesinger & Yron 1969).

2 *The maturation of immune response, 'self recognition' and tolerance*

The theory of clonal selection first put forward by Burnet & Fenner (1949) and since developed by Burnet (1959) to apply to a wide range of immunological phenomena can be summarized as follows:

a There exists in the body a population of cells differentiated for immune function by their ability to produce antibody and react in this and other ways to contact with specific antigen.
b Cells comprising this population are termed immunocytes and comprise small lymphocytes and plasma cells.
c The specific pattern of antibody is determined by the genetic endowment of the cell which produces it.
d The diversity of the immune pattern arises as a result of somatic mutation or gene recombination.

During the development of this theory in 1949, these authors directed their attention to two naturally occurring examples of immunological non-reactivity which the theory could not explain as presented above. The first was Owen's discovery that bovine dizygotic twins commonly possessed two blood groups, and that as adults these animals tolerated the two red cell populations throughout life.

These animals are chimeras, that is they each have their own and their partners red cell antigens. During foetal life the twins are synchorial, or share the same placenta, and thus exchange foetal blood. Anderson *et al* (1951) compared the skin graft reactions of identical and dizogotic cattle twins and found that grafts were tolerated between members of the dizogotic as well as the identical twin groups. The ability of the recipient to reject skin from other (non-twin) siblings remained unimpaired—thus showing the high degree of specificity of this effect. It appeared that natural tolerance had occurred as a result of exposure of the foetus to foreign antigen during the stages of lymphoreticular development. At the time of Owen's experiments Traub also demonstrated that congenital infection of mice with lymphocytic choriomeningitis virus produced long-lasting but asymptomatic infection. Both these phenomena are examples of acceptance by the young animal of material which a normal adult would regard as foreign, and the concept of auto-censorship leading to deletion of clones active against the individual's own tissues, during immunological maturation, was introduced.

It followed that if the foetus' own tissues induced immune non-reactivity then the introduction of foreign material into the foetus at the time of maturation would produce permanent tolerance in adult life to donor tissues of the same origin. This 'classical immune tolerance' was confirmed by Billingham and his colleagues in 1954, when they injected foetal mice of one pure line with homologous lymphoid tissue from another pure line strain; they demonstrated that subsequent skin homografts from syngeneic donors were accepted indefinitely whereas grafts from a third strain were rejected. Tolerance could also be induced to skin grafts by injection of donor kidney cells in embryonic life, indicating acceptance of individual-specific rather than tissue-specific antigen by the host.

While long-lasting, often permanent tolerance occurred if injection of donor cells was undertaken before birth, the same effect could be obtained if the injections were carried out during the first 24 h of neonatal life, however after 72 h antigen produced immunity, as evidenced by accelerated rejection of grafts from the donor strain.

B Experimental aspects

1 *Adoptive immunity*

As has already been described, the response in the regional lymphatic centre to a homograft in the area drained by the centre entails the generation of a line of immunologically competent cells specifically committed to the graft and the release of the cells into the circulation.

These immunologically competent cells constitute a population of recirculating small lymphocytes whose life span is 3 to 4 months. They originate in the paracortical area of the node and pass via efferent lymphatics and thoracic duct to the blood stream whence their contact with foreign antigen occurs by their random distribution. These cells appear to be active in graft rejection, a property demonstrated by the induction of 'adoptive immunity' to grafts, as shown by Mitchison (1953). Lymphosarcoma tissue from one pure mouse strain was rejected by another strain and the speed of rejection could be increased by prior skin grafting from the donor strain. Mitchison revealed that by injecting the recipient with syngeneic lymph node cells taken from animals previously immunized against the tumour, an accelerated type of rejection of primary tumour tissue grafts occurred, similar in timing to that observed in recipients immunized with skin.

Adoptive immunity to skin grafts was likewise induced by Billingham *et al* (1951) who demonstrated accelerated skin graft rejection after transferral of lymph-node cells from syngeneic mice previously immunized to skin grafts of the same donor strain. Such immunity could not be induced by the administration of antibody from the sensitized mice. In tolerant animals first-set skin graft rejection could be induced by injecting lymphocytes from unsensitized normal recipient strain mice; the administration of cells from sensitized mice led to rapid (second-set) destruction of the grafts. Similar effects were observed by the injection of thoracic duct cells (a pure population of small lymphocytes) into tolerant recipients, thus implicating these cells as the immunological effector cells in rejection.

2 *The graft-versus-host reaction*

Another preparation which reveals the immune reactivity of the lymphocyte is the reaction of living lymphocytes to host allogeneic tissue (the graft-versus-host reaction). If lymphoid cells from an allogeneic strain of rodent are injected into a host which possesses antigens not present in the donor, they react against the host, causing a wasting disease. The severity of this reaction depends on the degree and direction of antigen disparity (Simonsen 1962; Billingham & Brent 1959). The graft-versus-host reaction is well illustrated by the results of exchanging lymphoid cells between pure-strain mice and their hybrid offspring.

The cross-mating of two pure lines of rodent, for example AA × BB, produces a hybrid possessing antigen absent in both parents:

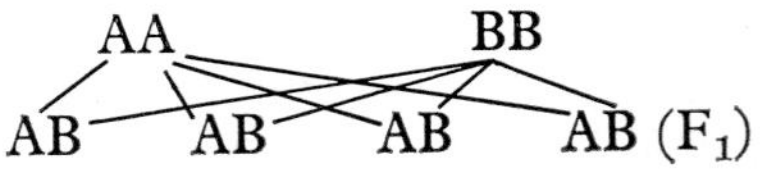

If parental strain lymphoid cells are injected into the hybrid offspring, (e.g. BB cells → AB recipients) the donor cells, lacking some of the host antigens, react against them producing a usually fatal wasting condition, known as ‘runt disease’.

Ford *et al* (1966) have used this preparation to demonstrate the participation of small lymphocytes in graft-verus-host reaction and their identity with the pyroninophyllic cells seen in rejection. Rat (xenogeneic) thoracic duct lymphocytes were injected into irradiated and therefore immunologically unresponsive mice. These lymphocytes were labelled beforehand with an isotope and autoradiographic examination of the host spleen after 24 h revealed the appearance of large pyroninophillic cells in the spleen which carried the isotopic label and therefore were presumed to be derived from the rat lymphocyte which had transformed to a type of cell which was active in the graft-versus-host attack. Furthermore, transplantation of these labelled cells back to isogeneic rats resulted in the appearance of radioactive lymphocytes in the thoracic duct. In this preparation 'recirculating' lymphocytes therefore appear to be capable of transformation to an active form in response to an antigenic stimulus, and reversion to their original form when the stimulus is removed. Subsequent work on transformation of cells *in vitro*, mentioned in Chapter 3 confirms this ability in peripheral blood lymphocytes.

3 *The normal lymphocyte transfer test*

Brent & Medawar (1967) have used a local version of the graft-verus-host response in guinea-pigs to demonstrate the correlation between lymphocyte activity and reactivity in terms of skin graft rejection. By injecting normal allogeneic lymphocytes isolated from peripheral blood intradermally a flare is produced within the first 36 h; this is thought to be due to lymphocyte proliferation on encountering antigen i.e. a local graft-versus-host reaction. This is followed occasionally by a late tuberculin like secondary erythema. By using multiple donors they showed by subsequent skin grafting from lymphocyte donors that there was a positive correlation between the speed of skin rejection and the magnitude of the early normal lymphocyte transfer reaction.

4 *Allogeneic inhibition*

This section has so far dealt with immune reactivity of immunocytes which shows patterns dependent on histocompatibility antigen differences between effector and target cells. In general the reactions obey the rule that reactivity occurs as a result of the presence of antigen on the target cell surface which is absent from the reactive cells. An important, possibly non-immune exception to this rule is the unexpected ability of cells to act in the opposite direction in tissue culture—a phenomenon known as allogeneic inhibition, or syngeneic preference, defined as target cell destruction triggered by contact with histoincompatible cells and first described by Hellstrom in 1963. The nature of allogeneic inhibition is illustrated in the Moller's experiments (1965, 1966): Lymphoid cells from F_1 hybrids were placed in tissue culture with pure strain parental (target) cells. These lymphoid cells would not generally be expected to react in culture as the parental strain did not possess any antigens foreign to the donor strain.

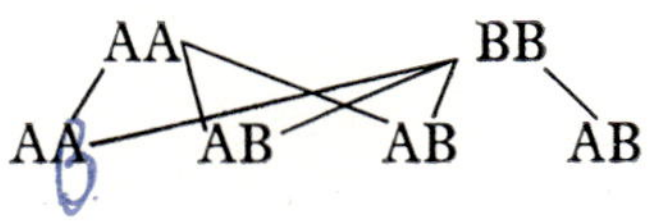

parental (target) cells

donor lymphoid cells

Somewhat surprisingly, damage to the target cells occurred. The absence of foreign antigen in the target cell suggested that this might be a non-immune phenomenon, and this view has been substantiated by the demonstration that the cytotoxicity is not antibody or complement mediated, and not altered by irradiation of lymphoid cells or treatment with prednisolone or antimetabolite drugs. Furthermore, not only lymphoid cells but a variety of neoplastic cells from lymphoid or non-lymphoid tumours can mediate allogeneic inhibition. The action of lymphocytes on target cells in the experiment described above may be blocked by treating donor cells with isoantibodies raised to donor cells of the target cell genotype; pretreatment with antibodies to an indifferent strain had no suppressive effect (Moller *et al* 1967). It is thus possible that geometrical or 'steric' differences in cell surface components between target and effector cells may be the stimulus to cell inhibition: masking of these differences by coating the cells with isoantibody thus abolishes the response which results in target cell inhibition.

The place of this phenomenon in the repertoire of reactivity of lymphoid cells to neighbouring cells is not known, but one may speculate in favour of the tumour suppressing function of lymphoid and other cells which encounter local difference in membrane structure in neoplastic cells. The role of allogeneic inhibition in transplantation, if any, is as yet obscure.

MODIFICATION OF ALLOGRAFT REJECTION

INTRODUCTION

From the foregoing review of the biological nature of the immune mechanisms in relation to allograft rejection, it would seem that interference with and disruption of the immunological reflex arc at one or more stages might modify the sequence of events and allow the allograft to survive. An understanding of the mechanism of immune rejection was derived from much experimental work designed to investigate the possible methods by which the reaction could be modified. The antigen or allograft, the afferent arc, the reaction and recognition centre, and the efferent arc have all been the targets of biological, physical and chemical assaults. The ways in which experimental workers have approached the problem at its different levels may be formally categorized as follows: (Calne 1967).

A Diminishing the antigencity of the graft.
B Prevention of antigenic material reaching the lymphoid system.

C Prevention of recognition of the antigenic material by the lymphoid system.
D Prevention of the central mechanism reacting against the antigenic material.
E Prevention of lymphoid cells reaching the graft.

It is worth stating at the outset that successful methods of immunosuppression used in clinical transplantation programmes fall into category D above, that is, they aim at preventing the central immune reaction centre from reacting against the antigenic material. A brief summary follows of experimental aspects of immunosuppression carried out under the other headings set out above.

A Diminishing the antigenic properties of the graft

Any attempt to destroy the antigenicity of the allograft is followed by cellular death. This is to be expected because tissue antigenicity is determined genetically in nucleated cells. However, there is evidence that some tissue is less antigenic than others, for instance, endocrine tissue (Woodruff 1959); it is possible that in some cases of free grafting of tissue to immunologically privileged sites some weeding out of antigenically potent material occurs leaving surviving cells of weaker antigenicity (Shaffer & Hulka 1969).

B Prevention of antigenic material reaching the lymphoid system

There is convincing evidence that implantation of tissue grafts to sites where lymphatic drainage is sparse or absent results in attentuation or absence of the rejection reaction because antigen is unable to reach the specific reactive centre to initiate the response. Such sites include the cornea, the hamster cheek pouch, the brain, the anterior chamber of the eye. Thus skin placed in the brain will survive but if the animal has been presensitized by skin grafts from the same donor rapid destruction of the graft occurs (Medawar 1948). These experiments have suggested that although the tissue itself was incapable of stimulating a central reaction, presumably by the lack of lymphatic drainage, the centre, once stimulated, was capable of reacting against the tissue graft.

Hume & Egdahl (1955) found that by enclosing canine renal allografts in plastic bags, thus isolating them from regional lymphatics, typical allograft rejection reactions occurred showing that in the case of organ transplants the antigenic stimulus was transmitted centrally by the blood stream. Yet for skin the role of lymphatic drainage is of great importance in the transmission of antigenic material to the local centre, as illustrated by the experiments of Barker & Billingham (1967); patches of skin were prepared possessing a blood supply, but stripped of their lymphatics. On this prepared site allograft skin survived indefinitely but sensitization by prior skin grafts resulted in rejection of the otherwise privileged tissue.

It has also been said that steroids applied locally to skin grafts delay vascularization and can prolong their survival probably by preventing the release of antigen from the graft (Billingham *et al* 1951). Another biological method of inducing 'afferent arc block' is by using enhancement. This is a specific immunological concept, originally detected as a depressant effect of antitumour antibodies on host rejection response to transplanted tumour tissue, and is defined as 'the successful establishment of a tumour homograft and its progressive growth (usually to the death of the host) as a consequence of the tumour's contact with specific antiserum in the host' (Kaliss 1958). It was thought initially by Kaliss that protection arose due to a physiological alteration in the tumour cells as a result of antibody treatment; this theory has been negated by Snell *et al* who demonstrated that tumour cells 'passaged' through a host treated with enhancing antibody did not change the virulence of the tumour transferred to a third host. Because of the specificity of the enhancing effect it is assumed that graft survival results from the deposition of non-cytotoxic antibody on the surface of foreign cells with subsequent masking and non-recognition of the protein coated allogeneic cells by recipient lymphocytes. It is also likely that enhancing antibody acts on immune reactive centres in inhibiting the development of cellular immunity (Snell *et al* 1960; Brent & Medawar 1961).

This principle has been applied by several authors in the protection of homografts—notably by Stuart *et al* (1968). They demonstrated prolonged survival of rat kidney grafts transplanted across a known histocompatibility barrier following injection of antibody and cellular antigen (donor spleen cells) 24 h before transplantation. Subsequently, French & Batchelor (1969) initiated enhancement 'passively' in parental strain rats bearing kidneys from F_1 hybrid donors. This was induced by intravenous injection of antiserum raised against donor strain lymphocytes, and in the F_1 situation 100% 6 month survival was achieved following removal of the animals own kidneys. Partial protection of kidney grafts in dogs, allegedly due to enhancement, has been reported by Wilson *et al* (1969). The injection of soluble splenic antigen at the time of the transplant enabled reduction in the dosage of immunosuppressive agents, with good renal function persisting.

C Prevention of recognition of the antigenic material by the lymphoid system

The reacting and recognition centre which is presumed to be situated in the lymphoreticular tissue and possibly the thymus, can recognize antigens as 'self' and 'non-self'. In order to accept an antigen as self, the centre must have had experience of it before reaching full maturity, i.e. by injection during embryonic life or soon after birth. This crucial period during which this effect may be induced varies from species to species. As has been described above, specific immune tolerance may occur following an injection of cells of one rodent strain into the foetus of another strain, which in adult life remains tolerant to skin grafts from the donor strain. This observation has prompted investigation of the possibility of inducing similar specific immune tolerance to homograft tissue in immunologically mature adults. Tolerance may be induced by a variety of antigens and the foundation of this work was laid down by Mitchison (1964, 1965, 1967) who introduced the concept of two zones of antigen dosage capable of inducing tolerance. Using repeated injections from bovine serum albumen in adult mice and assessing the animals' immune status by measuring the response to a maximal challenge of bovine serum albumen in adjuvant, he has shown that complete or partial tolerance may be induced in the very low range (10 μg) and very high range (10 mg) of antigen dose. In the intermediate range (e.g. 500 μg) immunity manifested by antibody formation is apparent. A possible explanation for these two zones of tolerance is that antigen sensitive cells may be driven towards tolerance or towards immunity —the tendency to immunity being a threshold phenomenon requiring a minimum concentration before antibody formation occurs. Thus a subimmunogenic dose leads to inactivation of the immunocyte with respect to the antigen concerned while a threshold dose leads to immunity; paralysis of, or inactivation of a population of cells sensitized to an antigen requires a very much higher concentration of antigen. Inactivation of such cells is believed to occur in high zone tolerance and is termed immunological paralysis. There is still much uncertainty as to the nature, necessary dosage, route of administration and fate of the antigen molecules concerned in tolerance induction and it is not surprising that research into this field has dealt mainly with tolerance to humoral antigen using pure antigen preparations in accurately controlled experiments. Extrapolation of data derived from these experiments to the allograft situation is difficult due to the increased complexity inherent in tissue transplantation. However, the principle of desensitization (probably analogous to low zone tolerance) has been employed by Owen (1969) who has shown that in a variety of species, microgramme quantities of specific antigen may render recipients tolerant to subsequent grafts from the same donor without the need for immunosuppression in the recipient. In fact final acceptance of this phenomenon as tolerance must await the demonstration of loss of specific activity against donor tissue by the recipient lymphoid cells in culture with donor cells. A form of graft protection which may well be partial tolerance is evident in Calne's experiments using pig liver allografts (Calne *et al* 1969). It was found that orthotopic liver allografts survived indefinitely without evidence of significant rejection. In addition to protecting its own tissue from rejection, liver was also capable of protecting renal, cardiac, and to some extent, skin, if the donor material was taken from the same animal and transplanted at the same time as the liver. Furthermore, auxiliary liver grafts removed at 24 h have been shown to exert a long-lasting protective effect on renal allografts from the same donor. One possible explanation for this could be that antigen produced by the liver in a tolerogenic form interacts with pig lymphoid tissue before sensitization occurs. The unique acceptance of liver in the pig may reflect a peculiarity of antigen release from pig liver or oddity of the pig's lymphoreticular system. It has also been shown that some degree of non-specific protection of donor organs may be induced by grafting the liver and kidney from two different individuals into the same recipient. No general immunosuppressive action of crude homogenate has yet been demonstrated so this protective effect appears to be a property of an intact functioning liver graft. If tolerance is found to be induced in these experiments by the release of histocompatibility antigen then the possibility of rendering human recipients tolerant of allografts by the administration of a suitable antigen fraction may be considered. But it is likely that consistent induction of artificial tolerance to allograft tissue without the risk of immunogenesis must await suitable extraction techniques which will enable purification of the tolerogenic form of histocompatibility antigen and preparation of the correct dose. If this is achieved then the application of tolerance induction to allograft and even heterograft tissue becomes a distinct possibility.

D Prevention of the central mechanism reacting against the antigenic material

1 *X-irradiation*

It has been known since the beginning of the century that antibody production was suppressed in animals exposed to ionizing irradiation and Dempster *et al* (1950) showed that skin grafts survived twice as long in irradiated as opposed to non-irradiated rabbits.

Total body irradiation. X-irradiation is particularly lethal to the lymphocyte family and as these cells were known to play an important role in the rejection reaction, it was not surprising that X-irradiation was one of the early methods used for immunosuppressive purposes. However, the dose of irradiation required to suppress the immune responses and allow allografts to be accepted usually results in almost complete depletion of the small lymphocyte population of the blood. Also lymph node germinal centres and bone marrow lymphocytes diminish. If the animal can be kept alive, histological recovery can be expected in the lymphoreticular tissues within 4–6 weeks. In man, however, the blood lymphocyte population may not return to normal after total body radiation for months or years (Cronkite & Chanana 1968).

The toxic effects of radiation of the gastrointestinal tract and haematopoietic system made the control of the immune response very difficult. centres that had used X-irradiation (Murray *et al* 1960; Hamburger 1965) reported two long-term survivals from dizygotic twin transplants but as other less dangerous methods of immunosuppression became available total body irradiation was discontinued.

LOCAL IRRADIATION

a The recipient bed: Stark *et al* (1955) employed this technique prior to skin grafting and reported slight prolongation of graft survival. Woodruff *et al* (1963) irradiated the iliac fossa prior to renal transplantation but found no beneficial effect on graft survival.

b Irradiation of arterial and venous blood was performed by Wolff & Hume (1965) and prolongation of some canine renal allografts was obtained only with very large doses.

c Parenteral radioactive isotopes; intralymphatic, intravenous and intra-arterial administration of radioactive isotopes have been used experimentally. Usually a transient lymphopenia was observed and there have been some claims that allograft survival has been prolonged.

d Local irradiation to the allograft: this has been used both immediately after transplantation and later in the treatment of rejection reactions. The beneficial effect of this method claimed by some workers may be due to

- i altering the antigenicity of the graft—this is highly unlikely;
- ii destroying the lymphatic tissues in the graft bed and surrounding lymphatics;
- iii an anti-inflammatory effect;
- iv destroying the small lymphocytes invading the graft.

e Extracorporeal irradiation: the concept of irradiating blood during its passage through an extracorporeal circuit was devised by Cronkite *et al* (1962) to deplete peripheral lymphocyte population and this has been used in the treatment of certain types of leukaemias. It has been investigated experimentally and clinically in attempts to prolong allograft survival but as yet its value is not certain (Maginn & Bullimore 1968).

2 *Corticosteroids*

Suppression of antibody formation by steroid drugs in rabbits is very effective but much less so in man and guinea-pigs. They are also capable of inhibiting the allograft response in a variety of mammals and there is a wealth of experimental evidence with skin grafts to support this. Whole organ grafts are less well protected and Dempster (1953) failed to prolong canine allografts with large doses of cortisone. He found nevertheless that swelling of the graft and cellular infiltration were much less marked than in the untreated dogs. Zukoski *et al* (1965) reported prolonged renal allograft function in a dog treated with 30 mg prednisolone daily. Evidence that steroids on their own prolong allografts in man is very slim, but their value in conjunction with other agents is undoubted.

MECHANISMS OF ACTION

1 They may inhibit the phagocytic activity of reticuloendothelial cells. It has been shown also that small doses may enhance phagocytic activity.

2 They may suppress the generation of lymphoid tissue and induce lymphocytolosis. There has been no evidence though that a sustained fall in circulating lymphocyte counts occurs when steroids have been used to prolong allograft survival.

3 By anti-inflammatory action they may interfere with the consequences of tissue destruction brought about by the antigen–antibody reaction. This anti-inflammatory action may be the result of interference with glucose metabolism.

4 By inhibiting protein synthesis and hence antibody production.

3 *Purine analogues*

In 1952 Elion *et al* developed an analogue of hypoxanthine which proved to be a powerful antimetabolite—this substance was 6-mercaptopurine. It interferes with the synthesis of nucleic acids probably at two different stages.

a In the synthesis of purines from the simple precursors e.g. glycine and formate.

b In the cell, 6 MP is converted to thioinosinic acid which inhibits the conversion of inosinic acid to adenylic and guanylic acids of ribonucleic and deoxyribonucleic acids.

Later, an imidazolyl substituted purine azathioprine (Imuran) was produced. This substance appeared to have a higher therapeutic index in mice than 6 MP even though *in vivo*, the molecule was split to produce 6 MP and the imadazolyl fraction. This may in part be due to the fact that the imidazolyl radical may have its own antimetabolite properties.

Both these drugs were extensively studied and were found to suppress the primary immune response in a variety of species including humans provided they were administered on the same day as the antigenic stimulus.

IgG synthesis seems to be almost invariably suppressed whereas IgM synthesis seems virtually unaffected and in general cells elaborating IgM are relatively resistant to immunosuppressive agents. Delayed hypersensitivity is also suppressed by 6 MP and azathioprine. The prolongation of skin graft survival in rabbits by 6 MP was demonstrated by Schwartz & Dameshek (1960) but second set rejection was unaffected. Skin grafting in rats gave inconsistent results Calne (1960) and Zukoski *et al* (1960) showed that canine renal allograft survival was prolonged by 6 MP and in 1961 Calne reported similar results with azathioprine which was less toxic to the bone marrow than 6 MP.

4 *Folic acid antagonists*

Methrotrexate has been shown to block antibody synthesis in the mouse, guinea-pig and in the dog, provided it was given within 48 h of the antigen. It has also been found to be a powerful immunosuppressive agent in man. Delayed hypersensitivity is suppressed in the guinea-pig and skin grafts in guinea-pigs and mice were markedly prolonged by it. The drug was ineffective in the rabbit presumably by its rapid detoxification by the species.

5 *Alkylating agents*

Cyclophosphamide, a nitrogen mustard derivative, is a powerful immunosuppressive agent with a high therapeutic index in mice, rats, guinea-pigs and in man. It probably acts by preventing differentiation, division or both in immunologically competent cells (Frisch & Davies 1965). Pre-existing delayed hypersensitivity is not suppressed by cyclophosphamide even when lymphopenia is produced but it is highly effective in preventing skin graft rejection in mice, rabbits and rats but not in the guinea-pig.

6 *Drug induced tolerance*

Rabbits treated with 6 MP can be rendered tolerant to human serum albumin (HSA) provided the 6 MP treatment is started on the day of antigen injection (Schwartz & Dameshek 1959). These results were confirmed by Nachtigal & Feldman (1963) who showed that rabbits made HSA tolerant by treatment with 6 MP could still respond normally to bovine serum albumin (BSA) challenge. Schwartz & Dameshek (1963) further showed that the proportion of rabbits rendered tolerant to BSA as a result of 6 MP treatment was directly related to the dose of antigen used. Cyclophosphamide has also been shown to induce tolerance to antigens in the guinea-pig. Tolerance to allograft tissue in mice treated with anti-metabolites combined with antigen administration was achieved by Uphoff (1961) and Hohen (1965)—the ease by which it was produced depending on whether donor and recipient shared the same H^2 allele. The long continued acceptance of renal allografts in dogs and man receiving minimal or even no immunosuppressive therapy has been observed. It has been suggested that this phenomenon is the result of chance histocompatibility (Calne *et al* 1962) or to the replacement of certain elements of long-term grafts by host tissues (Woodruff 1959). The mechanism of this drug induced tolerance of canine allografts was studied by Shiel *et al* (1967) and they demonstrated that dogs with long surviving renal allografts and who were maintained on immunosuppressive therapy had impaired immunological capabilities but were able to reject specific donor and indifferent skin whilst maintaining normal renal allograft function. Kidney donor skin survived longer than indifferent skin, but when the former rejected it caused greater impairment of renal allograft function than the latter.

Furthermore, dogs in whom drug therapy was stopped, rejected indifferent skin in first-set fashion and donor skin in accelerated fashion and the reaction against the renal allograft was increased though it was still capable of functioning.

Second renal allografts were accepted if transplanted relatively soon after the first when drug therapy was maintained, but if second renal allografts were transplanted after cessation of drug therapy, they were violently rejected, whilst the first graft from the same donor was unaffected. Thus a change, possibly due to enhancing antibody, had occurred in the first graft.

Finally the antigenicity of the long surviving allograft was not completely impaired for when transplanted into a third party it was rejected in normal fashion. It seems likely that chance histocompatibility, impairment in immune response with decreased reactivity against the resident kidney are the important mechanisms underlying acceptance of long surviving renal allografts.

7 *Antibiotics*

Actinomycin C, a toxic combination of three antibiotics isolated from Streptomyces chrysomallis, is too poisonous to use as an antibiotic but has been widely used in small doses (400–600 μg) during rejection crises. When used on its own experimentally it was found to be ineffective in prolonging skin graft survival but it added to the immunosuppressive effects of azathioprine in dogs with renal allografts (Calne *et al* 1962).

8 *Lymphocyte depletion*

a THYMECTOMY

The thymus is important in the development of the lymphoreticular system in mice and thymectomy performed soon after birth had a marked depressive effect on immunity responses (Martinez *et al* 1962) and will permit lifetime survival of allogeneic skin grafts and even skin grafts from rats (Miller 1962). Graft-versus-host reactions are usually produced in neonatally thymectomized mice.

The effect of thymectomy in the rabbit has less influence on immunity and on the development of the lymphoid system, but it was found that at birth the rabbit often possessed significant splenic lymphoid tissue which is probably capable of stimulating normal lymphoid development even in the absence of the thymus. It is also probable that the appendix and Peyer's patches play an important part in fostering the development of peripheral lymphoid tissues. Calne (1963) in a study of canine renal allografts treated with azathioprine and Actinomycin C found no prolongation of graft survival by performing thymectomy.

b THORACIC DUCT DRAINAGE

McGregor & Gowans (1963) showed that external drainage of thoracic duct lymph in rats was associated with a marked fall in circulating lymphocytes and this was associated with an inability to form antibodies against a variety of antigenic stimuli. Survival of rat skin homografts was significantly prolonged by chronic thoracic duct drainage. Similar results have been observed in dogs. Tilney & Murray (1966) studied 19 patients with renal transplants who were on conventional immunosuppressive therapy. Their thoracic ducts were cannulated 2 to 3 days before transplantation and cell free lymph was reinfused intravenously. Lymphopenia developed and rejection episodes were observed to be less severe than in a control group. Graber *et al* (1969) showed that immunological competence could be depressed in patients with thoracic duct fistulae after subjecting the lymph to dialysis and reinfusing it into the patients. They found that total lymphocyte counts were depressed and serum and lymph complement levels declined and the patients failed to produce primary or secondary antibody responses to antigen.

Sarles *et al* (1970) however found that lymph dialysis was an impractical method of controlling uraemia and reverted to haemodialysis in conjunction with thoracic duct drainage and reinfusion of lymphocyte free lymph after centrifugation. Depletion of lymph and blood lymphocyte population resulted in simultaneous depletion of lymphocytes from lymph nodes, spleen and intestinal wall, loss of delayed hypersensitivity skin reactions to a variety of antigens but there was no change in immunoglobulin concentration in the sera. Immunosuppressive drugs were withheld initially until rejection occurred and in five cases this period was as long as 32–78 days. Sixty-four per cent of these patients have maintained good renal function for up to 27 months.

9 *Antilymphocyte serum*

Antilymphocyte serum (ALS) suppressed cutaneous hypersensitivity reactions of the delayed type (Wilhelm *et al* 1958). Waksman *et al* (1961) produced significant results with first and second-set skin grafts in guinea-pigs treated with rabbit anti-guinea-pig lymph node sera. In 1963 Woodruff & Anderson showed that ALS and thoracic duct drainage prolonged skin homografts in rats.

The preparation of ALS has been reviewed by James (1969). Briefly, several doses of the antigen from the species to be treated e.g. thoracic duct lymphocytes, peripheral blood leucocytes or viable cell suspensions from the thymus, lymph nodes or spleen, is injected subcutaneously or intravenously into an animal of another species at suitable time intervals with or without Freund's adjuvant. The animal is bled after acceptable titres of antilymphocytic activity have been produced, the complement in the serum is inactivated by heating to 56°C and after removal of fibrinogen, it is adsorbed on erythrocytes and thrombocytes. The active IgG fraction of ALS is prepared on (G200) Sephadex columns and by salt precipitation. Sterilization by Seitz filtration is then performed and the serum is stored at −20°C.

Methods of assaying the *in vivo* activity of antilymphocytic preparations are difficult as they are species specific. The use of human volunteers would be highly undesirable to test antihuman lymphocyte serum and this led Balner *et al* (1968) to make use of the closely related subhuman primates. Chimpanzees share HL-A antigens with man and would be the obvious choice but they are rare and very expensive so that other members of the primate family—rhesus monkeys and baboons—have been used. The results however are not as clear cut. *In vitro* testing of antilymphocytic products until recently were confined to leuko-agglutination, cytotoxicity tests and immunoprecipitation but none gave good correlation between the effect of ALS and graft survival. Bach *et al* (1969) tested antilymphocyte globulin *in vitro* by means of a 'rosette test'. The basis of this test lies in the ability of an effective immunosuppressive agent to suppress the formation of spontaneous rosettes when lymphocytes are incubated with heterologous red blood cells. The results of this *in vitro* test on 50 specimens of ALG correlated well with Balner's *in vivo* tests on skin grafted monkeys.

The possible modes of action of ALS are as follows:

a Lymphocyte depletion. The acute administration of ALS leads to a rapid fall in peripheral leucocyte count probably by a cytotoxic effect and affects the delayed type of hypersensitivity in response to an antigenic challenge.

b Passive interference by masking the recognition sites by a coat of foreign protein (Levey & Medawar 1966).

c Active interference. ALS has the characteristics of an antibody but it also acts as an antigen for which every lymphocyte in the body has receptors. It therefore can compete with other antigens and attaches itself to all lymphocytes with which it comes into contact, thus altering the immunological commitment of such lymphocytes.

d Sterile activation. Levey & Medawar (1966) found the antibody converts the lymphocytes into sterile blast forms which cannot react normally to antigenic stimuli.

e ALS has a depressant effect on a thymus-dependent lymphoid system. Chiba *et al* (1965) suggested that lymphocytes may accquire autoantigenic properties after coupling with ALS.

Many questions are still left unanswered in regard to antilymphocyte serum. Here is an exciting approach to immunosuppressive therapy, which is of undoubted value in prolonging graft survival in rodents and small animals but its effect in human allografts is as yet inconclusive. Many centres are producing their own brand of ALS, so that not only do methods of preparation vary widely but also the immunosuppressive activity and toxicity of the products. A valid comparison is therefore impossible. There has not so far been a constructive attempt at running a controlled trial using uniform batches of ALS or ALG on a scale large enough to draw statistical conclusions—this is a much needed exercise if a fair evaluation of ALS is to be made.

The antihuman lymphocyte preparations have mainly been raised in the horse but is this the ideal animal? Antisera of various types have for many years been prepared from horses and are well tolerated by most humans but with fractionation of IgG thus eliminating most other protein elements it may be possible to use other large animals. Further problems in preparation lie in finding the ideal route of injection, the right dose of lymphocytes necessary, the frequency of injections and the optimum time for harvesting the serum.

E Prevention of lymphoid cells reaching the graft

First set tissue allografts become infiltrated with small lymphocytes during rejection crises. Corneal grafts however, unless they become vascularized, survive presumably because they are inaccessible to immunologically committed lymphocytes.

By enclosing allograft tissues in porous envelopes, Weaver *et al* (1955) were able to prevent rejection of the grafted tissues by using an envelope with pore sizes smaller than the diameter of the lymphoctyes. By increasing the dimension of the pores, thus allowing the passage of lymphocytes, normal rejection patterns occurred.

Canine renal allografts implanted in the neck and with the vascular pedicle surrounded by a skin tube were used as experimental models by Wolff & Hume (1965). Sources of ionizing radiation were applied to these pedicles in order to destroy the small lymphocytes invading the grafts but they found that even when a large dose of irradiation (7200 r) was used, the grafts were only protected in 50% of cases.

Clinical applications

The methods of immunosuppression in current use for organ transplantation have changed very little during the past 10 years—corticosteroids and azathioprine providing the mainstays with the addition of Actinomycin C during rejection crises. The promise of ALS has not yet been fulfilled but with standardization in techniques of preparation, purification and overall evaluation, an effective and valuable immunosuppressive effect may still be possible. During this time techniques in dialysis, surgery and in the day-to-day support of patients on these drugs has markedly improved so that the most experienced centres have almost achieved optimal success. Many other factors including histocompatibility matching, the quality and preservation of organs and the control of infection, however, leave much to be desired and it is only by continued search for more specific and less toxic immunosuppressive agents and the development of biological and immunological knowledge that further success will be achieved.

REFERENCES

Anderson D., Billingham R.E., Lampkin G.H. & Medawar P.B. (1951) The use of skin grafting to distinguish between monozygotic and dizicotic twins in cattle. *Heredity*, **5**, 379.

Bach J-F., Dardenna M., Dormont J. & Antoine B. (1969) A new *in vitro* test evaluating antilymphocyte serum potency. *Transplantation Proc.* **1**, Part II, 403.

Balner H., Eysvoagle V.P. & Cleton F.J. (1968) Testing of antihuman lymphocyte sera in chimpanzees and lower primates. *Lancet*, i, 19.

Barker C.F. & Billingham F.R. (1967) The role of regional lymphatics in the skin. *Transplantation*, **5**, 962.

Billingham R.E., Krohn P.L. & Medawar P.B. (1951) Effect of cortisone on survival of skin homografts in rabbits. *Br. med. J.* i, 1157.

BILLINGHAM R.E. & BRENT L. (1959) Quantitative studies on tissue transplantation immunity. Part 4 Induction of tolerance in new born mice. Studies on the phenomenon of runts disease. *Phil. Trans.* (*B*), **242,** 439.

BRENT L. & MEDAWAR P.B. (1961) Quantitative studies on tissue transplantation immunity. V. The role of antiserum in enhancement and desensitization. *Proc. Roy. Soc.* B, **155,** 392

BRENT L. & MEDAWAR P.B. (1967) Cellular immunity and the homograft reaction. *Br. med. Bull.* **23,** 55.

BURNET F.M. (1959) The clonal selection theory of acquired immunity. Cambridge University Press.

BURNET F.M. & FENNER F. (1949) The production of antibodies. 2nd Edition. Melbourne: Macmillan.

CALNE R.Y. (1960) The rejection of renal homografts. Inhibition in dogs by 6-mercaptopurine. *Lancet*, i, 417.

CALNE R.Y. (1961) Inhibition of the rejection of renal homografts in dogs by purine analogues. *Transpl. Bull.* **28,** 65.

CALNE R.Y., ALEXANDRE G.P.J. & MURRAY J.E. (1962) A study of the effect of drugs in prolonging survival of homologous renal transplants in dogs. *Ann. N.Y. Acad. Sci.* **99,** 743.

CALNE R.Y. (1963) Thymectomy in dogs with renal homografts treated with drugs. *Nature, Lond.* **199,** 388.

CALNE R.Y. (1967) *Renal Transplantation*, 2nd edition, p. 15. London: Edward Arnold.

CALNE R.Y., WHITE H.J.O., BINNS R.M., HERBERTSON B.M., MILLARD P.R., PENA J., SALAMAN J.R., SAMUEL J.R. & DAVIS D.R. (1969) Immunosuppressive effects of the orthotopically transplanted porcine liver. *Transplant. Proc.* **1,** i.

CHIBA C., ROSENBLATT M., YAMANAKA J., WOLF P.L., BASSENGE E. & BING R.J. (1965) Immunologically produced lymphopenia. *Arch. int. med.* **115,** 558

CRONKITE E.P., JANSEN C.R., MATHER G., ADAMICK E.A. & SIPE C.R. (1962) The induction of a prolonged lymphopenia by E.C.I. of blood. *Radiation Research*, **16,** 586.

CRONKITE E.P. & CHANANA A.D. (1968) In *Human Transplantation*, ed. DAUSSET J. & RAPAPORT, E., p. 424. Grune & Stratton.

DEMPSTER W.J. & LENNOX B. & BOAG J.W. (1950) Prolongation of survival of skin homotransplants in the rabbit by irradiation of the host. *Br. J. exp. Path.* **31,** 670.

DEMPSTER W.J. (1953) The effects of cortisone on the homotransplanted kidney. *Arch. Int. Pharmacol.* **95,** 253.

ELION G.B., BURGI E. & HITCHINGS G.H. (1952) Studies on condensed pyrimidine systems. IX. The synthesis of some 6-substituted purines. *J. Amer. Chem. Soc.* **74,** 411.

FORD W.L., GOWANS J.L. & MCCULLAGH P.L. (1966) *The Thymus: Experimental and Clinical Studies*, ed. WOLSTENHOLME G.E. & PORTER R., p. 58. London: Churchill.

FRENCH M.E. & BATCHELOR J.R. (1969) Immunological enhancement of rat kidney grafts. *Lancet*, ii, 1103.

FRISCH A.W. & DAVIES G.H. (1965) Inhibition of haemagglutinin synthesis by cytoxan. *Cancer Res.* **25,** 5.

GRABER C.D., FITTS T., WILLIAMS A.V., ARTZ C.P. & HARGEST T.S. (1969) Immunological competence in the lymph dialysed patient. *Surg. Gynec. Obst.* **128,** 1.

HAMBURGER J., GOSNIER J. & DORMONT J. (1965) Experience of 45 renal homotransplants in man. *Lancet,* i, 985.

HARDY M.A., QUINT J., FRANCA D.J. & MONACO A.P. (1969) Modification of immunosuppressive effects of antilymphocyte serum by a thymic humoral factor, Thymosin. Presented at a joint meeting of the Surgical Research Society, Society of University Surgeons and European Society of Experimental Surgery, London, 1969.

HELLSTROM K-E. (1963) Differential behaviour of transplanted mouse lymphoma lines in genetically compatible homozygous and F_1 hybrid mice. *Nature, Lond.* **199,** 614.

HOHEN R.J. (1965) Induction of tolerance to mouse tail skin homografts by combining paired immunosuppressive agents and cellular antigens. *Transplantation,* **3,** 131.

HUME D.M. & EGDAHL R.H. (1955) Progressive destruction of renal homografts isolated from the regional lymphatics of the host. *Surgery,* **38,** 194.

JAMES K. (1969) The preparation and properties of antilymphocytic sera. *Progr. Surg.* **7,** 140.

KALISS N. (1958) Immunological enhancement of tumour homografts in mice: a review. *Cancer Res.* **18,** 992.

LEVEY R.H. & MEDAWAR P.B. (1966) Some experiments on the action of antilymphoid antisera. *Ann N.Y. Acad. Sci.* **129,** 164.

MCGREGOR D.D. & GOWANS J.L. (1963) Antibody response of rats depleted of lymphocytes by chronic drainage from the thoracic duct. *J. exp. Med.* **117,** 303.

MAGINN R.R. & BULLIMORE J.A. (1968) Extracorporeal irradiation of the blood in renal homograft rejection. *Br. J. Radiol.* **41,** 127.

MARTINEZ C., DALMASSO A.P., BLAESE M. & GOOD R.A. (1962) Runt disease in thymectomized F_1 hybrid mice injected with parental strain lymphoid cells. *Proc. Soc. exp. Biol. Med.* **111,** 404.

MARTINEZ C., KERSEY J., PAPERMASTER B.W. & GOOD R.A. (1962) Skin homograft survival in thymectomized mice. *Proc. Soc. exp. Biol. Med.* **109,** 193.

MEDAWAR P.B. (1948) Immunity to homologous grafted skin. III. Fate of skin homografts to subcutaneous tissue and to the anterior chamber of the eye. *Br. J. exp. Path.* **29,** 58.

METCALF D. (1960) The effect of thymectomy on the lymphoid tissue in the mouse. *Br. J. Haemat.* **6,** 324.

MILLER J.F.A.P. (1962) Effect of neonatal thymectomy on the immunological responsiveness of the mouse. *Proc. Roy. Soc. Biol.,* **156,** 415.

MITCHISON N.A. (1953) Passive transfer of transplantation immunity. *Nature, Lond.* **171,** 267.

MITCHISON N.A. (1964) Inductions of immunological paralysis in two zones of dosage. *Proc. Roy. Soc. Biol.* **161,** 275.

MITCHISON N.A. (1965) Recovery from immunological paralysis and the relation to age and residual antigen. *Immunology,* **9,** 129.

MITCHISON N.A. (1967) Proceedings of symposium on the regulation of the antibody response. Ed. Cindader B.

MOLLER G. & MOLLER E. (1965) Plaque formation by non-immune allogeneic and semi-isologous lymphoid cells on monolayer culture of embryo cells. *Nature, Lond.* **208,** 260.

MOLLER G. & MOLLER E. (1966) Interaction between allogeneic cells in tissue transplantation. *Ann. N.Y. Acad. Sci.* **129,** 735.

MOLLER G., ZUKOSKI C., LUNDGREN G., BECKMAN V. & MOLLER E. (1967) *In vitro* cytotoxicity by non-immune lymphoid cells. Differential mechanisms of actions between various cell types. In *Advance in Transplantation* (Proceedings of the 1st International Congress of Transplantation Society, Munksgaard, Copenhagen), p. 67.

MURRAY J.E., MERRILL J.P., DAMMIN G.J., DEALEY J.B. Jr., WALTOR C.W., BROOKE M.S. & WILSON R.E. (1960) Study on transplant immunity after total body irradiation. Clinical experimental investigation. *Surgery,* **48,** 272.

NACHTIGAL D. & FELDMAN M. (1963) Immunological unresponsiveness to protein antigens in rabbits exposed to X-irradiation or 6 MP treatment. *Immunology,* **6,** 356.

OORT J. & TURK J.L. (1965) A histological and auto radiographic study of lymph nodes during the development of contact sensitivity in the guinea pig. *Br. J. exp. Path.* **46,** 147.

OSABA D & MILLER J.F.A.P. (1963) Evidence for a humoral thymus factor responsible for maturation of immunological faculty. *Nature, Lond.* **199,** 653.

OWEN E.R. (1969) Preventing the rejection of transplanted organs *Ann. R. Coll. Surg.* **45,** 63.

SARLES H.E., REMMERS A.R. Jr., FISH J.C., CANALES C.O., THOMAS F.D., TYSON K.R.T., BEATHARD G.A. & RITZMANN S.E. (1970) Depletion of lymphocytes for the protection of renal allografts. *Arch. Int. Med.* **125,** 443.

SCHLESINGER M. & YRON I. (1969) Antigenic changes in lymph node cells after administration of antiserum to thymus cells. *Science, N.Y.* **164,** 1412.

SCHLESINGER M. & YRON I. (1969) Antigenic changes in lymph node cells following thymectomy. *Israel J. Med. Sci.* **5,** 445.

SCHWARTZ R.S. & DAMESHEK W. (1959) Drug induced immunological tolerance. *Nature, Lond.* **183,** 1682.

SCHWARTZ R.S. & DAMESHEK W. (1960) The effects of 6 MP on homograft reactions. *J. Clin. Invest.* **39,** 952.

SCHWARTZ R.S. & DAMESHEK W. (1963) The role of antigen dosage in drug induced immunological tolerance. *J. Immunol.* **90,** 703.

SHAFFER C.F. & HILKA J.F. (1969) Ovarian transplantation—graft-host interactions in corneal encapsulated homografts. *Am. J. Obstet. & Gynec.* **103,** 1.

SHIEL A.G.R., MITCHELL R.M., DAMMIN G.J. & MURRAY J.E. (1967) Analysis of the mechanism of drug induced tolerance to renal allografts in dogs. *Proc. 1st Int. Congr. of Transpl. Soc.,* Paris, ed. DAUSSET J. & HAMBURGER J., p. 599. Copenhagen: Munksgaard.

SIMONSEN M. (1962) Graft versus host reactions. Their natural history and applicability as tools of research. *Prog. Allergy,* **6,** 349.

SNELL G.D., WINN H.J., STIMPFLING J.H. & PARKER J. (1960) Depression by antibody of the immune response to homografts and its role in immunological enhancement. *J. exp. Med.* **112,** 293.

STARK R.B., CONWAY H. & CEDAR J.D. (1955) Observation on the circulation of homologous grafts of skin to recipients treated with sodium salicylate, h stadyl and irradiation. *N.Y. Acad. Sci.* **59,** 343.

Stuart F.P., Saitoh T. & Fitch F.W. (1968) Rejection of renal allografts: specific immunological suppression. *Science, N.Y.* **160,** 1463.

Thomas L. (1959) In *Cellular and Humoral Aspects of the Hypersensitive State,* ed. Lawrence H.S. New York: Hoeber. In a discussion following P.B. Medawar's paper on reactions to homologous tissue antigens in relation to hypersensitivity, p. 529.

Tilney N.L. & Murray J.E. (1966) Thoracic duct fistula in human being renal transplantation. *Surg. Forum,* **17,** 234.

Uphoff D.E. (1961) Drug induced immunological tolerance for homotransplantation. *Transpl. Bull.* **28,** 110.

Waksman B.H., Arbouys S. & Arnason B.E. (1961) The use of specific lymphocyte antisera to inhibit hypersensitive reactions of the delayed type. *J. exp. Med.* **114,** 997.

Weaver J.M., Algire G.H. & Prehn R.T. (1955) The growth of cells *in vivo* in diffusion chambers. II. The role of cells in the destruction of homografts in mice. *J. Nat. Cancer Inst.* **15,** 1737.

Wilhelm R.E., Fisher J.P. & Cooke R.A. (1958) Experimental depletion of mononuclear cells for the purpose of investigating reactions of the allergic contact type. *J. Allerg.* **29,** 493.

Wilson R.E., Rittin A., Rifaat K.D., Kinneart P. & Busch G.J. (1969) Prolonged canine renal allograft: surgical intervention after pre-treatment with solubilized antigen. *Transplantation,* **7,** 360.

Wolff J.S. & Hume D.M. (1965) Prolongation of renal homograft survival by external radiation of renal arterial blood. Abstract—*Fed. Proc.* **24,** 573.

Woodruff M.F.A. (1954) The effect of cortisone and thyrotropin in thyroid transplants in the guinea-pig. *J. Endocr.* **11,** 1.

Woodruff M.F.A. (1959) *Biological Problems of Grafting,* ed. Albert F. & Medawar P.B., p. 83. Springfield, Ill.: Charles C. Thomas.

Woodruff M.F.A. & Anderson N.A. (1963) Effect of lymphocyte depletion by thoracic duct fistula and administration of antilymphocyte serum on the survival of skin homografts in rats. *Nature, Lond.* **200,** 702.

Woodruff M.F.A., Robson J.S., Nolan B., Lambie A.T., Wilson T.I. & Clark J.C. (1963) Homotransplantation of kidney in patients treated by preoperative local irradiation and post-operative administration of an antimetabolite (Imuran). *Lancet,* ii, 675.

Zukoski C.F., Lee H. & Hume D.M. (1960) The prolongation of functional survival of canine renal homografts by 6-mercaptopurine. *Surg. Forum,* **11,** 470.

Zukoski C.F., Callaway J.M. & Rhea W.G. Jr. (1965) Prolonged acceptance of a canine renal allograft achieved with prednisone. *Transplantation,* **3,** 380.

CHAPTER 3

Organ Preservation

V.C. Marshall

INTRODUCTION

Cadaver organs are increasingly used in clinical transplantation of the kidney, heart and liver. This has highlighted the urgent need for clinically applicable, and effective long-term organ preservation. This ultimate aim is as yet unachieved. Progress towards it will be reviewed in this section, and methods of organ storage in current clinical practice will be considered.

In the special instance of kidney transplantation, living donors also are frequently used. The procedure is then an elective one. The organization of personnel and facilities, the provision of a compatible tissue match, the appropriate clinical screening and informed consent of the participants, the careful preparation of the recipient so that his condition is optimum for the operation—all of these necessary items can be prearranged at comparative leisure. Under such circumstances the interval between organ removal and revascularization is usually short, and immediate function of the graft is expected. There are hazards of immunological rejection, but other physiological effects are largely those of denervation and of interruption of lymphatic drainage of the organ. Re-establishment of lymphatic pathways occurs rapidly, and of nervous connections more slowly. No ill effects of denervation of grafted organs are apparent except in the case of the heart and perhaps of the lung (Shumway *et al* 1967; Hardy & Alican 1966).

Organ preservation is thus of little clinical import in relation to the living donor, although simple cooling during the transition period has been used with advantage (Starzl, 1964).

With the cadaver donor, matters are quite different. Time is required to contact relatives, and to arrange consent for organ removal from all the appropriate parties. Time is required to mobilize operating teams for donor and recipient. Time is required for tissue typing and cross-matching, and for the exclusion of disease in the donor which would make grafting inadvisable. Such exclusion must often be made in the haste of urgent organ removal, without the immediate safeguard of a comprehensive autopsy aided by histological and bacteriological studies. Time is required to find the most suitable recipient from a local or national pool, to arrange admission and to prepare him for operation, and time is required to transport organs over long distances to the appropriate centre.

The smooth integration of all these necessary measures has in the past determined the success or failure of a cadaver transplant programme. Cumulative loss of time at each step resulted often in inability to use organs which would otherwise have been suitable. Time, rather than carefully co-ordinated treatment, can all too readily become the crucial and overriding issue.

Extension of the allowable time limits, with adequate protection of the organ between removal and implantation, is therefore essential if all available organs are to be used to best advantage. The gaining of several hours immeasurably assists the clinical programme, and the gaining of days of time would solve many of the present problems, and would make international transport of organs feasible.

True long-term storage for weeks, months or years, has only been achieved thus far with individual cells such as erythrocytes and spermatozoa (Huggins 1964, 1966; Sherman, 1965). Solution of problems of long-term organ storage seems at least as far from present realization as solution of the process of organ rejection.

The exigencies of clinical transplantation surgery have meant that techniques of organ preservation have often developed empirically. The numerous variable factors in cadaver organ transplantation, many of them incapable of control or of analysis, make interpretation of the efficacy of differing techniques difficult. In recent years evidence from the experimental animal has clarified some aspects, but the unqualified application of these findings to human transplantation has its own problems. The fact that the relatively crude techniques currently used function as well as they do is clinically fortunate, and emphasizes both the resistance of many organs to ischaemic damage and their marked recuperative powers.

Points considered pertinent to clinical organ preservation, which will be discussed in this brief review, are as follows:

1 Diagnosis and prevention of organ damage during the agonal stage;
2 Methods of extracorporeal organ preservation and storage between removal and transplantation;
3 Assessment of viability of the stored organ prior to transplantation;
4 Effects of preservation on antigenicity;
5 Resuscitation of organs after death.

1 Diagnosis and prevention of organ damage during the agonal stage

Cadaver organ transplantation is now a widely practised and reasonably effective method of treatment of advanced disease. This fact has highlighted something long known, but of little importance prior to the development of transplant surgery. It has long been evident that death, rather than being a moment in time as prescribed by law, is often a continuing process affecting different tissues and organs serially and in differing degree. Each successful cadaver organ transplant exemplified this principle of death by degree.

The organ most sensitive to ischaemia is the brain, and absence of cerebral circulation at normal temperature for more than a few minutes causes permanent loss of brain function. Diagnosis of irreversible loss of brain function (or brain death) is thus often crucial in deciding to abandon resuscitative measures which could otherwise maintain circulation and respiration for some time before inevitable death of the individual. Other organs and tissues show a spectrum of sensitivity to ischaemia.

Nail and hair growth may continue for a short period in the corpse, and similarly skin or cornea may be removed several hours after death and used subsequently as a successful allograft. Transplantable organs are much more susceptible to anoxia, and occupy various intermediate positions between brain and skin in their sensitivity.

Normothermic ischaemia of the kidney of less than 1 h is tolerated with likelihood of early return of function, ischaemia from 1 to 2 h is likely to cause severe temporary loss of function, and of more than 2 h causes permanent and irrecoverable damage (Friedman *et al* 1954). The times apply to absolute ischaemia after death or from complete vascular occlusion. Resuscitation of the heart has been possible after 30 to 60 min of normothermic anoxia in dogs (Angell & Shumway 1966; Koga *et al* 1968)

The liver, if deprived of blood supply, suffers severe damage very quickly at normal body temperature. Severe depression of function as determined by tests of cellular metabolism occurs within 15 min at normothermia, but the period can be extended by cooling for several hours (Sicular & Moore 1961). Blockage of the vascular inflow to the canine liver *in situ* for 30 min resulted in survival in all cases, for 45 min in two of three cases, and for 60 min in one of three cases. No survivals occurred when hepatic ischaemia exceeded 60 min (Fonkalsrud *et al* 1969). Hepatic functions are so varied and embracing that it is not surprising to find that differential loss of metabolic function occurs after death or vascular occlusion. Certain functions such as ammonia and bromsulphthalein excretion are relatively resistant to ischaemia, bile excretion is more sensitive and more subtle enzymatic activities may begin to deteriorate almost immediately (Van Wyk *et al* 1965a, b).

The maximum tolerated times of normothermic or warm ischaemia of the three major transplantable organs, kidney, heart and liver are thus in the order of 60 to 120 min, with a gradation of increasing sensitivity from kidney to liver. However, while early poor function in renal allografts is allowable and is known in fact to have given ultimately satisfactory recovery, with heart and liver allografts early function must be life-sustaining from the moment of grafting, so that minimizing agonal damage and ischaemic times is of particular importance in these cases.

Particularly is this so, as a variable period of relative ischaemia due to a gradually failing circulation pre-mortem must be added to the absolute ischaemia after death in most instances of cadaveric organ transplantation. The effects of pre-mortem ischaemia must be presumed to cause additional damage, damage to the kidney for example often being manifest as anuria in the donor after prolonged hypotension. Much of this agonal damage is uncontrollable and unpredictable and assessment of preservation methods in clinical practice with human cadaver organs is made correspondingly more difficult.

Minimizing agonal damage depends upon the following circumstances fortuitous to transplantation. Brain death must have been diagnosed with certainty by the attending clinicians. The decision to cease resuscitation and ventilatory support having been made on these grounds, notification of the transplant team at this time enables consent to be obtained, and tissue typing and mobilization of surgical teams to begin prior to donor death. The criteria of diagnosis of brain death in patients with documented overwhelming brain damage, were of course familiar to clinicians prior to the development of transplantation surgery and are discussed in Chapter 10. They include deep coma with apnoea, absence of pupil reactions and absence of response to atropine and caloric testing, isoelectric encephalograms on repeated study, and absence of cerebral circulation on angiography (Fig. 1). Sometimes direct visualization of brain necrosis will have been made at operation. No single feature is infallibly diagnostic and the difficulties of interpretation of isoelectric encephalograms in patients with barbiturate overdosage, in encephalitis or in cases of deep hypothermia are well known (Juul-Jensen 1970). Such patients are usually excluded from consideration as donors.

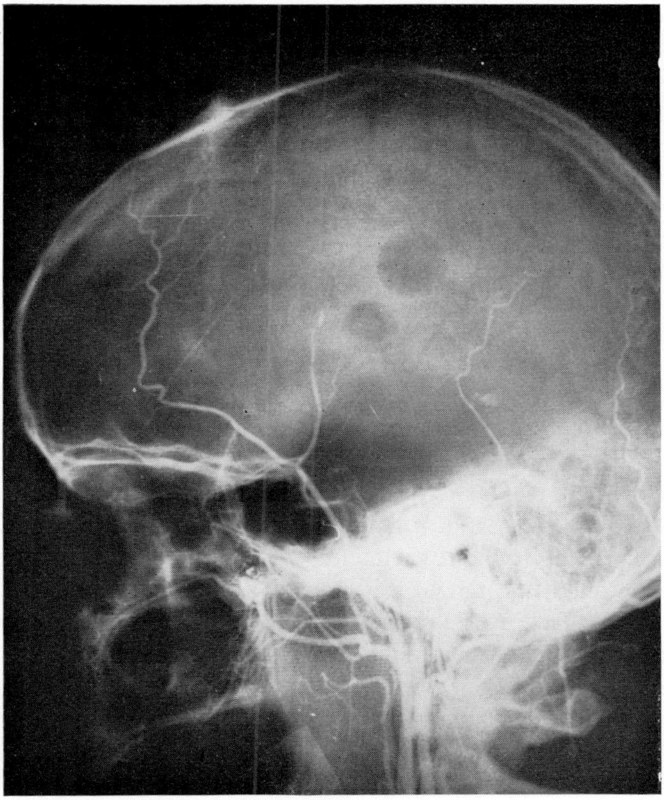

FIG. 1. X-ray picture of cerebral angiogram in patient with coma and assisted ventilation after head injury. No intracerebral circulation is visible, although facial and scalp vessels are perfused.

The diagnosis of brain death and the decision to cease resuscitation should be and invariably is made independently of the needs of transplantation, and involvement of the transplantation team begins only when the decision has been made. Under such circumstances, the timing of cessation of resuscitation can be such as to allow prior mobilization of facilities—the crucial decision has already been made and ultimate death of the donor is inevitable. It has seemed reasonable to many concerned with transplantation surgery that the time from this decision until ultimate death—this twilight zone between life and death—be utilized in minimizing the effects of agonal organ damage. This section will therefore consider only such protection of organ function between diagnosis of permanent loss of brain function and certification of ultimate death by the attending physician. In these specifically defined circumstances, all possible measures on the donor's behalf have already been used to no avail, and subsequent non-maiming measures to protect organs for cadaveric transplantation are justified in the interests of the recipient. It is also realized that many clinicians do not hold these views, and would feel that death of the prospective donor even in these circumstances must occur without cognizance or consideration of subsequent transplantation.

Current practice in many, although not all, transplant centres under circumstances of irretrievable brain death as described above, has therefore been as follows:

Resuscitation is stopped, and after the respirator has been turned off the clinician in charge certifies death at the appropriate time along standard and long-established lines (final cessation of cardiac activity, often with electrocardiographic monitoring). Donor organ removal then begins. Times of warm ischaemia in such circumstances can be very short and immediate function of heart, liver or kidney grafts can usually be anticipated. This combination of events, fortuitous for early graft function, may involve transferring the appropriate recipient to the hospital containing the donor. With kidney and liver grafting this involves no particular surgical problems, but the special facilities required for the surgery of heart transplantation make such transfer less commonly possible.

Although perhaps only a minority of the national population requiring organ grafts can be treated in the above manner, such an organization can provide organs from cadavers with very excellent early results, even without prospective tissue typing (Marshall *et al* 1968).

It would seem perhaps a logical extension of the above reasoning to remove organs for transplantation once diagnosis of brain death (*coma dépassé*) had been made, thus utilizing the advantages of an intact circulation to preserve organ function until the moment of removal. In several transplant centres, notably with heart transplantation, this has become in fact routine (Cooley *et al* 1969) and the procedure has also been employed with liver (Starzl & Putnam 1969) and kidney grafts (Alexandre 1966). The protection of organs from agonal damage is carried to its logical extreme but the ethical and legal problems of transplantation have been highlighted in the public mind by such practice, and it has understandably contributed to diminishing public and professional confidence in transplantation of all organs. Ready acceptance of the procedure by public and medical majority seems therefore unlikely in the near future. It is however relevant to note that the removal of organs for transplantation from the decerebrate individual with an intact circulation returns us to the equivalent of a living donor graft, and correspondingly simplifies or makes unnecessary organ preservation techniques.

Reverting to the standard procedure of removal of organs after circulatory arrest, we can consider possible ways of minimizing agonal damage from the time of diagnosis of loss of brain function until ultimate death. Damage pre-mortem is potentiated by prolonged hypotension in the dying patient. Fluid and electrolyte depletions, vasoconstrictor agents such as norepinephrine, and a normal or elevated body temperature are also deleterious (Gettler *et al* 1961). Pre-existing occult disease of the donor organ is likely to render it more susceptible to ischaemic damage.

The harmful effects of agonal changes may be mitigated by body cooling, by fluid and electrolyte replacement, by diuretic agents (mannitol, frusemide) by anticoagulants (heparin) and by vasodilator drugs (isoproterenol, phenoxybenzamine). Some of these measures have been demonstrated to be effective in producing better early function in grafts from living donors (Najarian *et al* 1966a) and also from cadavers. Measures such as body cooling, control of fluid and electrolyte balance, solute diuretics, steroids and supportive vaso-active drugs may often have been utilized already, in the attempted resuscitation of the donor neurosurgical patient. In our experience with cadaveric renal grafts these protective measures if continued have preserved measurable urine flows until death, even in the presence of prolonged hypotension. Under such circumstances of cadaver organ procurement prolonged acute tubular necrosis has not been seen. Contrariwise, the reverse has not necessarily applied, and in many instances if supportive treatment has been adequate, anuria in the donor for several hours has been compatible with immediate and sustained graft function if warm ischaemia has been minimal.

The primacy of prolonged warm ischaemia in causation of agonal damage is apparent experimentally and clinically.

Belzer *et al* (1968a) found dog kidneys could be uniformly well preserved for 24 h by continuous cold perfusion. The addition of 1 h of warm ischaemia caused survival to fall from 100% to 40%. No survivors occurred with 2 h of warm ischaemia.

Clinical support is given from analysis of clinical cadaveric renal transplant series in several centres. In centres using cadaveric renal allografts with a strict donor selection and relatively short times of warm and total ischaemia, early function of grafts has been usual, and the incidence of acute tubular necrosis and post-transplant dialysis has been low. In centres with less stringent criteria of donor selection, and with longer times of warm ischaemia, early tubular necrosis has been more common (Pletka *et al* 1969; Calne *et al* 1968; White *et al* 1968).

Gibson *et al* (1969) in a series where premortem cooling and induced diuresis had been used in most donors and where warm ischaemia was below 1 h and total ischaemia below 3 h in all cases, found immediate function in 64 of 67 grafts (95%). Dialysis after operation was required in only eight of the patients (12%).

Marshall *et al* (1969) compared early graft function in double cadaver grafts, where the same donor provided grafts for two separate recipients. Early graft function occurred in 45 of 52 grafts (87%) and only eight patients required post-operative dialysis (15%). Four other patients with acute tubular necrosis did not require post-transplant dialysis. Total ischaemia times were up to 3½ h.

The incidence of acute tubular necrosis rose with increasing times of warm ischaemia (Table 1). On three occasions tubular necrosis developed in each of the two recipients of the kidneys from the same donor. In each instance the longer period of oliguria occurred in the recipient who received the second kidney. Table 2 illustrates this in one pair where warm ischaemia times differed by 22 min with comparable times of total ischaemia.

TABLE 1. Warm ischaemia times and development of acute tubular necrosis in the recipient

Time hours	No. of patients	Patients with acute tubular necrosis
Less than ½	21	3
½–1	17	4
1–2	14	5

TABLE 2. Course of recipient pairs from single donor

	Warm ischaemia (min)	Total ischaemia (min)	Duration of acute tubular necrosis
Recipient of first kidney	38	147	5 days
Recipient of second kidney	60	153	9 days

With care in donor selection and appropriate protective measures pre-mortem, early function is thus possible in a high proportion of cases, where periods of warm ischaemia are less than 2 h and when total ischaemia is below 4 h. Bergentz *et al* (1969) also compared the function of double cadaver transplants. With short periods of warm ischaemia (15 to 60 min) prolonged cold ischaemia of up to 10 h was tolerated without significant further impairment of early function. No non-viable kidneys were grafted in the three groups considered but in other series of cadaveric renal allografts there has been a moderate incidence of grafts which have never functioned after operation—in one series of 76 grafts, 12 showed no function at any time (Pletka *et al* 1969).

Careful selection of donors, the use of protective agonal measures, and prevention of prolonged warm ischaemia can thus result in a high incidence

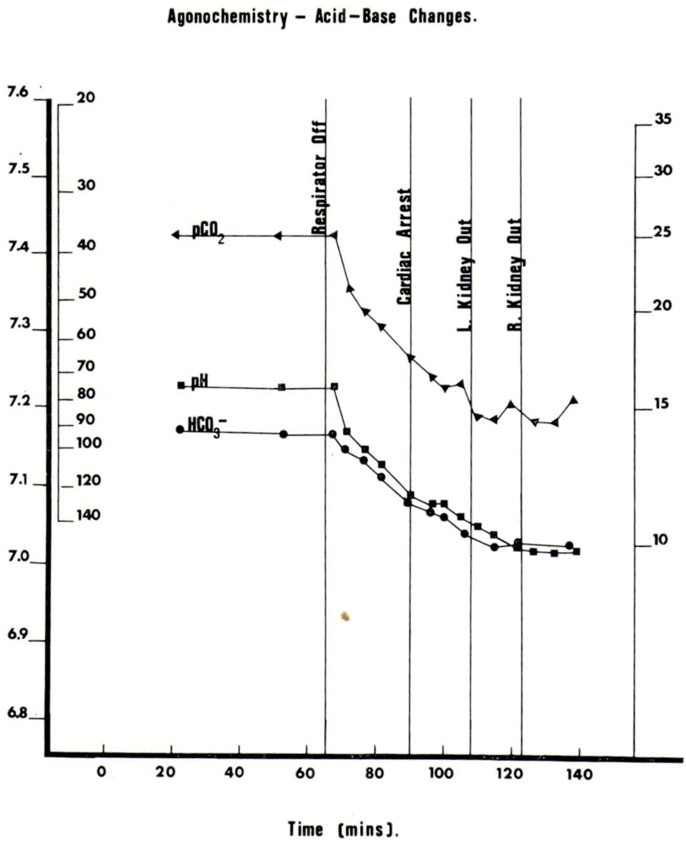

FIG. 2. Chemical changes occurring in arterial blood after cessation of artificial ventilation.

of early function in renal allografts from cadavers. These measures are of even greater importance in liver and heart allografts, and will be discussed further in the appropriate sections (Chapters 6 and 7).

Chemical changes in the agonal state

The resistance of transplantable organs to agonal damage is striking and fortunate. Certainly the chemical changes accompanying the agonal state are dramatic and would be expected to contribute to deleterious effects.

In a group of cadaver donors where acid-base monitoring was performed during the terminal stages of the illness, arterial blood-gas analysis was continued after the respirator was turned off until the time of kidney removal after death (Eremin & Marshall 1969). It was found that respirator support maintained adequate acid-base homeostasis in most instances prior to cessation of resuscitation, with a tendency to overventilation and a mild respiratory alkalosis.

The rapid development of a gross acidosis was apparent after the respirator was stopped (Fig. 2), as was the severe hypoxia during the agonal period. The time from cessation of respirator support to ul imate cardiac arrest was quite variable, from a few minutes to an hour in this small series. The timing of ultimate cardiac arrest was unrelated to the degree of acidaemia or hypercapnoea. It did however correlate well with the time taken for arterial oxygen tension to fall below 25 mmHg (Fig. 3). This correlation has also been seen in studies performed at death on other respirator patients not used as donors, when the PO_2 was found consistently to be below 25 mmHg, although acid-base changes were variable.

The disquieting sequel of a patient beginning spontaneous respiration after the respirator has been switched off with the diagnosis of brain death is an occasional finding in most units. This usually means that hypocapnoea from overventilation is the cause of temporary apnoea. It is a disturbing and distasteful event, which should be avoidable by serial agonal blood gas analysis to exclude apnoea from this cause. Although ultimate death of such patients is invariable, they are usually unsuitable as donors as the agonal period is often prolonged and hypotension severe.

2 Extracorporeal organ preservation and storage between removal and transplantation

General consideration of methods

The extracorporeal period, as we have seen, can vary from a few minutes with living donors to many hours in clinical transplantation of cadaver organs. To the cryobiologist, long-term organ preservation aims at storage

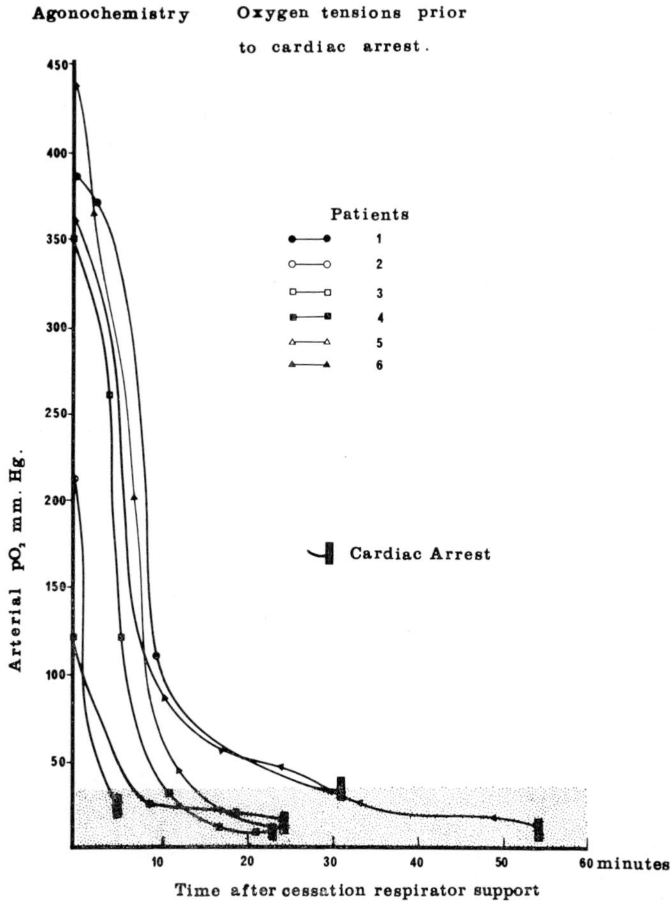

FIG. 3. Changes in PO_2 after cessation of artificial ventilation. The time at which cardiac arrest occurred correlates with the time taken for PO_2 levels to fall below 25 mmHg.

of organs for months or years, with organ banking a reality. This has only been feasible thus far with storage of individual cells and true long-term preservation of organs appears fairly remote from the present day reality of cadaver organ transplantation.

A less ambitious clinical aim would be reliable storage without deterioration of function over a few days; which would facilitate world wide organ transport. For national transfer between centres; organization of the various aspects of tissue matching, recipient selection, mobilization of teams and patients, and transport of organs can usually be performed within 12 to 24 h. Organizations such as Eurotransplant, Scandiatransplant and similar American and British arrangements have demonstrated the feasibility of simple storage methods over these time limits.

Extracorporeal storage in any form attempts to strike a balance between metabolic demand and its supply. If successful, minimal functional loss occurs over prolonged periods. Less successful methods result in gradual loss of function which is initially reversible, and later irreversible.

Inhibition of metabolic requirements is achieved by cooling or by various additives. Nutrients are supplied by the blood remaining in the organ, or this can be flushed out and replaced by another fluid. Oxygenation can be increased further by hyperbaria.

Storage by continuous perfusion attempts to mimic more closely the situation *in vivo*, and an alternative to artificial perfusion devices is to use an intermediate host for perfusion.

A classification of methods in clinical practice or under laboratory investigation is therefore as follows:

A Simple ice cooling (0°C and above).
B Freezing of organs.
C Organ perfusion.
D Ancillary methods—metabolic inhibitors
hyperbaric oxygenation.

Final evaluation of any method experimentally requires reimplantation of the organ as an autograft or allograft. Autotransplantation has been extensively used in investigation of kidney preservation. Immune problems are eliminated and specific early and late functional effects of prolonged ischaemia and of the storage procedure can be assessed. Late deterioration in function may occur (Milton & Craddock 1969), and progressive hypertension may also be seen. The difficulties of differentiation between ischaemic and immunologic damage after allotransplantation using cadaver organs are highlighted by these observations in autografts (Calne *et al* 1963).

With unpaired organs (heart, liver) support of the animal during the time of extracorporeal storage usually makes autotransplantation impractical for any prolonged storage study and allografting must be used.

A SIMPLE ICE COOLING

The maintenance of a constant body temperature is an efficient and exceedingly important homeostatic mechanism. The success of cold preservation of organs considered against this background may thus seem a singularly happy chance. Certainly hypothermia has been the cornerstone of clinical organ preservation—analogous to the place of azathioprine in clinical immunosuppression. Many ancillary aids have enhanced the effect of cold, but hypothermia remains the single most important method of organ preservation.

Brief consideration of the effects of cooling is therefore necessary. Cooling acts as a metabolic brake, but not uniformly on each metabolic process. As an over-simplification, the action of cooling is two-fold.

Firstly a number of physico-chemical functions, such as osmotic pressures, are dependent on colligative properties of matter in solution (i.e. properties related to the number of molecules rather than to their chemical nature). These functions are directly, and linearly, related to absolute temperature.

Secondly, many metabolic processes dependent on chemical reactions are temperature related but in a different manner. Chemical reactions vary directly with temperature but not in a linear fashion. They show an exponential decrease with cold, at a rate specific to each particular reaction (the Q_{10} number). Thus oxygen consumption decreases exponentially with cold (Semb *et al* 1960) and it reaches less than 5% of normal at 5°C (Levy 1959). Active renal tubular transport of water at this temperature is immeasurable (Harvey 1959).

This varying braking effect may have important implications in organ storage. A drop of 10°C from normothermia can be calculated to lower osmotic pressure of body fluids by about 3%. However, the normal maintenance of ionic gradients of marked degree across the cell membrane, although incompletely understood, is presumed to involve chemical reactions, the rate of which may be reduced by 50% by the same fall in temperature. If osmotic ion pressures are reduced by only 3%, while reactions responsible for maintaining ion gradients are halved, a new equilibrium would be anticipated, which can be calculated to produce a loss of potassium and magnesium from the cell and passage of sodium into the cell. These findings have been confirmed experimentally, although less predictably than may be expected from the oversimplified example given.

Cooling to temperatures above 25°C *in situ* is relatively ineffective in protecting against experimental ischaemia (Moyer *et al* 1957) but at 15–25°C 2 h of ischaemia of the kidney *in situ* is readily tolerated (Mitchell & Woodruff 1957); at 5–15°C 6 h of ischaemia is tolerated (Stueber *et al* 1958) and at 0–5°C 8 h (Schloerb *et al* 1959).

The efficiency of whole organ cooling is enhanced by cold perfusion, which allows rapid heat exchange over the large vascular surface area and also allows instillation of an appropriate flushing and preservative fluid. Substances can be added to prevent infection, vascular spasm and coagulation of blood within the organ, or to maintain stability of biological membranes.

Of the many different fluids which have been used for flushing out the organ in an attempt to enhance its cold preservation, some have not been demonstrably better than blood and some have been clearly worse as will be discussed later with specific organs (Keeler *et al* 1966). Fluids used have included plasma and serum, dextrans and synthetic plastics, electrolyte solutions mimicking extracellular or intracellular fluid, or even gases.

Additives have included antibiotics, heparin, procaine and papaverine, steroids, vasoactive drugs such as phenoxybenzamine and chlorpromazine, diuretics such as mannitol and frusemide, glucose, insulin and alkalis. The lipid content of the perfusate has been reduced by cryoprecipitation and filtration of β-lipoproteins (Belzer *et al* 1968) and platelets have been thought beneficial (Gimbrone *et al* 1967) or harmful (Vetto *et al* 1967). The relative importance of individual components becomes difficult to assess with so many variables. It is apparent that comparable results with ice preservation have been achieved by using widely different solutions, as will be discussed later with specific organs, but the flushing solution with best results thus far in kidney preservation has been an attempted replica of intracellular fluid.

B Freezing of organs

Techniques of storage by freezing have been outstandingly successful in preservation of individual cells. With preservation of whole organs, the problems are increased greatly and thus far little success has been achieved, although in the view of many, truly long-term survival will only be possible by such a method. As the method has little place in clinical transplantation at present, only a brief discussion will be undertaken, and the interested reader is directed to more detailed reviews of current techniques (Robertson & Jacob 1968; Pegg 1970).

Freezing involves ice crystal formation, with resultant cellular and organ damage. It is probable that damage is occasioned from removal of water as ice crystals, with consequent increase of solutes and hypertonicity in the remaining aqueous phase. Progressive freezing will thus cause progressive hypertonicity and cell damage. Direct cellular damage from intracellular ice crystal formation is likely to be of lesser importance. Damage may also occur by a direct toxic effect of the increasing intracellular concentrations of specific solutes, and by alteration in ion concentration gradients. The addition of solute to aqueous solutions, and increases in ambient pressure both depress the freezing point. Temperatures can then be lowered below 0°C without freezing and its potentially harmful effects.

A striking advance in cryobiology occurred when it was found that certain substances protected against the harmful effects of freezing (Polge *et al* 1949). Cryoprotective solutes include glycerol and dimethyl sulphoxide, and have been used successfully in storage of frozen blood and other tissues. With larger organs such as kidney, heart and liver, problems of uniform freezing and problems during the thawing phase are compounded by the bulk of tissue to be dealt with; and adequate delivery of cryoprotectives uniformly to the organ during graded perfusion with freezing has been difficult without exceeding toxic concentrations.

Thus freezing has been unsuccessful for 24 h storage of any transplantable organ, despite proven viability of individual cells and of various functions. Damaging effects of freezing in clinical practice as observed in frost bite are known to be associated with severe vascular damage. The effects of freezing on the microcirculation may thus be a formidable barrier to whole organ storage by this means (Barner 1965).

C Organ perfusion

Continuous extracorporeal organ perfusion has appealing advantages as a method of organ preservation.

Nutrients can be continuously supplied and potentially toxic waste metabolites can be removed. Conditions *in vivo* are approximated by including a pump, an oxygenator, a filter and a temperature regulator in the circuit. Continuous sterility is essential. Increasing sophistication of the apparatus usually increases its compexity. The risk of complications is correspondingly increased. The rewards are however also greater and the longest successful periods of extracorporeal storage of organs have been with perfusion techniques.

The requirements of a successful perfusion were set down by Alexis Carrel in 1938. He pointed out that the fluid must be free of floating particles or agglutinated cells which would act as emboli. The temperature, osmotic pressure and pH of the perfusate, the pulse rate and pressure ranges all needed exact adjustment. Chemical composition of the medium and its oxygenation were of capital importance, as was complete exclusion of bacteria.

He concluded 'Even if all conditions except one are satisfactory, the result of the experiment is utter failure'.

More than 30 years later, no more concise summary of the progress of perfusion research could be given.

The choice of perfusate has extended over a very wide range. Whole blood seemed an obvious empirical choice which would be expected to supply necessary but unclassified nutrients as well as oxygen. The dissociation curve of oxyhaemoglobin is displaced in hypothermia so that the percentage saturation of haemoglobin is increased by the lowered

6

temperature. Presumably the extraction of oxygen from blood by the tissues would also be reduced by hypothermia, although perhaps not to the same extent that oxygenation is facilitated. Blood however becomes much more viscous at low temperatures and increased resistance to perfusion occurs, making adequate flow rates difficult to achieve. Plasma is also twice as viscous at 10°C as at 37°C, but is still less than half as viscous as blood. Blood is therefore commonly diluted when used in combination with hypothermic perfusion. Considerable success has in fact attended the use of blood perfusates, in preservation of the kidney (Feemster & Lillehi 1969), liver (Brettschneider *et al* 1968a) and heart (Angell *et al* 1968) over periods of 24 h or longer. There are however many practical difficulties attending the use of blood perfusates.

Incompatibilities and clotting must be avoided. Aggregation of the formed elements (red cells and white cells and platelets) may cause emboli with decrease in tissue perfusion. Blood taken from donor animals under varying conditions of anaesthesia and injury may contain, or cause to be liberated, humoral vasoconstrictor agents such as histamine, epinephrine and serotonin. Prolonged exposure of blood to non-physiological surfaces, augmented by damage from pumps, oxygenators and heat exchangers also predisposes to haemolysis and to aggregation and emboli. Inclusion of the donor's lung or spleen in the circuit has thus been shown to act as a filter and to reduce microemboli (Hemingway 1931; Swank & Porter 1963). When kidneys were perfused with whole blood, Belzer *et al* (1964) showed that the rate of rise of perfusion pressures could be reduced by incorporating a glass wool filter in the circuit, and also demonstrated a secondary rise in perfusion pressures controllable by antihistamines and serotonin antagonists.

Much attention has therefore been focussed on the vital minutiae of perfusion technology, in an attempt to minimize damage to perfusate components by the perfusion apparatus itself. Tubing and connections must be finely machined and must possess a uniformly smooth internal surface. Surfaces in contact with perfusate must be of non-toxic materials. Stainless steel, glass, silicone rubber and a variety of plastics have been used and the surfaces have been modified by siliconization of glass, polishing of metals and coating of cannulae with graphite—benzalkonium-heparin.

Reduction of perfusate—air interfaces in the oxygenator has also seemed important. Oxygenators with a large blood-gas interface (bubble, screen and disc oxygenators) seem particularly prone to cause harmful effects which include erythrocyte and platelet aggregation, release of serotonin and histamine and denaturation of plasma proteins with release of unstable soluble lipoproteins, which may coalesce to form fat emboli (Lee *et al* 1961).

Membrane oxygenators with minimal blood-gas interfaces have been shown to minimize these effects (Wright *et al* 1963). If blood can be successfully eliminated from the perfusate, many of the above problems are simplified both in experimental and clinical practice. In terms of oxygen supply, oxygen solubility is increased by hypothermia, so that plasma or artificial perfusates can carry greater volumes of oxygen and of carbon dioxide in solution. As tissue oxygen needs are decreased by hypothermia along with increased oxygen solubility, adequate oxygenation should be possible with a perfusate free of erythrocytes.

Plasma has therefore been widely used as a perfusate base, either whole or diluted. It has been mentioned that plasma lipids may be denatured by oxygenators, and the work of Belzer *et al* (1968b) demonstrated that although this process could be minimized by incorporating a membrane oxygenator, soluble lipoproteins were still prone to damage by decreasing temperature, by changes in pH and by exposure to interphases. Such lipoprotein aggregates produced fat emboli and were the cause of increasing vascular resistance in prolonged kidney perfusion. The lipoproteins were accordingly deliberately denatured and removed by freezing and rapid thawing to produce a lipoprotein precipitate. The flocculent deposit was then removed by microfiltration through millipore filters down to 0·22 μ. This resulted in removal of 30–35% of the total lipid content, primarily low density lipoprotein. The residual more stable lipoprotein was apparently unaffected by prolonged perfusion, and no rise in perfusion pressures occurred over a 72 h period.

Confirmation of these findings has convincingly shown that at present, at least with kidney perfusion, best results are obtained with such cryoprecipitated filtered homologous plasma.

Of recent interest has been the suggestion that platelet-rich plasma was more effective in preserving histologic integrity in perfused organs than plasma poor in platelets (Gimbrone *et al* 1967). Such a finding contrasts with the previously described harmful effects of particulate emboli in organ preservation. The effects of platelet-rich plasma on reimplantation of organs after perfusion will be of great interest and early findings have suggested that no advantage occurs in 24-h renal preservation (Slapak, 1970).

Apart from blood and plasma, many synthetic perfusates have been used clinically and experimentally. Success with these has been moderate and has allowed kidney preservation for 24 h with immediate life-sustaining function after reimplantation. In none, however, has results been achieved excelling or equalling the prepared plasma perfusate.

Low molecular weight dextran (Dextran 40) has frequently been used, either alone or as a diluent for blood or plasma (Ackerman & Barnard

1966). The rheological properties of Dextran 40 make it potentially useful in improvement of uniform tissue perfusion, as flows throughout the microvasculature must be uniform and optimal if organ preservation is to be successful. Although widely and successfully used the specific benefits of Dextran 40 as distinct from other components are difficult to assess. In some instances it has been suggested to be detrimental (Collins *et al* 1969b).

Organic fluids (McCullough *et al* 1969) balanced electrolyte solutions and tissue culture media have also been used. In general, organs may be sustained by perfusion for periods up to a few days if the system provides oxygen and carbohydrate for metabolic need and if electrolyte and colloid concentrations are such as to maintain normal osmotic and ionic balance across capillary and cellular membranes. The use of simple electrolyte solutions without colloid osmotic agents is usually followed rapidly by oedema and rising vascular resistance (Pegg & Farrant 1967, 1968). However, Humphries *et al* (1968c) used a tissue culture medium successfully in kidney perfusion. Reimplantation with immediate contralateral nephrectomy was successful in four of four kidneys after 24 h, and in three of 12 kidneys preserved for 3 days. Survival occurred in one of four kidneys perfused for 4 days, with delayed contralateral nephrectomy. These results were as good as those previously reported by the same author at 1, 3 and 5 days with dilute blood or plasma (Humphries *et al* 1968a, b).

Synthetic fluids used to substitute for erythrocyte function include silicone and fluorocarbon fluids. Emulsified fluorocarbon fluids can be used as blood substitutes (Geyer *et al* 1968), forming homogeneous particles about 2 μ in diameter. They are effective in oxygen and carbon dioxide transport and permit rapid diffusion of these gases. So imitative are they that they exhibit the biconcave shape and potential for crenation of red cells. High molecular weight nonionic detergents can be used to emulsify the fluorocarbon and to act as oncotic agents. This combination can minimize some of the problems of prolonged perfusion of organs.

While still at an early stage of development, a few successful storages of kidneys for 24 h with immediate contralateral nephrectomy have been obtained with these ingenious techniques (McCullough *et al* 1969).

Equally important to the initial perfusate composition may be maintenance of constant composition during prolonged perfusion. This may be done by periodic replenishment of fresh perfusate, by appropriate additions to a closed perfusate system, or by purification of the perfusate by a dialyser which can serve as oxygenator as well.

Given the particular perfusate, simple or elaborate circuitry is used to provide optimal perfusion (Fig. 4). Pumps of roller or piston type powered by electricity or gas provide the *vis à tergo*. Damping devices can reproduce intermittent pulsatile flow, and a range of physiological pressures and flows is attainable. Pulsatile flows have been considered by many to give preferable results. Where a double blood supply must be provided as in the liver, split flows can provide pulsatile (arterial) and non pulsatile (portal) components, again at physiological pressures and flow rates. The organ is suspended, floated or supported in a suitable chamber and venous resistance can be simulated in a closed circuit, or the venous effluent can be unrestricted into the chamber and can then drain into a venous reservoir.

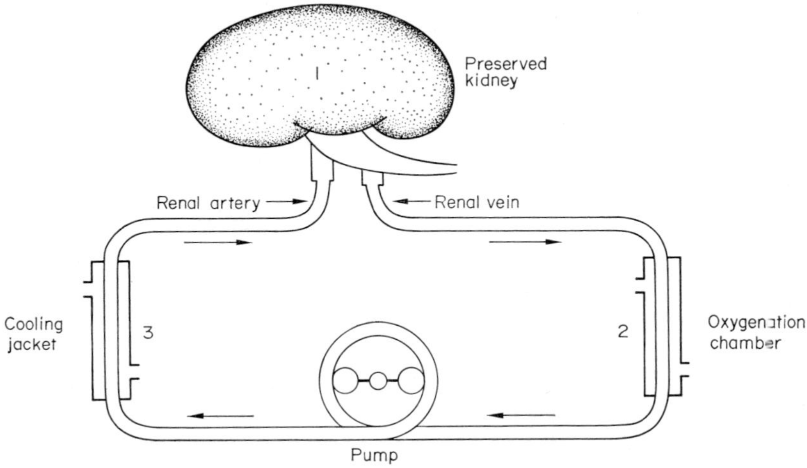

FIG. 4. Diagram of organ preservation by continuous cold perfusion. The organ being preserved, a kidney (1) is protected within a sterile container. Physiological fluid is oxygenated (2), cooled (3), and pumped into the renal artery. The effluent from the renal vein completing the circuit.
By Courtesy of the Medical and Technical Publishing Company Ltd.

An oxygenator is required if hyperbaria is not used, and membrane oxygenators have been increasingly used. They depend on the porosity of silicone rubber to oxygen and carbon dioxide. A suitable heat exchanger and thermostat, filters and various monitoring devices usually complete the circuit.

Each fresh component is a potential source of complication and careful monitoring throughout perfusion is essential.

A particular problem which has attended prolonged organ perfusion has been increasing vascular resistance during perfusion. A common sequel has been inexorably increasing perfusion pressures, progressive congestion and weight gain of the organ and lack of venous drainage with outflow block. Attempts to maintain physiological flow rates under these circumstances have been followed by organ damage and failure of perfusion.

The causes of the syndrome are very probably multiple. It can be minimized by dilution and careful filtering of blood or plasma perfusates, by care in perfusate buffering and in avoidance of rough surfaces and oxygenators involving a large air-perfusate interface. Lowering of flow rates and perfusion pressures also often minimizes but does not ultimately prevent the syndrome. Diversion of urine and bile from perfusate, and additives to the perfusate seeking to neutralise various humoral factors have also been helpful. Causes are thus likely to be partially mechanical from emboli (erythrocyte or platelet aggregates or lipoprotein conjugates), and partially humoral due to release of vasoconstrictor agents from perfusate and organ damage.

Removal of unstable β-lipoprotein fractions from plasma perfusates, combined with careful perfusion technology, has eliminated the problem in kidney perfusions lasting 3 days (Belzer *et al* 1967; Humphries 1969).

Perfusion by intermediate host

It has been seen that extracorporeal perfusion has tended to mimic various of the functions of the host by addition of substitutes for circulatory, respiratory, metabolic and excretory functions. Most studies involving preservation and reimplantation have been with hypothermia but normothermic perfusion for prolonged periods has also been possible and has provided considerable information on control of organ function. A rather bizarre but logical extension of this mimicry has been to use an intermediate host for temporary storage of the organ, with the view that optimal function will now be seen in surroundings more physiological than any perfusion circuit. Further attractions are that function can be assessed in the intermediate host before replantation, and that if temporary loss of function has occurred from agonal damage, it is given time to recover in the new host.

If complete abrogation of the rejection response between species was possible, such an approach with cadaver organs would be more directly applicable, but the problems of exposure of the organ to the severe hazards of immunological rejection while in the intermediate allograft or xenograft situation are formidable. The procedure has been utilized as simple extracorporeal perfusion from an arteriovenous shunt for kidneys in the dog, primate and man (Lavender *et al* 1968) with very limited success; and for the heart in dogs with considerable success (Angell *et al* 1968). The more exacting operative procedure of replantation of the organ after removal from the intermediate host has also been performed with kidneys and heart (Angell *et al* 1968). Conventional immunosuppression was unsuccessful in preventing rejection between primate species; but lethal total body irradiation went some way towards providing a temporary living xenobank using monkeys and baboons over 10 days, and goats and sheep for 4 days (Dupree *et al* 1968; Stevens *et al* 1968).

D Ancillary measures of organ preservation

1 Metabolic inhibition by drugs

Various drugs and chemical agents have been used in combination with hypothermia to enhance preservation.

Some agents have specific effects on a particular organ. In the case of the kidney, renal ischaemia has long been known to be potentiated by anti-diuresis and to be mitigated by a previously induced solute diuresis (Owen *et al* 1953). Mannitol, frusemide and ethacrynic acid have accordingly been used in pretreatment of the donor and as perfusate additives, with apparent improvement in results of preservation (Collins *et al* 1969a, b). These agents are relatively free of toxic effects of overdosage. A number of osmotic diuretic agents, including glucose, fructose and mannitol, have been shown to cause histological renal tubular vacuolation in high dosage (Doberneck *et al* 1962), but no functional renal damage has been demonstrated.

Other agents with a more general action applicable to preservation of all organs have been investigated. These agents have been thought to act by suspending biochemical processes, and by increasing the stability of biological membranes.

Webb *et al* (1966) used the isolated rat heart as a test organ, and investigated the effects of fluoride, adrenochrome, magnesium and potassium ions, and acetylcholine. Improved storage was found with fluoride and adrenochrome and particularly with magnesium ions. Normothermic storage for 6 h was followed by return of activity in some hearts.

Intracellular organelles, including mitochondria and lysosomes, undergo disruption following prolonged ischaemia, and the release into the circulation of enzymes normally contained within these organelles has been correlated with the degree of ischaemic organ damage (Fonkalsrud *et al* 1969). Particular attention has focussed on the lysosomes, which are intracellular inclusions containing a variety of lytic enzyme systems enclosed in a lipoprotein envelope. Disruption of the envelope occurs in anoxia, and cellular autolysis due to the released intracellular enzymes follows. Lysosomes have thus been described picturesquely as the suicide bags of the cell (De Duve, 1963). The damage which can occur to lipoproteins under hypothermia has already been alluded to, and ischaemia and endotoxin can also damage the lysosome membrane. Stabilization of the lysosome membrane has been described with cortisone, phenothiazides and phenoxybenzamine (Weissman, 1964).

Experimental evidence of improved preservation by these agents is increasing. Chlorpromazine has been shown to enhance preservation of heart and small bowel (Eyal *et al* 1965a, b). Chlorpromazine was the most successful of several agents investigated by Turner *et al* (1969) in kidney preservation. Addition of chlorpromazine to the serum used for initial flushing of ice-stored kidneys resulted in successful 24 h preservation, using delayed contralateral nephrectomy, in nine of ten animals. Chlorpromazine was demonstrated to improve the hepatic tolerance to ischaemia *in situ* by Fonkalsrud *et al* (1969). No control dogs survived more than 60 min of hepatic ischaemia, and only one of three dogs survived 60 min of ischaemia. Chlorpromazine pretreatment resulted in consistent survival after 90 min of ischaemia, and two of three animals survived after 120 min of ischaemia. Phenoxybenzamine was found to be equally effective in prolonging tolerance to hepatic ischaemia. Both drugs minimized hepatic outflow block following hepatic ischaemia or transplantation. The release of intracellular enzymes into the circulation after hepatic ischaemia was also minimized by drug pretreatment, and elevations of acid phosphatase and β-glucuronidase after induced ischaemia correlated well with mortality.

The precise action of these and other agents in protection from ischaemic damage and in enhancement of preservation is speculative.

Apart from their effect on biological membrane stability, agents such as phenoxybenzamine, chlorpromazine and steroids have vaso-active properties, which may well influence organ perfusion and preservation. Addition of various agents to perfusing fluids has been used to improve perfusion of the micro-circulation. Schalm *et al* (1969) demonstrated elimination of outflow block in canine hepatic transplants by the addition of procaine to the flushing fluid. Papaverine and low molecular weight dextran have also been used to aid vascular perfusion.

Drugs acting on α- and β-vascular receptors such as phenoxybenzamine, chlorpromazine and isoproterenol may have important circulatory effects in organ perfusion (Gayle *et al* 1968). Further improvement in results of long-term organ preservation may well require more precise dissection of the rheology of organ perfusion, and of the effects of vaso-active agents. A variety of physical and chemical measures may then be employed optimally to lower metabolic requirements, and to provide uniform and controlled circulatory sustenance throughout perfusion.

2 Hyperbaric oxygen

Oxygen solubility is increased by increased pressure as well as by cold. Hyperbaric oxygen has therefore been used extensively to improve oxygenation of stored organs. Combinations of hyperbaria with simple hypothermia and with perfusion circuits have each been used.

Results have been both encouraging and conflicting. Diffusion of oxygen across the capsule of the organ even under hyperbaria is limited (Matloff *et al* 1966), so that the effect of hyperbaric oxygenation in improving storage of hypothermic organs is unclear. Increased ambient pressure and increased oxygenation may have separate effects. Viability of dog hearts stored for 24 h under hyperbaria with nitrogen and helium at 4 atm was better than at normal pressures (Lyons *et al* 1966), and successful preservation of kidneys for 48 h has been claimed with hyperbaric helium (McBride *et al* 1967).

Oxygen at very high pressures may in fact be toxic (Norman *et al* 1966), so that slowing of metabolic processes by hyperbaria or by increased oxygenation may be partly responsible for improved preservation.

Hyperbaric oxygen at 3 atm combined with surface cooling was shown to improve function and survival of kidneys stored for 24 h by Manax *et al* (1964). Ladaga *et al* (1968) also demonstrated survival after 24 h of hyperbaric cold storage. Late renal function was well maintained. In both the above experiments delayed contralateral nephrectomy was used. On the other hand Matloff *et al* (1966) could not demonstrate improved renal function nor increased viability after induced renal ischaemia *in situ* over 1 or 2 h; and other workers have not demonstrated improvement in 24-h renal preservation by surface cooling combined with hyperbaria (Calne *et al* 1963; Collins *et al* 1969a, b). Hyperbaria has also been used in organ perfusion, where it inevitably adds to the complexity of the apparatus Monitoring of the perfusion and access to the organ during perfusion is also more difficult. Rapid decompression is inadvisable and may cause cellular damage and gas emboli (Brettschneider *et al* 1968a).

Successful kidney preservation with immediate contralateral nephrectomy in all of 12 experiments after 24 h perfusion has been achieved using hyperbaria at 3 atm and hypothermic perfusion with dilute blood (Ackerman & Barnard 1966). Ackerman *et al* (1968) also demonstrated normal function after perfusion of kidneys for 24 h under 4 atm, with reimplantation and immediate contralateral nephrectomy in ten of ten experiments.

Improved perfusion methods in recent years have resulted in equally satisfactory kidney preservation without hyperbaria (Belzer *et al* 1968; Humphries 1969; Scott *et al* 1969; Bauditz *et al* 1968), but in liver preservation best results have been achieved with hyperbaric hypothermic perfusion with diluted blood (Brettschneider *et al* 1968a, b).

Pancreatic preservation for 24 h has also been possible by a combination of hypothermia and hyperbaria (Idezuki *et al* 1968).

Results with specific organs

Progress in experimental and clinical preservation of each of the major transplantable organs by the various means will now briefly be reviewed and summarized. The present status of clinical preservation of the various organs will be discussed.

A **Kidney**

The most stringent test system is replacement as an autograft after preservation, with immediate removal of the remaining kidney. This will give the time limits for any method at which minimal and recoverable damage occurs. It will allow assessment of early function after preservation, and assessment of the severity of initial decrease in function.

Delayed removal of the contralateral kidney has several disadvantages. The function of the preserved kidney cannot easily be assessed until the other kidney is removed and the presence of a normal kidney may theoretically modify the early response of the reimplanted kidney, and also affect its subsequent function. Delayed contralateral nephrectomy is however useful in determining the potential for later recovery after severe initial damage, which would not be compatible with early survival; and in assessment of the late results of severe ischaemia. As the time of removal of the other kidney has varied from weeks to months, differing preservation techniques are less easy to compare by this method.

Results of organ preservation studies, particularly if early function of a solitary life-maintaining organ is impaired, may also be modified by variations in experimental technique and particularly by standards of preoperative, intraoperative and postoperative care of the experimental animals.

Such variations have been demonstrably important in other experimental procedures. For example, lowering of protein intake, minimizing protein catabolism by providing calories from carbohydrate and fat, and careful replacement of fluid and electrolyte losses from vomiting were highly effective in prolonging survival after renal allografts in dogs. Average survival time was extended from 9 to 13 days in a series by Halasz (1968)

Recent marked improvement in results from simple surface cooling in kidney preservation (Collins *et al* 1969a, b) may have been at least partly due to such meticulous attention to detail of experimental method.

Surface cooling

Surface cooling in ice at 0–1°C can certainly prevent severe deterioration of function for up to 12 h, after which time gradual deterioration occurs.

Calne *et al* (1963) found that 12 h ischaemia was the maximum consistently tolerated period of storage with immediate contralateral nephrectomy, and that between 12 and 17 h damage was sometimes partially reversible. With 24 h of storage severe and irreversible damage resulted. Addition of hyperbaric oxygen did not result in improvement. Ladaga *et al* (1967), using surface cooling alone found that 24 h of ischaemia was tolerated with survival after delayed contralateral nephrectomy. They found improvement when hypothermia was combined with hyperbaric oxygen; four of 11 dogs survived after storage for 48 h with delayed contralateral nephrectomy.

Manax *et al* (1964) also demonstrated successful 24 h preservation with delayed contralateral nephrectomy, using simple hypothermia combined with hyperbaria, and considered that hyperbaria had a marked additional beneficial effect over cooling alone.

Surface cooling was reappraised recently by Collins *et al* (1969a). They found only a small rise in serum creatinine after 12-h ice storage and autografting with immediate contralateral nephrectomy. With care in pretreatment of dogs during removal and reimplantation, the period of storage could be extended to 16 and 24 h with surface cooling alone; four of five dogs survived 24 h of storage and immediate contralateral nephrectomy, with early function and with considerable but reversible early damage. Factors contributing to early function were adequate hydration during operation, and the administration of a solute diuretic (mannitol) and vaso-active drugs (papaverine, phenoxybenzamine) during removal and reimplantation. Hyperbaric oxygen did not improve the results.

Surface cooling after initial perfusion

Replacement of the blood in the kidney by a perfusate, which can enhance the rate of cooling and also can provide a medium for addition of protective agents, has been demonstrated in the dog to give improved results from surface cooling alone. Pegg *et al* (1964) found that the protection by surface cooling was most enhanced by replacing the blood in the kidney by cooled autologous heparinized blood. In two animals, 24 h preservation was successful after delayed contralateral nephrectomy. Karlson *et al* (1968) also demonstrated prolonged survival in some dogs after 24 h ice-storage of blood-filled kidneys, with delayed contralateral nephrectomy. Turner *et al* (1969) had survival of ten of 20 blood-free kidneys after storage at hypothermia for 24 h. The blood was replaced by homologous cryoprecipitated serum. Opposite nephrectomy was delayed 2 weeks. Addition of chlorpromazine to the perfusate caused survival in nine of ten animals. Other additives were not helpful.

The most impressive results thus far recorded have been by initial flushing with a solution mimicking intracellular fluid in its composition rather than extracellular fluid (Collins *et al* 1969b). Along with an impressive improvement over previous results from surface cooling alone (survival at 24 h with immediate contralateral nephrectomy), they demonstrated that renal damage could be substantially prevented up to 24 and 30 h by simple ice preservation after flushing with a solution rich in potassium, magnesium and phosphate ions, with a low concentration of sodium ions, and with added procaine, heparin and phenoxybenzamine. There was uniformly good preservation in seven kidneys stored for 24 h and in three kidneys stored for 30 h, with immediate contralateral nephrectomy. Other perfusates, such as Ringer's lactate, dextran and sugar and bicarbonate mixtures (Brunius *et al* 1968) gave results inferior to blood left in the kidney.

The possible basis for the beneficial effects of such a solution has been discussed. Kidneys perfused with saline have been shown to lose potassium and magnesium. The loss of these intracellular ions can be minimized by perfusion with solution containing them (Keeler *et al* 1966).

In clinical transplantation of the cadaver kidney, the most widely used techniques have been simple surface cooling in ice, usually augmented by initial flushing with a perfusate.

The presence of uncontrollable agonal factors adding to renal damage makes evaluation of the additional benefits of a particular perfusate, above that given by hypothermia alone, extremely difficult. Homologous plasma albumin in Hartman's solution, Dextran 40 in electrolyte solution, invert sugar and bicarbonate mixtures, are commonly used with varying additives The evidence suggests that severe damage is avoided by simple hypothermia for upwards of 9–12 h in man (Bergentz *et al* 1969), but usually the degree of inevitable warm ischaemia determines subsequent function, and is the probable cause of the distressingly high incidence of non-viable kidneys implanted in many cadaver allograft series. The longest period of total ischaemia followed by good late function in one British series was 16 h (Sells & Pena 1970).

The clinical effectiveness of intracellular-type perfusates will be obviously of great interest in view of the striking success obtained in the dog with such a solution. Additional warm ischaemic damage would be expected in the human, and has been demonstrated in the dog (Frost *et al* 1970) to reduce the period of tolerated ischaemia.

With minimal warm ischaemia in human grafts, immediate function has occurred after total ischaemic periods up to 9 h, but the relative importance of cation and anion components of the perfusate is as yet uncertain (Collins 1971).

Continuous renal perfusion

Renal preservation has also been possible for over 24 h by many perfusion techniques. Hypothermic perfusion with dilute blood or plasma, electrolyte and synthetic solutions, with and without hyperbaria, have each been successful at 24 h, with immediate contralateral nephrectomy. Best results have been with cryoprecipitated filtered plasma, which must be considered the optimal perfusate at present. Excellent early function after 3 days in the dog has been followed by clinical application with transplantation of a cadaver kidney after a total ischaemia of 36 h. Function was immediate and no post-transplant dialysis was required (Belzer *et al* 1968c). For storage over short periods of less than 8 h, perfusion has not been shown to confer benefit over simple surface cooling (Martin *et al* 1969).

Thus, surface cooling, combined with initial cold flushing, has preserved good early function after 24 to 30 h of ischaemia, and these time limits seem likely to be approaching the limits compatible with good early function from simple ice storage. The degree of early function achieved has compared very favourably with that found after more elaborate perfusion methods and the advantages of a simple technique for rapid transport of organs are obvious.

Perfusion without hyperbaria with filtered plasma has provided excellent storage for several days and has given the best results for storage approaching long-term levels.

Summary of preferred methods of clinical renal preservation

Several alternatives exist, depending on circumstances. The aim of clinical organ preservation is to use only those organs with minimal damage compatible with early and complete recovery.

a MINIMAL PRESERVATION

Fortuitous circumstances include minimal agonal damage, pre-mortem matching and coincidence of donor and recipient operations, with total ischaemic times under 4 h. Flush cooling and simple ice storage can predictably give early function not much inferior to living donor grafts.

b PRESERVATION FOR PERIODS UP TO 24 H

Flush cooling with intracellular-type perfusate and ice storage is recommended. Early function will depend on the degree of agonal damage. Transport of kidneys over long distances is possible.

c PRESERVATION EXCEEDING 24 H

Hypothermic perfusion with cryoprecipitated filtered plasma is preferable under these exceptional circumstances. Transport requires special arrangements between centres.

The unknown factor of agonal damage in many instances makes decision as to the advisability of grafting in any circumstance, and particularly with prolonged storage, an individual one. The final choice of method will vary with the local organization of the particular unit, and its liaison with a national registry. Extension of the storage interval is often mainly taken up with kidney transport aimed at improving the match between donor and recipient. If this occurs at the expense of viability of the graft due to inadequate preservation, then results of cadaver renal grafting will not be improved, and may actually be worsened.

B **Heart**

Assessment of function of a preserved heart may be by restoration of electrical activity or of contraction, and the graft may be replaced as a heterotopic allograft. The ultimate test is survival after orthotopic allografting. Simple surface cooling with storage for 8 h has been successful, even after a period of 30 min warm ischaemia after death of the donor dog (Cleveland & Lower 1967).

Even greater success has been obtained by normothermic cardiac perfusion via an intermediate host (Angell *et al* 1968). This combines the twin aims of storage and of resuscitation. Canine hearts were removed 60 to 90 min after death, and were then subjected to short-term extracorporeal perfusion from an intermediate dog host, or to long-term perfusion by implantation in the neck pouch of the intermediate host. Final evaluation was by orthotopic transplantation. Rapid recovery from previous anoxia occurred with intermediate host perfusion over 1 to 2 h, and success was obtained with removal of the heart 90 min after death and storage in the intermediate host for 3 days, followed by orthotopic transplantation.

Clinical heart transplantation has most commonly involved coincidence of operative procedures in donor and recipient, and minimal agonal damage. Short-term preservation has been aided by extracorporeal donor perfusion via a heart-lung machine (Barnard 1968; Cooley *et al* 1969). Simple short-term preservation for transport between hospitals by relatively simple surface cooling has been suggested for clinical use (Proctor 1969).

C **Liver**

Preservation of the liver involves problems far more formidable than with the kidney. An orthotopic liver graft must commence to function immediately as no supportive treatment comparable to dialysis exists. The liver in addition is exceedingly intolerant of ischaemia, more so than kidney or heart. Sicular & Moore (1961) showed that after death, canine liver cells showed deterioration of enzyme activity within 15 min but demonstrated that the deterioration could be minimized for 4 h by hypothermia. Many research workers have demonstrated a remarkable range of maintained functions over many hours in the perfused extracorporeal liver and this was followed by the use of extracorporeal liver perfusion as a method of treatment of acute hepatic insufficiency with occasional dramatic success (Eiseman, 1966). However, the maintenance of even elaborate cellular and excretory functions has not correlated with the ability of the perfused organ to maintain life as an orthotopic allograft. Starzl demonstrated that consistent survival in canine hepatic allografts was only possible when total ischaemia did not exceed 60 to 120 min (Starzl & Putnam 1969). Poor early liver function after transplantation was associated with hepatic congestion and outflow block, irreversible shock and massive operative and post-operative haemorrhage, and massive fluid loss from the grafted liver, which were the major causes of death.

Hepatic allografts under optimal experimental conditions can be performed with minimal warm ischaemia. Systemic hypothermia of the donor animal can be induced, and intraportal infusion provides a very large surface for heat exchange so that liver core temperature can be lowered to 10°C within 10 min of beginning infusion. Rewarming of the organ at body or room temperature is slow, so that intra-operative damage can be minimal with expeditious surgery (Fig. 5).

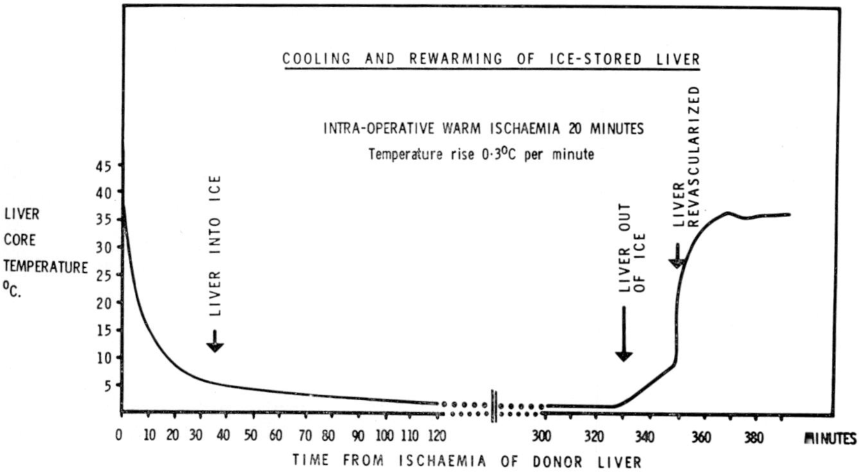

FIG. 5. Liver core temperature during cooling—rewarming of donor liver treated by intraportal infusion and ice storage.

Preservation by surface cooling

The results here are in marked contrast to kidney preservation. Preservation by surface cooling after intraportal infusion has not been successful in liver grafts for more than a few hours.

Schalm *et al* (1969) found in dogs that hepatic outflow block could be abolished by the addition of procaine to the flushing fluid. A buffered electrolyte solution with added low molecular weight dextran, heparin and procaine was used to flush the liver and was replaced by buffered plasma as a preserving fluid. Storage at 4°C after washing out the liver was possible for intervals up to $3\frac{1}{2}$ h, with life-sustaining function after heterotopic hepatic allografting and recipient hepatectomy. Early function was comparable to that of control animals subjected to the same procedure without organ storage.

Slapak *et al* (1970) used a similar technique of portal flushing and ice storage for a series of liver autografts in Rhesus monkeys. Storage for $2\frac{1}{2}$ h was occasionally successful, and attempts to prolong the period were made impractical by difficulties of maintenance of the anhepatic monkey during the storage period.

Initial attempts in Cambridge to prolong the preservation period possible with ice storage in the pig from 4 to 7 h were not successful (Marshall *et al* 1970). Pig hepatic allografts in control animals with intraportal electrolyte flushing and immediate transplantation have been consistently successful, with total ischaemic times usually under 60 min. There were no long-term survivors achieved with storage periods of over 4 h. Only one of 12 animals after 6 h ice storage survived for more than 24 h. Fluids left in the liver after flushing have included cooled autologous blood, cryoprecipitated filtered homologous plasma, unmodified plasma and balanced electrolyte solutions mimicking extracellular and intracellular fluid (Collins *et al* 1969b). Storage under hyperbaria at 2 ATA has not improved the results.

Outflow block has not been a problem, and a massive haemorrhagic tendency as occurs in the dog was also uncommon. Recovery from anaesthesia and early post-operative course were usually satisfactory, but death commonly occurred from 6 to 12 h after operation, after a latent period when the animals would often regain consciousness and appear well. Death occurred after sudden deterioration with twitching and convulsions, not relatable to treatable early complications (hyperkalaemia, hypoglycaemia and metabolic acidosis), and was presumably a manifestation of depletional or toxic hepatic failure. Similar post-operative courses have also been seen in recipients of preserved accessory liver grafts suggesting a toxic component of hepatic venous effluent as described by Fonkalsrud *et al* (1969). Attempted biochemical dissection of the syndrome has been unrewarding.

The initial hepatic venous effluent after transplantation of stored livers has been collected, and initially high levels of hydrogen and potassium ions have been consistently found, often causing marked systemic effects. These abnormalities often require early monitoring and correction, but over succeeding hours will usually diminish. The ischaemic liver may later act as a sump, taking up large amounts of glucose and potassium from the circulation, but correction of late hypoglycaemia and hypokalaemia has not prevented death.

Treatment of the donor with carbohydrate infusions and membrane stabilizers (steroids, chlorpromazine, phenoxybenzamine) did not have an obvious beneficial effect. However a further series of experiments has been more encouraging (Hadjiyannakis *et al* 1970). The donor animals were given 1 l Hartman's solution containing 25 g dextrose, 100 mg hydrocortisone, 100 mg phenoxybenzamine. The hepatic artery and portal vein were washed out with Hartman's solution containing heparin 1000 units/litre and Phenoxybenzamine 50 mg/litre. 450 ml of plasma were then infused containing 2% procaine 10 ml, 50% dextrose 8 ml, sodium bicarbonate 1·4% 20 ml. phenoxybenzamine 50 mg,. 1000 units heparine and in three of the six experiments 50 mg indomethacine. The liver was then stored in ice for between 5 and 8 h. When removed from ice it was washed out with a similar fluid of modified Hartman's solution to that used initially. Two animals after orthotopic transplantation of livers preserved 5 and 6 h respectively survived 31 and 37 days. One animal with a liver preserved for 7 h was alive and well 55 days after orthotopic transplantation. In the three experiments indomethacine was included in the perfusion fluid.

Surface cooling—clinical experience

Evaluation of techniques in man is difficult because of the extreme importance and unpredictability of agonal damage, but surface cooling in man after cold flushing of the liver was used in the early cases in the Denver series and in all of the 20 Cambridge cases. It has been apparent that such simple storage methods in man provided an extension of time of up to 5 h total ischaemia with recovery of function possible. In the Cambridge series, initial warm ischaemia from death of the donor until intraportal cold infusion has usually been brief. Apart from the first case, times have ranged from 3 to 22 min, and most have been less than 15 min (Table 3). In the first case, warm ischaemia was prolonged and adequate function of the graft never occurred.

The added intra-operative period of ischaemia during the anastomoses prior to release of vascular clamps has varied from 17 to 57 min. Increase in liver temperature occurs in this time. Total ischaemic times have thus

TABLE 3. Ischaemic times in human hepatic allografts (Cambridge—King's College Series)

No of grafts	19 (excluding Case 1)
	min
Times of initial warm ischaemia from death of donor till intraportal cold infusion	3–22
Times of cold ischaemia (ice storage)	52–290
Times of intra-operative warm ischaemia anastomosis time	17–57
Times of total ischaemia	83–321

ranged from a minimum of 83 min to a maximum of almost 5½ h, when air transport of the cooled liver was used. Although in this latter instance adequate function of the graft occurred for 7 days, the systemic effects of prolonged hepatic ischaemia were apparent. Serum potassium rose to 7·0 mEq/l and pH fell to 6·8 causing post-operative cardiac arrest. Orr *et al* (1969) also described adequate liver function following transplantation after 5 h of total ischaemia using ice storage.

The sensitivity to ischaemia of human, canine and porcine livers thus seems to be roughly comparable, with perhaps some favouring of the human liver. Livers preserved by surface cooling at the upper limit of the time period have in general showed problems from poorer early function, but premortem agonal damage was undoubtedly a contributory factor. Transport of the liver to the appropriate recipient is possible within such time limits and transport of the recipient to the donor hospital has also been used.

Liver perfusion

Techniques of liver perfusion are inevitably more complex than with kidney preservation and in most instances both artery and vein have been perfused (Hobbs *et al* 1968; Abouna 1968).

By far the best results have been those achieved by Brettschneider and his colleagues in dogs (Brettschneider *et al* 1968a, b). The combination of hypothermic hyperbaric perfusion with dilute blood was found to be most effective.

Using these techniques, consistent survival at 6 to 8 h of preservation was possible and occasional survival at 24 h. Variations in any of the constituents—absence of hyperbaria, lower perfusion rates or no perfusion, altering the perfusate to electrolyte solution in dextran, or cryoprecipitated plasma clearly worsened the results.

Clinical application of the method has followed and improved early function of human allografts was demonstrated with preservation times up to 7 h (Starzl & Putnam 1969; Brettschneider *et al* 1968c). Few other workers in the field have been able to achieve such outstanding results. Experience in Cambridge over the past 2 years with liver preservation in the pig has provided qualitative confirmation of these principles, but comparable times of preservation have not been possible (Marshall *et al* 1970). Our experience has suggested that survival after surface cooling beyond 4 h is extremely rare, and that perfusion has only marginally extended the time limits. Methods of perfusion investigated have been normobaric perfusion with filtered homologous plasma (Ashby 1969) using a machine similar to that developed for kidney preservation, and normobaric and hyperbaric perfusion with plasma and with blood using the Vickers mobile hyperbaric unit (Fig. 6). Occasional survival after 5 to 6 h of perfusion has

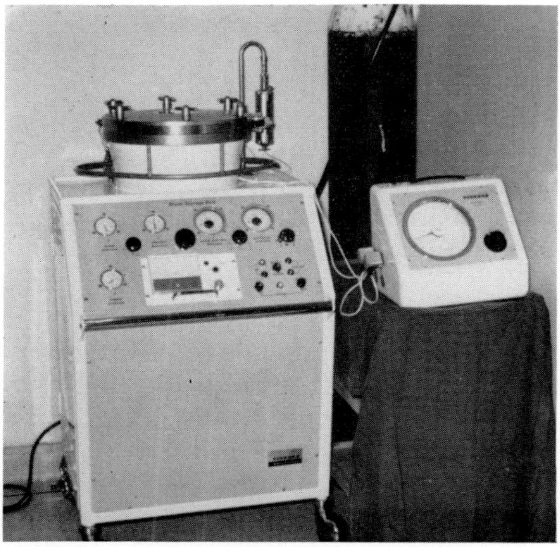

FIG. 6. Vicker's mobile hyperbaric perfusion used in liver preservation. The cylinder perfusion chamber is shown on top of the machine. On the right is the temperature gauge.

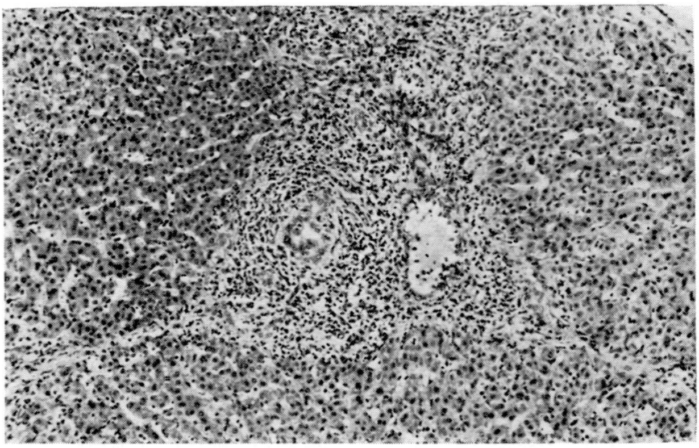

(a)

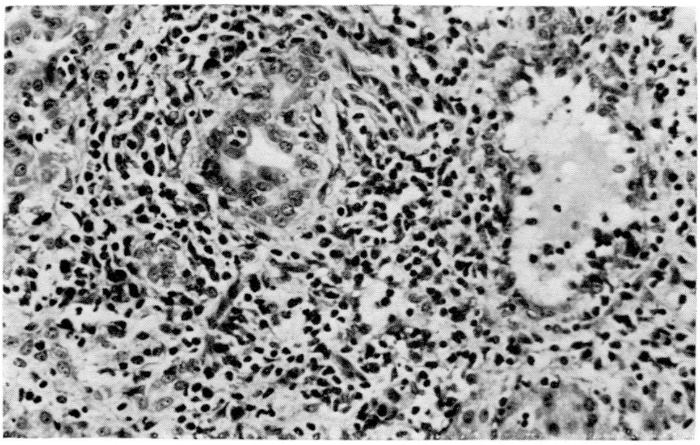

(b)

FIG. 7. Photomicrograph of an orthotopic liver allograft in the pig inserted after $5\frac{1}{2}$ h of cold preservation. Death from rejection 10 days after operation. (a) Low power. (b) High power.

been achieved but survival after extended perfusion up to 24 h has not been possible. Of great interest has been the occurrence of rejection in preserved livers (Fig. 7). Rejection in non-preserved porcine hepatic allografts has been exceedingly rare in our hands. The balance between the immunogenic effect and toleragenic effect of the pig liver may therefore depend upon degrees of hepatic ischaemia and damage of the allograft causing variable antigen release. Increase in antigen release from other ischaemic organs has been suggested (Najarian *et al* 1966b). It is possible that rejection of the allografted pig liver reported by other workers may have been influenced by variations in initial ischaemic damage. Prolonged

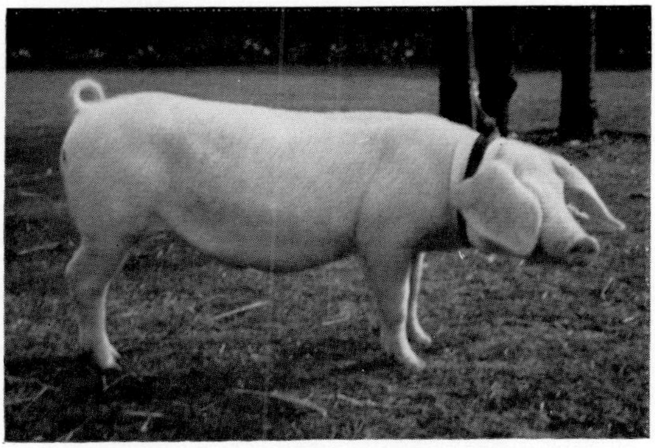

FIG. 8. Pig after orthotopic transplantation of liver preserved for 7 hours in the cold without perfusion. The animal was alive and well for three weeks after operation.

survival without immunosuppression is however possible, and Fig. 8 shows a pig surviving in good health with normal liver function for 3 weeks after an orthotopic liver graft preserved for 7 h in ice without perfusion, and other stored livers have shown normal function for many months.

Other agents

Hepatocytes are rich in lysosomes and protection from ischaemia has been demonstrated with pharmacologic membrane stabilizers. We have not been able to demonstrate improved survival with pre-treatment of donor and recipient by phenoxybenzamine, steroids or chlorpromazine but further exploration of the worth of these agents in liver preservation is obviously indicated.

LIVER PRESERVATION IN CLINICAL PRACTICE

Summary

Clinical liver allografting should only be performed when agonal damage can be minimal. Adequate donor selection is thus of prime importance in providing good early function. Systemic hypothermia, chlorpromazine and phenoxybenzamine probably are beneficial (see Chapter 21).

Coincidence of donor and recipient operations is potentially desirable, but the time required for recipient hepatectomy may be prolonged, and adequate protection of the donor liver over several hours may be required.

Surface cooling in man will provide a limited safe period of up to 4 to

5 h. Warm ischaemia times prior to cold flushing of the portal system should be only a few minutes, and the liver can then be stored in ice with a buffered plasma preserving solution (Schalm *et al* 1969). Extension of the total ischaemic period much beyond 5 h is likely to be associated with severe impairment of function.

In expert hands, hypothermic hyperbaric perfusion has extended the period of safety up to 7 h or more, with good early function. The degree of agonal damage remains the critical factor in determination of early function.

D **Lung**

Functional evaluation of preserved lung allografts suffers from the difficulty of distinguishing between ischaemic and immunological damage. Reimplantation as a pulmonary autograft avoids these problems but is technically more difficult.

Studies *in situ* have demonstrated that the canine lung is little affected by 2 h of ischaemia, and will survive after 6 h of vascular occlusion (Blades *et al* 1968). Simple hypothermic hyperbaric storage for 24 h was studied by reimplantation of the left lower lobe in the dog (Garzon *et al* 1968). Best results were obtained using 2 atm of oxygen.

Storage of the whole lung under hypothermia has occasionally allowed 24 h preservation to be tolerated (Hardy & Alican 1966). Progressive pulmonary damage is common in isolated perfusion of the lung (Stevens *et al* 1969). Perfusion with ACD blood at 25°C gave least damage (Veith *et al* 1968a). Elevation of pulmonary artery pressure and decreases in flow, compliance and gas exchange were sequential findings, suggesting pulmonary arteriolar vasoconstriction. Isolated perfused lungs and lungs after cardiopulmonary bypass and shock have similar pathological changes and a common humoral effect has been suggested in the three conditions.

3 **Assessment of viability of the stored organ prior to transplantation**

The ultimate proof of effective organ preservation in the experimental animal is life-preserving function as an allograft. Tests of effectiveness short of this are not uniformly predictive. Such an all-or-none test is obviously disadvantageous in clinical practice, but unfortunately clinical organ transplantation of cadaver organs still often represents a gamble in which the ultimate stakes may be life or death of the patient receiving the graft. The uncertainty of prediction of viability is illustrated by the incidence of non-viable transplanted kidneys; up to 10–20% of renal grafts from cadavers never function after grafting.

A simple and uniformly predictive test of function prior to grafting is obviously an urgent requirement for all transplantable organs. Such a test must be demonstrated to correlate precisely with ultimate function.

Tests which have been used include:

a *Gross appearance of the organ, or its response to initial and continued perfusion*

This will serve to eliminate some obviously non-viable and inadequately perfused organs. Any suspicion of defective perfusion should make one discard a prospective cadaver organ. Apart from such screening the response to perfusion is a very poor guide to subsequent function and apparently well-perfused organs may never function. Although temporary vascular spasm, for example in kidneys removed from donors who have received norepinephrine infusions prior to death, may be reversible and may be compatible with good subsequent function (Belzer *et al* 1970), it is probably safer to err on the side of conservatism in evaluation of organ perfusion. Initial or continued perfusion of the kidney and liver in clinical practice may also have the advantage of revealing vascular damage caused by removal—inadvertent injury to aberrant end arteries will be shown by failure of blanching of the involved segment, whereas surface cooling alone gives no guide to such accidents.

b *Histology and histochemical analysis of biopsy specimens*

The disadvantages of interference with the organ by biopsy are obvious but several tests have been evolved utilizing this approach. Histological examination may rarely reveal unsuspected systemic or local organ disease precluding transplantation, but normal gross histology gives little guide to subsequent function. It is customary to perform biopsies of transplanted organs at operation, and these are often exceedingly valuable in providing a baseline to compare with subsequent biopsies to diagnose transplant rejection (Kincaid-Smith *et al* 1968; Evans *et al* 1969).

Tests studying enzymatic and other functions of biopsy slices such as respiratory capacity and substrate metabolism share the general disadvantages of interference with the organ. The tetrazolium dye test measures the capacity of the cortical renal fragments to reduce a blue dye, and has been evaluated by Terasaki *et al* (1967).

All of the above methods however are of very limited value as a discriminant in prediction of functional organ survival.

c *Electrometric tests*

Other tests dependent on cellular metabolism have been correlated with the degree of ischaemic damage. Renal surface pH has been used as an indicator of anaerobic glycolysis and lactic acidosis, and has been shown to correlate with ischaemic damage at various temperatures in the rabbit kidney (Couch *et al* 1967). Surface redox potential of ischaemic kidneys has also been shown to vary inversely with temperature (Couch *et al* 1968). Correlation of such monitoring with function after transplantation, and the effects of altering perfusate composition or oxygenation on the data have not yet been demonstrated.

Cell membrane potential has also been investigated as a method of evaluation of cellular damage under storage conditions. It remains to be seen whether retention of these and other cellular metabolic functions is sufficient to predict life-sustaining function of an organ graft.

d *Tests of organ function*

Tests of a more organized nature than cellular metabolic functions have also been found wanting. Urine or bile production by a perfused liver, and electrical and contractile function of a perfused heart are examples. Renal tubular function is minimal at low temperatures and any urine produced is merely an ultrafiltrate of the perfusate. Any test requiring tubular function necessitates rewarming of the organ, during which time additional damage may occur. Rewarming by temporary extracorporeal transplantation to an arteriovenous shunt of the proposed recipient has been used. This has had especial application to exclude acute rejection in one of a pair of kidneys from the same donor, the other kidney being transplanted if no rejection occurs over an observed interval and if function is judged adequate. Extension of this principle to temporary surgical implantation in an intermediate host has already been discussed. The excretory ability of a perfused liver, at hypothermia or normothermia, does not correlate with synthetic and other functions necessary to maintain life as a homograft, and similarly normal electrical and muscular activity of a heart in an abnormal situation may not correlate with its ability to withstand normal resistances to outflow and to resume function as an orthotopic allograft.

e *Tests relying on changes in perfusate composition*

Such tests can be done simply by analysis of isolated or repeated perfusate samples. The method is potentially attractive as interference with the organ or with the storage system is minimal. Metabolic functions such as oxygen consumption and carbon dioxide excretion are depressed by hypothermia and are not helpful. Of many methods, the release of intracellular enzymes into the perfusate has shown most encouraging correlation with organ damage, and with subsequent function.

In kidney perfusion, lactic dehydrogenase release has been shown to correlate with subsequent function. The initial level of enzymes and the maximum levels reached appear to be of less importance than the rate of rise from the original level during the first few hours of perfusion. A discriminating test may thus be available some time after the beginning of perfusion (Belzer *et al* 1968a).

Similar correlations have been shown in liver preservation. The release of intracellular mitochondrial and lysosomal enzymes has been shown partially to correlate with ischaemic damage (Grana *et al* 1968; Fonkalsrud *et al* 1969). Enzymes studied have included glutamic-oxalacetic transaminase and glutamic-pyruvic transaminase, β-glucuronidase and acid phosphatase. In pancreatic preservation, insulin response of the perfused organ to induced hypoglycaemia has correlated with survival after 24 h of storage (Idezuki *et al* 1968).

4 Effects of preservation on antigenicity of grafted organs

Alteration of the state of antigenicity of a grafted organ by preservation, rendering it more or less susceptible to rejection, has been a recurring point of discussion and remains speculative despite considerable investigation.

Early fears of increased antigenicity after preservation were probably enhanced by difficulties in cadaveric or preserved allografts in distinguishing between ischaemic damage and that caused by rejection.

Tumour immunology suggested that strain specificity may be lost by frozen storage in transplantable animal tumours (Morgan *et al* 1956; Wodensky *et al* 1965). Most such evidence has been obtained with transplants not involving vascular anastomoses and in organ grafting the evidence is both conflicting and uncertain.

Rejection patterns in dog renal allografts have showed no difference between fresh kidneys and ischaemic ones (Robertson & Jacob 1968). Other workers have suggested that ischaemia may potentiate antigen release from the kidney (Najarian *et al* 1966b).

In clinical practice again the evidence is conflicting. Kidney grafts from unrelated cadaver donors have in the past given better results than those from unrelated living donors. Many other causes apart from alteration of renal antigenicity by the agonal state could have explained this, and such favouring has not occurred in more recent analyses.

The results for cadaver kidney grafts with early acute tubular necrosis have been thought to be better than those without tubular necrosis (Williams *et al* 1967). Most other centres have found merely that cadaveric grafts with acute tubular necrosis appear to represent a cross section of all grafts, with results neither improved nor worsened (Peart 1970; Marshall *et al* 1969).

Experimentally, liver grafts in the dog after preservation appeared similarly neither more nor less prone to rejection (Brettschneider *et al* 1968a). In pigs, rejection of severe degree in allografts, apart from accessory livers, has only been found in preserved livers in our hands, and the immunological significance of this finding has been mentioned.

In summary, the evidence for alteration of antigenicity in either direction by ischaemia is far from conclusive, and application to clinical transplantation is unproven.

Workers in organ preservation and in immunology may be encouraged or depressed by the apparent likelihood that significant alterations in antigenic structure of organs after preservation is not consistent with functional integrity of the organ. Attempts to modify graft rejection by altering graft antigenicity have long been thwarted by this fact.

5 Resuscitation of organs after death

A recurrent problem alluded to in this review has been the unpredictability of agonal damage suffered by the transplantable cadaver organ. The degree of such damage is of major importance in determining the degree of subsequent function obtained after transplantation, regardless of immunological hazards and of preservation methods. Early functional losses in transplants may be completely recoverable and are compatible with good long-term function and survival; but diagnosis and treatment of rejection episodes, and exclusion of mechanical and infective complications in the early period after operation are immeasurably easier if early function is optimal. Ways of minimizing agonal damage have been discussed, including the most radical, of organ removal from a donor with an intact circulation after brain death has been diagnosed. The adequate supply of suitable cadaver organs for transplantation may well remain a formidable problem even after solution of problems of immunological rejection. Future preservation techniques may thus demand methods of improving organ function after death, so that normal function can be assured prior to allografting.

Regrettably no method of ex-vivo preservation has been demonstrated capable of *improving* organ function during storage—the most achieved has been to delay deterioration of function. In-vivo preservation using a xenobank, with storage in the intermediate host allowing gradual recovery of function, may thus be of future clinical promise.

Resuscitation of the organ *in situ* within the cadaver donor is another possible method. No immune problems exist, and the cadaver provides his own perfusion circuitry. Many variations of this approach are currently used in clinical practice. The simplest has been attempted restoration of circulation by cardiac massage and ventilation during organ removal (Nakamoto *et al* 1965).

More elaborate and effective, but more time-consuming methods of donor perfusion, have also been used experimentally and clinically. Cannulae are inserted into a large peripheral artery and vein rapidly after death, and perfusion as for cardio-pulmonary bypass procedures is begun with an external heart-lung machine. Fairly rapid whole-body cooling is possible using this technique. Physiological flow rates and pressures may be difficult to achieve without organ damage. The vascular bed to be perfused can be limited to the appropriate organ—by clamping thoracic aorta if abdominal organs are to be used, and by isolated perfusion of the heart through suitable occluding aortic and venous cannulae for cardiac grafts. Such limitation of the perfused area has made it easier to obtain adequate pressures with smaller flow rates (Marchioro *et al* 1963). Such extracorporeal donor perfusion has been used to obtain livers for clinical transplantation (Starzl & Putman 1969). Perfusion with cooling was instituted after cardiac arrest, or could provide mechanical assistance to a failing circulation if brain death was used as the criterion for organ removal. Donor liver removal could then be performed with less urgency. Cardiac perfusion has been used for experimental and clinical heart transplantation (Parulkar *et al* 1968). Viability of heart grafts is said to be maintained if perfusion starts within 40 min of death, and best results are obtained if heart beat of the donor can be restored. Clinical application of a similar principle has been the use of organs for grafting from patients who have died while on cardiopulmonary bypass undergoing cardiac surgery. Prolongation of bypass until organ removal can result in immediate function of kidney grafts removed 7 h after death (Veith *et al* 1968b).

Extracorporeal perfusion is relatively elaborate and time-consuming with a risk of bacteraemia from poorly perfused bowel. In each instance the problem is to assess whether function will be aided by these means, or whether time could more profitably be spent in minimizing warm ischaemia by rapid organ removal. In the case of kidneys, the time taken for kidney removal may be not much different from that taken to insert the necessary cannulae and to begin perfusion. The techniques are at present, therefore, more applicable to allografts of heart and liver or to instances where multiple organ removal for transplantation is to be done.

A more direct approach to provide the driving pump for an *in vivo* cadaver perfusion system, has been to place a pneumatic device over the ventricles of the heart. Such a device can provide mechanical circulatory assistance and continued perfusion for several hours after death. This method of mechanical cardiac massage, if begun promptly after death in the dog, can provide optimal pressures and flows for 7 h, and organs then removed (lung, kidney and liver) have functioned immediately as allografts (Veith *et al* 1968b). Total body or specific organ perfusion can be performed. Maintenance of circulation in man has been possible for up to 4 h after death by similar means (Baue *et al* 1968). Use of the donor as his own heart-lung and perfusion apparatus is thus a logical clinical extension of preservation techniques, and sophistication of resuscitative devices may be expected to improve further. Conflict between objectives of resuscitation of the donor, and of resuscitation of his organs for transplantation must be avoided. If public and medical uneasiness of interference with the sanctity of death is increased by such measures, then much harm could be done.

It is however apposite to conclude this account of clinical organ preservation techniques where we began—with the cadaver donor. At present a variety of techniques of preservation has been demonstrated to be effective for short-term storage. This extension of time may seem miniscule in terms of future hopes for organ banking, but overall results of cadaver allografts should now be capable of considerable improvement with the better tissue matching possible within this time scale.

This capacity could readily be nullified by the indiscriminate use of organs with excessive agonal damage. At present the state of the donor organ at the time of its removal is often the most crucial factor in prognosis, rather than its subsequent treatment. Better means of diagnosis of the amount of organ damage induced by the agonal state, and improved means of reversing such damage, may thus prove as important in future progress as further extension of the extracorporeal storage period.

REFERENCES

ABOUNA G.M. (1968) Extracorporeal liver perfusion using a new perfusion chamber. *Lancet*, ii, 1216.

ACKERMANN J.R.W. & BARNARD C.N. (1966) Successful storage of kidneys. *Br. J. Surg.* **53**, 525.

ACKERMANN J.R.W, HOPKINSON W.I., MURPHY D.M.G. & KENYON J.R. (1968) Successful 24–48 hour canine kidney preservation. *Proc. 1st Intern. Congress Transplant Soc. (Paris)*, p. 743. *Advance in Transplantation.*

ALEXANDRE G.P.J. (1966) In *Ethics in Medical Progress with Special Reference to Transplantation*, ed. WOLSTENHOLME G.E.W. & O'CONNOR M., p. 54. Boston: Little Brown.

ANGELL W.W. & SHUMWAY N.E. (1966) Resuscitative storage of the cadaver heart transplant. *Surg. Forum*, **17**, 224.

ANGELL W.W., RIKKERS L., DONG E. & SHUMWAY N.E. (1968) Canine Cadaver Heart Procurement, Resuscitation and Storage. In *Organ Perfusion and Preservation*, ed. NORMAN J.C., p. 363. Appleton-Century-Crofts.

Ashby B.S. (1969) Unpublished observations.

Barnard C.N. (1968) Human cardiac transplantation. An evaluation of the first two operations performed at the Groote Schuur Hospital, Cape Town. *Amer. J. Cardiol.* **22,** 584.

Barner H.B. (1965) The vascular lesion of freezing as modified by dimethyl sulphoxide. *Crybiology*, **2,** 55.

Bauditz W., Olsson C.A., Kiser W.S., Nose I.Y. & Nakamoto S. (1968) 24-hour preservation of canine kidneys with pulsatile perfusion. *Trans. Amer. Soc. Artif. Intern Organs*, **14,** 134.

Baue A.E., Tragus E.T., Anstadt G.L. & Blakemore W.S. (1968) Circulatory Support by Mechanical Cardiac Massage in Potential Donors for Organ Transplantation. In *Organ Perfusion and Preservation*, ed. Norman J.C., p. 425. Appleton-Century-Crofts.

Belzer F.O., Park H.Y. & Vetto R.M. (1964) Factors influencing renal blood flow in isolated perfusion. *Surg. Forum*, **15,** 222.

Belzer F.O., Ashby B.S. & Dunphy J.E. (1967) 24-hour and 72-hour preservation of canine kidneys. *Lancet*, ii, 536.

Belzer F.O., Ashby B.S. & Downes G.L. (1968a) Lactic acid dehydrogenase as an index of future function of cadaver kidneys during isolated perfusion. *Surg. Forum*, **19,** 205.

Belzer F.O., Ashby B.S., Huang J.S. & Dunphy J.E. (1968b) Aetiology of rising organ pressure in isolated organ perfusion. *Ann. Surg.* **168,** 382.

Belzer F.O., Ashby B.S., Gulyassy P.F. & Powell M. (1968c) Successful 17-hour preservation and transplantation of human cadaver kidney. *New Eng. J. Med.* **278,** 608.

Belzer F.O., Reed T.W., Pryor J.P., Kountz S.L. & Dunphy J.E. (1970) Cause of renal injury in kidneys obtained from cadaver donors. *Surg. Gynec. & Obst.* **130,** 467.

Bergentz S.E., Brunius U., Claes G.L., Gelin L-E. & Lewis D.H. (1969) Double cadaver renal transplantations. An analysis of 21 pairs with special reference to the effects of variations in ischaemia time. *Ann. Surg.* **170,** 996.

Blades B., Beattie E.J., Hill R.P. & Thistlethwaite R. (1952) Ischaemia of the lung. *Ann. Surg.* **136,** 56.

Brettschneider L., Daloze P.M., Huguel C., Porter K.A., Groth C.G., Kashiwagi N., Hutchison D.E. & Starzl T.E. (1968a). The use of combined preservation techniques for extended storage of orthotopic liver homografts. *Surg. Gynec. & Obst.* **126,** 263.

Brettschneider L., Kolff J., Smith J.V., Martin A.J., Taylor P. & Starzl T.E. (1968b) An evaluation of perfusion constituents in liver preservation. *Surg. Forum* **19,** 354.

Brettschneider L., Groth C.G. & Starzl T.E. (1968) Experimental and clinical Preservation of Orthotopic Liver Homografts. In *Organ Perfusion and Preservation*, ed. by Norman J.C., p. 271. Appleton-Century-Crofts.

Brunius U., Bergentz S-E., Ekman H., Gehlin L-E. & Westberg G. (1968) The cadaveric kidney in clinical transplantation. *Scand. J. Urol. Nephrol* **2,** 15.

Calne R.Y., Pegg D.E., Pryse-Davis J. & Brown F.L. (1963) Renal preservation by ice-cooling: an experimental study relating to transplantation from cadavers. *Br. med. J.* ii, 651.

CALNE R.Y., EVANS D.B., HERBERTSON B.M., JOYSEY V., MCMILLAN R., MAGINN R.R., MILLARD P.R., PENA J.R., SALAMAN J.R., WHITE H.J.O., WITHCOMBE J.F.R. & YOFFA D.E. (1968) Survival after renal transplantation in man. An interim report on 54 consecutive transplants. *Br. med. J.* **2,** 404.

CARREL A. & LINDBERGH C.A. (1938) In *The Culture of Organs*. New York: P.B. Hoeber.

CLEVELAND R.J. & LOWER R.R. (1967) Transplantation of canine cadaver hearts after short term preservation. *Transplantation,* **5,** 904.

COLLINS G.M. (1971) Personal communication.

COLLINS G.M., BRAVO-SHUGARMAN M. & TERASAKI P.I. (1969a) Kidney preservation for transportation. II. A simple technique for 12-hour storage and air transport. *Transplantation,* **8,** 821.

COLLINS G.M., BRAVO-SHUGARMAN M. & TERASAKI P.I. (1969b) Kidney preservation for transport. Initial perfusion and 30 hours ice storage. *Lancet,* ii, 1219.

COOLEY D.A., BLOODWELL R.D., HALLMAN G.L., LEACHMAN R.D., NORA J.J. & MILAM J.D. (1969) Cardiac transplantation—general considerations and results. *Ann. Surg.* **169,** 892.

COUCH N.P., MAGINN R.R., MIDDLETON M.K., APPLETON D.R. & DMOTHOWSKI J.R. (1967) Effects of ischaemic interval and temperature on renal surface hydrogen ion concentration. *Surg. Gynec. & Obst.* **125,** 521.

COUCH N.P., LEMIEUX M.J. & MIDDLETON M.K. (1968) Effect of temperature and ischaemia on the surface redox potential of rabbit kidney. In *Organ Perfusion and Preservation,* ed. NORMAN J.C., p. 527. Appleton-Century-Crofts.

DE DUVE C. (1963) The lysosome. *Scientific American,* **208,** 64.

DOBERNECK R.C., SCHWARTZ F.D. & BARRY K.G. (1962) On the nature of the non-specific nephropathy attributed to mannitol. *Proc. Soc. Exp. Biol. Med.* **110,** 795.

DUPREE E.J., ABBOTT W.M. & SELL K.W. (1968) A xenobank for the storage of organs. In *Organ Perfusion and Preservation,* ed. NORMAN J.C., p. 397. Appleton-Century-Crofts.

EISEMAN B. (1966) Treatment of hepatic coma by extracorporeal liver transfusion. *Ann. Roy. Coll. Surg. Eng.* **38,** 329.

EREMIN J. & MARSHALL V. (1969). Unpublished observations.

EYAL Z., MANAX W.G., BLOCH J.H. & LILLEHEI R.C. (1965a) Successful *in vitro* preservation of the small bowel, including maintenance of mucosal integrity with chlorpromazine, hypothermia and hyperbaric oxygenation. *Surgery,* **57,** 259.

FEEMSTER J.A. & LILLEHEI R.C. (1969) Physiological responses of the preserved autotransplanted canine kidney. *Brit. J. Surg.* **56,** 622.

FOLEY E.J. (1953) Attempts to induce immunity against mammary adenocarcinoma in inbred mice. *Can. Res.* **13,** 578.

FONKALSRUD E.W., RANGEL D.M., BYFIELD J., BRUCKNER W., STEVENS G.H. & DINBAR A. (1969) Hepatic preservation with chlorpromazine and phenoxybenzamine; application to liver transplantation. *Surgery,* **66,** 23.

FRIEDMAN S.M., JOHNSON R.L. & FRIEDMAN C.L. (1954) The pattern of recovery of renal function following renal artery occlusion in the dog. *Circ. Res.* **2,** 231.

FROST A.B., ACKERMANN J., FINCH W.T. & MANTOVE A. (1970) Kidney preservation for transportation. *Lancet,* i, 620.

GARZON A.A., MINKOWITZ S., CHENG C. & KARLSON K.E. (1968) Twenty-four hour lung storage. In *Organ Perfusion and Preservation,* ed. NORMAN J.C., p. 665.

GAYLE W.E., WILLIAMS G.M. & HUME D.M. (1968) Control of hepatic sphincters by sympathetic amines: β-receptors. In *Organ Perfusion and Preservation*, ed. NORMAN J.C., p. 805.

GETTLER D.T., COLIP F.M. & SCHLOERB P.R. (1967) Effect of kidney hyperthermia on renal tolerance to total ischaemia. *Surg. Gynec. Obst.* **112,** 559.

GEYER R.P., MONROE R.G. & TAYLOR K. (1968) Survival of rats totally perfused with a fluorocarbon detergent emulsion. In *Organ Perfusion and Preservation*, ed. NORMAN J.C., p. 85.

GIBSON G.R., STOREY B.G., ROGERS J.H., MAY J. & SHEIL A.G.R. (1969) Early function in renal allografts from cadaver donors. *Aust. New Z. J. Surg.* **39,** 35.

GIMBRONE M.A., ASTER R.H., COTRAN R.S., CORKERY J., JANAL J.H. & FOLKMAN J. (1969) Preservation of vascular integrity in organs perfused *in vitro* with a platelet-rich medium. *Nature*, **222,** 33.

GRANA L., AHRENS J., DONNELLAN W.L. & SWENSON O. (1968) Enzyme patterns after hepatic ischaemia. In *Organ Perfusion and Preservation*, ed. NORMAN J.C., p. 551.

HADJIYANNAKIS E.J., CALNE R.Y., MARSHALL V.C. & DAVIS D.R. (1970) Successful preservation of pig's liver for 5–8 hours by simple ice storage. (In press.)

HALASZ N.A. (1968) Renal allografts in dogs: the effects of postoperative management in survival. *Surgery*, **63,** 954.

HARDY J.D. & ALICAN F. (1966) Lung transplantation. In *Advances in Surgery*, ed. WELCH C.E., **2,** 235. Year Book Medical Publishers.

HARVEY R.B. (1959) Effect of temperature on function of isolated dog kidney. *Amer. J. Physiol.* **197,** 181.

HEMINGWAY A. (1931) Some observations on the perfusions of the isolated kidney by a pump. *J. Physiol.* **7,** 201.

HOBBS K.E.F., HUNT A., PALMER D.B., BADRICK F.E., MORRIS A.M., MITRA S.K., PEACOCK J.A., IMMELMAN E.S. & RIDDELL A.G. (1968) Hypothermic low flow liver perfusion as a means of porcine hepatic storage for 6 hours. *Brit. J. Surg.* **55,** 696.

HOPKINSON B.R. & SCHENK W.G. (1968) The electromagnetic measurement of liver blood flow and cardiac output in conscious dogs during feeding and exercise. *Surgery*, **63,** 970.

HUGGINS C.E. (1964) Frozen blood. *Ann. Surg.* **160,** 643.

HUGGINS C.E. (1966) Frozen blood: clinical experience. *Surgery*, **60,** 77.

HUMPHRIES A.L. JR., RUSSELL R., STODDARD L. & MORETZ W.H. (1968a) Three day perfusion: perfusion of kidneys with hypothermic diluted blood or plasma. *Surgery*, **63,** 646.

HUMPHRIES A.L. JR., RUSSELL R., STODDARD L. & MORETZ W.H. (1968b) Successful five day kidney preservation. Perfusion with hypothermic diluted plasma. *Invest. Urol.* **5,** 509.

HUMPHRIES A.L. JR., RUSSELL R., STODDARD L. & MORETZ W.H. (1968c) Perfusion of dog kidneys with cooled medium 199 followed by auto or allotransplantation. In *Organ Perfusion and Preservation*, ed. NORMAN J.C., p. 13.

HUMPHRIES A.L. JR. (1969) Problems with various perfusates for kidney preservation. *Cryobiology*, **5,** 447.

IDEZUKI Y., GOETZ F.C., DIETZMAN R.H., KAUFMAN S. & LILLEHEI R.C. (1968) Functional testing and allotransplantation of the preserved canine pancreatic graft. In *Organ Perfusion and Preservation*, ed. NORMAN J.C., p. 621.

JOSEPH W.L., FONKALSRUD E.W. & LONGMIRE W.P. (1968) Vasodepressive effects of the venous effluent following canine liver allotransplantation. *J. Surg. Res.* **8,** 367.

JUUL-JENSEN P. (1970) *Criteria of Brain Death—Selection of Donors for Transplantation.* Munksgaard.

KARLSON K.E., DORMONT J. & HAMBURGER J. (1968) 24-hour kidney storage at 4°C with the vascular bed filled with arterial blood. In *Organ Perfusion and Preservation,* ed. NORMAN J.C., p. 687.

KEELER R., SWINNEL J., TAYLOR R.M.R. & ULDALL P.R. (1966) The problem of renal preservation. *Brit. J. Urol.* **38,** 653.

KINCAID-SMITH P., MORRIS P.J., SAKER B.M., TING A. & MARSHALL V.C. (1968) Immediate renal graft biopsy and subsequent rejection. *Lancet,* ii, 748.

KOGA Y., CARSTENSEN H.E., SUJANSKY E. & KANTROWITZ A. (1968) Resuscitation and preservation of canine cadaver hearts. *Trans. Amer. Soc. Artif. Intern. Org.* **14,** 140.

LAGADA L.G., GAULD M.H., SHELDON H. & MACLEAN L.D. (1968) Preservation of the dog kidney. *J. Surg. Res.* **8,** 495.

LAMBOTTE L. & SACY A. (1969) Liver cell resting membrane potential as a direct viability assay of preserved organs. (Abstract.) *Brit. J. Surg.* **56,** 693.

LAVENDER A.R., FORLAND M., RAMS J.J., THOMPSON J.S., RUSSE H.P. & SPARGO B.H. (1968) Laboratory and clinical studies in perfusion of the isolated kidney. In *Organ Perfusion and Preservation,* ed. NORMAN J.C., p. 339.

LEE W.H., KRUMHAAR D., FONKALSRUD E.W., SCHEIDE O.A. & MALONEY J.V. (1961) Denaturation of plasma proteins as a cause of morbidity and death after intracardiac operations. *Surgery,* **50,** 29.

LEVY M.N. (1959) Oxygen consumption and blood flow in the hypothermic, perfused kidney. *Amer. J. Physiol.* **197,** 111.

LEWIS M.R. & APTEKMAN P.M. (1952) Atrophy of tumors caused by strangulation and accompanied by development of tumour immunity in rats. *Cancer,* **5,** 411.

LYONS G.W., DIETZMAN R.H. & LILLEHEI R.C. (1966) On the mechanism of preservation with hypothermia and hyperbaric oxygen. *Tr. Am. Soc. Artif. Intern. Organs,* **12,** 236.

MCBRIDE C.M., HEALEY J.E., IBANEZ M.L. (1967) Effect of extracorporeal storage on canine kidney. *Trans. Am. Soc. Artif. Int. Org.* **13,** 364.

MCCULLOUGH W.B., JACOBS J.R. & HALASZ N.A. (1969) Renal perfusion and preservation with fluorocarbon emulsion. *Surg. Forum,* **20,** 308.

MANAX W.G., BLOCH J.H., LONGERBEAM J.K. & LILLEHEI R.C. (1964) Successful 24 hour *in vitro* preservation of canine kidneys by the combined use of hyperbaric oxygenation and hypothermia. *Surgery,* **56,** 275.

MANAX W.G., HIDALGO F., LYONS G.W., DUTZMAN R. & LILLEHEI R.C. (1966) Canine 'cadaver' kidneys: their procurement and application to clinical homotransplantation. *J.A.M.A.* **195,** 1010.

MARCHIORO T.L., HUNTLEY R.T., WADDELL W.R. & STARZL T.E. (1963) Extracorporeal perfusion for obtaining postmortem homografts. *Surgery,* **54,** 900.

MARSHALL V., KINCAID-SMITH P., MORRIS P.J. & EREMIN J. (1968) Cadaveric renal transplantation. *Lancet,* ii, 927.

MARSHALL V., BROWN R.B., EREMIN J., KINCAID-SMITH P. & MORRIS P.J. (1969) Early function and tubular necrosis in 'double-header' cadaveric renal allografts. *Aust. & New Z. J. Surg.* **39,** 38.

Marshall V., Ashby B.S., Hadjyannakis V. & Lines J. (1969) Unpublished observations.

Martin D.C., Smith G.A. & Fareed D.O. (1969) Experimental renal preservation. *Surg. Forum*, **20**, 529.

Matloff D.B., Mobiey T.L. & Schwartz S.I. (1966) Hyperbaric oxygenation and renal ischaemia. *Arch. Surg.* **92**, 83.

Mieny C.J. & Eiseman B. (1968) Liver preservation: unperfused cold storage and continuous cold preservation. *Surgery*, **63**, 923.

Milton S.H. & Craddock G.N. (1969) Logarithmic time: a new dimension in organ preservation. *Brit. J. Surg.* **56**, 614.

Mitchell R.M. & Woodruff M.F.A. (1957) The effects of local hypothermia in increasing tolerance of the kidney to ischaemia. *Transplantation*, **4**, 15.

Morgan J.F., Guerin L.F. & Morton H.J. (1956) The effect of low temperature and storage on the viability and mouse strain specificity of ascitic tumour cells. *Cancer Res.* **16**, 907.

Moyer J.H., Heider C., Morris G.C. & Handley C. (1957) Hypothermia III. The effect of hypothermia on renal damage resulting from ischaemia. *Ann. Surg.* **146**, 152.

Najarian J.S., Gulyassy P.F., Storey R.J., Duff G. & Braunstein P. (1966a) Protection of the donor kidney during homotransplantation. *Ann. Surg.* **164**, 398.

Najarian J.S., May J., Cochrum K.C., Baronberg N. & Way L.W. (1966b) Mechanism of antigen release from canine kidney homotransplants. *Ann. N.Y. Acad. Sci.* **129**, 76.

Nakamoto S., Straffon R. & Kolff W.J. (1965) Human renal homotransplantations, with cadaver kidneys. *J.A.M.A.* **192**, 302.

Nanninga J.B., Deam M., Holland J.M. & Grayhack J.T. (1969) Adjuncts to renal preservation. *Surg. Forum*, **20**, 527.

Norman J.N., Smith G. & Douglas T.A. (1966) The effect of oxygen at elevated atmospheric pressure and hypothermia on tissue metabolism. *Surg. Gynec. & Obst.* **122**, 778.

Orr W.McN., Charlesworth D., Mallick N.P., Jones C.B., Harris R., Jones A.W., Keen R.I., McIver J.E., Testa H.J. & Turnberg L.A. (1969) Liver transplantation in man after an extended period of preservation by a simple technique. *Brit. med. J.* **4**, 28.

Owen K., Desautels R. & Walter C.W. (1953) Experimental renal tubular necrosis —effect of pitressin. *Surg. Forum*, **4**, 459.

Parulkar G.B., Liotta D., Panday S.R., Sen P.K., Bloodwell R.D., Hallman G.L. & Cooley D.A. (1968) Closed chest partial extracorporeal perfusion for preservation of cardiac grafts. In *Organ Perfusion and Preservation*, ed. Norman J.C., p. 439. Appleton-Century-Crofts.

Peart W.S. (1970) Cadaveric renal transplantation. In *The Biology and Surgery of Tissue Transplantation*, ed. Anderson J.M. Blackwell Scientific Publications.

Pegg D.E., Calne R.Y., Pryse-Davies J. & Brown F.L. (1964) Canine renal preservation using surface and perfusion cooling techniques. *Ann. N.Y. Acad. Sci.* **120**, 506.

Pegg D.E. & Farrant J. (1967) *In vitro* perfusion of the rabbit kidney. *Cryobiology*, **3**, 373.

Pegg D.E. & Farrant J. (1968) Some effects of colloids and dimethylsulphoxide on the perfusion of isolated rabbit kidneys. *Cryobiology*, **4**, 264.

PEGG D.E. (1970) Organ storage: A review. In *The Biology and Surgery of Tissue Transplantation*, ed. ANDERSON J.M. Blackwell Scientific Publications.

PLETKA P., COHEN S.L., HULME B., KENYON J.R., OWEN K., THOMPSON A.E., SNELL M., MOWBRAY J.F., PORTER K.A., LEIGH D.A. & PEART W.S. (1969) Cadaveric renal transplantation. An analysis of 65 cases. *Lancet*, i, 1.

POLGE C., SMITH A.U. & PARKES A.S. (1949) Revival of spermatozoa after vitrification and dehydration at low temperatures. *Nature*, **164**, 666.

PROCTOR E. (1969) Storage and transport of organs. *Brit. J. Hosp. Med.* **2**, 29.

ROBERTSON R.D. & JACOB S.W. (1968) The preservation of intact organs. In *Advances in Surgery*, Vol. 3, ed. WELCH C.E., p. 75. Chicago; Year Book Medical Publications.

SCHALM S.W., TERPSTRA J.L., DRAYER B., VAN DEN BERG C. & VELTKAMP J.J. (1969) A simple method for short-term preservation of a liver homograft. *Transplantation*, **8**, 877.

SCHLOERB P.R., WALDORF R.D. & WELSH J.S. (1959) The protective effect of kidney hypothermia on total renal ischaemia. *Surg. Gynec. & Obst.* **109**, 561.

SCOTT D.F., MORLEY A.R. & SWINNEY J. (1969) Canine renal preservation following hypothermic perfusion and subsequent function. *Brit. J. Surg.* **56**, 688.

SELLS R.A. & PENA J.R. (1970.) Paper presented at Surgical Research Society Meeting, Glasgow,

SEMB G., KROG J. & JOHANSEN K. (1960) Renal metabolism and blood flow during local hypothermia, studied by means of renal perfusion *in situ*. *Acta chir. Scand.* Supplement no. 252, p. 196.

SHAFEY O.A. & HASSAB M.A. (1968) Experimental study on haenodynamics of hepatic arterial and portal venous flow. *Surgery*, **63**, 962.

SHERMAN J.K. (1965) Practical applications and technical problems of preserving spermatozoa by freezing. *Fed. Proc.* **24**, S-288.

SHUMWAY N.E., LOWER R.R. & STOFER R.C. (1967) Transplantation of the heart. In *Advances in Surgery*, Vol. 2, ed. WELSH C.E. Chicago; Year Book Medical Publishers.

SICULAR A. & MOORE F.D. (1961) The postmortem survival of tissues. I. A standardized glucose oxidation procedure for assessing tissue viability after death of the host. *J. Surg. Res.* i, 9.

SLAPAK M., WIGMORE R.A. & MACLEAN C.D. (1967) Twenty-four hour liver preservation by the use of continuous pulsatile perfusion and hyperbaric oxygen. *Transplantation*, **5**, 1154.

SLAPAK M., WIGMORE R.A., WEXLER M., GILES G., LATZINA A. & McDERMOTT W.V. (1969) Normobaric and hyperbaric preservation of the liver, kidney and heart in a manually portable apparatus. *Trans. Amer. Soc. Art. Intern. Org.* **15**, 225.

SLAPAK M., WEXLER M., MIZUMOTO R., LATZINA A., GILES G. & McDERMOTT W.V. (1970) 2½–6 hour preservation of the primate liver by simple cooling and orthotopic autotransplantation. Surg. Res. Soc. Meeting, Glasgow. Abstract: *Brit. J. Surg.* **57**, 392.

SLAPAK M. (1970) Personal communication.

STARZL T.E. (1964) *Experience in Renal Transplantation*. Philadelphia: W.B. Saunders Co.

STARZL T.E. & PUTNAM C.W. (1969) *Experience in Hepatic Transplantation*. Philadelphia; W.B.Saunders Co.

Stevens G.H., Joseph W.C., Rangel D.D.M., Yakushi Y., Sanchez M.N. & Fonkalsrud E.W. (1968) Evaluation in dogs of various techniques of perfusion to preserve the lung. In *Organic Perfusion and Preservation*, ed. Norman J.C., p. 229.

Stevens L.E., Iverson B.M., Freeman J.S., Moor B.J. & Reemtsma K. (1968) Storage of kidneys in an intermediate heterologous host. In *Organ Perfusion and Preservation*, ed. Norman J.C., p. 417.

Steuber P., Kovacs G., Koletsky S. & Persky L. (1958) Regional renal hypothermia. *Surgery*, **44**, 77.

Swank R.C. & Porter G.A. (1963) Disappearance of micro-emboli transfused into patients during cardio-pulmonary bypass. *Transfusion*, **3**, 192.

Swenson O., Grana L., Inonye T. & Donnellan W.L. (1967) Immediate and long-term effects of acute hepatic ischaemia. *Arch. Surg.* **95**, 451.

Terasaki P.I., Martin D.C. & Smith R.B. (1967) A rapid metabolic test to screen cadaver kidneys for transplantation. *Transplantation*, **5**, 76.

Turner M.D., Hicks F.F., Hicks J.S. & Warren R.B. (1969) The use of metabolic inhibitors in hypothermic kidney storage. *J. Surg. Res.* **9**, 665.

Van Wyk J., Liem D.S. & Eiseman B. (1965a) Function of cadaver liver. *Surgery*, **58**, 120.

Van Wyk J., Tait I. & Eiseman B. (1965b) Function of livers left for graded periods within the cadaver. *Surgery*, **58**, 374.

Van Wyk J. & Eiseman B. (1966) Cold preservation of excised asanguinous livers. *Gastroenterology*, **51**, 207.

Veith F.J., Panossian A., Nehlsen S.L., Deysine M., Thelmow L., Becker N.H. & Hagstrom J.W.C. (1968a) Factors influencing morphologic and functional integrity in isolated perfused lungs. In *Organ Perfusion and Preservation*, ed. Norman J.C., p. 45.

Veith F.J., Attai L., Panorrian A., Bogartz L., Swain B., Dougherty J., Buchberg A. & Gliedman M.L. (1968) Perfusion techniques for lung, liver and kidney transplantation with immediate functional adequacy. In *Organ Perfusion and Preservation*, ed. Norman J.C., p. 453.

Vetto R.M., Folkert O., Belzer M.D., Rogers R.C. & Park H.Y. (1967) Rapid flow and isolated renal perfusion. *J. Surg. Res.* **7**, 520.

Webb W.R., Dodds R.P., Unal M.O., Karow A.M., Cook W.A. & Daniel C.R. (1966) Suspended animation of the heart with metabolic inhibitors. *Ann. Surg.* **164**, 343.

Weissman G. (1964) Labilization and stabilization of lysosomes. *Fed. Proc.* **23**, 1038.

Weir D.M. (1967) The immunological consequences of cell death. *Lancet*, ii 1071.

White H.J.O., Evans D.B. & Calne R.Y. (1968) Function of cadaver renal homografts in relation to age of donor, cause of death and ischaemia time. *Brit. med. J.* **4**, 739.

Williams G.M., White H.J.O. & Hume D.M. (1967) Factors influencing the long-term functional success rate of human renal allografts. *Transplantation*, **5**, 837.

Wodinsky I., Meaney K.F. & Kensler C.J. (1965) The strain specificity of transplantable neoplasms after freezing and storage in liquid nitrogen. *Cryobiology*, **2**, 44.

Wright E.S., Sarkozy E., Dobell A.R.C. & Murphy D.R. (1963) Fat globulinaemia in intracorporeal circulation. *Surgery*, **53**, 500.

CHAPTER 4

Tissue Typing*

V.C. Joysey

INTRODUCTION

Tissue grafts are not rejected when the donor and recipient are genetically identical, as for example between monozygotic twins and between members of isogenic lines of laboratory animals. Under these circumstances no immunosuppression is necessary and the foreign material is tolerated as well as an isograft. However, a genetically identical individual is not normally available as a donor, and most early work on tissue grafts was performed between individuals in which the degree of genetic disparity between the donor and recipient was unknown. The use of immunosuppressive drugs enables some grafts to be retained despite genetic disparity between donor and recipient. Many grafts, however, are either inexorably rejected despite vigorous immunosuppressive therapy, or the patients succumb to the therapy, either by direct intoxication, or more usually by overwhelming infection by a variety of viral, fungal or bacterial organisms (Evans 1969), against which the heavily immunosuppressed patient is incapable of mounting an effective defence because of non-specific depression of the immune mechanism.

Histocompatibility relationships in man have been greatly illuminated by

---

* Some of the material in this chapter has also been produced in 'Tissue Typing in Relation to Transplantation' in *Int. Rev. Exp. Path.* Vol. 9, p. 233.

the comparative study of skin grafts and kidney transplants between members of families. Skin grafts are normally applied without immunosuppression; the grafts are small and the connection between the graft and the recipient is built up at the capillary level. In contrast, thereapeutic kidney grafts are protected by immunosuppression; the size of the graft is very much greater than that of an experimental skin graft, and the connection with the host is by large vessels.

Ceppellini *et al* (1966) performed skin grafts between individuals of three genetic categories, (1) unrelated U/U (2) parent to child P/C (3) sibling to sibling S/S. Mean survival times for the three categories were U/U 12·1 days, P/C 14·1 days, S/S 16·6 days respectively. The survival curves for the ABO compatible members of the three categories of skin graft are similar in course to those of the same three categories of kidney grafts, but with a different time scale, such that survival in days for skin grafts is roughly equivalent to survival in months for kidney grafts. Therefore for experimental work, skin grafts form a valuable testing ground for antigenic disparity between individuals.

ABO antigens in graft survival

The marked role of compatibility of the ABO red cell antigens on skin graft survival was demonstrated in the same series of skin graft experiments by Ceppellini *et al* (1966). Survival times of ABO compatible grafts were significantly greater than ABO incompatible grafts in both the unrelated (compatible 12·1/incompatible 9·1) and the sibling categories (compatible 16·6/incompatible 13·0). The relevance of ABO compatibility to skin graft survival has also been demonstrated by Dausset & Rapaport (1966) who obtained accelerated rejection of ABO incompatible skin grafts after pre-sensitization with red cell stroma of corresponding group to the donor.

The significant reduction of survival time of skin grafts between ABO incompatible individuals is borne out by the clinical kidney transplant data. Gleason & Murray (1967) using data from the kidney transplant registry, found that 46% of transplants with ABO incompatibility failed to function at all, compared with 9% in the ABO compatible group. In recent literature, reference to ABO incompatible kidney grafts is rare, as most transplant centres now make ABO compatibility a *sine qua non* of transplantation. However, Shiel *et al* (1969) reported two cases of group B donor kidneys in group A_2 recipients. Both grafts, after initially producing urine, had to be removed because of acute rejection with 6 h and 4 days respectively.

Suggestive, but not conclusive, results from both skin and kidney transplant data may implicate the P red cell antigens as relevant to rejection (Ceppellini 1968).

Tissue typing

Tissue typing tests are based on the assumption that the isoantigens detected on the test cells are characteristic of the antigens present on the other tissues. This is not always a valid assumption as tissue specific iso-antigens are known e.g. TL antigen in mice (Boyse *et al* 1964) and De R. antigen in man, which is confined to the neutrophils (Lalezari & Bernard 1965).

Production of antisera

Antisera used for tissue typing are normally of human origin as antisera obtained from animals tend to be complicated by species specific antibodies. Some antisera produced in the chimpanzee have roughly the same specificity as those produced in man, but as yet these do not form suitable reagents for routine typing. Human tissue typing antisera may be produced in several ways. (1) By recipients of skin grafts and/or injections of leukocytes. Careful matching of donor and recipient for all antigens, except the one against which it is desired to make an antibody can result in the production of antibody of limited specificity (Thorsby & Kissmeyer-Nielsen 1968, 1969; Shanbrom *et al* 1968). The production of high titre antibody in volunteers could create the hazard of nonhaemolytic transfusion reaction, should the volunteer need a blood transfusion at some future date. (2) By recipients of kidney grafts who have rejected their kidney and who may produce antibody of narrow specificity if there was little antigenic disparity between donor and recipient (Morris *et al* 1969). (3) By multiparous women who have been sensitized by pregnancy (Payne & Rolfs 1958; Van Rood *et al* 1958).

Technique

A number of tests are available for tissue typing. Leukoagglutination and cytotoxicity are the most widely used, and these will be described briefly. The complement fixation and the immune adherance techniques are also available but are not yet in general use for routine tissue typing. The four tests have different sensitivities which, in order of decreasing sensitivity are usually immune adherance, cytotoxicity, leukoagglutination, complement fixation. Differences in sensitivity are of great importance in that the extrapolation of results from one test to another is hazardous, as a serum deemed monospecific by an insensitive test may appear polyspecific by a more sensitive test.

1 *Leukoagglutination*

A suspension of leukocytes is incubated with an equal volume of antiserum for 1 or 2 h at 37°C. Clumping of the leucocytes indicates a positive reaction. The clumping is not a true agglutination as it is dependent upon the viability of the granulocytes. Hence, accurate results can only be obtained with very fresh samples of blood. If the leukocyte suspension is either a few hours old, or is obtained from a moribund individual, or from a normal individual who is under physiological stress, then false positive or negative results may be obtained (Zmijewski *et al* 1967), so making a number of replicate tests desirable. The leukoagglutination test is carried out either in the presence of complement (Dausset 1965) or in the presence of EDTA (Van Rood & Van Leeuwen 1965). These two techniques have different degrees of sensitivity, the former giving the larger number of positives.

2 *Cytotoxic test*

This test also has a number of variants according to the practising laboratory. A purified suspension of lymphocytes is incubated with an equal volume of antiserum in the presence of serum complement. Combination of antibody with the cells is manifested by cytolysis of the lymphocytes. The differential cell death is determined by one of several methods. (a) Staining dead cells by trypan blue (Walford *et al* 1965). (b) Staining dead cells by eosin Y and examination by phase contrast microscopy (Terasaki *et al* 1967). (c) Staining dead cells by trypan blue and examination by phase contrast microscopy, Plate 1 (Joysey 1969). (d) Labelling the lymphocytes before testing with ^{51}Cr and evaluationg the chromium release from the lysed cells by comparison with control negative and 100% positive lysed lymphocytes (Rogentine 1967).

Terasaki & McClelland (1964) described a microcytotoxic test that utilizes 1 μl volumes of test reagents. This test has been modified and is now performed in disposable plastic trays (Mittal *et al* 1968). Variants of this test are now used by most tissue typing laboratories. As will be seen in the next section, it is of the greatest importance that laboratories collaborating on tissue typing should use identical antisera. Hence, a test using micro volumes is now essential. As the microcytotoxic test enables 1000 tests to be performed with 1 ml of serum, even valuable well characterized sera can be widely distributed.

Speed and accuracy are at a premium in prospective tissue typing for transplantation from cadaver donors. It is desirable to perform the test rapidly so that ischaemia time may be kept as short as possible and, as there is usually no time for repeat tests, it is necessary that tests should be performed initially at least in duplicate.

Characterization of antisera

Before sera are used for tissue typing it is essential that they should be well characterized. It is desirable to use sera which are monospecific. Walford *et al* (1967) coined the phrase 'operationally monospecific' for a serum which, after absorption by the leukocytes of any of 30 positively reacting individuals, contained no antibody detectable by the stimulating antigen. The labour involved in demonstrating operational monospecificity is considerable. A somewhat different criterion of monospecificity may be obtained on the basis of factor analysis by computer (Van Rood 1962). If two sera have limited and identical specificity when tested on a large panel of cells then it is likely that they contain a common monospecific antibody. However, an anomaly that arose in the Histocompatibility Workshop 1970 is that some sera which according to some workers were monospecific by absorption (e.g. 4a and 4b of Van Rood), appeared to be multispecific by computer analysis. This may indicate the complexity of the problem. Antibodies are known to exist which are cross reactive with two antigens. These, being cross reactive, may be extracted as 'a unit' in absorption studies, but show the population distribution appropriate to the two antigens, suggesting a mixture of two antibody specificities.

Some leukocyte antigens are detectable with accuracy because good sera are readily available e.g. HLA2 (previously known as Mac or antigen 1 Dausset, 8a van Rood, La2 Payne/Bodmer and Kissmeyer-Nielsen, Lc2 Walford, To9 Ceppellini, 1 Amos, 2 Terasaki, 5 Batchelor, P1GrLy^{B1} Shulman). The rationalized notation devised by the WHO committee on nomenclature (1968) will be used throughout the rest of this article.

When several antisera defininining a particular antigen are tested on a panel of cells, although a high degree of correlation may be present between the different sera, the reactions are usually not identical, and so, for the definition of a given antigen in tissue typing it is desirable to include a number of sera of the 'same' specificity. In the event of organ exchange between different transplant centres, it is essential that evaluation of specificities should be carried out using identical sera in the different testing laboratories.

Inheritance of HLA antigens

Over the last 5 years all the major tissue typing laboratories have contributed to an understanding of the mechanism of the inheritance of the HLA antigens but details of the steps towards its elucidation will not be given here. In 1969/70 a Fourth International Histocompatibility Workshop was held, during which an attempt was made to clarify the genetics of the histocompatibility antigens. The cells of members of 298 families were examined by 15 collaborating laboratories using the cytotoxic test, and the results have been published in Histocompatibility Testing 1970.

A large measure of agreement now exists on the genetic relationships of the antigens. The HLA antigens are conveyed from parent to offspring as a linkage group similar to the Rh antigens. Each parental chromosome bears its own characteristic pattern of antigens which are conveyed to the offspring *en bloc*. Hence, for any one mating the two paternal (AB) and the two maternal (CD) chromosomes can be arranged in only four combinations in the offspring i.e. AC, AD, BC, BD, and only four combinations of HLA antigens are therefore possible in full siblings. Thus, identity of HLA antigens can occur in 25% of siblings, and where live donors are used for kidney transplantation an HLA identical sibling is the donor of choice, as will be discussed subsequently (Fig. 1).

The HLA antigens are now regarded by many workers as being controlled by two closely linked segregant series of genes. The first series contains the antigens HL-A 1, 2, 3, 9, 10 and 11 and the second series contains HL-A 5, 7, 8, 12 and 13. Other antigens are present in both the first and second series, but these have not yet been given WHO nomenclature. (The first series is also known as the LA series, and the second series as the 7 or 4 series after previous notations which could probably with advantage now be allowed to lapse.) Within each series, the constituent antigens appear to be controlled by allelomorphic genes, i.e. to be true genetic alternatives. If this is true, then (1) an individual can have no more than two antigens from the first series, and two from the second series, e.g. HLA1, HLA5/HLA2, HLA7, i.e. four HLA antigens should be the maximum number that a normal individual can exhibit, and (2) a parent can pass on to any one child only one antigen from each series. The haploid complement of HL-A antigens, such as would be represented in the gametes, is known as the haplotype, and on the two locus theory, the haplotype can contain only one antigen from the first series, and one from the second. Each normal individual therefore possesses two haplotypes. An individual with antigens HL-A1, 2, 5, 7 might have the halotypes HL-A1, 5 and HL-A2, 7 or HL-A2, 5 and HL-A1, 7, which could be passed on to the offspring as units, but antigens HL-A1 and 2 could never be conveyed from that parent to the same offspring, as they are on different haplotypes (Fig. 1).

The serological difficulty of definition of some of the antigens, such as HLA5 and HLA7, makes rigorous genetic assessment of the antigens difficult. Although sera classified as anti-HL-A5 are strongly positively correlated, a wide range of reactivity is found, which may be due either to contamination with other specificities or to cross reactivity. The same is true of HL-A7. However, the concept has emerged that the serum with

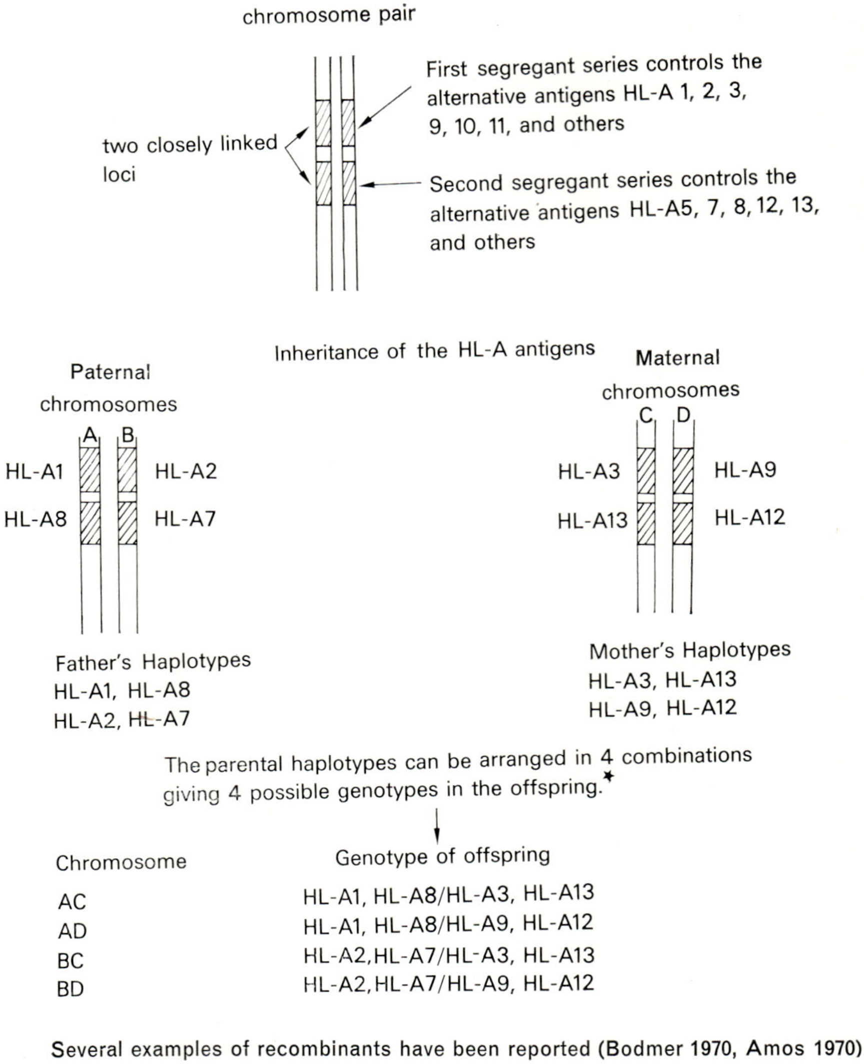

FIG 1. To illustrate the inheritance of the HLA antigens.

the lowest frequency of reaction forms the best tool for the identification of an antigen.

Although the Workshop results obtained were broadly in agreement with the hypothesis that the antigens are controlled by multiple alleles at two closely linked loci, caution in interpretation was advocated by Amos, who accepted that true allelism probably exists for HLA1, 2 and 3, and for some antigens of the second series, but emphasized that occasional individuals do appear to bear more than two antigens from either the first or the second series. Cross reactivity certainly occurs between some HL-A antigens within each segregant series e.g. HL-A3 and HL-A11. When present together with another member of the same series e.g. HL-A2, this could give the appearance of the simultaneous presence of three antigens of one segregant series. Likewise undetected duospecificity of typing sera could simulate the presence of three antigens in one series, but these problem cases have not yet been resolved. Furthermore, Yunis & Amos (1970) have found that treatment of the test lymphocytes by the enzyme neuraminidase can reveal in the cytotoxic test, the presence of an antigen that is normally demonstrable only by absorption. (CYNAP phenomenon: CYtotoxic Negative Absorption Positive, Ceppellini 1965; Walford 1965. Cells of some individuals possess an antigen, as demonstrated by their ability to absorb the appropriate antibody, but are not killed by that antibody in the cytotoxic test.) As the cytotoxic test was standardly used for the workshop some of the weak reactions might subsequently be revealed as being true positives. Should it become a certainty that more than two antigens of a series can be present in an individual, then the concept of the arrangement of antigens in only two series will require reappraisal.

It is, therefore, essential at the present stage of knowledge on the HL-A antigens to keep an open mind on the genetic situation. The conceptual framework of tissue typers should be sufficiently elastic to allow apparently heretical anomalies, such as the presence of three antigens at one locus, to appear on their charts. The supernumerary reactions may be the crucial evidence to the comprehension of the nature of the interaction of the HL-A antigens. The presence of two closely linked subloci each with the multiple alleles, as previously stated, forms a useful working hypothesis, but should not be allowed to form a conceptual straight jacket.

Van Rood's antigens 4a and 4b are demonstrated more readily by leuko-agglutination than by the cytotoxic test. Antisera are available which for practical purposes may be regarded as monospecific, and the antigens behave approximately in a Mendelian fashion in family studies. However, according to Kissmeyer-Nielsen *et al* (1968) the specificities HLA12, HLA5 and HLA13 are almost completely included within 4a, and HLA7 and some other lower frequency antigens within 4b. Hence, they regard 4a and 4b as being a cross reactive complex of other antigens of lower frequency. As some individuals have the same phenotypes for the second series but differ on the 4a and 4b phenotypes, Van Rood *et al* (1970) regard them as being more than the sum of antigens of the second sublocus, and consider them to be controlled by a third sublocus. That this is not merely an academic discussion will be seen when compatibility between donor and recipient is discussed subsequently. Kissmeyer-Nielsen *et al* (1970) have described a different third sublocus, closely linked with the first and second subloci, which so far is defined by a single antigen AJ. Other leukocyte antigens 5a and 5b, which form an allelomorohic pair, and 9a are known not to be closely linked with the HLA locus (Van Rood *et al* 1967), and are not currently regarded as having great significance in relation to transplantation. However, until most tissue typing laboratories type for these antigens, proof on this point will be difficult to obtain.

Although an individual who receives a skin graft from an HLA identical sibling retains that graft for an extended period of time, the skin graft is finally rejected, and so it seems that other loci such as 5a, 5b and 9a could be relevant to late rejection.

Population distribution of the HLA antigens

The HLA antigens are grossly polymorphic. Kissmeyer-Nielsen *et al* (1969) calculated that 1008 different HLA phenotypes were possible on the assumption that there were seven alleles at the first sublocus and eight at the second sublocus. They calculated that a random chance of finding two unrelated individuals with identical tissue types is about 1 in 1000.

Some antigen combinations are rare, e.g. HLA2, HLA13 and a patient with a phenotype which has a low population frequency may have to wait for a considerable length of time before an antigenically suitable donor becomes available.

The gene frequencies, and most of the serology and genetics of the HLA antigens have been worked out on Caucasians. The gene frequencies are known to be very different in different races, for example, the HLA1 antigen is present in 22·5% of Caucasians (Kissmeyer-Nielsen *et al* 1968), but has not so far been detected among Asians. Furthermore, the HLA antigens may be qualitatively different in different races. Dausset *et al* (1965, 1967) described the reactions of some anti-HL-A2 sera on the leukocytes of French, Japanese and Malian people. The frequency of HLA2 is very much lower in the Malians, and two sera, which on the French population acted as anti-HLA2, failed to react with nearly all Japanese and Malian HLA2 positive individuals. These observations could be important in tissue matching, if the donor and recipient have different racial origins.

Assessment of compatibility of donor and recipient

Compatibility between donor and recipient can be assessed in a variety of ways, e.g. by test skin grafting, by mixed lymphocyte culture (see chapter by Dr Festenstein) and by serological tests. Test skin grafts from potential donors on to the potential recipient to find the longest graft survival time form a reliable but unacceptable method, as the test graft sensitizes the recipient to donor antigens and any further grafts from the same donor are rejected in an accelerated fashion. Amos *et al* (1969) have used skin grafting in order to assess the degree of compatibility of members within families. Using serological and mixed lymphocyte culture tests it was sometimes possible to find a sibling who was HL-A identical with the potential recipient. The healthy sibling then received skin grafts from the potential donors and the order of compatibility between different family members was evaluated without sensitizing the potential recipient. This technique is a valuable research tool but not ideal for routine work even within families, and is useless for evaluation in cadaver transplantation.

Assessment by serological tests. A battery of antisera is tested against the lymphocytes of the recipient and the donor. Then a direct comparison is made between the reactions of each. An antigen present in the donor and lacking in the recipient was called a major incompatibility by Stickel *et al* 1967; and an antigen present in the recipient but lacking in the donor was called a minor incompatibility. Theoretically, the presence of a minor incompatibility should not evoke an immune reaction. However, Van Rood & Eernisse (1968) have emphasized that, within families, identity between donor and recipient is essential in order to significantly improve prognosis of kidney grafts. Furthermore, the range of sera at present available does not cover all the antigenic specificities that exist, and individuals are known who do not appear to possess any antigens of either the first or alternatively the second segregant series. Therefore, the antigens that these individuals do possess can not yet be demonstrated. If a recipient reacts with HLA1 and HLA2 and the donor only reacts with HLA2, this is a minor incompatibility on HLA1. The donor could have the constitution HLA2/HLA2 at the first sublocus which would not constitute a hazard to the graft, as no antigen would be present in the donor which was lacking in the recipient. However, the donor could have the constitution HLA2/X, with X representing an unknown allele. The minor incompatibility at HLA1 would in this case represent a major incompatibility at X, which would constitute a hazard to the graft. Hence, until we have sera representing the complete range of antigens, identity is likely to remain superior to compatibility. (On the two sublocus theory, if two antigens are present at either the first (or the second) sublocus then it is possible to fix the genotypes of that individual as further antigens could not be present at that locus) (Fig. 1).

The characterization of the test sera is of the greatest importance if tissue typing is to be valid and to correlate with the results of grafting.

Specificity of sera

As previously stated, batteries of monospecific sera of the 'same' speciffcity are desirable in order to define the presence of an antigen. In this way a 'majority verdict' on the presence of an antigen can be obtained. If sera are used that are duo, or multispecific, errors in evaluation of incompatibility can result. For example, if a serum contains antibody of two specificities anti-X and anti-Y and both donor and recipient give a positive reaction, this must not be taken to indicate compatibility, as the donor might possess antigen X and the recipient antigen Y and therefore a major incompatibility could be present at X. However, if the donor reacts with a multispecific serum and the recipient does not, then this can be regarded as a major incompatibility, even though its specificity may not be known. Most tissue typing laboratories have in use antisera which, although not fully characterized, are none the less useful in discriminating between family members. In the evaluation of incompatibility between two individuals, two possible courses are open; (a) assessment of incompatibility on the known antigenic groups. This may ignore some incompatibilities demonstrable with other sera. However, the well characterized antigens are those where a number of examples of antibody are available and, therefore, demonstrably immunogenic; (b) assessment of the number of incompatibilities on the whole battery of sera available. This could be subject to error consequent upon the frequency of antibody specificities within the battery of test sera, as incompatibility on one antigen whose specificity was represented a number of times could appear to represent a number of incompatibilities. There is a particular likelihood of error if unknown specificities and cross reactive antibodies are present in the sera.

The genetic perspective has considerable bearing on the evaluation of the incompatibilities between unrelated individuals. If the first and second subloci control all the main histocompatibility antigens then the maximum number of incompatibilities possible is four, two at the first sublocus and two at the second. If the 4a and 4b antigens are products of cross reactivity of the antigens at the second sublocus, as considered by Kissmeyer-Nielsen, then incompatibilities of these antigens should not be added to those manifested at the second sublocus. If, however, as Van Rood believes the 4a and 4b antigens are not the result of cross reactivity at the second sublocus but represent another sublocus, then incompatibility at 4a and 4b should be added to that of the first and second sublocus. As Van Rood has found individuals that are identical at the second sublocus but differ on 4a and 4b, it would seem wiser to err by counting the 4a and 4b incompatibilities separately. If multiple loci are involved, as Amos believes, then a larger number of incompatibilities is possible.

Dausset (1970) has suggested that the immunogenicity of an antigen is reduced in a recipient who bears an antigen which cross reacts with the donor antigen. If this were so, it might render some antigen incompatibilities less nocuous than others. At present the relative effect of mismatches of the different antigens is not known but, as discussed subsequently, there is a cumulative effect of multiple incompatibilities

Transplantation between related individuals

Since the HLA antigens are conveyed as a linked group, in family studies the demonstrable antigens act as chromosomal markers for other antigens within the linkage group which cannot yet be demonstrated. Therefore, it may be possible with relatively few sera to assign the appropriate parental haplotypes to a family of siblings, and to indicate which siblings are HLA identical. The patterns of reactivity of the siblings fall into no more than four groups, members of which have identical antigen profiles. Absolute monospecificity of the test sera is not essential as identity of overal antigen profile is being sought. Siblings that are HLA identical do not normally mutually stimulate in the MLC test, regardless of ABO group (Bach *et al* 1969). Amos *et al* (1969) have assessed the rejection time in days of a series of skin grafts between siblings of the three categories, those with identical alleles, those that differ by two alleles, and those that differ by one allele. When sibling donor and recipient differed by two alleles, graft rejection had always occurred by 15 days post grafting (range 6–15 days, mean $11{\cdot}6 \pm 5{\cdot}4$ days). When the siblings were HLA identical the rejection had never occurred by the 15th day, there being no overlap with the previous category (range 16–41 days, mean $24{\cdot}9 \pm 1{\cdot}1$). Those that differed by one allele had a range of 6–24 days (mean $14{\cdot}4 \pm 3{\cdot}4$), and overlapped the ranges of the other categories, but fell 16 days short of the longest rejection time for the HLA identical pairs. Extrapolating from the skin graft survival data within the family, the best donor is an HLA identical sibling, and second to best is a parent or a sibling who shares one haplotype with the recipient.

Amos *et al*, Biegel *et al*, Jonasson *et al* and Wonham *et al* (all 1970, in press), have reported selection of sibling donors who are ABO compatible, HLA identical with the recipient. The recipients from HLA identical donors up to 24 months after transplantation have excellent renal function, and receive minimal immunosuppression. The recipients appear to be healthy normal people!

Singal *et al* (1969) evaluated the role of compatibility of specific HLA antigens in kidney transplants from sibling to sibling and parent to child. They evaluated the matching using antisera to five antigenic groups HLA1,

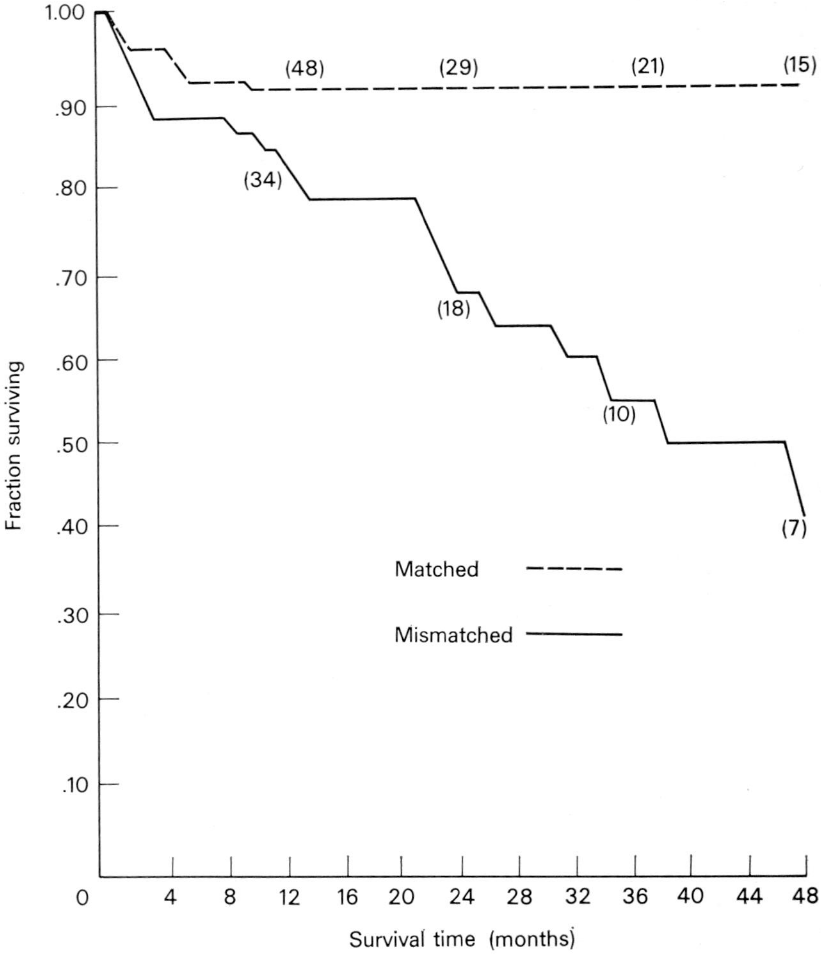

Fig. 2. Survival curves for matched and mismatched sibling kidney transplants. Roughly one-half of the recipient-donor pairs were tissue-typed retrospective and the other one-half prospective to grafting. The numbers alongside each curve indicate the number of patients at risk. The cumulative proportion of survivors was calculated by actuarial methods.

(Reproduced by permission from Singal *et al.*, 1969)

2, 5, 7 and Te 3 (4a), and classified the donor recipient pairs into 'matched' and 'mismatched' on the presence of any of these antigens in the donor, lacking in recipients (major mismatch). They plotted survival curves for matched and mismatched sibling transplants, and found a very marked correlation between clinical rank and leukocyte matching (Fig. 2). They state 'The level of significance between matched and mismatched sibling transplants was very high ($P < 0{\cdot}001$), while the difference in the survival of matched and mismatched parent/child transplants fell short of statistical significance ($P = 0{\cdot}16$). The anomaly of this second result is discussed elsewhere (Joysey 1970).

Singal *et al* had a number of survivors of 4 years duration who definitely had mismatched kidneys and, therefore, they concluded that incompatibility at any of the five antigens studied, with present immunosuppressive therapy, does not inevitably lead to graft rejection. They described the antigens as being of intermediate strength, and suggested that incompatibilities for the 'major' antigens are deleterious for only a proportion of the patients. This will be discussed in a later section.

Van Rood *et al* (1968) and Van Rood & Eernisse (1968), using antisera to nine HLA antigens have analysed the compatibility of the donor and recipients of the 18 survivors of 40 sib/sib transplants. From random family data, the number of 'identical', 'compatible' and 'incompatible' pairs to be expected in 40 transplants was calculated. This was then compared with the number of actual survivors in each category. From this data it seems likely that all the identicals have survived, while in the compatible and incompatible group all but 25% have died. These figures are significant $P = 0{\cdot}025$. Van Rood *et al* also found no significant difference between the compatible (those with minor mismatches), and incompatible group. This they attributed to the fact that a minor mismatch (compatibility), for an antigen we can detect, may represent a major mismatch (incompatibility) for an antigen we cannot yet detect (see assessment of serological tests). Van Rood *et al* used the same technique as was used with siblings, for comparison of the number of observed and expected surivors in the 'identical' and 'nonidentical' categories of the parent/child grafts, and found a significant excess of 'identical' to 'nonidentical' survivors ($P = 0{\cdot}05$). It should be noted, however, that true HLA identity normally occurs only in HLA identical siblings, as evidenced by lack of stimulation in the MLC test, and by the positive result obtained in all other categories. Van Rood *et al* 1969 postulate 'operationally identical' alleles and individuals, i.e. those that type 'identically' in serological tests with defined antisera and between which there is prolonged graft survival (Eijsvogel *et al* 1970 have subsequently found a pair of unrelated individuals who typed identically and who did not mutually stimulate.)

Transplantation from unrelated donors

Prolonged survival of operationally identical parent/child grafts renders it likely that extended survival might occur between unrelated individuals who have operational identity of tissue type. For this reason, van Rood inaugurated the organization Eurotransplant for the typing and distribution of organs of a donor to the most compatible recipient. Organization of such a scheme is discussed by Oliver, Sachs & Festenstein elsewhere in this volume.

Since the advent of Eurotransplant and the consequent improved proportion of well matched kidneys from cadaver donors, Van Rood *et al* (1969) have studied the survival of 37 kidney grafts. These were divided into categories on tissue typing of donor and recipient. (1) 'Identical', or nearly identical on HLA antigens. (2) Mismatched on two to three antigens i.e. major and minor incompatibilities added. (3) Four or more mismatches. After 1 year there was a marked difference ($P > 0{\cdot}02$) in the proportion of functioning grafts in the three categories, such that:

0–1 mismatches had 75% functioning
2–3 mismatches had 60% functioning
4 or more mismatches had 30% functioning

Hence, on this small series there is a markedly improved prognosis for well matched grafts.

Similarly, Kissmeyer-Nielsen *et al* (1970) have studied the relationship between tissue matching, and survival and clinical rank, in Scandinavian transplants for related and unrelated donors. They used sera recognizing up to 18 antigens of the first and second series. In their assessment of incompatibilities they have not taken into account the 4a and 4b antigens as they regard them as complexes of antigens of the second sublocus. Kissmeyer-Nielsen *et al* divide their serological data into categories:

A1 (sibling, true HLA identity)
A2 (related apparent identity)
A3 (apparent identity, unrelated cadaver)
B minor mismatches only
C one major mismatch
D two major mismatch
E three major mismatch
F antibody in the serum of the recipient reacting with donor cells.

Likewise clinical ranks are classified after Terasaki from 1 to 5.

1 having minimal rejection and normal function
2 having moderate rejection and good function
3 having moderate rejection and subnormal function
4 having frank rejection
5 having hyperacute rejection.

Kissmeyer-Nielsen *et al* have presented the Scandiatransplant data as survival curves, but as the scheme has been operative for only 12 months the data are short term. However, several facts clearly emerge. (1) In mismatched grafts a fall off occurs in graft survival during the 1st year. (2) The correlation between matching and survival improves if the worst possible match is computed on the theory that HLA antigens are controlled by multiple alleles at two closely linked subloci. Kissmeyer-Nielsen *et al* (1970) Table 6, includes all HLA typed transplantations, both related and unrelated, performed in Scandinavia since 1964. The cadaver data from Kissmeyer-Nielsen *et al* Table 6 is reproduced here by permission as Table 1.

TABLE 1. The correlation between clinical rank and serological match grade from Kissmeyer-Nielsen *et al* (1970) ($P=0{\cdot}005$)

		Clinical rank				
		1	2	3	4	5
Serological	A apparent identity	—	1	—	—	—
match	B minor mismatch	4	4	2	1	—
grade	C 1 major	5	8	—	3	—
	D 2 major	1	1	2	8	—
	F antibody	—	—	—	1	3

Similar evidence is adduced by Morris *et al* (1970) in analysis of 72 patients over a period of 3 to 30 months. Morris *et al* excluded 18 patients because of death or non-function of the kidney for reasons other than normal rejection. Again clinical evaluation was carried out on the number and severity of rejection episodes, and graded from (A) no rejection episodes, to (D) rejection requiring nephrectomy or causing death of the patient. Histological studies of the grafted kidney were also carried out at 3 weeks and 3 months after grafting. Serological assessment was made on ten antigens including 4a and 4b, and the evaluation made on the criteria of both non-identity (i.e. sum of major and minor mismatches) and in compatibility (major mismatches only). In this series they found no advantage of assessing non-identity over incompatibility, as both methods of assessment gave a comparable correlation between matching and rejection grade. They illustrated the relationship between compatibility and non-identity by a graph, which suggests that 0–1 incompatibilities are roughly equivalent to 0–2 non-identities, and hence they used incompatibilities in subsequent evaluation. However, it is essential to realize that their assessment of a major incompatibility involves counting two demonstrable minor mismatches at one locus as one major mismatch. Thus, if the donor has no demonstrable antigens at one locus and the recipient has two antigens at that locus, then this is counted as a major mismatch on the assumption that an incompatibility must be present for an antigen at that locus which is not yet demonstrable. When sera identifying all relevant antigens at the two subloci become available, it is likely to become unnecessary to take minor mismatches into consideration. However, this is based on the assumption that it is the individual antigens that are important in the transplantation situation, rather than the complex of antigens controlled by the genotype and this could be a false assumption.

Morris *et al* (1970) compared the number of donor/recipient incompatibilities (major mismatches) with the early rejection grade (3 months), and found significant correlation between them. (Table 2).

TABLE 2. A comparison between the number of HL-A incompatibilities between donor and recipient and the early course of the graft as judged by rejection grades

	No. of incompatibilities	Rejection grade	
		A+B	C+D
	0–1	23	11
$P<0{\cdot}02$	>1	15	23

(Table 2 reproduced by permission, part of Morris *et al*'s Table 3.)

Further evaluation, at a year after grafting, of recipients whose graft had survived beyond 3 months, showed correlation between the number of incompatibilities and fuction. Function was measured by serum creatinine. A good course was judged as having S Cr less than 1·8 and a bad course as S Cr more than 1·8, or death, or rejection between 3 months and 1 year (Table 3).

TABLE 3. A comparison between the number of incompatibilities between donor and recipient and the course of grafts which were functioning 3 months after transplant, at 1 year

	Incompatibilities	Good course	Bad course
	0–1	9	8
	>1	2	13
$P<0{\cdot}05$			

(Table 3 reproduced by permission part of Morris *et al*'s Table VII.)

As there is a significant correlation between histocompatibility matching and the survival and function of the graft at 3 months and 1 year after grafting, Morris *et al* suggest that 'a useful cut off point, from a practical

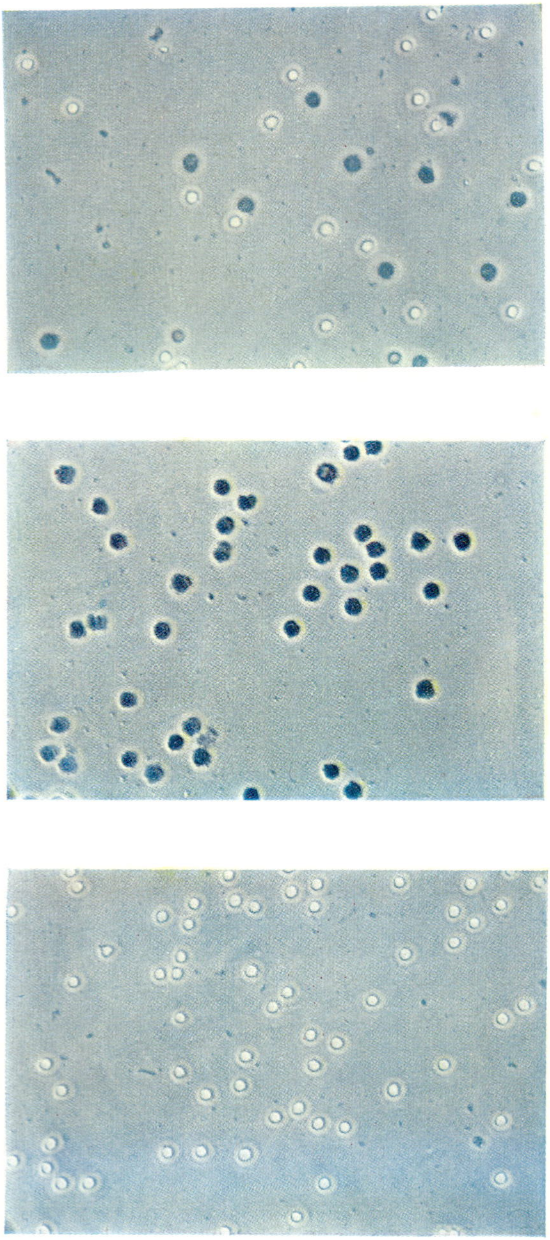

PLATE I Microcytotoxic test, stained by Trypan Blue and examined by phase contrast microscopy. All cells had been stored in liquid nitrogen.

i. Negative, all but one of the cells are alive.
ii. Strong Positive ++. All the cells are dead.
iii. Positive +. About half the cells are dead.

viewpoint between good and bad matches could be taken as more than one incompatible group or more than two non-identical groups'.

In their assessment Morris *et al* in common with Van Rood but unlike Kissmeyer-Nielsen, consider the 4a and 4b antigens to be of great importance in tissue matching as they include antigens that cannot yet be recognized by sera reacting with the second series. In Morris *et al*'s data the significance of association of rejection grade with the 4a and 4b antigens was $P > 0{\cdot}01$.

A similar picture of association between donor/recipient compatibility and recipient survival is presented by the results obtained from cadaver kidney transplantation from our own group in Cambridge. The results of Joysey & Calne (1968) are here brought up to date. Transplants that failed for technical or other obviously non-immunological reasons were eliminated leaving 38 donor recipient pairs which had been typed for the antigens HLA1, 2, 5, 7, 8 and 4a and 4b. The grafts were divided into two categories (1) those capable of supporting life up to 6 months post transplant; (2) those in which, within the first 6 months, rejection caused either death, or necessitated nephrectomy, or required increased immunosuppression which resulted in death by infection superimposed on rejection. The number of major mismatches was assessed and plotted on a histogram Plate 1 (Fig. III). The correlation between the match grade and survival is significant at the level $P = 0{\cdot}05$.

The results obtained independently by Van Rood, Kissmeyer-Nielsen, Morris, the present author and many others point inexorably to the conclusion that with cadaver transplantation, as with transplantation from a related donor, the degree of serological similarity of donor and recipient is correlated with survival. At present accurate correlation between the different authors is not possible, as there were differences in the number and specificity of sera used. However, agreement exists that operational identity, or failing this the presence of minor mismatches only, gives a better than average prognosis, and multiple major incompatibilities are usually associated with graft rejection. For example, in Kissmeyer-Nielsen's category D (2 major mismatches), 10/12 individuals had rejection (8) or subnormal function (2). Similarly, in Morris' category > 1 major mismatch, 13/15 had subnormal creatinine clearance or rejection, and in Joysey and Calne's category of 3 or more major mismatches, 5/6 grafts ceased to function by 6 months. These figures indicate that despite occasional success, which will be discussed subsequently, the prognosis for patients receiving such a graft is utterly unsatisfactory. Superficially, the good results obtained in the well matched categories of the authors quoted may seem to be at variance with the results of the Kidney Transplant Registry (1969), where the overall survival rate of transplanted cadaver kidneys has not greatly increased since the advent of tissue typing. This is not really surprising, however, in view of the fact that some centres still perform random grafts, either because of a lack of conviction of the value of tissue typing or because of the inadequate supply of kidneys available for transplantation, which often necessitates the grafting of kidneys which are poor matches, the majority of which predictably fail.

Factors affecting graft survival

The rejection of a grafted organ is controlled by a number of factors, including size, site of graft, organ grafted, and the immunosuppressive therapy applied, but the antigenic relationship between the donor and recipient is a dominant factor. Grafts differing from the recipient by several major mismatches may sometimes function for a number of years, but this is the exception rather than the rule. Other grafts, apparently well matched, may be promptly rejected, but this could be due to incompatibility for an antigen as yet undetected. Likewise, response by different patients to multiple blood transfusions varies greatly, some producing a detectable leucocyte antibody after a few transfusions, whereas others do so only after many transfusions.

Amos *et al* (1969) performed a series of skin grafts on members of a family who had been HLA typed. Three offspring were identical for one HLA type (AD) and two for another (BD). The two categories differed by one haplotype. Skin grafts were exchanged between the siblings and their mother. These skin grafts were rejected in the same sequence by two HLA identical siblings (Ev and Ma), and the rejection times were correlated with the HLA relationship, but in any given genetical situation sibling Ev rejected 6 to 9 days before sibling Ma. This is illustrated in Table 4 which is constructed by permission from the data in Amos *et al* (1969) Fig. 2.

TABLE 4. Skin graft survival time between family members. Data from Amos *et al* (1969)

Donor	Rejection time in days of graft to AD sibling recipients	
	Ev	Ma
AD	30	36
AD	30	37
CD mother	18	24
BD	13	21
BD	12	21

The BD sibling pair in the same family also showed a marked difference in reactivity. Ward *et al* (1970) have extended these observations and described other families showing similar differences in reactivity of HLA identical siblings under identical HLA stimulation. The authors postulated the existence of a gene controlling the immunological responsiveness to some HLA specificities. By analogy this suggests a possible basis for some of the variability which occurs in kidney grafting. For instance, the long term survivors who have multiple mismatches might be genetically slow rejectors, and therefore at an advantage in any grafting situation. A further variable that may affect survival of a mismatched graft is the phenomenon of enhancement which will be discussed at the end of the next section.

Transplantation in the presence of antibody against the graft

Cochrum *et al* (1969) in the goat, infused high titre cytotoxic antibody into autografted kidneys against which the antibody was reactive. This initiated rejection of the autografts, which with one exception became anuric 36 to 72 h later.

In man Kissmeyer Nielsen *et al* (1966); Williams *et al* (1967); Starzl *et al* (1968); Terasaki *et al* (1968); Jeannet *et al* (1970), have described hyperacute rejection of the grafted kidney associated with the presence of pre-existing cytotoxic antibody in the recipient, reactive against donor cells. The kidney is rapidly rejected, the time of rejection being measured from minutes to days. In one of our own patients (Evans *et al* in preparation), the kidney became flaccid and cyanosed within minutes of completion of the vascular anastomoses. Hence, it is imperative to test the sera of all potential recipients for the presence of cytotoxic antibodies against the donor. Cytotoxic antibody in potential recipients may be stimulated by (1) Isoimmunization of pregnancy. Multiparous women form one of the best sources of tissue typing antibody, but antibody can be produced after only one pregnancy. (2) Blood transfusion. Leukocytes in transfused blood can form a powerful antigenic stimulus. Repeated transfusions are often necessary for the patient awaiting kidney transplantation and, being derived from many different donors, they may sensitize the patient to a wide spectrum of antigens. Hence, in a multitransfused patient it may be virtually impossible to obtain a negative cross match test. Evans *et al* (in preparation) have reported a patient who received two grafts; the first was rejected within 6 weeks, the second was rejected hyperacutely in the presence of circulating antibody against the graft. Subsequently, in the serum of this patient antibody was demonstrated to be reactive against 99% of the population. Although neither kidney graft contained antigen HL-A2, antibody of specificity anti-HLA2 was demonstrated in the patient's serum by absorption studies. About 50% of the many blood transfusions that the patient had received would have contained the HLA-2 antigen, and as the patient is a male, these blood transfusions are the most likely source of stimulation to produce the anti-HLA2.

The unpredictability of the fluctuations of antibody titre makes it essential that monitoring of the antibody should be performed at frequent intervals, as suggested by Van Rood. Any rise in titre consequent upon transfusion can then be noted. The serum titre may 'peak' after a gross antigenic stimulus, such as a kidney graft or massive blood transfusion; therefore, in this laboratory, two serum samples are used for cross matching, the 'peak' sample (if any), and the most recent sample. In this way it is hoped also to exclude as donors those individuals who give a positive cross match on the 'peak' sample, on the grounds that this indicates a previous sensitization with donor antigens, and the likelihood of accelerated rejection.

Hattler *et al* (1966) demonstrated cytotoxic antibodies in 29% of patients who had received massive blood transfusions during open heart surgery. They also observed that volunteers rejected skin grafts in an accelerated fashion 2 weeks after receiving one unit of fresh whole blood from the same donor and therefore the authors questioned the advisability of giving fresh whole blood to potential organ graft recipients. The blood transfusions that are essential to the survival of the patient may prejudice the survival of the graft. The relevant histocompatibility antigens are carried by the leukocytes and platelets, and are also present in the plasma in sufficient quantity that infusion of plasma prior to grafting can cause accelerated rejection of skin grafts (Van Rood *et al* 1970).

While it is theoretically desirable that potential graft recipients should only be given white cell free, washed red cells, the effective removal of all leukocytes presents a practical problem. Washing of dextran sedimented red cells, or of red cells from stored blood in which the leukocytes have deteriorated is not completely effective at removing leukocytes, as some are still present in both types of preparation (Dr D.C.L. James personal communication). However, while not completely preventing sensitization, it should greatly reduce it. Dr M.Berah has suggested the use of blood compatible on the main leukocyte groups with the recipient. It is perhaps worthy of thought, in the context of sensitization, that the multiple blood samples taken from transplant patients for investigative purposes tend to make the patient anaemic and, therefore, should be kept to the minimum in order to obviate frequent transfusions.

Cytotoxic antibodies are often demonstrable in patients who have had allograft nephrectomy. (Morris *et al* (1969) found that 13/24 such patients had antibody; Joysey (unpublished) found 7/8). Hence, in a second graft the possibility of hyperacute rejection is high, but this may be rendered less likely by the performance of a cross match test. However, Heale *et al* (1969) have reported a single case of survival of the graft in the presence of a positive cross match and Morris *et al* (1969) have reported hyperacute rejection in the presence of an apparently negative cross match. Here the sensitivity of the cross match test is at a premium, and in the future it may be desirable to use a more sensitive test for cross matching than for ordinary tissue typing.

The presence of antibody *per se* need not be prejudicial to graft survival, but can enhance it, as has been shown by Rowley *et al* (1969) and French & Batchelor (1969). Rowley *et al* (1969) treated Lewis rats which had received renal allografts from Lewis XBN F_1 donors with antiserum to the allograft and also with living donor lymphoid cells. The antibody alone enhanced graft survival (untreated 13/14 died within 30 days, treated 7/7 survived longer than 60 days), but the additional injection of donor cell antigen immediately before grafting, potentiated graft survival, as the BUN level was significantly lower in rats that had received the dual treatment.

French & Batchelor (1969) grafted inbred AS rats with an AS X August kidney. In untreated rats the kidney was rejected in 12 days. However, when antibody against the donor was injected into the recipient at intervals after grafting, so that a low level of circulating antibody was produced, the graft survival was enhanced. In the absence of other immunosuppression the graft survived with good function for more than 120 days. This treatment had not induced tolerance as the rats could still make antibody when challenged with donor cells, and such antibody production was considered to continue graft protection. When the donor and recipient had a greater antigenic disparity, the enhancement was less marked. Enhancement of graft survival can sometimes therefore be obtained by means of circulating antibody in experimental animals. The features of the antibody which cause enhancement of the graft rather than hyperacute rejection are at present unclear. In the human situation, however, the demonstration of preformed antibody has usually been associated with hyperacute rejection.

Second kidney grafts

The complexity of the polymorphism of the HLA antigens makes it theoretically likely that second grafts will have a lower chance of success than the first, because some of the antigens in the second graft are likely to have been encountered before. On the other hand, Van Rood *et al* (1969) quoted their observations that 'our sib/sib and parent/child series have shown clearly that the adverse effect of leukocyte group incompatibility only become apparent after 1 to 2 years'. It is possibly dangerous to transfer conclusions based on living related donors to the situation of unrelated cadaver donors as is illustrated by their further statement that: 'as already mentioned, (that) the adverse effect of lymphocyte group incompatibility only becomes apparent after 1 or 2 years. A mismatched kidney transplant can therefore be used until a kidney with a better fit becomes available'. The data from cadaver donors, quoted previously, leaves no doubt that a

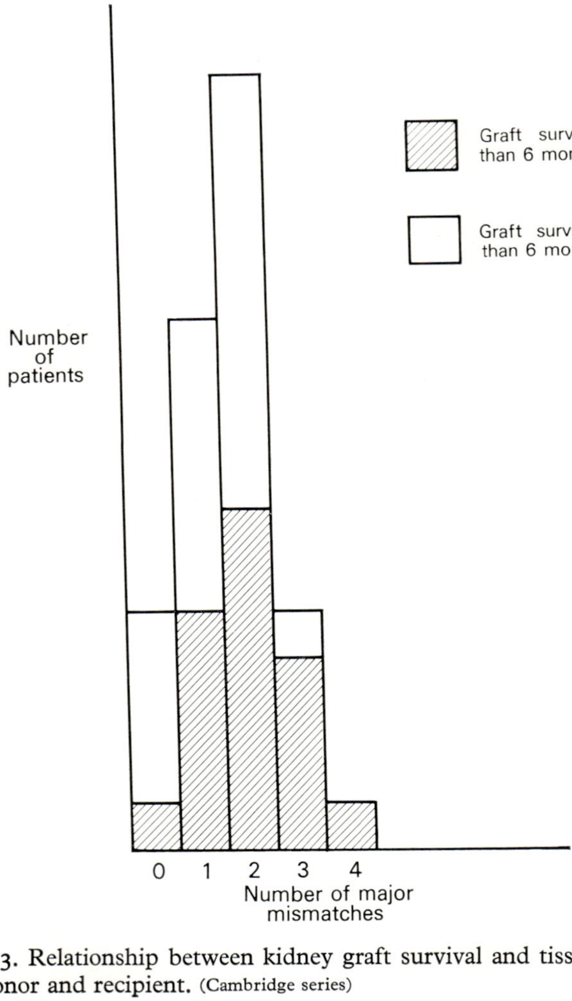

Fig. 3. Relationship between kidney graft survival and tissue matching of donor and recipient. (Cambridge series)

strong adverse selection occurs on multiply mismatched grafts during the first 6 months post transplant.

As described in the previous section post allograft nephrectomy serum frequently contains antibody directed against the graft. Even when no antibody is demonstrable, the patient has still been sensitized to the antigens contained in the graft, and if presented with the same antigens at a subsequent graft, is liable to reject the graft in an accelerated fashion (Medawar 1946). This may be particularly unfortunate as a relatively well matched second kidney, differing from the recipient by only one major mismatch, may be promptly rejected if the mismatched antigen has been encountered before. Hence, it is not advisable to use a badly mismatched kidney until a better match becomes available, as a multiply mismatched cadaver kidney is likely to be rejected within 6 months, and this will result in sensitization of the recipient, which may prejudice the survival of a subsequent graft. In this context it is worthy of note that of the six patients in the Cambridge series who had antibody, and received a second transplant, two had a weak positive cross match and rapidly rejected, four had a definately negative cross match and, of these, two have rejected and two survive at 2 and 6 months respectively. One patient has received and rejected three kidney grafts. Subsequently to grafting, the recipient and her donors have been reassessed using sera from the 1970 Histocompatibility Workshop, kindly donated by other laboratories. Incompatibilities on the three grafts were (1) HLA1, HLA2, HLA8; (2) HLA2, HLA3, HLA7, FJH; (3) HLA3. Previous tests on the third donor using 50 sera of 17 specificities, including anti-HLA3 serum Storm, failed to demonstrate incompatibility of HLA3, possibly due to the CYNAP phenomenon: it is likely that even before grafting the patient had been sensitized to common HLA antigens, e.g. HLA2. The first and second kidneys shared an incompatibility on HLA2, and the second and third shared an incompatibility on HLA3. It is theoretically possible that in the third graft, as well as HLA3 two other undetectable incompatibilities could also have been present. The thrice grafted patient now gives a positive cross match with virtually all bloods tested, and if a future graft is to succeed, she will need an HLA identical donor.

Xenografts or heterografts

The serum of most species of mammal contains 'naturally occurring' antibody to the cells of most other species. This is normally present between members of different orders of mammals, but even between species within the same family strong species antibodies may occur, e.g. between rabbit and hare (Joysey unpublished). Considering the apparent role of preformed cytotoxic antibody in hyperacute rejection, it is not surprising that grafts between different orders of mammal are rejected speedily. Calne (1961) found that a goat kidney transplanted to a dog became cyanosed and flaccid in 90 min. Gerwurz *et al* (1966) quote 10 min as the rejection time of kidneys from sheep to dog. McKenzie *et al* (1968) found that all of the 20 human sera tested had cytotoxic activity against sheep and pig lymphocytes and therefore, by analogy with other situations in which cytotoxic antibody is present, they recommended caution in the use of xenografts in man.

On the grounds of phylogenetic similarity, if heterografts are to be considered for use in man, those from higher primates are the obvious source. Chimpanzee, which is phylogenetically man's closest primate relative, has been used as a kidney donor for man, the longest survivor reported by Reemtsma (1969) being 9 months. Chimpanzees have antigens reacting like human A and O, and also bear many leukocyte antigens similar to, but not identical, with those in man (Balner *et al* 1967). Problems of tissue matching using chimpanzee donors are not likely to be less than in man and would almost certainly be greater. In addition, approximately 50% of people possess a haemagglutinin to chimpanzee red cells, which could cause intravascular agglutination should any chimpanzee red cells remain in the renal blood vessels. Serological considerations, therefore, make the chimpanzee a potentially worse candidate than the human cadaver for organ donation. Immunosuppression is not yet sufficiently advanced to reliably overcome the incompatibilities present within our own species and therefore the superimposition of species incompatibilities seems undesirable.

Comment

The leukocyte antigens are grossly polymorphic, and the frequency of the haplotypes is such that prolonged search may be necessary before an acceptable match can be found.

The evidence is now unequivocal that tissue match between donor and recipient is a dominant factor in graft survival between unrelated as well as between related pairs. It is also evident that while a patient waits for a kidney it is advisable to keep stimulation with foreign tissue antigen to a minimum, and that 'stop gap' grafting may prejudice the survival of a later well matched graft.

The present inadequate supply of donors in the United Kingdom sometimes necessitates the use of ill matched kidneys which might, in unknown circumstances, succeed even though statistically their chance of survival is low. If all the victims of fatal road casualties could be used as donors, then true selection of donors would be possible, and true selection involves the rejection by the surgeons of unsuitable tissue matches. Experience has shown that even with the antisera at present available, early rejection is rare in the group with no major mismatches. The amount of immunosuppression necessary is less, consequently the incidence of infection is reduced and the patient lives longer. The present shortage of donors therefore directly and adversely affects the success of those transplants that are performed.

The criterion of 'success' which is currently used in transplantation is short term; the latest kidney transplant registry data gives the survival rate for cadaver transplants as 42% at 1 year. Ceppellini (1968), using the evidence of the different survival time of three categories of skin grafts (sib/sig, parent/child, unrelated/unrelated) postulated that 'with time a greater number of potentially incompatible donor-recipient combinations, requiring a longer induction period, express their immunogenicity. Thus, the effective histocompatibility system changes with time . . .' This is in agreement with the kidney graft data, where gross antigenic discrepancies normally exert their deleterious effect first, and other antigens, many of which we probably can not yet detect, exert their effect later.

Both tolerance induction, and graft enhancement, are easier to produce across small antigenic barriers than across large ones. In the future, therefore, good tissue matching should enable these phenomena to be deliberately exploited as an added method of immunosuppression. When logistics allow each kidney recipient to receive a kidney well matched for the major antigens, with improved immunosuppression and tolerance induction it may be possible to achieve true success i.e. a graft that will serve the new host for a term approximating to his or her normal life span.

REFERENCES

AMOS D.B., SEIGLER H.I., SOUTHWORTH J.G. & WARD F.E. (1969) Skin graft rejection between subjects genotyped for HLA. *Transplantation Proc.* **1**, 342.

AMOS D.B. *et al.* (1970) (In preparation).

BACH F.H., ALBERTINI R.J., AMOS D.B., CEPPELLINI R., MATTIUZ P.L. & MIGGIANO U.C. (1969) Mixed leukocyte culture studies in families with known HLA genotypes. *Transplantation Proc.* **1**, 339.

BALNER H., VAN LEEUWEN A., DERSJANT H. & VAN ROOD J.J. (1967) Defined leukocyte antigens of chimpanzees: use of chimpanzee isoantisera for leukocyte typing in man. *Transplantation* **5**, 624.

BIEGEL A. *et al* (1970) (In preparation).

BOYSE E.A., OLD L.J. & LUELL S. (1964) Genetic determination of the TL (thymus leukaemia) antigen in the mouse. *Nature, Lond.* **201**, 779.

CALNE R.Y. (1961) Observations on renal homotransplantation. *A. Brit. J. Surg.* **48**, 384.

CEPPELLINI R. (1968) The Genetic Basis of Transplantation. In *Human Transplantation*, ed. RAPAPORT F.T. & DAUSSET J., p. 29. Grune & Stratton.

CEPPELLINI R., CURTONI E.S., MATTIUZ P.L., LEIGHEB G., VISETTI M. & COLOMBI A. (1966) Survival of test skin grafts in man. Effects of genetic relationship and blood groups incompatibility. *Ann. N.Y. Acad. Sci.* **129,** 421.

COCHRUM K.C., DAVIS W.C., KOUNTZ S.L. & FUDENBERG H.H. (1969) Renal autograft rejection initiated by passive transfer of immune plasma. *Transplantation Proc.* **1,** 301.

DAUSSET J. (1965) Technique for Demonstrating Leukocyte Agglutination. In *Histocompatibility Testing* (Report of Conference and Workshop June 1964), p. 147.

DAUSSET J. (1970) Subdivision of the HL-A locus. In *Biology and Surgery of Tissue Transplantation*, ed. Maxwell Anderson.

DAUSSET J., IVANYI P. & IVANYI D. (1965) Tissue alloantigens in Humans. Identification of a complex system (Hu-1). *Histocompatibility Testing* 1965, p. 51.

DAUSSET J. & RAPAPORT F.T. (1966) Role of ABO erythrocyte groups in human histocompatibility reactions. *Nature, Lond.,* **209,** 209.

DAUSSET J., IVANYI P., COLOMBANI J., FEINGOLD N. & LEGRAND L. (1967) The Hu-1 system. *Histocompatibility Testing* 1967, p. 189.

EIJSVOOGEL U.P., SCHELLEKENS P.T.A., BREUR-URIESENDORP B., VAN LEEUWEN A., KOCH C. & VAN ROOD J.J. (1970) HL-A identity and one-allelic differences in families and unrelated individuals. *Histocompatability Testing* 1970, p. 523.

EVANS D.B. (1969) Infectious complications of transplantation surgery. *Proc. roy. Soc. Med.* **62,** 597

EVANS D.B. *et al* (1971) (In preparation.)

FRENCH M.E. & BATCHELOR J.R. (1969) Immunological enhancement of rat kidney grafts. *Lancet,* 1103.

GERWURZ H., SCOTT CLARK D., FINSTAD J., KELLY W.D., VARCO R.L., GOOD R.A. & GABRIELSON A.E. (1966) Role of the complement system in graft rejections in experimental animals and man. *Ann. N.Y. Acad. Sci.* **129,** 673.

GLEASON R.E. & MURRAY J.E. (1967) Report from kidney transplant registry. Analysis of variables in the function of human kidney transplants. I. Blood group compatibility and splenectomy. *Transplantation,* **5,** 343.

HATTLER B.G., GLENN YOUNG W., AMOS D.B., HUTCHIN P. & MACQUEEN M. (1966) White cell antibodies. Occurrence in patients undergoing open heart surgery. *Arch. Surg.* **93,** 741.

HEALE W.F., MORRIS P.J., BENNETT R.C., MORTENSEN P.J. & TING A. (1969) Leukocyte antigens in renal transplantation. Successful renal transplantation in the presence of a positive cross match. *Med. J. Aust.* **2,** 382.

JEANNET M., PINN V.W., FLAX M.H., WINN H.J. & RUSSELL P.S. (1970) Humoral antibodies in renal allotransplantation in man. *New Eng. J. med.* **282,** 111.

JONASSAN *et al.* (In preparation.)

JOYSEY V.C. (1969) A modified microcytotoxic test for lymphocyte typing using siliconed glass slides and ordinary phase contrast microscopy. *Proceedings of the Symposium on Transplantation Antigens and Tissue Typing, Oswestry* 1968. Ed. ELVES M.W. & NISBET N.W. Robert Jones and Agnes Hunt Orthopaedic Hospital Management Committee, Oswestry, England.

JOYSEY V.C. (1970) Tissue typing in relation to transplantation. *Int. Rev. Exp. Path.* **9,** 233.

JOYSEY V.C. & CALNE R.Y. (1968) Preliminary results of tissue typing in relation to clinical transplantation. *Proceedings of the Symposium on Transplantation Antigens and Tissue Typing, Oswestry* 1968. Ed. ELVES M.W. & NISBET N.W. Robert Jones and Agnes Hunt Orthopaedic Hospital Management Committee, Oswestry, England.

KIDNEY TRANSPLANT REGISTRY (1969) Seventh report of the human kidney transplant registry. *Transplantation,* **8,** 721.

KISSMEYER-NIELSEN F., OLSEN S., PETERSEN V.P. & FJELDBORG O. (1966) Hyperacute rejection of kidney allografts, associated with pre-existing humoral antibodies against donor cells. *Lancet,* ii, 662

KISSMEYER-NIELSEN F , SVEJGAARD A. & HAUGE M. (1968) Genetics of the human HLA transplantation system. *Nature, Lond.* **219,** 1116.

KISSMEYER-NIELSEN F., SVEJGAARD A. & HAUGE M. (1969) The HLA system defined with lymphocytotoxic and platelet antibodies in relation to kidney transplantation. *Transplantation Proc.* **1,** 357.

KISSMEYER-NIELSEN F., STAUB NIELSEN L., LINDHOLM A., SANDBERG L., SVEJGAARD A. & THORSBY E. The HL-A system in relation to human transplantations. *Histocompatibility Testing* 1970. P. 105

LALEZARI P. & BERNARD G. (1965) Distribution of leukocyte antigens in various blood cells and body tissues. *Histocompatibility Testing* 1965, p. 167.

MCKENZIE I.F.C., STOCKER J., TING A. & MORRIS P.J. (1968) Human lymphocytotoxic and haemagglutinating activity against sheep and pig cells. *Lancet,* ii, 386.

MEDAWAR P.B. (1946) Immunity to homologous grafted skin. I. The suppression of cell division in grafts transplanted to immunised animals. II. The Relationship between the antigens of blood and skin. *Br. J. exp. Path.* **27,** p. 9 and p. 15.

MITTAL K.K., MICKEY M.R., SINGAL D.P. & TERASAKI P.I. (1968) Serotyping for homotransplantation. XVIII. Refinement of microdroplet lymphocyte cytotoxicity test. *Transplantation,* **6,** 913.

MORRIS P.J., WILLIAMS G.M., HUME D.M., MICKEY M.R. & TERASAKI P.I. (1968) Serotyping for homotransplantation. XII. Occurrence of cytotoxic antibodies following kidney transplantation in man. *Transplantation,* **6,** 392.

MORRIS P.J., KINCAID-SMITH P., MCKENZIE I.F.C., MARSHALL V.C. & TING A. (1969) Leukocyte antigens in renal transplantation. VII. Immediate renal allograft rejection with a negative cross match. *Med. J. Aust.* **2,** 379.

MORRIS P.J., MICKEY M.R., SINGAL D.P. & TERASAKI P.I. (1969) Serotyping for homotransplantation. XXII. Specificity of cytotoxic antibodies developing after renal transplantation. *Br. med. J.* i, 758.

MORRIS P.J., TING A. & KINCAID-SMITH P. (1970) Leukocyte antigens in renal transplantation. X. A clinical and histological evaluation of matching for HL-A in cadaver renal transplantation. *Histocompatibility Testing* 1970, p. 371.

PAYNE R. & ROLFS M.R. (1958) Fetomaternal leukocyte incompatibility. *J. clin. Invest.* **37,** 1756.

REEMTSMA, K. (1969) Heterotransplantation. *Transplantation Proc.* **1,** 251.

ROGENTINE G.N. (1967) Detection of isoantigens on human lymphocytes and tissue culture cells by ^{51}Cr cytotoxicity assay. *Histocompatibility Testing* 1967, 371.

VAN ROOD J.J. (1962). Leucocyte grouping. A method and its application. Thesis, University of Leiden.

VAN ROOD J.J., EERNISSE J.G. & VAN LEEUWEN A. (1958) Leukocyte antibodies in sera from pregnant women. *Nature, Lond.* **181,** 1735.

VAN ROOD J.J. & VAN LEEUWEN A. (1965) An agglutination technique for the demonstration of leukocyte antigens in man using leukocytes from EDTA blood. *Histocompatibility Testing*. (Report of Conference and Workshop, June 1964), p. 153.

VAN ROOD J.J., VAN LEEUWEN A., SCHIPPERS A.M.J., PEARCE R., VAN BLANKENSTEIN M. & VOLKERS W. (1967) Immunogenetics of the group four, five and nine systems. *Histocompatibility Testing* 1967, 203.

VAN ROOD J.J. & EERNISSE J.G. (1968) The detection of transplantation antigens in leukocytes. *Seminars in Haematology*, **5**, 187.

VAN ROOD J.J., VAN LEEUWEN A., BRUNING J.W. & PORTER K.A. (1968) The Importance of Leukocyte Antigens in Renal Transplantation. A Study of Patients of: G.R.J.Alexandre, J. van Geertruyden, W.D.Kelly, J.P.Merrill, J.Morelle, J.P.Mowbray, J.Murray, P.S.Russell, T.E.Starzl, Ch.Toussaint and M.F.A.Woodruff. *Advance in Transplantation*, ed. DAUSSET J., HAMBURGER J. & MATHÉ G., p. 213. Copenhagen: Munksgaard.

VAN ROOD J.J., VAN LEEUWEN A., PEARCE R. & VAN DER DOES J.A. (1969) Leukocyte typing and kidney transplantation in unrelated donor recipient pairs. A study of the patients of Drs' S. Peart, J.F.Mowbray and G.R.J.Alexandre. *Transplantation Proc.* **1**, 372.

VAN ROOD J.J., VAN LEEUWEN A., KOCH C.T. & FREDERIKS E. (1970) HL-A inhibiting activity of serum. *Histocompatibility Testing* 1970, p. 483.

VAN ROOD J.J., VAN LEEUWEN A., KOOISTRA P.T. & VAN SANTEN-SCHROTEN M.C.T. (1970) The 4a and 4b antigens; do they or don't they?. *Histocompatibility Testing* 1970, p. 93

ROWLEY D.A., FITCH F.W., SAITCH T. & STUART F.P. (1969) Specific suppression of cell mediated immune responses. *Transplantation Proceedings*, **1**, 580.

SHANBROM E., FEINGOLD E., SHEPHERD L. & WALFORD R.L. (1968) Antisera for tissue typing. The production of cytotoxic and agglutinating antibodies following intradermal leukocyte injections in man. *Blood*, **32**, 402.

SHIEL A.G., STEWART J.H., TILLER D.J. & MAY J. (1969) ABO blood group incompatibility in renal transplantation. *Transplantation*, **8**, 299.

SINGAL D.P., MICKEY M.R. & TERASAKI P.I. (1969) Serotyping for homotransplantation. XXIII. Analysis of kidney transplants from parental versus sibling donors. *Transplantation*, **7**, 246.

STARZL T.E., LERNER R.A., DIXON F.J., GROTH C.A., BRETTSCHREIDER L. & TERASAKI P.I. (1968) Schwartzman reaction after human transplantation. *New Engl. J. Med.* **278**, 642.

STICKEL D.L., AMOS D.B., ZMIJEWSKI C.M., GLENN J.F. & ROBINSON R.R. (1967) Human renal transplantation with donor selection by leukocyte typing. *Transplantation*, **5**, 1024.

TERASAKI P.I. & MCCLELLAND J.D. (1964) Microdroplet assay of human serum cytotoxins. *Nature, Lond.* **204**, 998.

TERASAKI P.I., VREDEROE D.L. & MICKEY M.R. (1967) Serotyping for homotransplantation. X. Survival of 196 grafted kidneys subsequent to typing. *Transplantation*, **5**, 1057.

TERASAKI P.I., THRASHER D.L. & HAUBER T.H. (1968) Serotyping for Homotransplantation. XIII. Immediate Kidney Transplant Rejection and Associated Preformed Antibodies. In *Advance in Transplantation*, ed. DAUSSET, J., HAMBURGER J. & MATHÉ, pp. 225–229. Copenhagen: Munksgaard.

THORSBY E. & KISSMEYER-NIELSEN F. (1968) Lymphocytotoxic antisera of limited iso-specificity after skin grafting in man. *Vox Sang.* **14,** 417.

THORSBY E. & KISSMEYER-NIELSEN F. (1969) HL-A antigens and genes. III. Production of HL-A typing antisera of desired specificity. *Vox Sang.* **17,** 1.

WALFORD R.L., GALLAGHER R. & TROUP G.M. (1965) Human lymphocyte typing with isologous antisera; technical considerations and a preliminary study of the cytotoxic reaction system. *Transplantation,* **3,** 387.

WALFORD R.L., SHANBROM E., TROUP G.M., ZELLER E. & ACKERMAN B. (1967) Lymphocyte grouping with defined antisera. *Histocompatibility Testing* 1967, 221.

WARD F.E., SEIGLER H.F., SOUTHWORTH J.G., ANDRUS C.H. & AMOS D.B. (1970) Immunogenicity of HLA antigens. *Histocompatibility Testing* 1970. (In press.)

WHO COMMITTEE ON NOMENCLATURE (1968) *Bull. Wld. Hlth. Org.* **39,** 483.

WILLIAMS G.M., HUME D.M., HUDSON R.P., MORRIS P.J., KANO K. & MILGROM F. (1967) Hyperacute renal homograft rejection in man. *New Eng. J. Med.* **279,** 611.

WONHAM *et al.* (In preparation.)

YUNIS E.J. & AMOS D.B. (1970) Observations on the CNAP phenomenon. *Histocompatibility Testing* 1970, p. 315

ZMIJEWSKI C.M., MCCLOSKEY R.V. & ST. PIERRE R.L. (1967) The effect of environmental extremes on the detectibility of leukocyte isoantigens in normal humans with inference to tissue typing of prospective donors. *Histocompatibility Testing* 1967, 397.

ACKNOWLEDGEMENTS

My thanks are due to the Medical Research Council, and the East Anglian Regional Hospital Board for support, and to Dr D.G. Chalmers and Professor R.I.N. Greaves for provision of research facilities. I also wish to thank colleagues for valuable discussion, especially Professor D.B. Amos, Professor R.Y. Calne, Dr D.B. Evans and Mr A. Smellie, and others who gave me access to their work prior to publication; also Mr C. Bland for technical assistance and Dr K.A. Joysey for criticism of the manuscript.

CHAPTER 5

Lymphocyte Transformation in Transplantation

Hilliard Festenstein

When transplants are carried out, small lymphocytes are stimulated by the foreign transplantation antigens in the grafts to transform into large pyrinophilic blast cells which then divide. This recognition process eventually leads to graft destruction and rejection although little is known about the precise mechanisms involved.

Medawar (1944) first suggested that lymphoid cells play an important role in allograft rejection processes—an idea which was fully substantiated in cell transfer experiments by Mitchison (1953) and Billingham *et al* (1954). In addition, large pyrinophilic blast cells were found in the regional lymph nodes of rabbits and sheep following skin allograft rejection (Scothorne & McGregor 1955; Hall 1967), and in rejected kidney allografts in dogs, rat and man (Porter & Calne 1960; Feldman & Lee 1967; Porter 1967).

Definitive proof that small lymphocytes transform into pyrinophilic blast cells came from experiments by Gowans *et al* (1962) using a modification of Simonsen's graft versus host technique. Simonsen (1967) had previously shown that the intravenous injection of a suspension of adult allogenic spleen cells into immunologically unresponsive chick embryos caused gross splenomegaly and similar changes in other organs. It was presumed that the grafted lymphocytes responded to the foreign antigens of the host by proliferation into pyrinophilic blast cells as the latter were seen in histological sections of the host spleens. It is also possible to render an animal unresponsive to graft antigens artificially by irradiation. Following irradiation, the injected foreign lymphocytes can proliferate in response to the host's tissue antigens, without being rejected themselves. Gowans *et al* (1962) injected a pure suspension of small lymphocytes from the thoracic duct of rats into lethally irradiated mice. Thirty-seven to 60 h following cell transfer pyrinophilic blast cells could be demonstrated in the spleen. A number of these cells were seen in mitosis and by chromosome analysis could be shown to be of rat origin and hence that they had arisen from small lymphocytes. Other workers obtained similar results from further graft versus host experiments in which paternal allogenic rat thoracic duct lymphocytes were injected into genetically unresponsive F_1 hybrid female rats (Porter and Cooper 1962).

TRANSFORMATION *IN VITRO*

The need for an *in vitro* model which would parallel the *in vivo* proliferative response of lymphocytes to transplantation antigens was satisfied following a series of accidental discoveries. The first observations concerned the effect of phytohaemagglutinin (PHA) on cultured peripheral blood lymphocytes. PHA, an extract of the red kidney bean (*phaseolus vulgaris*), was originally used by Dorset & Henley (1916) to agglutinate red blood cells in the preparation of therapeutic serum and by Li & Osgood (1949) for separating leucocytes from erythrocytes. Although Hungerford *et al* (1959) observed the development of blast cells and mitosis in cultures of peripheral blood lymphocytes, Nowell (1960) was the first to attribute these changes to PHA. One of the important immediate applications of this discovery was its use in the study of human karyotypes. The transformed cells were at first believed by these workers and others (Cooper *et al* 1963) to have originated from monocytes or large lymphocytes rather than from small lymphocytes. Carstairs (1961, 1962) corrected this view and Marshall & Roberts (1965) were able to observe visually human small lymphocytes transforming into blast cells in the presence of PHA. Furthermore, it was shown that only thymic influenced lymphocytes are transformed by PHA (Davies *et al* 1968; Festenstein *et al* 1969; Doenhoff 1970).

Morphology

The *in vitro* morphological changes occurring in the presence of PHA are identical to those that occur *in vivo* in response to graft antigens. The first observable change is in the nucleus which becomes euchromatic and develops nucleoli. The cells enlarge and the cytoplasm becomes deeply basophilic and pyrinophilic (Fig. 1). Electron micrographs of transformed cells show them to be rich in ribosomes with a poorly developed endoplasmic reticulum (Johnson & Roberts 1964; Inman & Cooper 1963). Similar morphological changes were also found when peripheral blood lymphocytes were cultured with various other nonspecific mitogenic agents including pokeweed (Farnes *et al* 1964) and a variety of bacterial

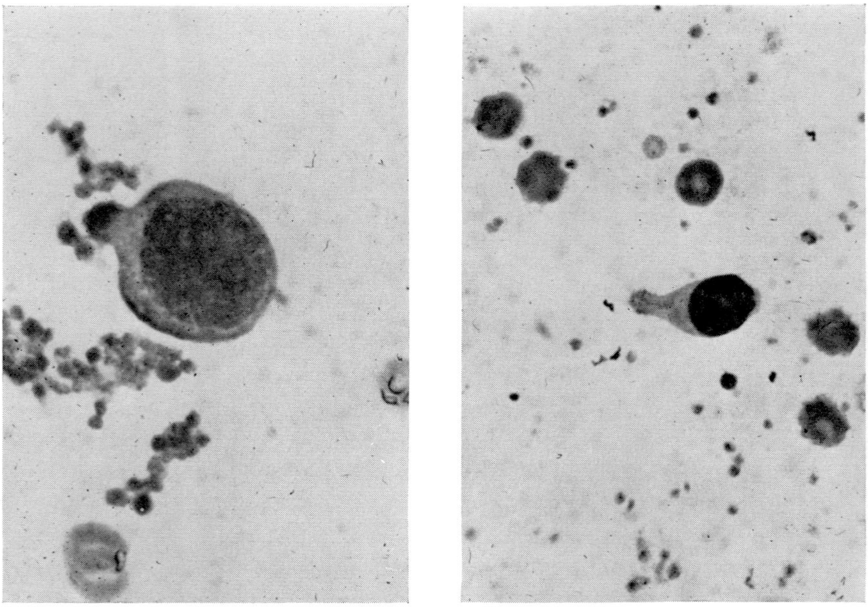

(a) (b)

FIG. 1. (a) PHA transformed lymphocyte showing nucleoli and uropod. (b) Small lymphocyte showing uropod. This cell is starting to transform. (Moorhead).

toxins (Hirschhorn *et al* 1964; Ling & Husband 1964). The mode of action of the agents responsible for proliferation and blast transformation discussed so far, have all been non-specific. However, it was also shown that specific stimulation involving antigen could be demonstrated; it was found to follow exposure to various antigens, e.g. tuberculin and smallpox vaccine as well as by allogenic lymphoid cells. The morphological changes induced by allogenic lymphocytes were found to be essentially the same as have been described for PHA.

Mixed lymphocyte culture in histocompatibility

Whilst culturing human lymphocytes Schrek & Donnelly (1961) inadvertently mixed peripheral blood lymphocytes, from two unrelated individuals. They noted after a few days that the cultured cells had been mutually stimulated to transform into pyrinophilic blast cells and to divide. This finding was further investigated by Bain *et al* (1963), Bain & Lowenstein (1964) and Bach & Hirschhorn (1964) who cultured mixtures of lymphocytes from twins, and from related and unrelated individuals. Mixtures from identical twins consistently failed to stimulate while those from unrelated individuals always did. Those from related individuals resulted on the average in an intermediate degree of stimulation. These results supported the idea that there is an immunogenetic basis for this phenomenon. To establish this concept, it was necessary to study the mixed lymphocyte reaction in human families and in various inbred genetically defined models including the mouse, rat and chicken.

Method of culturing lymphocytes

Many techniques of culturing human and animal lymphocytes have been described. The techniques vary in detail but in principle follow a general pattern. Lymphocytes are obtained from blood by first removing the red cells by sedimentation and centrifugation procedures. Most granulocytes are removed by exposure to foreign surfaces to which they adhere. The lymphocytes are washed and resuspended in nutrient culture media including serum. Cell concentrations are adjusted and the stimulating cells pretreated (see below) prior to mixing. The cells are then mixed and in parallel with unpaired and PHA controls dispensed into tubes and cultured in a CO_2 enriched atmosphere. In addition rodent cells survive and transform better when the oxygen content of the atmosphere is reduced (Festenstein 1966a, b, 1968). In some methods the culture medium is frequently changed. Individual cultures are terminated at various intervals. The assays for stimulation vary from morphological assessment of autoradiographs and the percentage of transformed cells to the measurement of incorporation of radioactive tracers, e.g. thymidine, uridine, leucine. In addition, various chemical methods of assay are now being developed. Detailed descriptions of the various methods of culture can be found in the works of Adler *et al* (1970); Bach & Voynow (1966); Bach *et al* (1970); Bain *et al* (1963); Bain (1970); Elves (1967); Festenstein (1965a, 1968, 1969, 1970); Hirschhorn *et al* (1963); Hirschhorn (1969); Ling *et al* (1968); Schellekens & Eijsvoogel (1968); Schellekens *et al* (1970); Skopinska & Skamene (1968); Sorensen *et al* (1969a, b); Tridente *et al* (1967); Wilson *et al* (1967).

Problems inherent in the cultural technique

Since the stimulation of the cell populations in culture was reciprocal, it was not possible to easily ascertain how much of the total response could be attributed to each one. In addition Festenstein (1966a) in his work on 'two-way' mixed spleen cell cultures in mice showed that mutual cell killing, which was particularly marked in the 'strongly' differing combinations studies, followed stimulation. Such phenomena undoubtedly gave rise to misleading results and incorrect interpretations of antigenic strength. Methods of rendering the stimulating lymphocytes incapable of synthesizing DNA in mixed cultures, were developed by Kasakura & Lowenstein (1965) by exposing them to ionizing irradiation by Bach & Voynow (1966) by pretreating them with Mitomycin C or N-mustard derivatives (Cepellini *et al* 1965). Elves (1969) compared pretreatment with X-irradiation and Mitomycin C and concluded that the former method was the better. In this way it was possible to carry out 'one-way' mixed lymphocyte cultures and to define histocompatibility differences between individuals. It may be necessary to vary the proportion of stimulating and responding cells when setting up the mixed cultures. Albertini & Bach (1968) have reported failure of stimulation between known incompatible individuals using equal proportions of cells. By using increasing numbers of stimulating cells a positive reaction was always produced. In contrast Sorensen and Kissmeyer-Nielsen (1969) always demonstrated positive reactions in culture when they used equal proportions of cells from known HL-A incompatible individuals.

Quantitation of results

Quantitation of the mixed lymphocyte reaction is most often carried out by measuring radiothymidine incorporation at a time when the response is believed to be maximal, e.g. day 7, Albertini & Bach (1968). Festenstein (1966a) pointed out that measuring the response on a single day might be misleading, due to the fact that the peak response day varied and suggested that kinetic experiments should be carried out each time. A false negative result obtained by assaying too late could thus be avoided. In addition, ranking orders of several mixed cultures could be more accurately determined in this way. Sorensen & Kissmeyer-Nielsen (1969) maintained that because of the inhibiting influence of suboptimal cultural conditions an index of reactivity based on the results of assay on days 2, 3, and 4, proved more reliable than any based on either single measurements (e.g. day 7), or peak responses. It is best, therefore, to measure the reaction during the early phase of culture which is exponential.

Kinetic experiments during this period allow a more precise method of quantitation (Festenstein 1970) (Fig. 2). Other investigators have since modified their methods to assay on the 3rd day of culture (Bach *et al.* 1970).

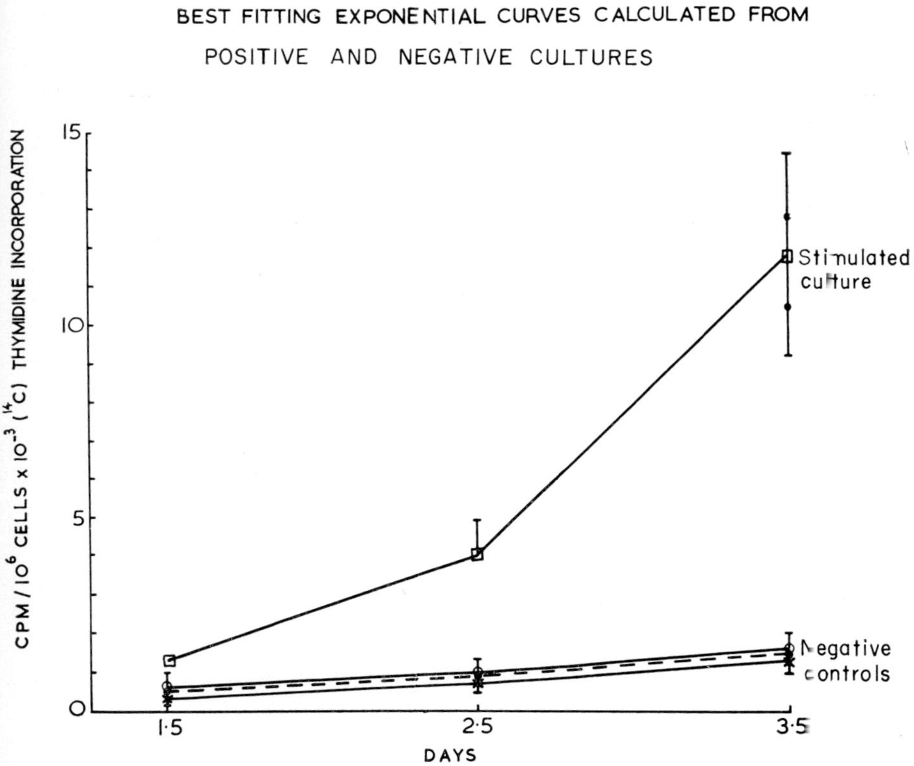

FIG. 2. (Festenstin, H. 1970, *Transplantation Reviews*)

'One-way' stimulation in genetically defined models

In an inbred genetic model, such as the mouse or rat, it is possible to culture mixtures of lymphocytes from two populations, one of which should theoretically be unresponsive to the antigens of the other. F_1 (A × B) hybrid lymphocytes carry all the antigens of both parents and should therefore be incapable of being stimulated in culture by lymphocytes from either parent strain (A or B). Mixed culture experiments were carried out, in which chromosomal markers were present in either the parent or F_1 lymphocytes. Wilson *et al* (1967) observed that in mixed lymphocyte cultures in the rat, mitoses occurred predominantly among cells of parental origin. Some F_1 mitoses were observed on the 6th and

7th day of culture but as there was some background mitotic activity in the unpaired control cultures, they concluded that the mitoses in the mixed cultures were not the result of specific proliferative activity against parental cells but to non-specific factors in the culture medium. Similarly, Festenstein & Davies (1969) found in mixed cultures of a 'strong' (H-2) incompatible parent-F_1 combination in the mouse, that only parental cells divided. Other investigators working with parent-F_1 mixed cultures in the mouse model were able to show some F_1 cells in division (Adler *et al* 1970; Doenhoff 1970; Nisbet 1970) but these were usually a relatively small proportion of the total number of dividing cells.

The fact that few F_1 cells are usually found in division in mixed cultures must mean that the non-specific recruitment of 'innocent bystanders' by specifically dividing cells must be negligible.

Validity of the mixed lymphocyte culture test as a measure of histocompatibility and antigenic strength

The influence of major and minor histocompatibility loci

Each species so far studied including man, has a single strong genetic locus which is of overriding importance in transplantation (Simonsen 1965; Palm 1964; Shierman & Nordskog 1963; Snell *et al* 1953). Incompatibility at this locus is reflected in a positive mixed lymphocyte culture test and prompt graft rejection; human siblings and inbred rats on the other hand, who are identical at this major locus usually give a negative mixed lymphocyte culture test (Amos & Bach 1968; Sorensen & Kissmeyer-Nielsen 1969; Elves 1967), and retain organ allografts for long periods (Silvers *et al* 1967; Singal *et al* 1969; Bildsoe *et al* 1970). This occurs despite the presence of additional multiple minor histocompatibility differences which can nevertheless initiate the rejection of skin allografts (Silvers *et al* 1967; Silvers & Billingham 1969; Hildemann 1970).

Neither in man nor rat is there conclusive evidence that histocompatibility loci other than the strongest—HL-A and H-1—ordinarily influence the mixed lymphocyte reaction (Bach *et al* 1970; Sorensen 1970; Silvers *et al* 1967); in contrast there is evidence that they may do so in mice (Festenstein 1966a, b, 1969; Häyry & Defendi 1970; Tridente *et al* 1967; Rychlikova & Ivanyi 1969). Rychlikova & Ivanyi found stimulation with strain pairs differing at more than 12 non H-2 loci; they presumed it to be due to their combined influence as experiments with strong H-2 identical strain pairs differing at a few specified non H-2 loci failed to react. The possibility that unspecified individual non H-2 loci acting alone were implicated was not excluded. Festenstein (1970) studied the MLC stimulating, H-2 identical

Balb/c and DBA/2 strains in depth and showed that stimulation was governed by a single histocompatibility locus. If this locus proves to be H-2 linked and codes for antigens which are poor antibody producers (see below) this will not radically alter the current concept of a dominant single strong locus controlling the outcome of organ transplants. If, on the other hand, the locus is shown to segregate independently of H-2 and has a human homologue it may call for a reassessment of our present concept of matching donors and recipients for transplantation. Another locus in addition to ABO and HL-A whose products are difficult to detect serologically might also have to be taken into consideration.

Subliminal quantities of various non-specific lymphocyte stimulating agents can render normally non-stimulatory cultures in humans and mice positive (Plate & Ward 1970; Adler *et al* 1970). The biological significance of these findings is not clear.

The effect of the ABO blood group antigens on the mixed lymphocyte reaction

Sorensen (1970) carried out seven one-way mixed lymphocyte culture tests with lymphocytes from family members who were identical at the HL-A locus but incompatible for ABO blood group antigens. Proliferation did not occur even when the stimulating cells carried the A^1 antigen and the responding lymphocytes were from an individual of blood group O. He concluded that the ABO system must therefore be regarded as weak in the transplantation sense. However, the presence of naturally occurring cytotoxic antibodies may nevertheless give rise to acute rejection phenomena in renal transplantation (see p. 100).

Quantitative differences in the mixed lymphocyte culture test in human siblings and its application to the selection of family donors in renal transplantation

If the paternal chromosomes on which the HL-A genetic region is located are designated a and b and the maternal chromosomes c and d (see p. 103) then the siblings can be shown to be either identical, e.g. ac/ac, differing with respect to one chromosome, ac/bc, or two chromosomes ac/bd. Mixtures of lymphocytes from siblings who can be shown to be identical at the HL-A locus by serological means almost always fail to elicit a proliferative response in culture (Amos & Bach 1968; Sorensen & Kissmeyer-Nielsen 1969). This mixed lymphocyte culture test can therefore be directly employed in the selection of HL-A identical live sibling donors for renal transplantation or as a check on the serological diagnosis of identity at the

HL-A locus (van Rood & Eijsvoogel 1970). On the other hand cultures carried out with lymphocytes from siblings differing with respect to one (ac/bc) and two chromosomes (ac/bd) always stimulated. Furthermore those differing with respect to two chromosomes (ac/bd) usually stimulated to a greater extent than those differing with respect to one chromosome (ac/bc) (Sorensen & Kissmeyer-Nielsen 1969; Albertini & Bach 1968; Schellekens *et al* 1970). Proliferation in mixed lymphocyte culture is, therefore, not only a reliable indication of incompatibility at the strong histocompatibility locus but can also be used to measure the degree of antigenic differences; these degrees of incompatibility are also reflected in the results of renal transplantation between family members differing with respect to 2, 1 and 0 chromosomes carrying the HL-A locus (Singal *et al* 1969).

Investigation of the HL-A system by the mixed lymphocyte reaction

The mixed lymphocyte culture test can be used as a check on the diagnosis of serological identity at the HL-A locus. It is currently held by most workers in the field that the HL-A system consists of two segregant series, each with a large number of mutually exclusive alleles (see p. 104). Most of the characterized HL-A antigens can be shown to be associated with either the LA or the FOUR series. Although sera recognizing all the HL-A specificities governed by these series have not yet been discovered, it is nevertheless possible to find unrelated individuals who are completely matched on this basis. Mixed lymphocyte cultures have been performed with cells from such individuals. A serologically unrecognizable HL-A incompatibility would be reflected by a positive mixed lymphocyte culture test. Sorensen (1970) tested lymphocytes in culture from eight pairs of unrelated individuals who had identical typings for the HL-A antigens at the LA and FOUR series and in all cases significant stimulation was observed indicating that none of the eight pairs was in fact HL-A identical. He suggested that this could be explained by unknown possible heterogeneity of the antigens involved but favoured the explanation that there are additional HL-A antigens not contained either in the LA or FOUR series. Although these results point to the existence of at least one additional segregant series, it is nevertheless possible to find parent-child and unrelated pairs who type identically and whose lymphocytes fail to stimulate in mixed culture (Sorensen 1970; van Rood & Eijsvoogel 1970). The reason for this may be as Walford (1969) suggests that the LA and FOUR series of HL-A are characterized by mutually exclusive specificities probably none of which are 'null' factors while other factors, e.g. those of an hypothetical third segregant series may have 'null' opposites like D in the RH system (where 'd' has never been shown to exist.)

Poor antibody producing antigens of the major histocompatibility locus and their effect on mixed lymphocyte culture and organ transplantation

Several HL-A antigens have been shown to be notoriously poor antibody producers following skin graft experiments between unrelated volunteers (Thorsby 1970). Mixed lymphocyte culture tests with cells from such HL-A incompatible individuals would be expected to be positive. Many of the undiscovered HL-A antigens may also be poor antibody producers, since extensive screening of pregnancy sera and repeated immunization of volunteers have still left many HL-A antigens undiscovered. These antigens would also be expected to give a positive MLC test.

In the mouse model too, strong mixed lymphocyte culture reactions have been observed with lymphocytes from the DBA/2 and Balb/c strains. The available evidence indicates that they are identical at the strong H-2 locus. No antibodies which could detect such a difference serologically can be raised by direct cross-immunization. However, genetic experiments have shown that this mixed lymphocyte culture reactivity is probably due to a single locus. If, by linkage experiments, this locus can be shown to be H-2 or H-2 linked, this would be another example of a poor antibody producing, lymphocyte stimulating antigen associated with the major histocompatibility locus of a species (Festenstein 1970).

There is no evidence that the undiscovered poor antibody producing HL-A antigens in question are necessarily 'weak' in the transplantation sense. However, recent evidence from the rat model suggests that at least some antigens governed by the strong locus of this species may not easily initiate organ graft rejection. Salaman (1970) transplanted kidneys from AS to major locus incompatible AS/2 rats. The AS/2 rats do not easily produce antibody following repeated immunization with AS lymphoid cells and skin. Nevertheless, AS/2 lymphocytes readily stimulate AS lymphocytes in mixed culture and vice versa. The kidney transplants however were retained without immunosuppression for long periods. After kidney grafting, skin grafts from the same source were also tolerated whereas without prior transplantation of the kidney they were rejected in 14 days.

The effect of such antigens may therefore be to facilitate the induction of immunological tolerance in organ transplantation (Simonsen 1970). This view is supported by associated diminished reactivity of the recipient lymphocytes in mixed lymphocyte culture towards donor cells following renal transplantation in these rats (Salaman, Elves & Festenstein 1970).

INHIBITION OF *IN VITRO* LYMPHOCYTE TRANSFORMATION

Non-specific depression of transformation

Postoperative depression of the normal proliferative response of lymphocytes to PHA was observed by Riddle & Berenbaum (1967) in five patients undergoing a variety of surgical procedures. The percentage of lymphocytes in the peripheral blood undergoing transformation in response to PHA fell significantly 1 to 8 days following operation. Recovery occurred between 8 and 21 days post-operatively in most cases. They suggested that the depression may be due to substances released from tissues damaged by surgical trauma or by steroids released by the adrenals in response to stress. Similar non-specific depression of lymphocyte response to PHA was observed in 11 patients following cholecystectomy (Bergman *et al* 1969). Recovery was evident in most of those cases from the 6th to 10th post-operative day.

Lymphocytes from pigs undergoing liver allotransplantation were similarly found to have a non-specifically reduced response to PHA and allogenic lymphocytes during the immediate postoperative period (Festenstein *et al* 1970). Recovery was evident by the 5th post-operative day in most cases. A possible explanation for these findings is that antigen sensitive cells are withdrawn from the circulation into the liver. Alternatively there may have been a direct effect of the ischaemic autolytic products of the allografted liver on antigen-sensitive cells, an effect which may facilitate the induction of tolerance. However, there is no direct evidence at present for either of these explanations.

Reduced responsiveness in diseases

A reduced response of peripheral blood lymphocytes to PHA has been found in a variety of diseases with impaired immunological competence such as lymphoproliferative disorders (Damshek 1967), ataxia telangiectasia (Oppenheim *et al* 1966), and sarcoidosis (Hirschhorn *et al* 1964).

The effect of drugs

Various drugs including immunosuppressive agents have been shown to produce depression of lymphocyte transformation in culture, e.g. nitrogen mustards, salicylates, imuran, mercaptoethanol, puromycin, actinomycin, cyclohexamide, chloramphenicol, tetracycline and the antimalarial chloroquin (see Ling 1968).

Antilymphocyte serum

Lymphocytes taken from mice treated with antilymphocyte serum and antilymphocyte globulin showed a greatly diminished response to PHA *in vitro* and this was correlated with prolonged skin graft survival as well as reduced potency of the lymphocytes in graft versus host reaction (Thursi *et al* 1969; Tridente & Van Bekkum 1969). Mosedale *et al* (1968) have also been able to demonstrate depression of PHA responsiveness of human and mouse lymphocytes *in vitro* when incubated with antilymphocyte serum.

This method can therefore be used to assess the potency of antilymphocyte serum in primates or in human patients undergoing renal transplantation. It could also be used to assess the efficacy of immunosuppressive therapy generally in patients following organ transplantation.

Effect of serum and plasma factors

Serum factors causing non-specific depression of lymphocyte transforming ability to PHA and allogenic lymphocytes have been incriminated in various diseases. Lymphocytes from uraemic patients cultured with autologous serum showed such a non-specific depressed response (Elves *et al* 1966). Sorensen (1970) investigated the response of lymphocytes from five pairs of HL-A identical siblings (one from each pair being uraemic and one healthy) to allogeneic cells and PHA. He showed no consistent difference in reactivity between normal and uraemic lymphocytes. All culture media were supplemented with normal serum. The previously described depression was probably due to serum factors associated with uraemia rather than an intrinsic defect of the cells in disease.

A similar factor in the plasma of patients suffering from secondary syphilis has been demonstrated by Levene *et al* (1969).

Specific depression of transformation—in vitro *demonstration of immunological 'tolerance'*

When lymphocytes from immunologically tolerant rats, e.g. A (tolerant of B) were cultured with A × BF[1] hybrid cells bearing the appropriate antigen in mixed culture Wilson *et al* (1967) were able to show that they did not respond by proliferation in mixed culture, but were fully and quantitatively responsive to other antigenic systems, e.g. A × CF[1]. Amos & Bach (1968) have reported two cases of recipients of human kidney transplants who had received kidneys from unrelated donors. In each case HL-A antigens were detected on the donors' cells which were absent from the recipients'. After 2 years during which time the recipients were on immunosuppressive therapy, mixed lymphocyte culture tests were carried out and it was found that they did not respond to the donors' cells, but were able to respond to unrelated allogenic cells. The authors suggested that the recipients may have become immunologically 'tolerant' to donor antigens.

Calne *et al* (1969) have shown that pigs allografted with orthotopic livers survived for prolonged periods without immunosuppression. They suggested that immunological tolerance was induced in the pigs through the release of histocompatibility antigens in a tolerogenic form. Lymphocytes taken from these allografted pigs before operation and at various times postoperatively were set up in culture with PHA, irradiated donor and unrelated allogenic lymphocytes. Pre-operative samples of lymphocytes from the recipient pigs responded in MLC to irradiated donor and unrelated lymphocytes and to PHA. The post-operative response measured between 4 and 90 days gave more variable results. In one group, the recipients' lymphocytes behaved in a similar manner to those from tolerant rats (Wilson *et al* 1967) i.e. they failed to respond by proliferation in mixed cultures with donor lymphocytes but reacted to lymphocytes from unrelated pigs and PHA. These findings are consistent with the hypothesis that immunological tolerance had been induced. In contrast, the post-operative samples of lymphocytes from another group of recipients were found to be responsive to both unrelated and donor lymphocytes as well as to PHA; the *in vitro* proliferative response in mixed lymphocyte culture presumably parallels the *in vivo* division of lymphocytes in the presence of alloantigen, in this case it did not lead to tissue damage and graft rejection either because the lymphocytes became committed to the production of the wrong form of immune response or to the production of enhancing antibodies (Festenstein *et al* 1969). Tolerance and enhancement may perhaps be competing processes related to the differing inherent abilities of various antigens of the strong histocompatibility locus at eliciting humoral antibody formation and inducing tolerance (Simonsen 1970).

Pregnancy

Spensieri & Carnevale (1968) reported diminished responsiveness in culture of lymphocytes from pregnant women to their husbands' cells but not to lymphocytes from unrelated individuals. The percentage of blast transformation decreased with parity. There was however no difference between the stimulating ability of husbands' cells and unrelated individuals when the responding lymphocytes were from non-pregnant women. The authors conclude that pregnant women acquire specific tolerance to histocompatibility antigens of the foetus by the continuous passage of very small doses of foetal antigens into the mother and that this 'tolerance' has some bearing on the non-expulsion of the conceptus.

The proliferative response of small lymphocytes to allogeneic transplantation antigens in mixed lymphocyte culture, probably represents the best available *in vitro* model for the study of transplantation phenomena. Its applicability to the study of antigenic strength, problems of histocompatibility including the unravelling of the genetics of the HL-A system and its practical corollary of donor selection for transplantation are perhaps its most well known uses—all of which have been discussed in this chapter. However its use in the study of basic phenomenon such as immunological unresponsiveness and in the study of cell participation in immune responses has been no less significant. Future refinements and sophistication of the existing techniques are likely to lead to better understanding of the cellular and biochemical processes involved in immune response not only to transplantation antigens but also to various other antigens.

REFERENCES

ADLER W.H., TAKIGUCHI T., MARSH B. & SMITH R.T. (1970) *Cellular Recognition by Mouse Lymphocytes in vitro.* I, and II. *Stimulation by Histocompatibility Antigens in Mixed Cell Culture.* In press.

ALBERTINI R.J. & BACH F.H. (1968) Quantitative assay of antigenic disparity at HL-A—the major histocompatibility locus in man. *J. exp. Med.* **128,** 639.

AMOS D.B. & BACH F.H. (1968) Phenotypic expressions of the main histocompatibility locus in man (HL-A): Leukocyte antigens and mixed leukocyte culture reactivity. *J. exp. Med.* **128,** 623.

BACH F.H. & HIRSCHHORN K. (1964) Lymphocyte interaction: a potential histocompatibility test *in vitro. Science,* **143,** 813.

BACH F.H. & VOYNOW N.R. (1966) One-way stimulation in mixed leukocyte cultures. *Science,* **153,** 545.

BACH M.L., SOLLIDAY S. & STAMBUK B.A. (1970) Detection of Disparity in the Mixed Leukocyte Culture Test: A More Rapid Assay. In *Histocompatibility Testing.* Copenhagen: Munksgaard. In press.

BACH F.H., DAY E., LEBRUN A. & BACH M.L. (1970) Phenotypic Expression of HL-A: the Effect of Other Loci on Stimulation by and the Response to HL-A Antigens. *Histocompatibility Testing.* Copenhagen: Munksgaard.

BAIN B., VAS M.R. & LOWENSTEIN L. (1963) A reaction between leucocytes in mixed peripheral blood cultures. *Fed. Proc.* **22,** 428.

BAIN B. & LOWENSTEIN L. (1964) Genetic studies on the mixed leucocyte reaction. *Science,* **145,** 1315.

BAIN B. (1970) Tritiated-thymidine uptake in mixed leucocyte cultures: effect of specific activity and exposure time. *Clin. Exp. Immunol.* **6,** 255.

BERGMAN S., BORGSTRÖM S. & TÄRNVIK A. (1969) Lymphocyte response to phytohaemagglutin following cholecystectomy. *Acta Path. Microbiol. Scandinav.* **76**, 363.

BILLINGHAM R.E., BRENT L., MEDAWAR P.B. & SPARROW E.M. (1954) Quantitative studies on tissue transplantation immunity. I. The survival times of skin homografts exchanged between members of different inbred strains of mice. II. The origin, strength and duration of actively and adoptively acquired immunity. *Proc. Roy. Soc.* B. **143**, 43, 58.

BILDSØE PER., FREISLEBEN-SORENSEN S., PETTIROSSI O., & SIMONSEN M. (1970) Heart and kidney transplantation from segregating hybrid to parental rats. *Transplant Rev.* **3**, 36–45.

CALNE R.Y., SELLS R.A., PENA J.R., DAVIS D.R., MILLARD P.R., HERBERTSON B.M., BINNS R.M. & DAVIES D.A.L. (1969) Induction of Immunological Tolerance by Porcine Liver Allografts. *Nature, Lond.* **223**, 472.

CARSTAIRS K. (1961) Transformation of the small lymphocyte in culture. *Lancet*, ii, 984.

CARSTAIRS K. (1962) The human small lymphocyte: its possible pluripotential quality. *Lancet*, i, 829.

COOPER E.H., BARKHAM P. & HALE A.J. (1963) Mitogenic activity of phytohaemagglutinin. *Br. J. Haemat.* **9**, 101.

CEPPELLINI R., FRANCESCHINI P., MIGGIANO V.C. & TRIDENTE G. (1965) Directional Activation of Mixed Lymphocyte Cultures (a Preliminary Report). In *Histocompatibility Testing*, p. 13. Copenhagen: Munksgaard.

DAMESHEK W., (1967) Chronic lymphatic leukaemia—an accumulative disease of immunologically incompetent lymphocytes. *Blood*, **29**, 566.

DAVIES A.J.S., FESTENSTEIN H., LEUCHARS E., WALLIS V.J. & DOENHOFF M.J. (1968) A thymic origin for some peripheral blood lymphocytes. *Lancet*, i, 183.

DOENHOFF M.J. (1970) Unpublished work.

DORSET M. & HENLEY R.R. (1916) Production of clear and sterilized anti-hog cholera serum. *J. Agric. Res.* **6**, 1333.

ELVES M.W. (1967) The mixed leucocyte reaction in inbred strains of rat. *Vox Sang. (Basel)*, **13**, 1.

ELVES M.W. (1969) Comparison of mitomycin C and X-rays for the production of one-way stimulation in mixed leucocyte cultures. *Nature, Lond.* **223**, 90.

ELVES M.W., ISRAELS M.C.C. & COLLINGE M. (1966) An assessment of the mixed leucocyte reaction in renal failure. *Lancet*, i, 682.

FARNES P., BARKER B.E., BROWNHILL L.E. & FANGER H. (1964) Mitogenic activity in *Phytolacca Americana* (pokeweed). *Lancet*, i, 1100.

FELDMAN J. & LEE S. (1967) Renal homotransplantation in rats. *J. exp. Med.* **126**, 783.

FESTENSTEIN H. (1966a) Antigenic strength investigated by mixed culture of allogeneic mouse spleen cells. *Ann. N.Y. Acad. Sci.* **129**, 567.

FESTENSTEIN H. (1966b) Further studies in antigenic strength by the mixed spleen cell reaction. *Excertpa. Medica. Int. Congress Series* **131**, 214.

FESTENSTEIN H. (1968) Mouse peripheral blood lymphocytes in culture. *Lancet*, i, 182.

FESTENSTEIN H. (1969) Evaluation of the Mixed Leucocyte Reaction in the Mouse Model. Translantation Antigens and Tissue Typing. *Proc. of Symp. Robert Jones and Agnes Hunt Orthopaedic Hospital, England.* p. 165.

FESTENSTEIN H. & DAVIES A.J.S. (1969) Unpublished work.

FESTENSTEIN H., DAVIES A.J.S., LEUCHARS E., WALLIS V.J. & DOENHOFF M.J. (1969) Mouse Peripheral Blood Lymphocyte Origins Investigated by a Simple Cell Culture Technique. In *Lymphatic Tissue and Germinal Centers in Immune Response*, ed. FIORE-DONATI L. & HANNA M.G., p. 121. New York: Plenum Press.

FESTENSTEIN H. (1970) Strong and Weak Histocompatibility Antigens. In *Transplantation Reviews*, p. 76. Copenhagen: Munksgaard.

FESTENSTEIN H., LUBLING N., CALNE R.Y. & BINNS R. (1970) Unpublished work.

GOWANS J.L., MCGREGOR D.D., COWEN D.M. & FORD C.E. (1962) Initiation of immune responses by small lymphocytes. *Nature, Lond.* **196,** 651.

HALL J.G. (1967) Studies of the cells in the efferent and afferent lymph nodes draining the site of skin homografts. *J. exp. Med.* **125,** 737.

HAYRY P. & DEFENDI V. (1970) Allograft immunity *in vitro*. III. Induction of deoxyribonucleic acid synthesis in mixed cultures of mouse peripheral lymphocytes from inbred strains differing at non-H-2 loci. *Transplantation,* **9,** 410.

HILDEMANN W.H. (1970) Components and Concepts of Antigenic Strength. *Transplantation Reviews,* **3,** 5.

HIRSCHHORN K. (1964) *In vitro* studies of lymphocytes from patients with sarcoidosis and lymphoproliferative diseases. *Lancet,* ii, 842.

HIRSCHHORN K. (1969) In *Mediators of Cellular Immunity*, p. 3. New York and London: Academic Press.

HIRSCHHORN K., BACH F.H., KOLODNY R.L., FIRSCHEIN I.L. & HASHEM N. (1963) Immune response and mitosis of human peripheral blood lymphocytes *in vitro. Science,* **142,** 1185.

HIRSCHHORN K., SCHREIBMAN R.R., VERBO S. & GRUSKIN R.H. (1964) The action of Streptolysin S on peripheral lymphocytes of normal subjects and patients with acute rheumatic fever. *Proc. Nat. Acad. Sci. (Wash.),* **52,** 1151.

HUNGERFORD D.A., DONNELLY A.J., NOWELL P.C. & BECK S. (1959) The chromosome constitution of a human phenotype intersex. *Amer. J. Hum. Gen.* ii, 215.

INMAN D.R. & COOPER E.H. (1963) Electron microscopy of human lymphocytes stimulated by phytohaemagglutinin. *J. Cell. Biol.* **19,** 441.

JOHNSON F.R. & ROBERTS K.B. (1964) The growth and division of human small lymphocytes in tissue culture—an electron microscopic study. *J. Anat. Lond.* **98,** 303.

KASAKURA S. & LOWENSTEIN L. (1965) The Effect of Irradiation *In Vitro* on Mixed Leucocyte Cultures and on Leukocyte Cultures with Phytohaemagglutinin. In *Histocompatibility Testing* 1965. Copenhagen: Munksgaard.

LEVENE G.M., TURK J.L., WRIGHT D.J.M. & GRIMBLE A.G.S. (1969) Reduced lymphocyte transformation due to a plasma factor in patients with active syphilis. *Lancet,* ii, 246.

LI I.G. & OSGOOD E.E. (1949) A method for the rapid separation of leucocytes and nucleated erythrocytes from blood or marrow with a phytohaemagglutinin from red beans. *Blood,* **4,** 670.

LING N.R. & HUSBAND E.M. (1964) Specific and non-specific stimulation of peripheral lymphocytes. *Lancet,* i, 363.

LING N.R. (1968) *Lymphocyte Stimulation.* Amsterdam: North Holland Publishing Co.

MARSHALL W.H. & ROBERTS K.B. (1965) Continuous cinematography of human lymphocytes cultured with phytohaemagglutinin including observations on cell division and interphase. *Quart. J. Exp. Physiol.* **50,** 361.

Medawar P.B. (1944) The behaviour and fate of skin autografts and skin homografts in rabbits. *J. Anat.* **78,** 176.

Mitchison N.A. (1953) Passive transfer of transplantation immunity. *Nature, Lond.* **171,** 267.

Mosedale B., Felstead K.J. & Parke J.A.C. (1968) Effect of anti-lymphocyte serum on the response of human and mouse lymphocytes to PHA. *Nature, Lond.* **218,** 983.

Nisbet (1970) Personal communication.

Nowell P.C. (1960a) Differentiation of human leukemic leukocytes in tissue culture. *Exp. Cell. Res.* **19,** 267.

Nowell P.C. (1960b) Phytohaemagglutinin: An initiator of mitosis in cultures of normal leukocytes. *Cancer Res.* **20,** 462.

Oppenheim J.J., Barlow M., Waldman J.A. & Bloch J.B. (1966) Impaired *in vitro* lymphocyte transformation in patients with ataxia telangiectasis. *Br. med. J.* **2,** 330.

Palm J. (1964) Serological detection of histocompatibility antigens in two strains of rats. *Trans.* **2,** 603.

Plate J. & Ward F. (1970) Lymphocyte Stimulation by HL-A Identical Siblings Detected by a Modified Technique. In *Histocompatibility Testing.* Copenhagen: Munskgaard. In press.

Porter K.A. & Calne R.Y. (1960) The origin of the infiltrating cells in skin and kidney homografts. *Transplant. Bull.* **26,** 458.

Porter K.A. & Cooper E.H. (1962) Recognition of transformed small lymphocytes by combined chromosomal and isotopic labels. *Lancet,* ii, 317.

Porter K.A. (1967) Rejection in treated renal allografts. *Symp. Tissue Org. Transplant* (*Suppl. J. Clin. Path.*) 518.

Rychlikova M. & Ivanyi P. (1969) Mixed lymphocyte cultures and histocompatibility antigens in mice. *Folia Biol.* (*Praha*) **15,** 126.

Riddle P.R. & Berenbaum M.C. (1967) Post-operative depression of the lymphocyte response to PHA. *Lancet,* i, 746.

Salaman J.R. (1970a) Personal communication cited by Festenstein H. in 1970(b). *Transplantation Reviews,* **3,** 93.

Salaman J.R., Elves M. & Festenstein H. (1970) *Transplantation Proceedings* (in press).

Scothorne R.J. & McGregor I.A. (1955) Cellular changes in lymph nodes and spleen following skin homografting in the rabbit. *J. Anat.* **89,** 283.

Schellekens P.Th. & Eijsvoogel V.P. (1968) Lymphocyte transformation *in vitro.* I. Tissue culture conditions and quantitative measurements. *Clin. exp. Immun.* **3,** 57.

Schellekens P.Th., Vriesendorp B., Eijsvoogel V.P., van Leeuwen A., van Rood J.J., Miggiano V. & Ceppellini R. (1970) Lymphocyte transformation *in vitro.* II. Mixed lymphocyte culture in relation to leucocyte antigens. *Clin. exp. Immun.* **6,** 241.

Schrek R. & Donnelly W.J. (1961) Differences between lymphocytes of leukemic patients with respect to morphologic features, motility, and sensitivity to guinea pig serum. *Blood,* **18,** 561.

Schierman L.W. & Nordskog A.W. (1963) Influence of the B blood group-histocompatibility locus in chickens on a graft versus host reaction. *Nature, Lond.* **197,** 512.

SILVERS W.K., WILSON D.B. & PALM J. (1967) Mixed leukocyte reactions and histocompatibility in rats. *Science*, **155**, 3763.

SILVERS W.K. & BILLINGHAM R.E. (1969) Influence of the Ag-B locus on reactivity to skin homografts and tolerance responsiveness in rats *Transplantation*, **8**, 167.

SIMONSEN M. (1957) The impact on the developing embryo and newborn animal of adult homologous cells. *Acta. Path. et Micriobiol. Scand.* **XL**, 480.

SIMONSEN M. (1965) Strong transplantation antigens in man. *Lancet*, i, 415.

SIMONSEN M. (1970) On the nature and measurement of antigenic strength. *Transplantation Reviews*, **3**, 22.

SINGAL D.P., MICKEY M.R. & TERASAKI P.J. (1969) Serotyping for homotransplantation. XXIII. Analysis of kidney transplants from parental versus sibling donors. *Transplantation*, **7**, 246.

SKOPINSKA E. & SKAMENE E. (1968) Stimulation of DNA synthesis in mixed lymphocyte culture of chickens. *Fol. Biol. (Praha)*, **14**, 289.

SNELL G.D., SMITH P. & GABRIELSON F. (1953) Analysis of the histocompatibility-2 locus in the mouse. *J.N.C.I.* **14**, 457.

SORENSEN S. FREISLEBEN (1970) *Transplantation Reviews*, **3**, 70, 78, 97.

SORENSEN S. FREISLEBEN, ANDERSEN V. & GIEGE J. (1969a) Studies on the quantitation of lymphocyte response *in vitro. Acta Path. and Micriobiol. Scand.* **76**, 259.

SORENSEN S. FREISLEBEN & KISSMEYER-NIELSEN F. (1969b) Studies on the quantitation of the lymphocyte response *in vitro*—a family study. *Acta. Path and Microbiol. Scand.* **77**, 117.

SPENSIERI S. & CARNEVALE A.E. (1968) Transformazione di linfociti in blasti in colture leucocitairie miste. I. Ricerca nella gravidanza fisiologica. *Quad. Clin. Ostet. Ginec.* **23**, 393.

THORSBY E. (1970) In *Transplantation Reviews*, **3**, 80.

TRIDENTE G. CAPPUZZO G.M. & CHIECO-BIANCHI L. (1967) Lymphocyte Interaction in Mixed Mouse Leukocyte Cultures. In *Histocompatibility Testing*. Copenhagen: Munksgaard.

TRIDENTE G. & VAN BEKKUM D.W. (1969) Effect of anti-lymphocyte serum on mouse lymphoid tissues *in vivo* and *in vitro. Adv. exp. Med. and Biol.* **5**, 371.

TURSI A., GREAVES M.F., TORRIGIANI G., PLAYFAIR J.H.L. & ROITT I.M. (1969) Response to phytohaemagglutinin of lymphocytes from mice treated with anti-lymphocyte globulin. *Immunology*, **17**, 801.

VAN ROOD J.J. & EIJSVOOGEL V.P. (1970) HL-A identical phenotypes and genotypes in unrelated individuals. *Lancet*, i, 698.

WALFORD R.L. (1969) The Isoantigenic Systems of Human Leukocytes: Medical and Biological Significance. In *Series Haematologica* II. Copenhagen: Munksgaard.

WILSON D.B., SILVERS W.K. & NOWELL P.C. (1967) Quantitative studies on the mixed lymphocyte interaction in rats. II. Relationship of the proliferative response to the immunologic status of the donors. *J. exp. Med.* **126**, 655.

CHAPTER 6

Collaboration in Transplantation

H. Festenstein
J. Sachs and
R.T.D. Oliver

Recently reported clinical and experimental results support the hypothesis (Simonsen 1965) that a single strong genetic locus is of overriding importance in the determination of organ graft survival in man and rat (Singal *et al* 1969; Bildsøe *et al* 1970; Sakai & Simonsen 1969). Apart from major blood group compatibility, donor and recipient matching for identity at the main histocompatibility locus (HL-A) should therefore form the basis for collaboration in organ exchange for transplantation.

BLOOD GROUP SYSTEMS IN RELATION TO MATCHING

ABO blood group compatibility between donor and recipient is of prime importance in renal transplantation as there is a high incidence of immediate failure for incompatible grafts. Fifty per cent of the ABO incompatible cadaver grafts reported to the Boston Kidney Transplant Registry never functioned (Gleeson *et al* 1967), and Khastagir *et al* (1969) reported that ten out of 11 ABO incompatible grafts were rejected. Nevertheless, there are isolated reports of prolonged renal graft survival (some for more than $2\frac{1}{2}$ years) in the face of ABO incompatibility (Starzl *et al* 1964, 1965;

Murnaghan *et al* 1967). There is therefore a need for more information on this problem.

Other blood group systems

There is at present no conclusive evidence that blood group antigens other than ABO are involved in organ graft rejection (Gleeson *et al* 1967). There is, however, suggestive evidence that incompatibility involving P and RH blood group antigens may influence skin graft survival (Ceppellini *et al* 1966; Legrand *et al* 1970 in press).

THE HL-A SYSTEM IN RELATION TO MATCHING

Many HL-A antigens have been discovered in laboratories throughout the world, 11 of which are clearly defined and have been given WHO International Designation (*Transplant Proc.*, 1969; *Histocompatibility Testing*, 1970). The inheritance of these HL-A antigens is controlled by genetic information on a single pair of chromosomes (Fig. 1). The chromosome region in question (locus) can be divided into two or more closely linked genetic units (subloci). At each of the two subloci so far analysed, multiple alleles, of which no individual can have more than two, determine the detectable antigens (Fig. 1); every individual will therefore have a

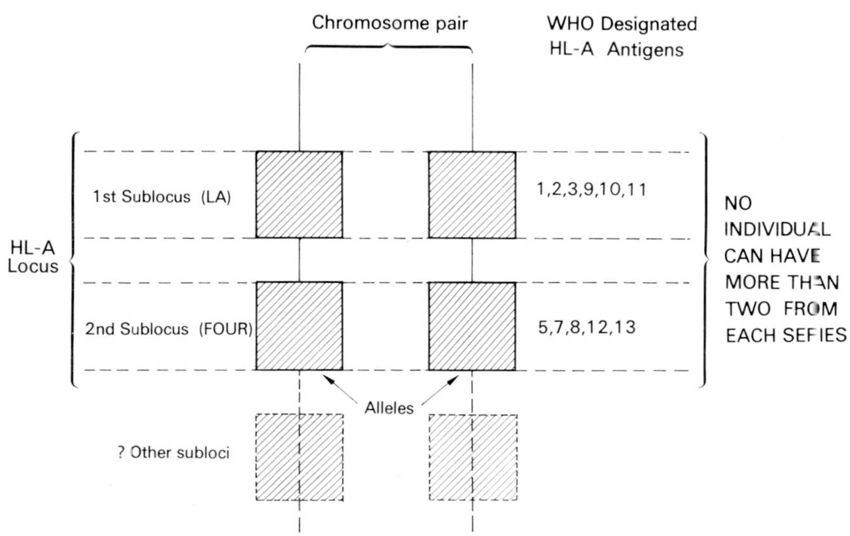

Fig. 1. HL-A locus in man.

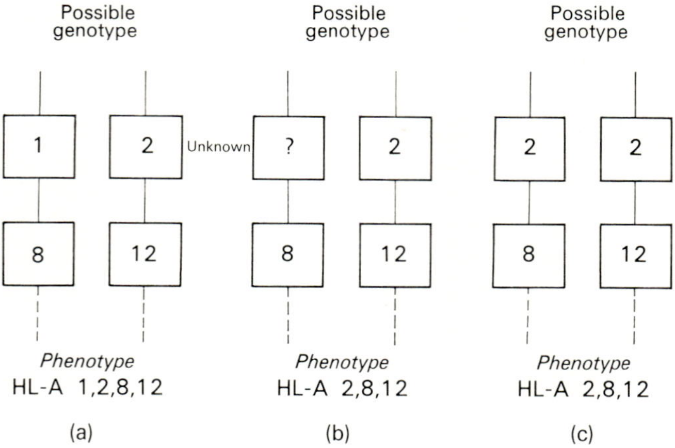

Fig. 2.

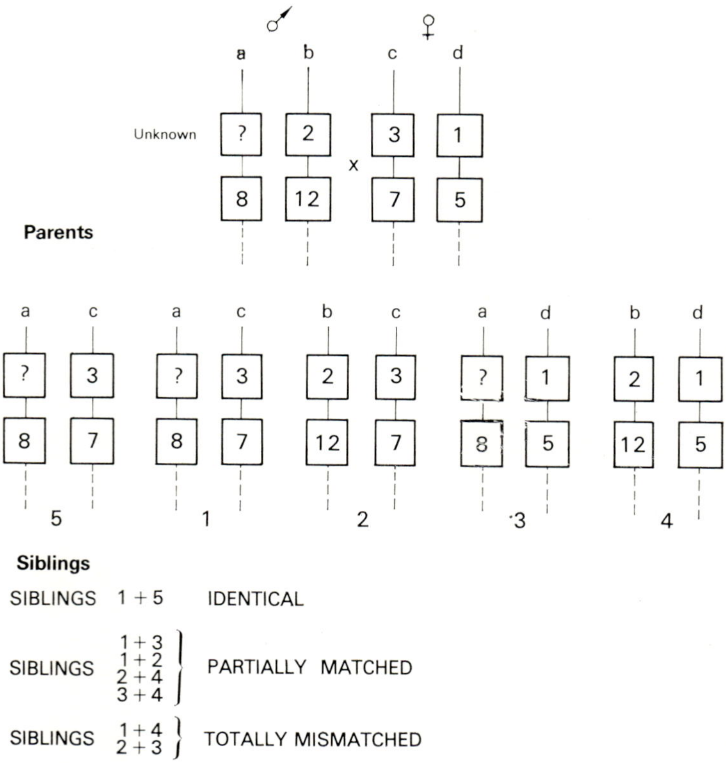

Fig. 3. Inheritance and matching of HL-A antigens within a family.

total of four antigens (Fig. 2a). Those individuals with less than the full complement are thought to have as yet undefined antigens (Fig. 2b) or to be homozygous for the antigen detected (Fig. 2c).

Studies of inheritance have shown that every individual receives from each parent alleles for the first and second sublocus, which determine corresponding antigens. If one designates the two paternal chromosomes carrying the HL-A locus as a and b, and the maternal chromosomes as c and d, four possible combinations can be inherited (i.e. ac, ad, bc, bd, Fig. 3). The probability of finding within any family a pair of siblings with the same four antigens (ac/ac) is 1 in 4 and for a pair who are partially matched with two parental antigens in common (e.g. ac/bc) it is 1 in 2 (van Rood *et al* 1967; Dausset 1969).

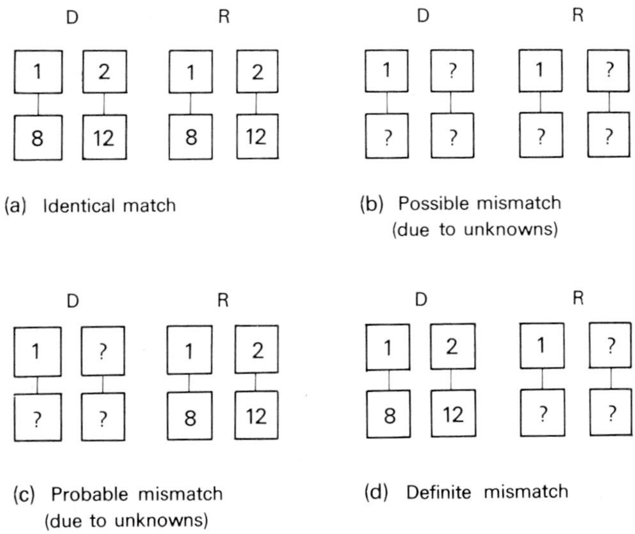

Fig. 4. Matching unrelated individuals.

When considering transplants between siblings the fact that the HL-A antigens are inherited *en bloc* makes it unnecessary to define all four HL-A antigens to achieve identical matching between donor and recipient (see ac/ac, Fig. 3). However, in unrelated individuals, identical matching is possible only when all four antigens are known in both donor and recipient (Fig. 4a). If all four donor antigens are known it is possible to define accurately the degree and nature of mismatch irrespective of whether the recipient antigens are known or not (Fig. 4d). Where there are unknown donor and recipient antigens the degree of mismatch becomes less well defined (see b and c, Fig. 4b and c).

This difficulty in finding identical matches amongst unrelated individuals is highlighted by van Rood *et al* (1967) who reported that only 17 out of 372 unrelated individuals had the same leucocyte antigens. He suggested (van Rood 1967) that it would therefore be possible to match closely the antigens of cadaver donors with those of potential recipients only by pooling all the tissue typing information of a large number of dialysis patients from different centres. At present it is not known what is the ideal pool size for close matching between donor and recipient. However, as the genetics of the HL-A system have become clearer, so has the understanding of what is a good match and what is the probability of obtaining it within a random population.

Assuming random distribution of the HL-A antigens, Dausset estimated on the basis of 20 antigens defined in his laboratory that the probability of finding two individuals with the same HL-A antigens was 1 in 10,000 (Legrand *et al* 1970). In practice, however, the antigens are not randomly distributed as certain of the antigens and antigen combinations occur more frequently than others (Dausset 1970). The analysis of Festenstein *et al* (1969) of 180 actual typings based on ABO blood groups and the seven then defined HL-A antigens and six other serological specificities takes these factors into account (Table 1). They concluded that a minimum

TABLE 1. Probability analysis

No. of mismatches	No. of recipients expected to be found in a recipient pool of size*			
	1	12	120	240
0	0·0041	0·04	0·49	0·98
1	0·0186	0·22	2·20	4·40
2	0·0527	0·63	6·30	12·60
3	0·0945	1·14	11·40	22·80

* This was worked out on the basis of comparing each of the 180 typings with the 179 others (Festenstein *et al*, *Lancet*, 1969).

pool size of 250 was required to match for identity. This, however, is a conservative estimate as many more antigens are now defined which were not used in this analysis. Nevertheless this figure may have some relevance as the antigens taken into consideration are the most frequently occurring and Legrand *et al* 1970, taking into account the recently demonstrated cross reactivity between many of the HL-A antigens (Kissmeyer-Nielsen *et al* 1968; Colombani *et al* 1970) has calculated that a pool size of 220 may be adequate to find an acceptable recipient for every donor.

Recently van Rood & Eijsvogel (1970) also found that a pool of approximately 250 patients would seem to be the minimum required to find an identical match for a random donor. They screened typings of 500 unrelated persons in order to select phenotypically identical individuals and found four who were serologically identical at the HL-A locus. However, only two of these proved to be truly identical according to the mixed lymphocyte culture test.

The London Transplant Group has an average of 300 patients actually fit and awaiting renal transplantation. There are probably more than 100 other suitable patients in Great Britain. Such a pool size for the whole of the country fulfils the minimum suggested requirements and is logistically feasible. Furthermore, collaboration with the other European schemes is practicable and will result in a combined pool size of approaching 1000. This would permit close matching for most donors and recipients and even those having less common phenotypes.

REQUIREMENTS FOR COLLABORATION

Recipient pool

A large number of patients awaiting renal transplantation is required. The selection and preparation of the patients for renal transplantation is dealt with in Chapter 12. However, from an immunological point of view certain categories of patient may have to wait a long time for a well matched donor kidney—those with rare combinations of HL-A antigens and those pre-immunized against transplantation antigens by previous pregnancies, blood transfusions or organ transplantation. As most patients on chronic haemodialysis may eventually be considered for transplantation, such patients could be dialysed at home while waiting for a suitable donor; as a general policy blood transfusion should be kept to a minimum.

Donor supply

At present the donor supply is always less than the demand and a first priority for all collaborating hospitals is to foster good relations with all other departments in their own and neighbouring hospitals. Contact can take the form of lectures, discussion and demonstrations to show the contribution each hospital can make, and should include medical and nursing personnel. In America there are already voluntary organizations to promote donation of organs run on the lines of blood banks. They distribute literature and arrange for individuals who wish to donate their organs to carry cards which give consent in the event of sudden death.

Donor supply could be greatly facilitated if the legislation concerning permission for consent is altered. In the first instance, it should be possible for any individual to will their body or parts thereof, as is the case in the United States. However, legislation permitting routine removal of organs, unless otherwise indicated by the individual, may in the future be considered.

Organ removal and preservation

This subject is discussed in full in Chapter 3. However, for successful interchange of cadaver kidneys it is essential that there is prior agreement between collaborating surgeons on methods of removal and preservation and an acceptable time limit for post mortem ischaemia. After completion of the donor nephrectomy, lymph nodes and spleen should be removed, and the latter perfused (Festenstein *et al* 1969). These provide an additional source of lymphocytes for tissue typing, pre-operative cross-matching, as well as for restrospective immunological studies.

To avoid unnecessary delays, the co-ordinating centre should relay clinical information about the age, blood pressure, renal function prior to death, the anatomy and ischaemia times of the donor kidney to the recipient hospitals. Further detailed information should be obtained by direct communication between the donor and recipient surgical teams. A brief resumé of the above information as well as tissue typing and ABO blood grouping results should accompany every kidney exchanged.

Co-ordinating centre and tissue typing laboratories

The establishment of tissue typing facilities requires considerable preliminary work before exchange of kidneys can occur. Collaboration is likely to involve several laboratories though, in densely populated areas with good communications, it may be possible to tissue type potential recipients from several hospitals in one central laboratory. In either case effective exchange will require:

a *Standardization of reagents*

For reliable matching each collaborating laboratory must use a panel of tissue typing sera defining the same HL-A antigens (see Chapter 4). Through international exchange of sera and histocompatibility workshops, many tissue typing sera have been accurately characterized. Some of these sera are held at the International Serum Bank at the National Institutes of Health, Bethesda, Maryland, USA and have acted as a nucleus in the establishment of panels of sera for collaborative schemes throughout the world. It is necessary to supplement such sera with others obtained from screening programmes organized within the collaborative scheme and by exchange of sera with other centres. In most circumstances sera are distributed frozen, either in bulk or dispensed into tissue typing plates, but it may be possible in the near future to distribute lyophilized sera. In Britain there is a National Tissue Typing Reference Laboratory set up by the Ministry of Health and Social Security to characterize and distribute a standard panel of tissue typing sera.

b *Standardization of technique*

Considerable experience is required in the reading and interpretation of the results of tissue typing. Within a large collaborative scheme, many individuals may be involved in the typing of donors and recipients To ensure reproducibility there must be a standard technique and method of interpretation and to achieve this:

i Technicians from collaborating hospitals should have a prolonged training period preferably at a central laboratory.

ii Tissue typing plates should have each serum dispensed in duplicate and where possible at least three sera recognizing each specificity.

iii All potential recipients should be tissue typed at least twice and donor tissue typing confirmed at the recipient hospital when possible.

iv Standard test cells with known HL-A groups should be distributed at regular intervals to act as internal laboratory controls.

c *Storage of information*

For matching of donors and recipients rapid access is required to both ABO and HL-A groups on large numbers of patients. Such information is complicated to record and subject to errors of transcription. For this reason carbon or photocopying of a standard tissue typing form should be used to transfer results from each tissue typing laboratory to the co-ordinating centre.

For storage of information and matching at least three systems are available:

i Direct visual assessment of wall charts with the recipient antigens arranged in columns. This is the simplest system but it is only possible to assess a small number of patients (40 to 80). Although it is easy to pick out an identical match where there are several recipients with only a few antigens mismatched, it is often possible to overlook one of them in the final selection.

ii Punch cards. In the marginal punch card system each patient has a card on which is punched the tissue typing and blood group. If all the cards are held together and a needle passed through the hole representing a particular antigen those positive for that antigen will be extracted. It is possible, by a series of such manoeuvres, to rapidly select the 4 or 5 best matched recipients from several hundred cases.

An optical coincidence non marginal punch card system (Ewertsen & Ericksen 1956) enables one to store the tissue typing information of up to 1000 recipients on less than 20 cards (Kissmeyer-Nielsen & Kjerbe 1970). Each card which corresponds to one antigen or an ABO group has 1000 punch-holes numbered from 0–999. The punch-hole corresponding to a recipient's serial number is punched out only on those antigen cards for which the recipient is positive. To match, the cards corresponding to the donor's HL-A antigens and ABO group are superimposed and those recipients with punch-holes on all the cards will be matched identically to the donor. In the event of no identical recipient being available one card is removed and it is then possible to find recipients only mismatched for that donor antigen.

The advantages of such systems are that they are portable, and matching can be performed very quickly but it can occasionally be unreliable if cards are lost or damaged.

iii Computers. From the point of view of storing large amounts of information computers have obvious advantages. They have been applied to the problem of matching for organ grafting in two principal ways.

The computer classifies the recipients according to their tissue groups and prints out a directory with an index of the pages on which recipients with a particular tissue grouping can be found (van Rood 1969). This system is particularly advantageous where collaboration involves long distances as copies of the directory can be distributed to each collaborating hospital and matching performed on the spot.

The computer can select the best match from any number of stored recipients using a step by step elimination of each less well matched recipient. The result may be printed on an output terminal giving alternative recipients if the one chosen was unfit for operation (Festenstein *et al* 1969). For this system to function there must be a direct link from the laboratory to the computer which should be available 24 hours a day as well as an alternative method of selection in the event of mechanical failure.

Whichever selection procedure is used reference should again be made to the original recorded serological reactions to ensure that errors of transcription have not occurred.

d *Distribution of sera for crossmatch*

Ideally each hospital providing donors should have aliquots of sera from all potential recipients in the collaborating hospitals. Additional or replacement samples should be distributed every three months or a few weeks after each transfusion.

e *Updating recipient pool*

At regular intervals the co-ordinating centre should contact all the collaborating hospitals to ascertain whether any patients have been added to or removed from the pool as well as checking to see if any recipients are temporarily unfit for transplantation.

f *Follow-up*

It is only by the detailed follow-up of the patients who have been transplanted that the benefit of collaboration can be demonstrated. Investigation into the effects of prolonged storage of donor kidneys, problems of rejection and the influence of different levels of matching on long term survival should be undertaken by the collaborating hospitals.

g *Screening for new antisera*

All laboratories should be involved in the evaluation of new sera for tissue typing. Depending on the facilities available, initial screening should be performed at a few reference laboratories; once useful sera have been discovered they should be distributed as widely as possible to be compared with standard sera. Regular interchange of information between laboratories will help to accelerate this process.

h *Finance*

The costs of a co-ordinating centre are high and adequate financial support is necessary for its efficient function. Expenses include salaries of personnel (administrative, nursing, medical, technical and computer staff), laboratory and computer facilities, telephone and telex expenses and transportation costs. Such a venture should be directly supported by the state or through contributions from participating hospitals.

PROCEDURE FOLLOWED WHEN DONOR BECOMES AVAILABLE

The authors have been responsible for organizing a matching and distribution centre for the London based collaborative scheme. The following is an outline of the function of the co-ordinating centre:

A 24 hour on-call rota is maintained at the co-ordinating centre with access to the computer. Individuals on call carry a complete set of recipient index cards and a comprehensive directory of telephone numbers for key personnel within the group, personnel of other transplant centres and for essential channels of communication such as taxi services, police, airports and stations.

Tissue typing is performed using lymphocytes from peripheral blood, lymph node or spleen. After approximately 2 hours the tissue typing is read, the two best matched recipients are selected and their sera cross matched with the cells of the donor. Where there is no serum of the selected recipient available, a lymphocyte suspension is sent to the recipient hospital in advance of the kidney. When hospitals outside the collaborative scheme contribute kidneys, the tissue typing may have to be repeated.

Where no suitable recipients are available within the pool, telephone calls are made to several different hospitals outside the collaborative scheme and the kidney sent to the first hospital to have a suitably matched recipient. This has proved a very effective way of making contact with other collaborative schemes and improving inter-regional exchange.

A large proportion of the time and energy of the staff of the co-ordinating centre is taken up by communicating with donor and recipient hospitals and arranging the actual carriage of the kidneys to the recipients. Existing public transport facilities are used for the majority of exchanges. When such services are not available, however, it has been necessary to resort to the use of private and/or emergency services and this gives rise to considerable expense. As the areas of collaboration extend it will be necessary to set up a central independent transport organization closely linked to the co-ordinating centre. Such an organization could be responsible for the movement of personnel, patients and lymphocytes as well as kidneys.

SOME EXPERIENCES IN COLLABORATION FOR RENAL TRANSPLANTATION

Since 1967 several collaborative schemes have been established in different parts of the world (Patel *et al* 1968; Sheils *et al* 1968; van Rood 1969; Festenstein *et al* 1969; Kissmeyer-Nielsen & Kjerbe 1970). The first two reported schemes began in Sydney and Los Angeles. In Sydney two surgical teams transplanted kidneys from four dialysis units and received donor kidneys from 12 other nearby hospitals. One central laboratory performed the tissue typing and selection of recipients; 96 transplants were performed in the first 2 years. In Los Angeles, Terasaki's Laboratory organized the tissue typing and matching for eight hospitals as well as several others in the nearby States of Washington, Oregon, Colorado and Arizona. Once selection had been made, the recipient hospital was responsible for organizing and financing the movement of the kidney. In $2\frac{1}{2}$ years this group was able to perform 150 kidney grafts mostly in the city, but recently the distance of exchange has increased.

Eurotransplant centred on van Rood's laboratory at the University of Leiden Hospital includes transplant centres in NW Germany, Belgium and the Netherlands with more than 300 dialysis patients in 28 hospitals. A classified printout of the tissue typing results updated monthly is distributed to the local tissue typing laboratories and used by the donor hospital personnel to perform the matching. They contact the recipient hospital and refer to the central laboratory only if there are difficulties in finding a suitable recipient. Van Rood (1969) has reported the results of the first thirty exchanges.

In Paris, the laboratory of Dausset acts as the co-ordinating centre for Eurotransplant West. This collaborative scheme includes transplant centres in ten major French cities as well as Barcelona, Madrid and Lisbon. There is a recipient pool of more than 125 and in the first year 39 transplants were performed.

The Scandinavian countries are served by Scandiatransplant centred on Kissmeyer-Nielsen's laboratory at Arhus (Kissmeyer-Nielsen & Kjerbe 1970).

In the British Isles there are regional schemes centred in London and the west and north of England. The London transplant group co-ordinates the exchange of kidneys between 14 transplant centres in London, central England and Ireland. The majority of the hospitals have their own tissue typing laboratories from where the donor and recipient information is sent to the central laboratory at the London Hospital which is responsible for the matching and selection of recipients. One hundred and sixty-eight kidneys have been exchanged during the 20 months (Festenstein 1971).

Although blood group compatibility and HL-A tissue typing has been the basis for selection in all the reported collaborative schemes, many centres have modified their selection according to local circumstances. In Los Angeles donating hospitals transplanted one of the kidneys themselves while the other was donated to the pool. In Sydney tissue typing was the basis for the selection of recipients but no kidney was excluded from use on this ground alone. Both groups accepted these procedures as a compromise while the donor supply was inadequate.

Three centres reported interchange of recipients to enable full use of all available donor kidneys. In one group (Sheil *et al* 1969) it was calculated that only 18 of the first 54 transplants would have been performed had this interchange not taken place.

The published results showed an overall reduction in the degree of mismatching by approximately 50%. However, in all centres the number of identically matched grafts was less than 10% and the authors concluded that considerably larger recipient pools were necessary to find identical recipients for each donor. To this end the areas of collaboration are now being extended and there are at least five groups in America and eight in Europe including four in Britain. Preliminary steps have been taken to link the European schemes by interchanging information about recipients with rare tissue groups and preformed cytotoxic antibodies.

CONCLUSION

While the superior results of renal transplantation between siblings, where donor and recipient are matched identically for antigens governed by the HL-A locus, cannot be disputed (Singal *et al* 1969) there is at present only suggestive evidence that this is so for unrelated (cadaver) transplants as until recently very few such identically matched grafts had been performed (van Rood *et al* 1969; Morris *et al* 1968; Batchelor & Joysey 1969; Kreisler *et al* 1970). The most important result of collaboration so far reported is that, as van Rood originally predicted, the larger the recipient pool size the easier it is to find an identical recipient for any random donors. Only when a large number of such identically matched grafts have been followed for more than a year will one obtain conclusive evidence for the importance of matching in cadaver renal transplantation.

Future prospects for the success of collaboration will depend on:

i Further clarification of the HL-A system and understanding of the problems of antigenic strength.

ii Larger areas of collaboration which can only be achieved by closer links between regional, national and international schemes.

iii Improved donor supply and techniques of organ preservation.

However, in the final analysis the viability of these schemes will depend on the financial support available.

REFERENCES

BATCHELOR J.R. & JOYSEY V. (1969) Influence of HL-A incompatibility on cadaveric renal transplantation. *Lancet*, i, 790.

BILDSØE P., FREIESLEBEN SØRENSEN S., PETTIROSSI O. & SIMONSEN M. (1970) Heart and kidney transplantation from segregating hybrid to parental rats. *Transplant. Rev.* **3**, 36.

CEPPELLINI R., CURTONI E.S., MATTIUZ P.L., LEIGHEB G., VISETTI M. & COLOMBI A. (1966) Survival of test skin grafts in man: effect of genetic relationship and blood group incompatibility. *Ann. N.Y. Acad. Sci.* **129,** 421.

CEPPELLINI R., CURTONI E.S., MATTIUZ P.L., MIGGIANO G., SCUDELLAR G. & SERRA A. (1967) Genetics of leukocyte antigens: A family study of segregations and linkage. In *Histocompatibility Testing*, eds. CURTONI E.S., MATTIUZ P.L. & TOSI R.M. Copenhagen: Munksgaard.

COLOMBANI J., COLOMBANI M. & DAUSSET J. (1970) Cross reactions in the HL-A system with special reference to Da6 cross-reacting group. In *Histocompatibility Testing*. In press.

DAUSSET J. (1969) Tissue typing and transplantation. *Vox Sanguinis*, **16,** 263.

DAUSSET J. (1970) Subdivision of the HL-A locus. In *Biology and Surgery of Tissue Transplantation*, ed. MAXWELL ANDERSON J.

EWERTSEN H.W. & ERICKSEN E. (1956) Universalhulkort I medicinens tjenste. *Nor. Med.* **56,** 1441.

FESTENSTEIN H. (1970) (in preparation).

FESTENSTEIN H., OLIVER R.T.D., HYAMS A., MOORHEAD J.F., PIRRIE A.J., PEGRUM G.D. & BALFOUR I.C. (1969) A collaborative scheme for tissue typing and matching in renal transplantation. *Lancet*, ii, 389.

GLEESON R.E., & MURRAY J.E. (1967) Report from kidney transplant registry: analysis of variables in the function of human kidney transplants. *Transplantation*, **5,** 343.

KHASTAGIR B., MONTANDON A., NAKAMOTO S. & KOLFF W.J. (1969) Early and late failures of human cadaveric renal allografts. *Arch. Intern. Med.*, **123,** 8.

KISSMEYER-NIELSEN F. & KJERBYE K. (1970) Scandiatransplant. A visual matching system. In *Histocompatibility Testing*. In press.

KISSMEYER-NIELSEN F., SVEJGAARD A. & HAUGE M. (1968) Genetics of the Human HL-A Transplantation System. *Nature, Lond.* **219,** 1116.

KREISLER M., SINGAL D.P., LINSCOTT JR.S., MICKEY M.R. & TERASAKI P.I. (1970) *Relative Strength of Individual HL-A Antigens and Haplotypes in* 614 *Kidney Transplants.* In press.

LEGRAND L., HORS J., COLOMBANI J., RAPAPORT F.T. & DAUSSET J. (1970) *Relative Strength of Individual HL-A Antigens and Haplotypes in* 614 *Kidney Transplants.* In press.

MORRIS P.J., KINCAID-SMITH P., TING A., STOCKER J.W. & MARSHALL V.C (1968) Prospective leucocyte typing in cadaver renal transplantation. *Lancet*, ii, 803.

MURNAGHAN G.F., JEREMY D., TRACE G.D., FARNSWORTH R.W. & MCCREDIE K.B. (1967) Successful human cadaveric renal homograft with major blood group incompatibility. *Lancet*, ii, 852.

PATEL R., GLASSOCK R. & TERASAKI P. (1969) Experience with an interhospital scheme of cadaver kidney sharing and tissue typing. *J.A.M.A.* **207,** 1319.

PATEL R., TERASAKI P. & BERGWERFF K. (1968) A city-wide scheme for cadaver kidney procurement, sharing and tissue typing. *Trans. Amer. Soc. Artif. Int. Organs*, **14,** 132.

REPORT OF W.H.O. WORKSHOP COMMITTEE (1969) Nomenclature for factors of HL-A system. *Transplant. Proc.* **1,** 368.

REPORT OF W.H.O. WORKSHOP COMMITTEE (1970) Nomenclature for factors of HL-A system. In *Histocompatibility Testing*. In press.

SAKAI A. & SIMONSEN M. (1969) Kidney transplantation in siblings. *Transplantation*, **7**, 444.

SHEIL A.G.R., JOHNSON J.R., STOREY B.G., CHARLESWORTH J.A., SHARP A., SANDS J.R., STEWART J.H., MAY J., ROGERS J.H., WRIGHT R., JOHNSTON J.M. & LOEWENTHAL J. (1969) Community treatment of end-stage renal failure by dialysis and renal transplantation from cadaver donors. *Lancet*, ii, 917.

SHEIL A.G.R., STEWART J.H., MAY J., JOHNSON J., TILLER D., GEORGE C.R.P., ROGERS J.H., STOREY B.G., MANI M.K., GIBSON G.R., SHARP A., WYATT, K.M., SANDS J.R. & LOEWENTHAL J. (1968) Renal transplantation from cadaver donors. *Med. J. Australia*. ii, 1079.

SIMONSEN M. (1965) Strong transplantation antigens in man. *Lancet*, i, 495.

SINGAL D.P., MICKEY M.R. & TERASAKI P.I. (1969) Serotyping for homotransplantation. XXIII. Analysis of kidney transplants from parental versus sibling donors. *Transplantation*, **7**, 246.

STARZL T.E., MARCHIORO T.L., RIFKIND D., HOLMES J.M., ROWLANDS D.T. & WADDELL W.R. (1964) Factors in successful renal transplantation. *Surgery*, **56**, 296.

STARZL T.E., MARCHIORO T.L., TERASAKI P.I., PORTER K.A., FARIS T.D., HERRMAN T.J., VREDVOE D.L., HUTT M.P., OGDEN D.A. & WADDELL W.R. (1965) Chronic survival after human renal homotransplantation. *Ann. Surg*. **162**, 749.

TERASAKI P., MICKEY M.R., SINGAL D.P., MITTAL K.K. & PATEL R. (1968) Serotyping for homotransplantation. XX. Selection of recipients for cadaver donor transplants. *New Engl. J. of Med.*, **279**, 1101.

VAN ROOD J.J. (1967) A proposal for international cooperation in organ transplantation: Eurotransplant. In *Histocompatibility Testing*, 451, eds. CURTONI E.S., MATTIUZ P.L. & TOSI R.M., p. 451. Copenhagen: Munksgaard.

VAN ROOD J.J. (1969) Tissue typing and organ transplantation. *Lancet*, ii, 1142.

VAN ROOD J.J., VAN LEEUWEN A., SCHIPPERS A.M.J., PEARCE R., VAN BLANKENSTEIN M. & VOLLERS W. (1967) Immunogenetics of group four, five and nine systems. In *Histocompatibility Testing*, eds. CURTONI E.S., MATTIUZ P.L. & TOSI R.M., p. 203. Copenhagen: Munksgaard.

VAN ROOD J.J. & EIJSVOOGEL V.P. (1970) HL-A identical phenotypes and genotypes in unrelated individuals. *Lancet*, i, 698.

CHAPTER 7

Infectious Problems in Transplantation

D.B. Evans

INTRODUCTION

THE ability of the human body to recognize and resist transplanted organs and invading material which are not identical to its own tissues is one of life's fundamental attributes. Everyone involved in the rapidly developing field of organ transplantation has experienced the frustrations and disappointments caused by infection. There is no doubt that the most important factor responsible for the uninhibited proliferation of micro-organisms in organ transplant recipients is the inevitable use of steroids and other immunosuppressive agents and reports of infective complications in patients with autoimmune, neoplastic and other diseases treated with immunosuppressive drugs lends confirmation to the hypothesis.

The actions of the immunosuppressive agents are unfortunately not directed specifically and singly against the immune response to transplanted tissue. Azathioprine, a derivative of 6-mercaptopurine interferes with the synthesis of purine nucleotides with the result that immunoglobulin synthesis is impaired. Gradual depletion of lymphoid tissue may occur, though peripheral lymphocyte counts are usually normal. Toxic dores often inhibit leucocyte and platelet production by the bone marrow and may interfere with the turnover of the rapidly dividing cells of the intestines.

Corticosteroids on their own are not particularly effective in controlling rejection but in association with azathioprine they play a very important role in basic immunosuppressive therapy and in the treatment of rejection crises. The way in which they work is open to conjecture—claims have been made that they inhibit lymphoid cell generation and the phagocytic properties of reticuloendothelial cells, they have anti-inflammatory properties and probably inhibit synthesis of proteins and hence antibodies.

Any patient considered for organ transplantation has to be admitted to hospital at some stage for assessment. This in itself may be a disadvantage in so far that hospital micro-organisms may be picked up. These organisms may prove to be of such a strain as to be resistant to the usual range of antibiotics, and in debilitated patients may carry a particularly high morbidity. Renal transplant candidates will require haemodialysis or peritoneal dialysis treatment in preparation for transplantation and these procedures carry their own infection risks e.g. peritonitis, shunt infections, septicaemias and viral hepatitis. Care is necessary to minimize such risks and postponement of any operation is essential until eradication of infection is achieved.

TABLE 1. Infections—sources

Endogenous	Nasopharynx G.U. tract G.I. tract Shunts Lungs
Exogenous	Allograft Atmosphere Staff, visitors etc. Dialysers, blood transfusion
Latent	Viruses Fungi Protozoans Parasites

In addition, organisms which are normally considered saprophytic in the general population may, in the presence of immunosuppressive drugs, take on the guise of pathogens and produce bizarre and often fulminating sepsis.

SOURCES OF INFECTIONS

1 Endogenous

Experience with nasal and pharyngeal carriers of staphylococcus pyogenes has shown that the rate of wound sepsis is doubled in those patients harbouring the organisms pre-operatively. Attempts to eradicate the carrier state by local therapy has usually resulted in temporary clearance only, and sometimes resistant organisms have replaced them.

The gastrointestinal tract normally harbours a host of bacteria ranging from *E. coli* to *Ps. aeruginosa* and in the event of biliary surgery associated with transplantation, the emergence of intestinal bacteria at the site of transplantation has been all too common.

The genito-urinary tract must be rendered sterile prior to renal transplantation—if not, the incidence of post-operative urinary sepsis is significantly increased and septicaemias and pelvic sepsis frequently follow. The indication for the removal of infected or potentially infected kidneys and ureters is absolute and a thorough investigation of the lower urinary tract in order to eliminate factors that might predispose to recurrent infection is desirable.

External arteriovenous shunts placed in forearm or leg vessels for purposes of dialysis or to facilitate blood taking should be cared for meticulously. Frequent swabbing of exit sites and culture should be performed as these are important potential sources of infection which may easily lead to bacteraemia or septicaemia. Similar care should be taken of internal fistulae for they may become sources of systemic infection.

2 Exogenous

Human beings, particularly those working in hospital environments, are probably the commonest vector for the spread of infection. Droplet infection or spread via fomites may constitute a hazard to potential recipients. Atmospheric carriage by infected dust and fungi such as *Aspergillus* spp. usually cause few problems for the healthy individual but they may be a particular hazard in the immunosuppressed patient. Influenza epidemics may pave the way in these patients to secondary bacterial infection and care should be taken to eliminate staff and visitors who might be carriers from transplant units.

Dialysed patients are specially at risk particularly from the point of view of recurrent blood transfusions. The transmission of the hepatitis virus via blood transfusions has brought dialysis and transplantation programmes almost to a standstill in many units throughout the country and cross infection from one patient to another may well be transmitted via 'shared' dialysers. Fresh blood transfusion carries an additional risk—that of cytomegalovirus—an organism particularly dangerous to foetuses, young children and to immunosuppressed patients. Better and more efficient methods of dialysis it is hoped might lessen the risk of these serious infections.

Perhaps the least thought of potential infection risk is the organ donor. Infection in the donor, often a result of long continued attempts at resuscitation may lead to respiratory, urinary and systemic infections, so that organs removed from such donors may harbour organisms at the time of death. The presence of any evidence of infection should therefore exclude such a donor. Ignoring such a practice will, in many cases result in catastrophic septicaemias and secondary haemorrhage in the recipient.

3 **Latent**

Latent virus infections are harboured by many individuals—the commonest being herpes simplex which is responsible for the common cold sore. The varicella-Zoster virus may also lurk in human tissues and normally may not be reactivated. *Candida albicans* and *Aspergillus* spp may live symbiotically in the GI and respiratory tracts and in any situation where the balance of bacterial flora is upset by antibiotics these organisms find themselves unrestricted and free to proliferate at will. If immunosuppressive drugs are present as well further proliferation can result.

Two very unusual latent organisms have been encountered by the author—leprosy and listeria monocytogenes. The former appeared in a Eurasian man who had received a cadaveric renal transplant 2 years previously—he developed erythema nodosum leprosum whilst on immunosuppressive therapy. He admitted to having suffered from leprosy nearly 20 years previously. The other patient developed a *L. monocytogenes* meningitis 2 months after renal transplantation. The condition responsed to Penbritin therapy but he died later of a cerebral haemorrhage. This unusual organism had probably been harboured in his body prior to transplantation and had multiplied in the presence of heavy immunosuppression.

PRE-EXISTING INFECTION

Of all the categories of infection by far the commonest clinical pattern has been the result of proliferation of pre-existing endogenous organsisms. Complete eradication of all sources of infection before embarking upon transplantation surgery is almost impossible particularly in the fields of transplantation other than the kidney. Life can be supported indefinitely by dialysis in the latter field, whereas in the case of other organs the opportunities for transplantation are much less and often have to be undertaken before optimal preparation has been achieved.

An intensive search should be made for infection in any potential recipient of an organ transplant. Swabs from the throat, nose and skin folds should be cultured frequently, and urine, sputum, faecal, vaginal and blood cultures should be taken if considered appropriate. Not only is it necessary to culture for bacteria but fungi should be sought for as well. If peritoneal dialysis is being performed, the dialysis fluid should be cultured daily and any wounds, shunts and other lesions swabbed and cultured. If a significant growth of organisms results from these investigations, appropriate narrow spectrum antibiotics should be prescribed in full doses, especial care being taken in cases of renal failure (Kunin 1967). Antifungal agents should also be given if indicated. In cases of severe gram negative infections where potentially toxic antibiotics may have to be used, it is highly desirable that blood levels of the antibiotic be checked frequently and the bactericidal activity of the serum to the particular organism measured. Intensive physiotherapy plays an important role in mobilizing these patients and in establishing good ventilation of the lungs. As soon as they are fit, patients should spend as much time as possible out in the open air and away from the hospital.

Surgical drainage of infected areas, the removal of pyelonephritic kidneys and bladder neck resection all help to lessen the chances of post-transplantation sepsis. Patients with chronic, irreversible infections such as bronchiectasis should not be considered as potential recipients. Quiescent tuberculosis of the lungs should be treated with antituberculous drugs lest the condition be reactivated in the presence of steroids. Renal tuberculosis should be treated surgically.

The presence of active viral hepatitis should probably be a contra-indication to immediate transplantation though liver transplantation has been performed for acute hepatic necrosis due to viral hepatitis. If possible, transplantation of other organs should be postponed for at least 6 months.

FACTORS PREDISPOSING TO POST-OPERATIVE INFECTIONS

1 Damage to the graft

Ischaemic damage to organs taken for grafting results in functional derangement which may be temporary or permanent. Temporary derangement can be tolerated provided some function remains or life can be supported artificially. Cellular ischaemic damage may however allow invasion of the devitalized tissue by micro-organisms resulting in abscesses and septicaemia. This is not usually a hazard in the kidney but transplanted livers and lungs may suffer seriously from such complications.

Considerable surgical skill is required to ensure swift and careful removal and transplantation of these organs in order to minimise ischaemic damage but better methods of preservation of these organs is necessary so that great haste becomes unnecessary.

2 Technical problems

Anatomical anomalies and the minuteness and sometimes inaccessibility of vascular and other anastomoses make organ transplantation a skilful but nevertheless a hazardous procedure. Kinking or thrombosis of blood vessels, ureters, bile ducts etc. may result in infarction of part of or the whole organ or its drainage system. Leakage of excretory products invariably leads to infection, initially localized but in the presence of immunosuppressive drugs, frequently disseminated. In renal transplantation these technical difficulties are nowadays rarely a problem but in far more difficult liver transplant operations, they may still occur.

3 Rejection and immunosuppressive drugs

As mentioned in the introduction the one common factor in all clinical organ transplantation work is the immunosuppressive therapy. An immune response to an allograft always occurs so that these drugs must always be given (until better alternatives have been found). In those patients fortunate enough to have received well matched grafts the immune response will usually be overcome easily by the basic regime described (see Chapter 5). Provided no significant nidus of infection is present those patients can expect an uneventful course. However, the vast majority of patients suffer one or more rejection crises and if they have in addition some technical or ischaemic problem, the chances of infection are high. With each successive course of antirejection therapy within a short space of time, the risk of infective complications escalates, so much so that our current practice is to abandon any kidney that does not respond to three courses of anti-rejection therapy (confirmed by biopsy). After every transplant operation great pains should be taken to look for infection and any significant growth coupled with clinical evidence for infection should be treated vigorously with the appropriate narrow spectrum antibiotic as indicated by sensitivity testing. Prophylactic antibiotics should not be given under any condition as they may produce drug resistant strains and may well allow the multiplication of saprophytic bacteria, fungi or viruses. This is, of course, a risk even when antibiotics are used therapeutically, but drug resistance and alteration in endogenous flora can be minimized by using narrow spectrum drugs. It is debatable whether prophylactic antifungal agents should be used—it is our policy to give daily Nystatin or Fungilin lozenges to all patients on immunosuppressive drugs and we have found as a result, a lowering in the incidence of oral thrush.

4 Bone marrow depression

This is usually a complication of azathioprine, Actinomycin C and sometimes antilymphocytic serum, though overwhelming septicaemias and other drugs e.g. phenytoin, chloramphenicol etc. may be responsible. Care must be exercised in prescribing these drugs in the presence of renal or hepatic malfunction for fear of marrow depression. This complication will further lower the host's chances of overcoming infections and in conjunction with rejection it usually indicates a very poor prognosis. Judicious use of antibiotics, reverse barrier nursing and abstinence from immunosuppressive therapy, even at the risk of losing the graft, may save the life of a kidney graft recipient but in the cases of more vital grafts, such a luxury is not possible. It is therefore of vital importance to prescribe drug therapy very carefully and only after measuring daily blood counts.

INVESTIGATION OF INFECTIONS

Routine search for infection pre-operatively has already been outlined. At operation foci of infection should be looked for and it is customary to swab anything that looks suspicious or that may be a potential site of infection e.g. the urinary bladder. The presence of significant though not previously diagnosed infection should be an indication for postponing the operation. Care to secure good haemostasis should be made and all potential dead spaces should be obliterated.

Post-operatively reverse barrier nursing should be practiced and in some units (Woodruff *et al* 1968) complete sterile nursing is performed. Clinical evidence of infection should be looked for daily and swabs from nose and throat cultured every few days or more often if the patient complains of a sore throat. Daily blood cultures are a wise precaution during the first fortnight and urine cultures should be taken thrice weekly. The development of wound infections, shunt infections or infections around drains should be promptly investigated. Drains should be removed as early as possible, bladder catheters are left *in situ* according to the discretion of the surgeon and wound stitches removed at 10–14 days. All catheter tips, drain tips and stitches should be submitted for culture.

Barrier conditions are usually lifted once catheters are removed and wounds are healed.

Post-operative chest complications should be largely avoided if physiotherapy is instituted before operation and continues immediately after. All sputum specimens should be sent to the laboratory for culture and where there is clinical suspicion of infection chest X-rays should be taken.

TYPES OF INFECTION

As in general medical practice many allograft recipients develop infections with common organisms, which seem to have a predilection for the correspondingly usual sites e.g. staphylococcal wound infections, coliform urinary tract infections, pneumococcal respiratory tract infections and coliform infections of the biliary system. However in more complicated situations, particularly where high immunosuppressive drug doses have had to be used, a far more bizarre pattern of infections develops and such organisms as *Proteus* spp and *Ps. aeruginosa* tend to appear in the sputum and urinary tract. Treatment with 'appropriate' antibiotics has often resulted in the emergence of a *Klebsiella* spp which is resistant to the antibiotics used. The similarity of organisms in the bile to those inhabiting the gut has been a marked feature in liver transplantation, with occasional dissemination of the same organism in the blood stream. Colonization and dissemination of normally considered 'nonpathogenic' organisms has also been frequently observed. Lung abscesses following pneumonia have produced multiple infections with both gram positive and gram negative organisms—in fact the colonization of devitalized tissue by gram negative organisms has been a marked feature of both renal and hepatic transplantation. Systemic infections with gram positive cocci (*staph. pyogenes*) has frequently followed shunt infections whereas gram negative septicaemias have followed urinary, peritoneal or biliary infections. The mortality in the latter group was significantly higher than in the former despite prompt antibiotic therapy.

Fungal, viral and protozoal infections have been common—the fungi usually affecting the respiratory tract, the brain, upper gastrointestinal tract and urinary systems whereas *H. Simplex* has been responsible for ocular, oral and respiratory infections. It has been suggested (Slapak *et al* 1968) that fungal and viral infections in the lung may develop following 'transplant pneumonitis'. Cytomegalovirus has been seen in the liver and kidneys and one case of fulminating varicella invaded almost every tissue examined at necropsy. *Pneumocystis carinii* lung infections have been reported but we have seen this protozoan in the lungs of only one of our cases. In American series Histoplasmosis, Coccydioidiomycosis etc. have also been reported.

Opportunistic infections with *listeria monocytogenes* and *mycobacterium lepri* have already been referred to. Tuberculosis may occur *de novo* in immunosuppressed patients but far commoner is the reactivation of a dormant pulmonary lesion. Antituberculous drug cover should be given whenever this condition is suspected.

CONCLUSIONS

From the foregoing discussion it would appear that in order to achieve a reasonable measure of success the following principles might serve as useful guidelines to those embarking upon organ transplantation:

a The potential recipient should be well prepared and sources of infection should be eradicated as far as possible. One has to remember that occasionally these sources can only be eliminated by the removal of the offending organ at the time of the transplant operation.

b Ideally, perfect preservation of the organ and uncomplicated surgery should be aimed at, if technical problems arise, prompt correction and drainage may reduce the spread of infection.

c Good histocompatibility matching will reduce the risk of rejection and therefore eliminate the need for very high immunosuppressive drug doses with the danger of marrow depression.

d Short but adequate courses of appropriate narrow spectrum antibiotics should be used in the event of a significant infection.

e In the event of severe infections developing, every attempt should be made to reduce immunosuppressive drug therapy as far as is possible, and in renal transplantation the allograft should be removed and the patient restored to intermittent dialysis.

REFERENCES

Kunin C.M. (1967) A guide to use of antibiotics in patients with renal disease. *Ann. Int. Med.* **67,** 151.

Slapak M., Lee H.M. & Hume D.M. (1968) Transplant lung—a new syndrome. *Br. med. J.* i, 80.

Woodruff M.F.A., Nolan B., Bowie J.H. & Gould J.C. (1968) The Nuffield Transplantation Surgery Unit. *Lancet*, i, 905.

ACKNOWLEDGEMENTS

I should like to thank Dr S.O.B. Roberts for dermatological advice; Mr D. Rosborough for orthopaedic advice; the Department of Medical Photography and Illustration (Addenbrooke's Hospital); Mrs J. Small for typing the chapter and Miss A. Trelogan for checking my proofs.

CHAPTER 8

Cancer and Transplantation

W.A.B. Smellie

Neoplasia is of practical importance in transplantation for a variety of reasons. Firstly, cancer cells may be transmitted unwittingly with the donor organ and may grow unchecked in the immunosuppressed recipient; secondly, neoplasia may develop *de novo* in the immunosuppressed patient; and thirdly, the question may arise of grafting an organ into a recipient previously suffering from a carcinoma, either of the organ to be replaced or elsewhere. Each of these aspects will be considered separately.

1 TRANSMISSION OF GROWTH WITH DONOR ORGAN

Numerous cases have now been reported of malignancy in a renal cadaveric donor being transmitted to the recipient. Sites of origin of these donor growths have included bronchus (Wilson *et al* 1968); breast (MacLean *et al* 1965), thyroid (Muiznieks *et al* 1968), larynx (McPhaul & McIntosh 1965) and liver (Zukoski *et al* 1970). The interval between transplantation and the appearance of growth in the recipient has varied from between several months to 2 years. Of particular interest among these reported cases has been the experience first of the Brigham group (Wilson *et al* 1968) and later of Zukoski (Zukoski *et al* 1970) of tumour regressing or indeed actually being rejected after the cessation of immunosuppressive therapy.

These unfortunate incidents have lead to the widespread exclusion as organ donors of all patients dying from neoplasia of organs other than the brain. Although secondary spread is exceptionally uncommon from tumours arising within the skull, either from the brain substance or from the meninges, it can indeed occur, and we have recently performed an orthotopic liver transplant for a patient whose own organ was largely replaced by meningioma, the primary tumour had been removed some 5 years previously. From a practical point of view however, patients dying from brain tumours are highly suitable organ donors, and there has been no recorded case of malignant disease transmitted by their use.

2 SPONTANEOUS DEVELOPMENT OF NEOPLASIA IN IMMUNOSUPPRESSED INDIVIDUALS

This has long been feared on theoretical grounds, and has now been reported on numerous occasions (Doak *et al* 1968; Woodruff 1968; Starzl *et al* 1970). The great majority of these growths have arisen in the reticulo-endothelial system, though others have occurred in skin, testis, cervix, and bowel (Starzl *et al* 1970) Whether neoplasia in sites other than the reticulo-endothelial system is statistically more common in immunosuppressed than normal individuals remains a matter of doubt; a prospective trial recently organized by the British Medical Research Council to follow the progress of immunosuppressed patients, both transplanted and otherwise, should produce a definite answer to this question. The classical explanation of neoplasia in immunosuppressed individuals is that immunosuppression inhibits a cellular mechanism normally responsible for the destruction of spontaneously arising tumours. This fails to explain why the reticulo-endothelial system itself should be the site most often affected; one would have expected that all tissues should be equally at risk. An alternative suggestion to satisfy this objection has been that chronic stimulation of the reticulo-endothelial system by the antigen of the graft, or by the immunosuppressive drugs themselves, can produce somatic mutation leading to malignant change. A further possibility is that immunosuppression allows unimpeded growth of neoplasia inducing viruses similar to the experimental viral tumours of chickens (Rous 1911) and rabbits (Shope 1932). As yet all these theories remain matters of conjecture with very little evidence to support any one of them.

3 NEOPLASIA IN THE PROPOSED RECIPIENT

Pre-existing cancer in the recipient has long been regarded as a contra-indication to organ transplantation and subsequent immunosuppression (*Lancet* 1969). Certainly, previously 'successfully' treated growths have 'reawakened' after the onset of immunosuppression, leading to the death of the recipient. Hume (Hume 1968) has described such a case, where recurrent Wilm's tumour caused death 2 years after transplantation and 2½ years after removal of the original tumour. The experience of Starzl (Starzl 1969) with local and distant malignant recurrence following hepatectomy and orthotopic liver replacement for juvenile hepatoma has been similarly disappointing. However, there have been clear exceptions to this gloomy expectation, for Woodruff (Woodruff 1969) has a case now alive and recurrence free 5 years after renal transplantation and immuno-suppression following the removal of bilateral hypernephromata. We have an adult case of hepatoma treated by hepatectomy and orthotopic liver graft in good health and recurrence free 23 months post-transplantation. Our experience with liver tumours, both cholangiocarcinomata and hepa-tomata, has been that malignant recurrence after hepatectomy and ortho-topic liver grafting is rather unpredictable, an observation confirmed by others (Fortner 1970). Provided that the primary tumour and any local spread can be removed *en bloc*, we feel that advanced malignancy is not an absolute contraindication to hepatic transplantation. Quite clearly, malig-nancy in a proposed recipient is a very unfavourable situation, but under special circumstances an organ transplant may be justifiable, and on occasion has produced results far superior to conventional therapy.

REFERENCES

DOAK P.B., MONTGOMERIE J.Z., NORTH J.D.K. & SMITH F. (1968) Reticulum cell sarcoma after renal homotransplantation and azathioprine and prednisone therapy. *Br. Med. J.* ii, 764.

FORTNER J.E., SHIV M.H. & BEATTIE E.J. (1970) Long term management of clinical orthotopic and heterotopic liver homografts. Unpublished data. Paper read to 5th Congress of European Society for Experimental Surgery Venice.

HUME D.M. (1968) In *Human Transplantation*, ed. RAPAPORT & DAUSSET, **10,** 112.

LANCET, Leading article Lancet i, 505 (1969) Immunosuppression and cancer.

MACLEAN L.D., DOSSETOR J.B., GAULT M.H., OLIVER J.A., INGLIS F.G. & MAC-KINNON K.J. (1965) Renal homotransplantation using cadaver donors. *Arch. Surg. Chic.* **91,** 288.

MCPHAUL J.J. & MCINTOSH D.A. (1965) Tissue transplantation still vexes. *New Eng. J. Med.* **272,** 105.

Muiznieks H.W., Berg J.W., Lawrence W. & Randall H.T. (1968) Suitability of donor kidneys from patients with cancer'. *Surgery St. Louis*, **64**, 871.

Rous P. (1911) Viral aetiology of cancer in birds. *J. exp. Med.* **56**, 198.

Shope R.E. (1932) Viral aetiology of cancer in the rabbit. *J. exp. Med.* **56**, 793.

Starzl T.E. (1969) *Experience in Hepatic Transplantation*, p. 350. W.B. Saunders.

Starzl T.E. *et al* (1970) Unpublished data submitted to *Surgery, St. Louis.*

Wilson R.E., Hager E.B., Hampers C.L., Corson J.M., Merrill J.P. & Murray J.E. (1968) Immunologic rejection of human cancer transplanted with renal allograft. *New Eng. J. Med.* **278**, 479.

Woodruff M.F.A. (1968) Quoted in *Lancet* annotation i, 1299.

Woodruff M.F.A. (1969) Immunosuppression and cancer. *Lancet* i, 672.

Zukoski C.F., Killen D.A., Ginn E., Matter B., Lucas D.O. & Seigler H.F. (1970) Transplanted carcinoma in an immunosuppressed patient. *Transplantation*, **9**, 71.

Part 2
Kidney Transplantation

CHAPTER 9

The Selection of Cadaver Donors and Removal of Kidneys for Transplantation

R.A. Sells

INTRODUCTION

Since kidneys are bilateral organs, it is possible to transplant a kidney from a live related or unrelated donor to a suitable recipient. The operations can be performed electively, and live donor nephrectomy and transplantation into a well prepared recipient provides a graft exposed to a short ischaemic time which should function immediately after implantation. There is also convincing evidence that grafts from related donors carry a higher success rate than cadaveric kidneys, a point discussed more fully elsewhere. Frequently however there is no suitable live donor and in order to treat patients dying of renal failure when long term dialysis is not available, cadaveric renal transplantation is obligatory.

SELECTION OF THE CADAVER KIDNEY DONOR

Before any decision is made to remove organs from a potential donor the situation and condition of the patient must be considered in relation to certain basic rules of transplantation, outlined here:

1. Legal requirements

In Great Britain the 'use of parts of bodies of deceased persons for therapeutic purposes' is governed by the Human Tissues Act of 1961. Contained in the same Act are regulations concerning the use of bodies for medical education, research and cremation of bodies after anatomical examination; no allowance is made for extra urgency involved in the removal of organs for grafting. The relevant parts of this Act are quoted below in full.

'1 (1) If any person, either in writing at any time or orally in the presence of two or more witnesses during his last illness has expressed a request that his body or any specified part of his body be used after his death for therapeutic purposes or for purposes of medical education or research, the person lawfully in possession of his body after his death may, unless he has reason to believe the request was subsequently withdrawn, authorize the removal from the body of any part or, as the case may be, the specified part, for use in accordance with the request.

'(2) Without prejudice to the foregoing subsection, the person lawfully in possession of the body of a deceased person may authorize the removal of any part from the body for use for the said purposes, if, having made such reasonable enquiry as may be practicable, he has no reason to believe:

'(a) that the deceased had expressed an objection to his body being so dealt with after his death, and had not withdrawn it; or
'(b) that the surviving spouse or any surviving relative of the deceased objects to the body being so dealt with.

'(3) Subject to subsections (4) and (5) of this section, the removal and use of any part of a body in accordance with an authority given in pursuance of this section shall be lawful.

'(4) No such removal shall be effected except by a fully registered medical practitioner, who must have satisfied himself by personal examination of the body that life is extinct.

'(5) Where a person has reason to believe that an inquest may be required to be held on any body or that a post-mortem examination of any body may be required by the coroner, he shall not, except with the consent of the coroner,—

'(a) give an authority under this section in respect of the body; or
'(b) act on such authority given by any other person'.

Therefore in the absence of permission having been given for organ removal by the dead person during his or her lifetime, the permission of the nearest relative must be sought before organ removal can be carried out. This applies to the majority of prospective donors, whose wishes are not known to the practitioner who certifies death. The possible exceptions to this are the occasions when sudden death occurs and the death certificate cannot immediately be issued. Under these circumstances the coroner will require a post-morten examination, and if every attempt to contact the relatives has been unsuccessful a Coroner may permit a member of the transplant team to carry out a preliminary examination which enables the removal of organs before irreversible damage occurs.

It is now widely accepted that in cases where death is certain to occur after withdrawal of support (e.g. in the case of decerebrate patient on a respirator, or with an artificially stimulated heart beat) consent of the relatives must of course be obtained. The diagnosis of irreversible brain damage, the decision that death is inevitable and that artificial support should be withdrawn, must be made by two experienced practitioners independent of the transplant team. One of these doctors should be registered for more than 5 years. It is important that the transplant team should be alerted to the situation so that minimal delay should occur between certification of death of the donor and removal of the organs.

Experience in the transplant unit at Cambridge, England, suggests that despite adverse publicity, public opinion now is in favour of transplantation. There is no doubt, however, that exposure of a donor's family by publication of intimate details in the national press can influence the relatives' decision. For this reason it is important to inform the relatives at the time of the interview that the details of the patient's identity will remain undisclosed.

2. Renal function

If possible an accurate assessment of renal function should be made prior to death. This is clearly impractical if the potential donor is brought to the hospital dead. A detailed questionnarie on the deceased person's previous diseases and bodily functions is obviously an unjustifiable burden to impose on the bereaved relatives, but enquiries should be made about the dead person's general health, in particular with respect to renal disease, chronic hypertension, diabetes and malignant disease, all of which will normally exclude the patient from being a donor. Patients maintained on respirators, however, usually have closely monitored renal function and blood pressure and more useful data is therefore forthcoming. The daily urine volume, specific gravity and urea output are good indices of renal function. Blood urea and creatinine levels are also useful, but a potential source of error in the judgment of kidney performance may arise in a patient with a head injury who has received a large intravenous dose of urea in whom kidney function is satisfactory despite a high blood urea level. Similarly, some patients suffering from intracerebral or subarachnoid haemorrhage may have a raised blood urea, which does not necessarily indicate impaired renal function.

In the investigation of prospective donors, unnecessary sampling of blood or tests which are not in the patient's own interest are best avoided: the interval between the decision that the prognosis is hopeless and turning off the respirator will usually be fairly short, so evidence regarding renal function (urinary output) will be ascertainable almost up to the time of death, without necessarily having to take extra blood samples. One possible exception to this is the taking of blood for tissue-typing. This is obviously not in the patient's own interest and the withdrawal of blood for such an investigation could, in some people's view, be a matter for litigation on the grounds of assault. No doubt any future revision of the law in respect of premortem investigation of potential tissue donors will include allowances for this sort of essential investigation.

Oliguria is common in patients who have been on a respirator for more than a day or two, because positive pressure ventilation causes hypotension with a subsequent fall in glomerular perfusion pressure and filtration fraction. This development does not necessarily prohibit the use of such kidneys, as the parenchyma other than the glomeruli is still being perfused with oxygenated blood, and recovery may occur when the kidney is perfused with recipient blood at a normal pressure. It seems that the prolonged administration of vasopressor agents (e.g. Noradrenaline) in the premortem phase does increase the incidence of irreversible renal damage, but little experimental work has been done on this topic. It is difficult to generalize on this subject, where so many uncontrollable variables operate, but a useful empirical rule is that anuria which has persisted for more than 12 hours renders the kidneys untransplantable.

3. **Infection**

One exceedingly important source of danger to the transplant recipient is transferred infection. Introduction of pathogens via the graft into the circulation of a patient on immunosuppressives may produce uncontrollable sepsis and death. Therefore all donors should be very carefully examined clinically and bacteriologically for evidence of sepsis. Prolonged positive pressure respiration in an unconscious patient usually leads to ciliary depression, mucus retention and bronchopneumonia, despite vigorous bronchial toilet. The infecting organisms are commonly gram negative bacteria (e.g. *E coli*, *pseudomonas pyocyanea*) and staphylococci; resistant strains may be present, resulting from prophylactic antibiotics. The presence of an indwelling catheter is also a source of infection causing both ascending renal tract infection and intermittent bacteraemia. In transplantation of organs from cases of respirator death, it is the practice at Cambridge routinely to give a recipient a single, intravenous dose of Ampicillin and Cloxacillin to cover the possibility of a transient bacteraemia at the time of the transplant operation.

4. Cancer in the donor

Patients dying from cancer of any system other than primary growths of the central nervous tissue should be excluded from consideration as donors because of the possibility of tumour transference. There is no doubt that transplantation of tumour cells in humans can be followed by uncontrollable spread of the disease in the recipient; the importance of this factor justifies the inclusion in this chapter of some case reports. Scanlon & Hawkins *et al* (1965) reported the death of a woman 4 months after the subcutaneous transplantation of a malignant melanoma from her daughter. The piece of tissue measured 0·5 cm in diameter and the condition of the daughter being hopeless, the transplant was carried out in order to obtain a serum antibody which might, when reinjected into the donor, cause remission of her disease: the recipient succumbed 4 months later with disseminated melanomatous carcinomatosis. Deaths due to widespread carcinomatous deposits derived from donor primary lesions have been reported in cases where the donor was found to be suffering from bronchogenic, mammary and laryngeal carcinomas. In one case where the donor suffered from breast cancer the graft was removed from the recipient 5 days after transplantation because of infection. Histological examination of the specimen revealed carcinomatous deposits in the kidney (MacLean, Dosseter *et al* 1965).

The same authors reported transplantation of a kidney removed from a man who had a known growth of the colon, who died of secondary deposits. The fate of the recipient has not been reported. Inadvertent transplantation of bronchogenic carcinoma occurred in a 46-year-old recipient of a kidney who died of dissemination of the carcinoma 5 months after the operation (Martin, Rubini *et al* 1965). A similar case, with a happier outcome, was reported by Wilson, Hager *et al* in 1968; 18 months after receiving a transplant the patient developed secondary deposits histologically similar to a carcinoma of the bronchus found in the donor, which was unsuspected at the time of the transplant. On the assumption that all homologous tissue would be rejected, immunosuppression was stopped but although the kidney homograft showed signs of rejection the tumour continued to grow. The homograft was then removed, following which the tumour regressed. The patient recovered and recently received another graft without sign of recurrence.

Zukoski *et al* (1970), showed a similar course of events in a patient who received his second renal allograft from a donor dying of a primary hepatic carcinoma; 29 months after the transplant radiological evidence of disseminated tumour was found in the recipient's lung. Immunosuppression was stopped, but the expected regression of the metastases did not occur. Finally the renal allograft was removed and the tumour growth continued unabated until 39 months after the transplant operation when it suddenly regressed. Two weeks later radiological appearances were normal. The patient subsequently received a third allograft and died shortly afterwards. Autopsy revealed no sign of disseminated cancer.

There are cases where malignant donor disease has not been transplanted, despite the existence of an occult primary diagnosed at post mortem examination of the donor. One recipient at St Mary's Hospital (Peart 1969) is alive and well after transplantation of a kidney taken from a man with carcinoma of the oesophagus.

From studying these case reports it is unjustifiable to assume that if vicarious transplantation of a tumour has occurred with a renal allograft its rejection will automatically follow if anti-rejection therapy is discontinued, particularly as donor-patient antigen disparity diminishes with the more widespread use of tissue typing. It is significant that in the two successfully treated cases, regression, probably rejection, of the tumour did not occur until the allograft was removed. In experimental tumour transplantation metastatic lesions have frequently been shown to regress following excision of the primary transplanted lesion. It seems fair to assume that in these clinical cases removal of a large proportion of the antigen mass, as well as cessation of suppression, is necessary for sufficient recovery of the host's immune responses to reject tumour tissue.

Occasionally a 'free' kidney may arise from a case of benign papilloma of the ureter, or bladder involving ureter, and where obligatory nephrectomy is the treatment of choice. It is known that the urinary epithelium in such patients is unstable and the possibility of further benign or malignant lesions subsequently developing in such a kidney must not be discounted. A patient of Ellis (1969) received such a graft which is functioning normally 2 years after the operation without sign of recurrent neoplasia.

The kidney is not an uncommon site for metastases to occur; following the detection of thyroid carcinoma deposits in a kidney which was removed 7 days after transplantation Muiznieks, Berg *et al* (1968) showed by analysing post-mortem data of patients who died of growths in the head and neck that 5% of carcinomas and 10% of sarcomas have detectable renal metastases; comparable figures are not available for primary cancers from other sites. On the other hand metastases of primary tumours of the central nervous system practically never occur outside the cranial cavity and victims of this type of growth may safely be considered potential donors.

5. Age of donor

The oldest donor kidney used so far at Cambridge came from a patient of 72 and the youngest was from a child of 4 years. In the case of the older age group, (i.e. over 50 years) so long as renal function has been satisfactory prior to death the kidneys may be used and overall comparison of kidneys function after grafting from young or old age groups does not reveal any significant difference. However, kidneys obtained from the older age group may not tolerate prolonged warm ischaemia time as well as do kidneys from the young donors (Tables 1 and 2) in an analysis of 93 cadaveric kidneys (Sells & Pena 1970). Comparison of the post-transplant oliguric period in

TABLE 1. The oliguric period of cadaveric kidneys from donors older than 50 years

Donor	Brought in dead	Died in the ward
Average total warm ischaemic time	97 min	58 min
Average	52 years	51 years
Average duration of transplant oliguria	21 days	11 days

TABLE 2. The oliguric period of cadaveric kidneys from donors younger than 40 years

Donor	Brought in dead	Died in ward
Average total warm ischaemic time	93 min	58 min
Average age	30 years	39 years
Average duration of transplant oliguria	13 days	9 days

kidneys taken from cases of over 50 years old, brought in dead from outside hospital, and after dying in hospital, showed that the average warm ischaemic time was 39 minutes longer in the former group. Diuresis of these kidneys occurred later than those kidneys which had a shorter warm ischaemic time (Table 1). Similar analysis of younger donors (Table 2) shows that kidneys from such donors tolerate a prolonged warm ischaemia better.

With regard to the extremely young donor it is technically difficult to transplant the kidneys from a child less than 2 years old. Kidneys from very young donors should be used with caution as the presence of hypertension in the recipient may cause oedema of the kidney with subsequent vascular and parenchymal damage.

PREPARATION FOR REMOVAL OF KIDNEYS

The efficient and rapid removal of cadaver kidneys for transplantation depends on smooth communication, co-operation between doctors and nurses responsible for the dying or dead individual, and operating facilities which can be rapidly mobilized. In the case of people brought in dead to the hospital one of the biggest problems is contacting the relatives and obtaining permission before the maximum permissible warm ischaemia time has elapsed. Early identification of the person and enlisting the co-operation of the police in transporting the relatives to the hospital will all help to shorten this interval.

1. The relatives

In the delicate and stressful situation which the transplant surgeon and relatives are faced with much depends on the tact of the doctor who is required to interview and obtain consent. In the case of the prospective cadaveric donor in whom death is inevitable it is essential that the physician looking after the case should leave the relatives in no doubt as to the precise nature of the prognosis and the reasons for which he is withdrawing artificial support. It is only after this ground has been prepared that the transplant surgeon can request permission of the relatives for the removal of organs without appearing to be in some way involved in the management of the patient. It is also important that the nursing staff involved in the terminal care of the donor should be informed of developments, in particular the decision for withdrawal of suport and the likelihood that the patient's organs will be used for transplantation. It is impossible to formulate the precise questions that the transplant surgeon should ask the relatives. Although relatives of patients who are dead or who are about to die are usually in a state of emotional confusion, personal experience suggests that people are usually quite capable of coming to a rational and humane decision. Most relatives will make the decision which they feel accords best with the wishes of the deceased individual.

2. Logistics

If brain death has been diagnosed and it has been decided to stop mechanical ventilation the transplantation team can be informed so that there will be no delay in removing the kidney when the circulation ceases. Clearly, however, the dead person brought into hospital poses a very different problem. Where a working arrangement exists between the casualty department and the transplant team one or two members of the team may be alerted after death has been certified. Long-range radio receivers are extremely useful in a situation where the casualty department may need to call the transplant team over fairly long distances. After certification of death, blood should be taken for grouping and tissue-typing and the appropriate departments notified that donor kidneys may shortly become available. After permission has been obtained the donor is taken to theatre, where pre-sterilized instruments and pre-cooled perfusion fluids are ready.

3. The operation

Cadaver donor nephrectomy should be carried out using standard aseptic precautions in an operating theatre with good illumination. The minimum staff required are a surgeon, one assistant and a scrub nurse. In addition

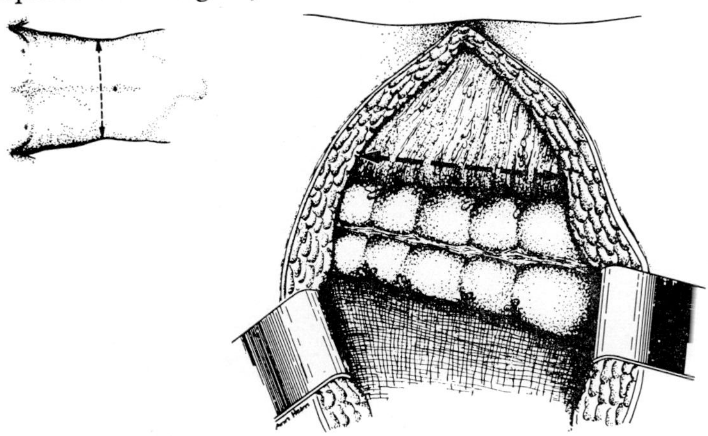

FIG. 1. Cadaver donor nephrectomy—the abdominal incision and mobilization of the left colon.

there should be one nurse who need not scrub who attends to the perfusion fluids, and one other person to fetch extra equipment, alter the lighting as necessary, and deal with the inevitable incoming telephone calls. It is difficult to achieve these ideal conditions at very short notice. Nevertheless it is important to aim at the ideal situation for the surgeon to carry out an accurate dissection of the renal vessels.

A bilateral subcostal incision is used (Calne 1969) extending across the abdomen joining both axillary lines in the coronal plane (Fig. 1). The muscles and peritoneum are divided with a knife, care being taken not to damage the bowel. The left kidney is approached from the left side by reflecting the descending colon forwards. This is achieved by dividing the peritoneum of the paracolic gutter, extending this incision up to the splenic flexure and down to the pelvic colon. The bowel can then be moved medially, exposing the perinephric fat. The plane between this tissue and the renal capsule is found by scissors dissection and this plane is best developed by blunt dissection, working the fingers upwards and downwards, freeing the kidney from the surrounding tissue.

The renal vessels are next dissected: the renal vein normally lies anterior to the artery and is a single trunk crossing the aorta and draining into the vena cava which lies to the right of the mid-line. The vein on the left is therefore rather longer than on the right. It is best approached by dissecting in the tissue 1 inch medial to the hilum of the kidney and it can be recognized as a broad vessel receiving two vertical tributaries, the adrenal vein from above and the gonadal vein from below. These vessels are divided between ligatures, the renal vein is dissected free posteriorly, great care

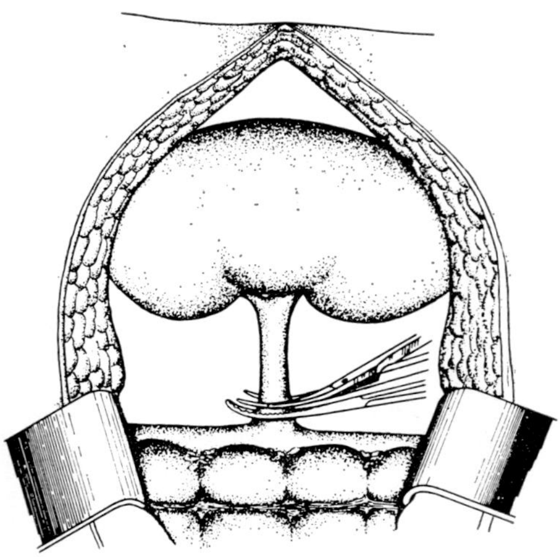

FIG. 2. Dividing the renal vein.

being taken not to damage the adjacent artery, a clamp is placed at its junction with the vena cava and the vein is divided cleanly (Fig. 2). Occasionally some variation of the venous drainage of the kidney is encountered, usually in the form of a small accessory vein draining separately into the vena cava. This may safely be divided, as collateral intra-renal anastomoses exist. If however two renal veins of equal size are encountered or a double renal vein which fuses near the vena cava to form a single trunk, it is best to take a cuff of vena cava with the renal vein or veins.

The dissection of the renal artery is more difficult because variation of the arterial supply to the kidney is commonly encountered, usually in the form of accessory vessels going to the upper pole: as the arterial supply to the kidney is segmental, each vessel is an end artery and intra-renal anastomosis does not occur. Division of a polar vessel will therefore result in infarction of the area supplied by this vessel. Bearing this in mind the surgeon next dissects the angle between the upper pole of the kidney and the aorta. By dissecting outside the capsule to the upper pole of the kidney the adrenal gland may be lifted off the capsule; the connective tissue is divided and a polar vessel can usually be detected with the finger and thumb placed medial to the upper pole of the kidney. By extending this dissection medially the upper part of the aorta is exposed and if a high polar vessel exists then a separate patch of aorta is taken bearing this vessel. The aorta is then cleaned down to the origin of the main renal artery and the patch of aorta from which this arises is excised. If a single renal trunk is found a Carrel patch is not mandatory for satisfactory

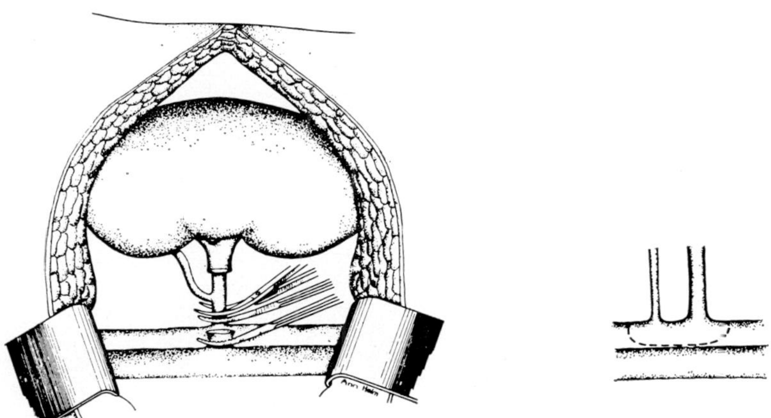

(a) (b)

FIG. 3. (a) Dividing the renal artery. (b) The extent of an aortic patch required when a polar artery is encountered.

anastomosis unless the kidney is small, and the artery may be divided at its origin (Fig. 3). Occasionally smaller vessels arise lower down the aorta and a careful examination for this abnormality should be made before dividing the connective tissue medial to the ureter.

The ureter is then identified, and the peritoneum stripped off it down to the pelvic brim. The ureter should not be cleaned of its adventitia as this tissue contains blood vessels supplying it from the renal artery. The ureter is divided cleanly at the pelvic brim and the kidney is removed and put straight into a bowl of ice cold saline (Fig. 5).

Removal of the right kidney is performed from the right side of the abdomen in a manner similar to that used on the left side. The relative lengths of the vessels is of course different: the renal vein, being fairly short, should be divided at its junction with the vena cava. The origin of the renal artery will be less accessible to the operator and this vessel has to be traced behind the vena cava to its origin from the aorta.

The kidney may then be perfused with an ice-cold fluid prior to storage on ice. At Cambridge, kidneys are perfused with a mixture described by Brunius *et al* (1968) consisting of 5% Rheomacrodex in a buffer/electrolyte solution and followed by a mixture of equal volumes of 10% invert sugar

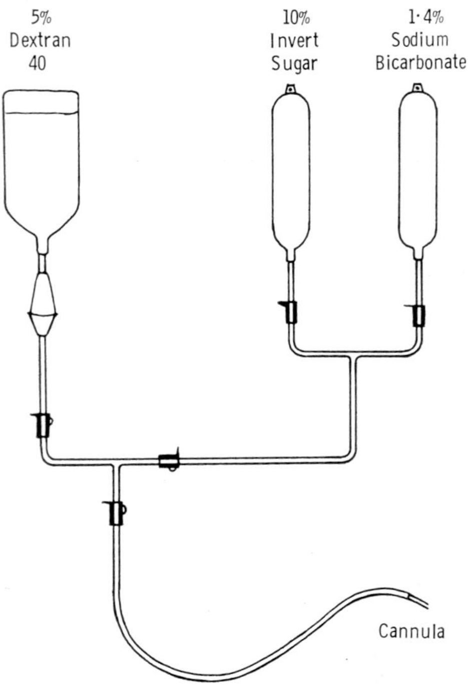

Fig. 4.

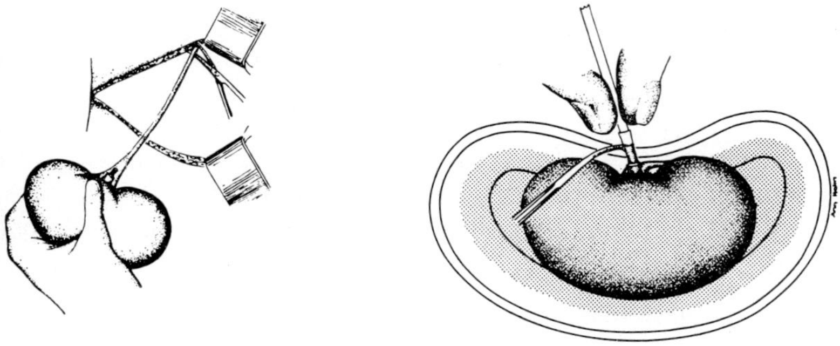

(a) (b)

FIG. 5. (a) Dividing the ureter. (b) Perfusing the kidney.

and 1·4% sodium bicarbonate solution. These solutions are kept cool in a domestic refrigerator and are administered through a pre-sterilized drip set (Fig. 4). The drip set nozzle (Fig. 5) is inserted into the renal artery osteum and approximately 200 ml of Rheomacrodex is infused until the renal vein effluent is clear. The solutions are then changed to the fructose/bicarbonate solution (mixed immediately before use) and about 200 ml are infused. A rapid and even passage of perfusion fluid through the kidney usually results in the cortex achieving a uniform pale colour within a few minutes of the perfusion starting. A diseased kidney or one which has undergone severe ischaemic damage and oedema will usually fail to perfuse easily and the cortex becomes blotchy and the kidney feels turgid. If a kidney fails to perfuse evenly it is not normally considered suitable for transplantation. Occasionally agonal release of noradrenaline or pre-mortem administration of vasoactive drugs causes profound constriction of the renal vessels in a kidney where the ischaemia time is low, which may lead to poor initial perfusion of the organ. In such cases the addition of procaine to the perfusate or the external application of 4% papaverine to the artery frequently improves the vascular spasm and enables satisfactory perfusion. The perfused kidney is put into a sterile plastic bag containing a little of the perfusion fluid to improve dissipation of heat and prevent damage from direct contact with ice, the bag is sealed with a rubber band and this is in turn placed in another sterile bag also containing fluid. This bag is sealed with a rubber band and placed in a vacuum flask containing crushed ice. A little more ice is put on top of the bag and the flask is gently stoppered.

The accidental division of a polar vessel may be immediately obvious to the surgeon after he has removed the kidney. If it is not obvious then it will become so after perfusing the kidney, for a discrete patch of persistently dark cortex will remain while the rest of the kidney achieves a homogenous pale colour (Fig. 6). Another less common cause of technical failure at the time of kidney removal is unsuspected damage to the intima of the renal artery by excessive traction, a complication to which atheromatous vessels are particularly prone (Fig. 7).

It is particularly important to recognize this complication at the time of perfusion, for the flow of arterial blood in such a vessel at the time of transplantation will lead to dissection and arterial occlusion. Atheromatous vessels should therefore be gently explored with a blunt probe before storage in ice.

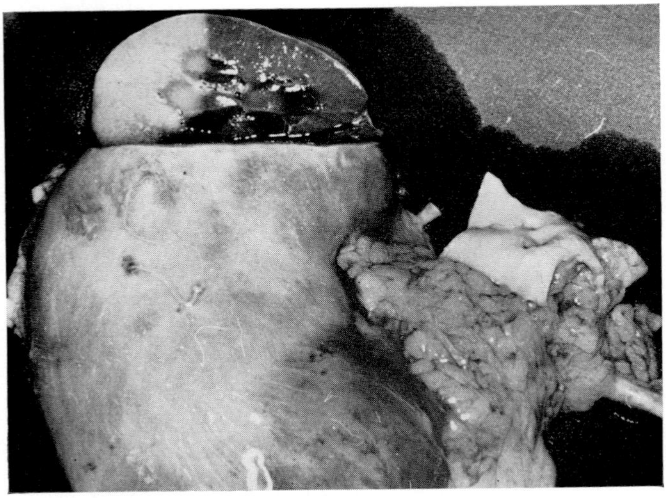

Fig. 6.

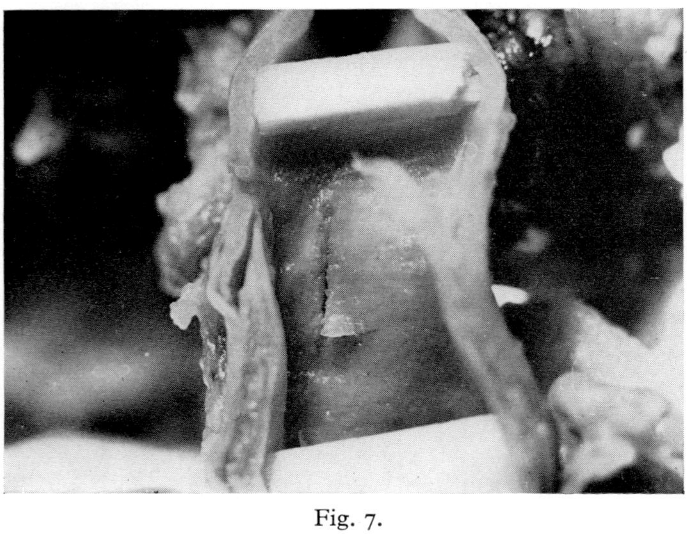

Fig. 7.

4 The en-bloc technique

An alternative technique to that described above is the en-bloc removal of both kidneys with a segment of aorta and vena cava without prior dissection of the renal vessels. The main disadvantages are two-fold. Firstly, to be absolutely certain that a high polar artery is not divided at the time of removal, the operator is obliged to dissect very carefully the area between the upper pole and the aorta; blind transection of the aorta cannot be carried out high enough or accurately enough to assure consistent safety of abnormal polar arteries. Secondly, the kidneys and their vessels will have to be dissected free of periaortic tissue removed with the renal axis and the ends of the vessels prepared for suturing. This is obviously not ideally performed whilst the kidney is being perfused, or immersed in a bowl of cold saline, and might just as well be done at the time of kidney removal.

The time taken for nephrectomy is not significantly reduced using this method, although cold perfusion of both kidneys in situ is possible through an aortic cannula inserted prior to dissection. The merits of this technique have not been assessed but would appear to confer a marginally reduced warm ischaemia time (Sells, unpublished data).

The former technique of cadaveric kidney removal has been used at Cambridge and other transplant centres with consistently good results, providing the proper facilities and opportunities for co-operative effort have existed. It has been found possible to enlist the help of outlying hospitals in obtaining donor organs; in these places the operation may be carried out by the resident surgical officer and provided the interval between death of the donor and cooling of the kidney is not more than 1 hour, the organ may be kept on ice long enough to allow tissue-typing and transport to the best recipient within the United Kingdom and Ireland. This means that the area from which donor kidneys are available need not be very close geographically to the transplant centre, and with a high degree of co-operation between general and neurosurgeons and the regional transplant centre, a large supply of donors should become available within any region. The practical aspects such as the supply of instruments to peripheral hospitals and instruction in removal and storage of kidneys are easily dealt with. Any difficulties encountered in this respect are small by comparison with the resistance to using cadaveric organs shown by many doctors in charge of respirator cases, and those who certify dead people. It is to be hoped that with a growing awareness of the flexibility of allocation of kidneys (enabled by the prolonged permissible ischaemic time) and the practicability of the removal technique, that co-operation of hospital doctors will improve and the number of wasted organs will diminish.

REFERENCES

BRUNIUS U. BERGENTZ S-E., EKMAN H., GELIN L.E., WESTBERG G. (1968) The cadaveric kidney in clinical transplantation. *Scand. J. Urol. Nephrol.* **2,** 15.

CALNE R.Y. (1969) Cadaveric kidneys for transplantation. *Br. med. J.* ii, 565.

ELLIS F.G. (1969) Personal communication.

HUMAN TISSUE ACT (1961) H.M.S.O.

MACLEAN L.D., DOSSETER J.B., GAULT M.H., OLIVER J.A., INGLES F.G. & MCKINNON K.J. (1965) Renal homotransplantation using cadaver donors. *Arch. Surg. Chicago,* **91,** 288.

MARTIN D.C., RUBINI M. & ROSEN V.J. (1965) Cadaveric renal homotransplantation with inadvertent transplantation of carcinoma. *J. Am. Med. Assoc.* **192,** 82.

MUIZNIEKS H.W., BERG J.W., LAWRENCE W. & RANDALL H.T. (1968) The suitability of donor kidneys from patients with cancer. *Surgery St. Louis,* **64,** 871.

OSGOOD E.E. (1959) Regulation of cell proliferation. In *The Kinetics of Cellular Proliferation,* ed. STOHLMAN F., p. 282. Grune & Stratton, New York.

PEART S. (1969) Personal communication.

SCANLON E.F., HAWKINS R.A., FOX W.W. & SCOTT SMITH W. (1965) Fatal homotransplanted melanoma—a case report. *Cancer N.Y.* **18,** 782.

SELLS R.A. & PENA J.R. (1970) Preservation of cadaveric kidneys for transplantation. *Lancet,* i, 539.

WILSON R.E., HAGER E.B., HAMPERS C.L., CORSON J.M., MERRILL J.P. & MURRAY J.E. (1968) Immunological rejection of human carcinoma transplanted with a renal allograft. *New Engl. J. Med.* **278,** 479.

ZUKOSKI C.F., KILLEN D.A., GINN E. & MATTER W. (1970) Transplanted carcinoma in an immunosuppressed patient. *Transplantation,* **9,** 71.

CHAPTER 10

Selection of Related Living Donors

W.A.B. Smellie

The results of renal transplantation from well matched related human donors are now so good that this method is likely to increase in popularity on both sides of the Atlantic. In Europe at present cadaveric donors outnumber related living donors by about three to one; in our own unit from a series of 142 transplants, related living donors have been used on seven occasions only. In America this trend is reversed, with the result that cadaveric and related living donors supply about equal numbers in the Transplant Registry's total analysis (Human Transplant Registry 1970). The reasons for this difference in attitudes on the two sides of the Atlantic are complex, but it may be significant that related living donors are least available in countries where the Welfare State is most strongly developed.

The motivation of the proposed donor is of extreme importance. He must not have been pressurized by the recipient, the remaining relatives, or the recipient's medical advisers. He must have the opportunity of frank discussion with an entirely independent physician, unconnected with the transplant programme, who can provide a convenient let-out if he considers that undue influences have been brought to bear on his patient. Twins are especially prone to emotional problems in this situation, and may indeed have a genuine sense of deprivation if not permitted to donate. Of interest here are the rulings of the Massachusetts Supreme Court on three occasions in 1956, allowing the donation of kidneys from minors to their identical twins, on the grounds that if the operations were not performed the deaths of the sick twins would result in 'a grave emotional impact' on the survivors (Louisell 1966). In general, however, the intended donor should have reached the age of consent to operation, which in England is 18.

The risks of the donor nephrectomy must be fully and frankly discussed with the intended donor and his adult dependents. Although slight, these risks are real. Several accounts are available of complications to the donor at or near the time of nephrectomy, including haemorrhage, fluid intoxication and pulmonary embolism. There have now been two unconfirmed reports of fatality following nephrectomy for transplantation, from more than 1600 operations performed.

The long-term hazard to a donor existing on one kidney alone has not yet been accurately defined, but appears to be very small, Trauma, infection and malignancy affecting the remaining kidney are the obvious risks, though there is not yet a report of serious morbidity arising in a donor as a result of any of these. There have been situations where the terminal renal disease of the proposed recipient is familial in nature and here of course the greatest care must be exercised in selection of a donor.

If a theoretically suitable donor is forthcoming it is sensible to undertake extensive physical examination supported by the necessary laboratory tests before accepting him for the programme. Several potential donors may be available from within the same family, and the one nearest the recipient in tissue typing is preferable. The donor must be in sound general health, over the age of 18, preferably under the age of 50, and with no past significant medical history, particularly of cardiovascular, chronic infective or malignant disease. A complete physical examination is undertaken, and provided no untoward signs are discovered special tests are performed. These entail:

1 Blood group and tissue-typing
2 Chest X-ray
3 Urine analysis
4 Urine culture
5 Creatinine clearance
6 Complete blood chemistry
7 Routine blood count
8 Blood clotting profile
9 Electrocardiogram
10 Intravenous pyelogram.

Incompatibility of blood groups between the intended donor and recipient is an absolute contra-indication to the proposed operation

(Starzl *et al* 1964). Differences in tissue-typing are more hard to evaluate. Some centres would insist on identity, as demonstrated by currently available typing methods, while others will not allow more than one major mismatch between donor and recipient. Each case here has to be judged on its own merits.

If the remaining investigations reveal no significant contra-indication, renal angiography is next performed. This must be of sufficient quality to exclude with certainty the presence of multiple renal arteries, a relative contra-indication to the use of that kidney as a donor organ (unlike the situation in a cadaveric donor when an aortic cuff, including the origin of both or all renal arteries may be excised).

If the donor has been passed as physically and mentally suitable he is transferred to the care of the surgeon who is to perform his nephrectomy and in whose clinical charge he should subsequently remain. Ideally this surgeon should not be a member of the transplanting team, so that his sole clinical responsibility is for the donor, and not for the recipient.

REFERENCES

8TH REPORT OF THE HUMAN TRANSPLANT REGISTRY (1970).

LOUISELL D.W. (1966) *Ethics in Medical Progress*. Ciba Symposium, p. 85.

STARZL T.E., MARCHIORO T.L., HOLMES J.H., HERMANN G., BRITTAIN P.S., STONINGH O.H., TALMAGE D.W. & WADDELL W.R. (1964) Renal Homografts in patients with major donor-recipient blood-group incompatibility. *Surgery*, **55**, 195.

CHAPTER 11

Living Donor Nephrectomy

J.F.R. Withycombe
W.A.B. Smellie

The donor is carefully investigated, as described in the previous section. The angiogram will have demonstrated the arterial supply to the kidneys, and a side with a single artery is selected. If both kidneys have a single artery the left is chosen for removal, because of the greater length of its vein.

The patient is anaesthetized with a standard intubation technique, using muscle relaxants. Great attention is paid to the state of hydration, and an intravenous infusion of 5% Dextrose should be started some hours before surgery. Mannitol 12·5 g should be given after the induction of anaesthesia and repeated 10 min before clamping the renal pedicle. By the time the kidney is removed, between $1\frac{1}{2}$–2 l of 5% Dextrose should have been given in the previous 5 hours, thus ensuring a moderate diuresis; this precaution has been shown in the laboratory and in transplanted patients to minimize the deleterous effects of renal ischaemia.

The patient is placed in the standard lateral position, and the kidney exposed through a long incision through the bed of the eleventh rib. Care is taken to handle the kidney as little as possible. The upper pole is mobilized first; here a very small artery arising from either the adrenal or the aorta itself may require ligaturing and dividing. The pedicle is next dissected, keeping as far away from the hilum as possible. The vein is best approached from in front; on the left the adrenal and gonadal veins must be identified and preserved if possible: on the right the vein may be very short, and its junction with the inferior vena cava must be clearly exposed. The kidney is now further mobilized and turned anteriorly and the ureter and renal artery identified. The course of the ureter is followed downwards towards the pelvis; if the hydration regime has been effective it will appear distended and with active peristalsis: on no account should it be stripped of its surrounding areolar tissue for fear of damaging the blood supply. The renal artery is now dissected as far away from the hilum as is possible. Care must be taken to avoid undue traction on the kidney, which may produce an intimal fracture within the artery. The kidney is now ready for removal.

When the recipient team have completely prepared their patient, a message is sent to the donor team. The renal artery is doubly ligatured in continuity with 00 silk and divided to produce as long a renal artery as is possible. The renal vein is now controlled with a Satinsky clamp; on the right this must be at the caval junction, but on the left may be just proximal to the adrenal and gonadal vein terminations. The vein is now divided and the kidney lifted into the wound. The ureter is followed downwards as far as possible, certainly to the pelvic brim and is ligatured with double 00 chromic catgut and divided at this level. The kidney is now removed with a considerable amount of periureteric areolar tissue and placed in a beaker of cold saline for delivery to the recipient team. All that now remains to be done is to oversew the renal vein stump with a continuous 5/0 arterial silk suture. The renal bed is drained and the incision closed in the routine way. The main renal vessels are irrigated with heparinized saline but the kidney is not normally perfused.

CHAPTER 12

Pre-operative Management of Patients

D.B. Evans

Until renal transplantation can guarantee an almost certain cure in patients with irreversible renal failure, it would not be justifiable to undertake this procedure until the patient has reached the terminal stages of renal failure, when survival cannot be further prolonged by conservative means.

MEDICAL MANAGEMENT

It is important first to establish the irreversibility of the condition in any patient with renal failure by excluding obstructive conditions of the outflow tract and salt and water losing states. Both these conditions if dealt with in time may allow useful renal function to return.

a **Dietary control**

Patients with severely impaired renal function may be satisfactorily managed conservatively for variable periods. Dietary restriction and control of electrolyte imbalance and infection may prolong life in slowly progressive conditions such as polycystic disease and pyelonephritis. Hypertension may accelerate the downhill progress so that adequate control with sodium restriction and hypotensive agents is important. Giordano (1963) and Giovanetti & Maggiore (1964) studied the effect of diets containing very low quantities of first class proteins and showed that nitrogen balance was improved and the blood urea levels were lowered in patients with minimal renal function with subsequent relief of gastrointestinal symptoms. Shaw *et al* (1965) adapted these diets to suit British palates—the main calorie source being low protein bread. Further work by Ford *et al* (1969) suggested that the rigorous control of protein and calories advocated by the previous workers was perhaps not necessary and found that approximately 0·5 g/kg body weight/day of protein (all classes) without high calorie intake would still allow the patients to remain in nitrogen balance. However, they emphasized that this form of treatment should only be a temporary measure and if prolonged unduly resulted ultimately in muscle wasting and deterioration in the general health of the patients. Uraemic complications (Table 1) will finally develop and unless dialysis or transplantation is available death of the patient is inevitable.

Ideally a prospective transplant recipient should be referred to a transplantation unit at a stage when regular medical supervision becomes necessary. In this way a psychological assessment can be made, the patient has an opportunity of acquainting himself with members of the transplantation team and gets used to the idea that when the time comes he will be prepared for transplantation before crippling complications supervene. If these complications do appear, dialysis can reverse them but at the cost of prolonged and expensive treatment.

b **Peritoneal dialysis**

Many patients will have been peritoneally dialysed before transfer to a transplantation unit. It is considered by most units as a valuable and life-saving form of treatment when haemodialysis facilities are not available. Peritoneal dialysis basically is a simple technique needing no capital expenditure and it can therefore be performed in the general wards of a hospital without the need of a special unit or specially trained nursing and technical personnel (Fig. 1). It has however certain disadvantages (see Table 2). Most transplant units consider peritoneal dialysis only as an interim treatment though transplantation programmes have been successfully supported (Cohen & Percival 1968) by the use of overnight peritoneal dialysis. Usually 48–72 h of peritoneal dialysis per week will maintain a patient in reasonable health for several months, but eventually hypoproteinaemia with wasting and peripheral neuropathies tend to develop. If haemodialysis is eventually contemplated, the insertion of a Teflon Silastic shunt (Quinton 1960) or the fashioning of a Brescia Cimino AV fistula can profitably be performed at this stage. Peritoneal dialysis can be performed

TABLE 1. Complications of 'Uraemia'

A	Cardiovascular	fluid and sodium retention leading to heart failure hypertension pericarditis and tamponade cardiomyopathy arrhythmias
B	Respiratory	'uraemic' pneumonitis haemoptysis
C	Gastrointestinal	peptic ulceration GI tract haemorrhage enterocolitis
D	Renal (metabolic) bone disease	osteoporosis osteomalacia (Rickets) hyperparathyroidism: secondary, tertiary osteosclerosis
E	Neurological	epileptiform convulsions cerebral haemorrhage peripheral neuropathy myopathy
F	Metastatic calcification	'pseudogout' arterial calcification
G	Chronic anaemia	
H	Endocrine	infertility and amenorrhoea loss of libido and potency
I	Skin	pigmentation pruritus
J	Growth	impairment in children

simply by the infusion of sterile dialysing fluid under gravity via a catheter (Trocath) into the peritoneal cavity and draining into a closed receptor bag slung under the bed. More sophisticated automatic cycling machines have been devised which incorporate large reservoirs of sterilized dialysis fluid and receptors (thus reducing the risk of infection) with monitoring equipment which economizes on nursing time. Control of electrolytes and acid-base balance can be achieved in this way. Potassium chloride needs to be added to the dialysing fluid in order that the patient's serum potassium level be kept at or around 3·5–4 mEq/l. Dialysis fluid is available containing

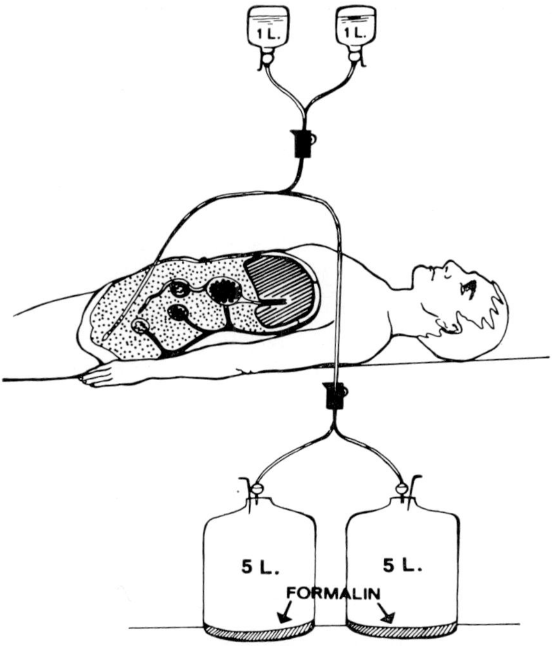

FIG. 1. Diagram to illustrate peritoneal dialysis.

either 1·36–1·5 g/100 ml or 6·36–7 g/100 ml of Dextrose. Under normal circumstances the former strength would be used, but if the patient is 'waterlogged', the solution containing the higher Dextrose concentration will facilitate the massive removal of excess extracellular fluid. Careful measurement of intake and output from the peritoneum and/or frequent weighing of the patient on a bed scale will provide a guide to the loss of weight achieved. With strict aseptic techniques a closed drainage system and the removal of the peritoneal catheter between dialyses, the risk of peritoneal infection is

TABLE 2. Disadvantages of peritoneal dialysis

Peritoneal infection and intestinal obstruction
Adhesions and loculation of dialysis fluid with loss of efficiency
Haemorrhage
Perforation of a viscus
Pain
Hypoproteinaemia
Hypo or hypervolaemia
Pulmonary collapse and infection
Rarely disequilibrium syndrome and lacticacidaemia

low. However, daily sampling of peritoneal fluid should be performed so that infection, if it occurs, can be treated early with appropriate systemic antibiotics.

c Haemodialysis

This is a more efficient and less traumatic form of therapy than peritoneal dialysis. The pioneer work of Kolff (1944) during the war developed haemodialysis as a treatment of acute renal failure and the work of Scribner (1960) made intermittent dialysis a life saving procedure for patients with terminal renal failure. Techniques have been simplified and automated so that haemodialysis is now considered a routine procedure which can be operated by a nurse and is available in most large hospital centres. Hospital dialysis facilities being limited, expansion into the field of home dialysis is increasing so that an integrated home dialysis training scheme running concomitantly with hospital dialysis and transplantation will be commonplace in the foreseeable future.

Two main haemodialysis systems are available currently:

1 modified Kiil dialysers (or disposable dialysers) run in conjunction with a warm (37°C) single pass dialysate supplied by either a tank or a proportionating system (Fig. 2). Monitoring and fail safe appliances render the system virtually 'foolproof' and with the development of heat sterilization and automation, the labours of the dialysis room assistant have been considerably lessened.

2 disposable coil dialysers incorporated in a recirculating system. The development of the Travenol Ultraflow coil using comparable membranes to those conventionally used in the Kiil dialyser and the reduction in the priming volume of the dialyser has improved considerably the efficiency of this type of dialyser.

Dialysis efficiency cannot be judged merely by the fall in the blood urea. Far more pertinent are the fluctuations in plasma creatinine, uric acid and phosphate, the improvement in patients' well being, muscle mass, renal bone disease, peripheral neuropathy and erythropoiesis. Experienced units therefore advocate a minimum dialysis period for patients of 28–30 h week (usually 14–15 h twice weekly). Further improvement has been found in patients dialysed thrice weekly for 10 h periods. This latter regime is eminently feasible for home dialysis but more difficult in hospital centres where dialysis space and staff are limited. The techniques of haemodialysis have been abundantly described by many workers and will not be considered here. The weakest link in the haemodialysis system has been the external AV shunt which may sometimes become infected and may suffer from recurrent clotting episodes necessitating repeated revisions. Some patients have little trouble and shunts may survive for 1–2 years, whereas others frequently have problems. The important contribution of Brescia *et al* (1966) in describing an internal AV fistula may prolong the life expectancy and allow greater freedom for patients on haemodialysis. The advantages of an internal fistula seem to outweight the disadvantages of needle punctures required at the beginning of dialysis. These AV fistulae should be

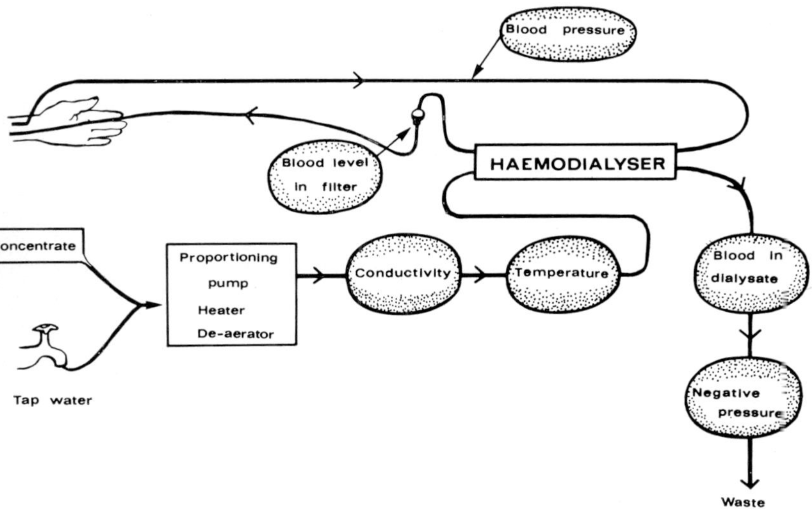

FIG. 2. Diagram to illustrate schematically a haemodialysis system.

performed by surgeons skilled in vascular work and care should be taken to make the anastomosis diameter 0·5–1 cm. Larger fistulae may cause significant shunting and lead to embarrassment of an already overburdened heart, with consequent precipitation of heart failure. Total heparinization of the dialysis patient is practiced where there is no evidence of bleeding, but in the presence of GI tract bleeding or pericarditis and during the first 14 days after a major operation, regional heparinization should be used—heparin being continuously infused by roller or syringe pump into the 'arterial line' and protamine sulphate infused via a similar pump, continuously into the 'venous line'. An attempt is made to keep the patient's clotting time as near normal as possible yet keeping the dialyser anticoagulated. This tends to be a tricky procedure requiring considerable care and monitoring by the nurse. It is often helpful to assess heparin/protamine doses by an *in vitro* assay beforehand. As soon as the patient is established on haemodialysis, a reappraisal of the hitherto strict dietary régime is made and the patient should be allowed a protein diet of at least 1 g/kg body weight, with vitamin supplements and sodium and potassium control depending on the presence or absence of hypertension and hyperkalaemia. A high calorie intake is encouraged. Fluid allowances can be judged according to urinary output and insensible loss (usually 400–500 ml plus previous day's urinary volume) and the use of hypotensive therapy should be practiced when necessary.

d **Transfusion**

The anaemia of chronic renal failure has been ascribed to several factors. Most patients are refractory to the usual haematinics though after a prolonged period of efficient haemodialysis, Crockett *et al* (1967) have found that by infusion of iron dextran, improved erythropoiesis can be achieved. However, many of our patients who are recipients of cadaver kidneys come to operation before reaching this stage. Multiple transfusions carry risks of transmitting hepatitis, cytomegalovirus (fresh blood) and of developing leucocyte antibodies. Ideally, in order to keep the haemoglobin at an acceptable level (arbitrarily 6 g%, PCV 20%) infusions of leucocyte free packed red cells should be administered during dialysis. Rendering the blood leucocyte free, however, is a tedious procedure and is not readily available in all centres.

e **Bilaterial nephrectomy**

The removal of the kidneys prior to transplantation is often a matter of personal choice. In some centres the indications are infected or potentially infected kidneys, ureteric reflux, polycystic disease, intractable hypertension and renal tumours. Other centres undertake bilateral nephrectomy routinely. In addition to eliminating infected or potentially infected foci, it may allow for a better interpretation of urinary findings after transplantation and possibly make the diagnostic problems of rejection a little less confusing. The removal of the kidneys through a transperitoneal approach as practised at this centre allows a careful examination of the whole of the intestinal tract. The presence of peptic ulceration, Meckel's diverticula, diverticular disease of the colon and foci of infection resulting from previous peritoneal dialysis can be detected and appropriate corrective procedures can be undertaken well before transplantation.

PREOPERATIVE COMPLICATIONS REQUIRING INVESTIGATION AND CORRECTION

1 Infections: bacterial, fungal, viral.
2 Peptic ulceration and/or GI tract bleeding.
3 Lower urinary tract abnormalities.
4 Hyperparathyroidism.
5 Hypertension.

1 A careful and extensive search should be made for infection in the recipient before transplantation. Routine culture of nose and throat swabs, faeces and urine for bacteria and fungi should be performed. Scribner shunt sites require great care and regular swabs are taken for culture. Appropriate antibiotic therapy or antifungal agents should be given whenever indicated. Physiotherapy preoperatively and cessation of smoking can reduce the risk of pulmonary infections in debilitated patients. The commonest post-operative infections usually arise from endogenous sources e.g. AV shunt sepsis may, in the presence of immunosuppressive drugs, result in septicaemia and metastatic abscesses and oral candidiasis may spread to produce painful candidal ulcers at the lower end of the oesophagus. Chronic urinary tract infection is an absolute indication for bilateral nephrectomy.

2 Peptic ulceration is a common accompaniment of chronic renal failure and may be aggravated by hyperparathyroidism (Barreras & Donaldson 1967). GI tract bleeding and a history of dyspepsia makes barium meal studies mandatory but this should probably be a routine investigation in all cases. Surgical correction of any abnormality should be performed well before transplantation is contemplated.

3 Cystography and cystoscopy are desirable to detect anatomical abnormalities such as ureterocoeles, bladder diverticula and bladder neck dysfunction and appropriate surgical procedures undertaken to correct these abnormalities.

4 Evidence of renal bone disease and metastatic calcification should be sought by careful skeletal survey and estimations of plasma calcium, phosphate and alkaline phosphatase. Primary hyperparathyroidsm may be the cause of renal failure and may be first diagnosed by observing the presence of nephrocalcinosis and bone pain or spontaneous fractures. Secondary hyperparathyroidism occurs commonly in association with renal failure and in many cases can be reversed by efficient haemodialysis with or without vitamin D. It has been clearly shown by Wing *et al* (1968) that dialysate calcium concentrations of 6 mg% will ensure calcium balance in these patients. If the hyperparathyroid state persists despite treatment an

autonomous state may have developed and it may be necessary to consider parathyroidectomy before embarking upon transplantation. Stanbury & Nicholson (1960) showed that subotal parathyroidectomy in a patient with severe secondary hyperparathyroidism allowed the bony lesions to heal with vitamin D therapy without producing hypercalcaemia. Ogg (1967) reported four cases with secondary hyperparathyroidsm complicating chronic renal failure who benefitted from parathyroidectomy.

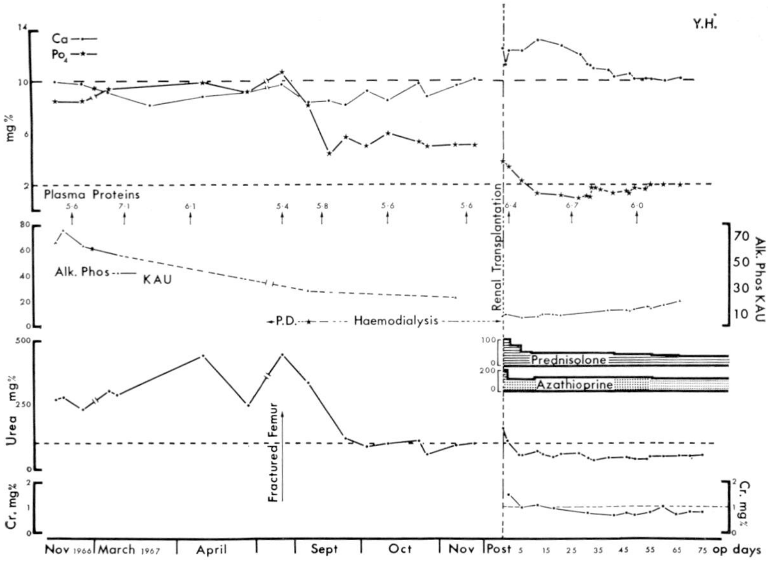

FIG. 3. Progress chart of a patient with chronic pyelonephritis and secondary hyperparathyroidism showing the effect of haemodialysis on plasma calcium and phosphate; an initial rise in plasma calcium to 14 mg% after successful renal transplantation followed by return to normal in 45 days. (The possibility of parathyroid autonomy was considered during the period of hypercalcaemia and hypophosphataemia but parathyroidectomy was not performed.)

In one of our cases thought to have had tertiary hyperparathyroidism due to chronic renal failure, healing of a femoral fracture occurred after successful parental renal transplant. There was an initial rise in plasma calcium levels during the first weeks of steroid therapy but this settled with time and parathyroidectomy was avoided (Fig. 3). Metastatic calcification and pseudo-gout can usually be controlled by dialysis and by control of plasma phosphate levels with aluminium hydroxide.

5 Many hypertensive patients with terminal renal failure can be controlled by rigid sodium restriction in conjunction with dialysis. Hypotensive

agents may be necessary initially but in many cases, these may be discontinued later. However, some patients have severe hypertension which cannot be controlled by sodium restriction and drugs and they tend to have high plasma renin levels. Bilateral nephrectomy usually has a dramatic effect in lowering the blood pressure in such patients.

A patient established on dialysis can be allowed to spend much of his time at home and after all the pre-operative investigations and preparatory measures have been undertaken he can be 'on call' for transplantation provided he can be reached by telephone at any time of day or night and can arrive at the transplant unit within 1–2 h of an alert. He may, however, have to make several unfruitful journeys to the unit before a suitable kidney is found, but despite this, the morale and well being of patients living at home is usually incomparably better and the risk of infection much lower than that of the chronically hospitalized individual.

PATIENT SELECTION

This can be a difficult and often emotional problem. In practice, most patients would be suitable but many workers have suggested certain criteria for selection because of the lack of facilities:

a a reasonable level of intelligence and psychiatric stability (often difficult to assess in the severely uraemic patient);
b willingness to co-operate (often apparent from the patient's behaviour on his dietary regime);
c absence of systemic disease of which renal failure is but one manifestation e.g. systemic LE, diabetes, polyarteritis nodosa;
d absence of severe coronary artery or cerebrovascular disease. Hypertension per se is not a contraindication;
e stable home background and occupation (if male) and zest for survival.

In the sphere of haemodialysis where the emphasis nowadays tends to be more towards home dialysis, the suitability of the home for installation of dialysis equipment and the ability and enthusiasm of the patient and his relatives to take on this responsibility have to be considered. As far as renal transplantation is concerned, many of these criteria would be considered desirable though in our experience they are not absolutely necessary.

Multisystem disease (e.g. diabetes mellitus and collagen diseases) involving the kidneys might make the post-operative management difficult. Steroid induced diabetes occurs not uncommonly after transplantation and in many cases does not make management too difficult. However, the long term effect on the graft is uncertain. It would seem possible that a combined pancreatic and renal transplant might in the future be a practical approach to the diabetic with renal failure.

Diseases of collagen tissue are being frequently treated with immunosuppressive drugs, so that a kidney transplant in a patient suffering from polyarteritis nodosa or SLE may be protected by this therapy. It would seem that such systemic conditions may in future not prejudice the patient's chance of grafting.

Secondary amyloid disease affecting the kidney should not be a contraindication to transplantation, provided the original condition is quiescent. In cases of amyloid due to longstanding tuberculosis, the use of prophylactic chemotherapy should probably be given even though the condition is quiescent. Renal failure due to gout should be devoid of hazards now that the xanthine oxidase inhibitor allopurinol is available.

Active glomerulonephritis may be transmitted to the graft even in the presence of immunosuppressive therapy; it would seem justifiable therefore to keep such a patient on dialysis until all signs of activity have disappeared as determined by serum complement estimations and detection of anti-kidney antibodies. The detection of antibodies against kidney tissue is not a readily available service and would necessitate the co-operation of an experienced and adequately motivated immunological department. In addition, a patient with his own kidneys *in situ* may 'mop up' any circulating antibodies and make their detection in the serum extremely difficult. By removing such kidneys, however, detectable levels may be released into the bloodstream. An additional advantage of such a procedure may also be the removal of the antigenic stimulus.

A normal lower urinary tract is highly desirable if transplantation is contemplated and patients with neurogenic bladders and ileal conduits may not be good transplant prospects because of the risk of infection. However, reports of successful transplants in patients with ileal bladders and with skin ureterostomies have been published. Any patient with bladder dysfunction should be investigated and the necessary correction performed prior to transplantation.

Patients with localized renal tumours have been successfully transplanted (Woodruff *et al* 1969). Patients with carcinoma in other sites are usually not suitable, for the neoplastic process is likely to disseminate under the influence of immunosuppressive therapy. The evidence for this is not very strong but Hume (1968) mentioned two cases in which neoplasia proliferated under the influence of immunosuppressive drugs.

An upper age limit of approximately 45–50 years is usually agreed upon because of the increased incidence of associated cardiovascular and cerebrovascular complications in the older age groups, but each patient should be considered on his or her mertis. As far as the lower age group, it is more difficult to know where to draw the line. Undoubtedly many young children will do well though the effect of steroid drugs on their development and appearance have to be considered. We feel that for prepubertal children, live related donor kidney grafts are desirable as histocompatibility is likely to be better than in cadaveric grafting. The dose of immunosuppressive drugs can therefore be kept at a minimum.

Most patients referred from physicians from other centres have already undergone some degree of selection. They tend to fall roughly into the accepted age groups and these with vascular and other complications have been excluded, so that one rarely has to turn anyone down. However, the ability of referring centres to keep the patients alive and well is often a problem, so that the co-operation between haemodialysis units who would take on temporary patients pending a space on a transplant programme is often greatly appreciated.

REFERENCES

Barreras R.F. & Donaldson R.M. (1967) Role of calcium in gastric hypersecretion, parathyroid adenoma and peptic ulcer. *New Eng. J. Med.* **276,** 1122.

Brescia M.J., Cimino J.E., Appel K. & Harwich B.J. (1966) Chronic haemodialysis using venipuncture and a surgically created arteriovenous fistula. *New Engl. J. Med.* **275,** 1089.

Cohen S.L. & Percival A. (1968) Prolonged peritoneal dialysis in patients awaiting renal transplantation. *Br. med. J.* i, 409.

Crockett R.E., Baillod R.A., Lee B.N., Moorhead J.F., Stevenson C.M., Varghese Z. & Shaldon S. (1967) Maintenance of 50 patients on intermittent haemodialysis without blood transfusion. *Proc. E.D.T.A.* IV, 17.

Ford J., Phillips M.E., Toye F.E., Luck V.A. & de Wardener H.E. (1969) Nitrogen balance in patients with chronic renal failure on diets containing varying quantities of protein. *Br. med. J.* i, 735.

Giordano C. (1963) Use of exogenous and endogenous urea for protein synthesis in normal uremic subjects. *J. Lab. Clin. Med.* **62,** 231.

Giovanetti S. & Maggiore Q. (1964) A low nitrogen diet with proteins of high biological value for severe chronic uraemia. *Lancet,* i, 1000.

Hume D.M. (1968) In *Human Transplantation* by Rapaport & Dausset. Chapter 10.

Kolff W.J., Berk H. Th. J. (1944) The artificial kidney: a dialyser with a great area. *Acta med. scan.* **117,** 121.

Ogg C.S. (1967) Total parathyroidectomy in treatment of secondary (renal) hyperparathyroidism. *Lancet,* iv, 331.

Quinton W., Dillard D. & Scribner B.H. (1960) Cannulation of blood vessels for prolonged haemodialysis. *Trans. Am. Soc. Artif. Int. Org.* **6,** 104.

Scribner B.H., Buri R., Caner J.E., Hegstrom R.E. & Burnell J.M. (1960) The treatment of chronic uraemia by means of intermittent haemodialysis: a preliminary report. *Trans. Am. Soc. Artif. Int. Org.* **6,** 114.

SHAW A.B., BAZZARD F.J., BOOTH E.M., NILWARANGKUR S., BERLYNE G.M. (1965) The treatment of chronic renal failure by a modified Giovanetti diet. *Quart. J. Med.* **34**, 237.

STANBURY S.W., LUMB G. & NICHOLSON W.F. (1960) Elective subtotal parathyroidectomy for renal hyperparathyroidism. *Lancet*, i, 793.

WING A.J., CURTIS J.R., EASTWOOD J.B., SMITH E.K.M. & DE WARDENER H.E. (1968) Transient and persistent hypercalcaemia in patients treated by maintenance haemodialysis. *Br. Med. J.* iv, 150.

WOODRUFF M.F.A., NOLAN B., ROBSON J.S. & MACDONALD M.K. (1969) Renal transplantation in man: experience in 35 cases. *Lancet*, i, 6.

CHAPTER 13

Anaesthesia for the Recipient Operation

D. Powell
J.R. Samuel

At first sight these patients may seem to present almost insuperable problems, but they may be anaesthetized with safety and with surprisingly few complications provided that extreme care is taken at all stages—not least in the selection of the most appropriate technique.

PREPARATION FOR TRANSPLANTATION

Although pre-operative preparation was the subject of the preceding section, and is not normally the responsibility of the anaesthetist, certain aspects of it should be discussed further because of their importance and immediate bearing on the anaesthetic to be administered. Even an optimally prepared patient remains one who would be regarded as an extremely poor risk by the standards of normal anaesthetic practice. Haemodialysis is usually successful in correcting the electrolyte imbalance and in lowering the blood urea. Transplantation should not be considered unless these two objects have been largely achieved.

The anaemia associated with uraemia is usually profound and is notoriously refractory. Its treatment is complicated by the danger of large transfusions in patients who may have incipient pulmonary oedema. Patients with haemoglobin levels entirely unthinkable in other fields of surgery have therefore to be accepted for anaesthesia. Nevertheless these patients with *chronic* anaemia if carefully handled usually tolerate major operations under general anaesthesia surprisingly well.

The average haemoglobin and serum electrolyte levels of 100 such patients after pre-operative medical preparation and at the time of anaesthesia for renal transplantation are shown in Table 1. Adequate preparation produces near normal serum electrolyte levels but the blood urea levels remain elevated and the degree of anaemia remains profound.

TABLE 1. Haemoglobin and blood biochemistry levels before induction of anaesthesia in 100 cases

		Patient range	
Investigation	Average	Low	High
Haemoglobin g/100 ml	7·6	4·3	11·8
Blood urea mg%	111	15	256
Serum Na meq/l.	129	117	156
Serum K meq/l.	4·4	3·0	7·2
Serum HCO_3 meq/l.	24	13	32

PRELIMINARY OPERATIONS

In preparation for transplantation patients may have a bilateral nephrectomy carried out some time beforehand. These patients may come to their preliminary nephrectomy in a much worse condition than to their eventual transplantation. For instance they may be severely hypertensive with incipient or actual heart failure, and be receiving anti-hypertensive agents and digitalis. Removal of the diseased kidneys often reduces the hypertension, relieving the heart failure and rendering the drugs unnecessary. Nevertheless the same principles should be followed, and the same techniques applied to both operations. Of the first 100 renal transplantations at Cambridge, 31 had had previous bilateral nephrectomy; and 39 had received anti-hypertensive agents (commonly methyldopa). Even in the absence of heart failure, uraemic patients are liable to develop pulmonary oedema. Pericardial and pleural effusions usually regress with improvement in the heart failure but if they persist they should be tapped before general anaesthesia is contemplated.

FACTORS AFFECTING THE CHOICE OF MAIN ANAESTHETIC AGENT

Reginal techniques

The use of regional techniques has been advocated (Vandam, Harrison *et al* 1962; Wynant 1967). In addition a covering general anaesthetic is recommended by these authors on some occasions. It is important, especially in patients on immunosuppressive therapy, to protect the tracheobronchial tree from the possibility of inhalation of stomach contents. This may occur without definite vomiting or obvious regurgitation. The psychological state of the recipient is seldom ideal for a prolonged procedure whilst still conscious (Lofstrom 1967). We feel therefore that a general anaesthetic technique incorporating endotracheal intubation is essential.

Inhalational agents

Some anaesthetists use an inhalational anaesthetic as the main agent for renal transplantation but certain contra-indications exist.

Cyclopropane and ether

Neither of these agents, being explosive, can be used in conjunction with surgical diathermy. Ether, also, causes depression of renal function and increased secretion of ADH. Neither has sufficient advantage to compensate for the interference with standard surgical technique and consequent prolonged operating time.

Halothane

This has been recommended (Strunin 1966). However, if used in concentrations suitable for its employment as the main anaesthetic agent, it is liable to cause unpredictable hypotension in patients with potentially abnormal plasma volumes following dialysis. We have used concentrations up to 0·5% as an intermittent supplement to nitrous oxide, and as an easily controllable antihypertensive agent.

Although profound relaxation is not essential for transplantation in the iliac region, it makes the surgical procedure quicker and easier. Such relaxation is not easy to achieve in young muscular patients with halothane alone.

Methoxyflurane

Because it has greater analgesic properties than halothane, it might be thought that there was a place for this agent as a supplement to nitrous oxide and oxygen. However there have been several reports of post-operative nephropathy from the use of methoxyflurane (Crandall & Macdonald 1968) and so its use must be contraindicated in renal transplantation.

Muscle relaxants

Suxamethonium

Although intermittent suxamethonium has been advocated as a maintenance agent of choice in renal transplantation, it has several theoretical disadvantages. Patients with chronic renal failure, unless recently and effectively dialysed, are often hyperkalaemic. It has been shown that there is a significant rise in the serum potassium level in patients given suxamethonium, although this rise is less after induction with thiopentone than with halothane, and it reaches its peak 60 min after injection (List 1967; Striker & Morrow 1968). Also it has been pointed out that cardiac irregularities, bradycardia and cardiac arrest are commoner after the second and subsequent injections of suxamethonium. In patients with potential hyperkalaemia it would seem advisable to avoid a technique which is known to raise the serum potassium, and which has been suspected of causing cardiac arrest, or arrhythmias (Roth & Wuthrick 1969). Even intravenous atropine 0·6 mg does not fully protect the patient from cardiac arrhythmia following subsequent doses of suxamethonium.

The employment of a single dose of suxamethonium following intravenous atropine is justified by the need for rapid intubation with a cuffed endotracheal tube to protect the patient from the possible consequences of a full stomach. Although a low pseudocholinesterase level has been described following dialysis, we have not encountered prolonged apnoea (Levine & Virtue 1964).

Gallamine

Feldman showed in dogs that gallamine is excreted entirely by the kidneys (Feldman *et al* 1969). In the absence of renal function a sustained level of gallamine was obtained.

Churchill-Davidson has quoted a case in which a boy was mistakenly given 380 mg of gallamine during an operation for exploration of a kidney transplant (Churchill-Davidson *et al* 1967). He remained apnoeic for

3 days until the situation was reversed by dialysis. Gallamine is not therefore a suitable agent for patients with reduced renal function.

d-Tubocourarine

The basis of our technique has always been the use of d-tubocourarine and positive-pressure ventilation. In the early days of renal transplantation curare was used cautiously, if at all, because the mechanism of its excretion was thought to be mostly renal, although some was metabolized in the liver.

Then it was shown in dogs, using tritated d-tubocourarine, that in the absence of renal function the liver was able to excrete up to 40% of a given dose of curare in the bile in a few hours (Cohen *et al* 1967). This alternative route of excretion helps to explain the absence of a prolongation of effect in the anuric patient.

Dhuner and his colleagues (1968) used d-tubocourarine and noted that when the same patients returned to theatre at a later date for bilateral nephrectomy when their transplanted kidneys were working well, their curare requirement was the same as when they had no renal function. Our experience has been similar, and there has been no case of prolonged action of curare or of difficulty in reversing its action at the end of operation.

Other relaxants

Pancuronium and alcuronium have not been used by the authors although they would probably produce equally good operating conditions. Pancuronium, particularly, seems to cause less fall in blood pressure than curare. However, the pharmacology of its termination of action has yet to be fully worked out.

ANAESTHETIC TECHNIQUE

As soon as operation is decided upon, the current haemoglobin concentration, serum electrolytes and blood urea must be made available.

Premedication

Because of the importance of keeping the donor kidney ischaemic time to a minimum, and the consequent short notice of impending operation, many patients for cadaveric transplantation come to operation with a full stomach and are totally unprepared for anaesthesia. Tissue typing may involve a delay of up to 2 h but the actual recipient is not known until these results are obtained. Although modern methods of preservation have succeeded in storing kidneys for several hours it is still desirable that the operation proceeds immediately the identity of the recipient is decided.

Emptying the stomach by gastric intubation is traumatic and not fully effective and is therefore not attempted, but the routine neutralization of the gastric juice by 30 ml of magnesium trisilicate mixture is recommended. All patients should be given atropine 0·6 mg intravenously at induction of anaesthesia. If there is time for other than intravenous medication, as in live donor transplantation, a sedative premedication such as a small dose of opiate is helpful and humane.

Apparatus

As far as possible the equipment used for transplant anaesthesia must be sterile because of the increased danger of infection. Most ventilators are difficult to maintain in a sterile condition and for this reason we have adopted the use of the East-Automaticvent, although any ventilator which can be easily sterilized would be suitable. With this we use sterile plastic cuffed endotracheal tubes, and the laryngoscope blades and connectors are autoclaved and kept ready for use.

Induction

Lack of superficial veins for intravenous induction and for transfusion may be a major problem. After long periods of frequent blood sampling for biochemical analysis, and following repeated replacement of shunts which have usually a limited life, the patient's arm may resemble a battle-field. Meticulous care should be taken to safeguard the shunt in use at the time of operation, because the patient's life may depend on it aftewards. Stasis and clotting may be prevented by wrapping the shunt in wool, placing the arm by the side of the patient, and by not applying the sphygmomanometer cuff to the same arm as the shunt. The shunt should not be used to administer drugs less this is made unavoidable by the absence of other veins.

In all cases an intravenous infusion should be set up before induction of anaesthesia, preferably in the back of the hand, to avoid spoiling valuable forearm veins.

Extra care must be taken in moving and positioning these patients as decalcification, due to their renal failure, is occasionally present and it is easy for the unwary to produce serious damage.

Preoxygenation for 5 min is carried out because of the severe anaemia usually present, and to eliminate the risks of positive-pressure ventilation during induction in patients with a full stomach. A sleep dose of a short-acting barbiturate, either thiopentone or methohexitone, is used for induction. This is followed by suxamethonium for intubation. Crico-thyroid pressure to prevent regurgitation and aspiration of stomach contents is mandatory because of the increased risks in patients on immunosuppressive therapy.

Maintenance

Maintenance doses of d-tubocourarine are given and the patient ventilated with nitrous oxide and oxygen. In patients who may well develop pulmonary oedema, positive pressure ventilation may prove preventative or therapeutic. Halothane is usually used to supplement the nitrous oxide but a concentration of more than 1% is seldom required. Alternatively a narcotic drug such as morohine or pethidine may be preferred.

Low blood pressure during operation has not been a problem, although many patients have been until recently on antihypertensive drugs. The use of vasopressors is seldom if ever required, most hypotension being caused by blood loss and treated by blood transfusion. An uncommon cause of low blood pressure is the 'supine hypotensive syndrome' usually associated with obstetric anaesthesia. Sometimes the kidneys are so large in polycystic disease that they may cause obstruction to the inferior vena cava, especially when displaced by the surgeon in order to dissect the renal pedicle; or they may hamper movement of the diaphragm and render ventilation difficult. A dangerous rise in blood pressure on release of the arterial clamps was described by Strunin (1966), but we have not often met it. It can be treated by giving a hypotensive agent (e.g. hexamethonium 15–40 mg) but this may not be needed when halothane has been used to control the blood pressure. Should a severe hypertensive episode be allowed to occur at this stage it may increase the blood loss or rupture the arterial anastomosis.

At the end of the operation neostigmine 2·5 mg with atropine 1·2 mg must be given to reverse the action of the curare. This has always been satisfactorily achieved even if the serum potassium was abnormal.

Non-anaesthetic drugs

Some drugs have been given by the anaesthetists the action of which is related more to the success of the transplantation than to the maintenance of anaesthesia. The drugs given have gradually changed and the reasons for this are discussed below.

Heparin

It was originally our practice to give an injection of 10,000 units (100 mg) of heparin in the average adult. At the end of the operation, it was reversed by giving 100 mg of protamine sulphate 1% slowly intravenously. More recently, following the occurrence of post-operative bleeding, the practice of systemic heparinization of the patient during the operation has been abandoned. No ill-effects have followed cessation of systemic heparinization. The technique of dialysis now utilizes regional heparinization within the machine and neutralization with protamine in the venous line for the first 14 post-operative days, to minimize the risk of secondary haemorrhage.

Patients who are taken off the dialysis machine to receive their transplant are already heparinized before operation, and should receive protamine sulphate at the end of the operation.

Mannitol

Earlier 100–150 ml of 20% mannitol were infused during the operation, to attempt to produce an osmotic diuresis in the transplanted organ, and to help reduce ischaemic damage. This procedure has two theoretical disadvantages:

Firstly, that hypertensive patients may have incipient cardiac failure and the sudden increase in blood volume caused by mannitol can cause acute heart failure and pulmonary oedema.

Secondly, a patient who has little or no urinary output will be unable to rid himself of the mannitol which will remain in his extracellular fluid.

No evidence was found that the use of mannitol protects the kidney from ischaemic damage, and so its use was abandoned (Salaman, Calne *et al* 1969).

Immunosuppression

Immunosuppressive therapy is not started before transplantation. All patients are given hydrocortisone hemisuccinate 200 mg by intravenous injection when the arterial clamp has been removed. Azathioprine (Imuran) may be given intravenously during or after operation at a dosage of 5 mg/kg.

Antibiotics

Patients on immunosuppressive therapy are especially liable to develop infections, and it has become increasingly common practice to give one dose of prophylactic antibiotics during the operation particularly where the donor patient has been maintained on a ventilator prior to death. The antibiotics most commonly used are ampicillin and carbenacillin. These are given intravenously when the anastomoses had been completed.

The dangers of interaction between antibiotics and anaesthetic agents must be remembered. Infections are a common feature of terminal renal failure, and many of these patients received antibiotics during their period of medical preparation for transplantation. It is well known that topical intraperitoneal or intrapleural streptomycin, neomycin and polymixin may give rise to prolonged apnoea after anaesthesia utilising non-depolarising relaxants. This phenomenon following injected antibiotics is less well known (Emery 1963; Perkins 1964). Patients with little or no urinary output (as after bilateral nephrectomy) have a greatly reduced requirement for these drugs, and so what in a normal patient would be a standard dose carries a greatly increased risk of potentiating, or causing, neuromuscular block. One such patient who had had a bilateral nephrectomy underwent laparotmy for intestinal obstruction. She had been given 3 megaunits of colomycin daily and a single dose of 1 g of streptomycin. Following a normal dose of d-tubocourarine she required artificial ventilation for 36 h.

BLOOD REPLACEMENT

In patients with severe chronic anaemia it is important to replace only the blood which is lost and this loss must therefore be measured accurately. With any arterial surgery one must be prepared for the occurrence of sudden severe haemorrhages and an adequate supply of cross-matched blood (6 units) must be readily available. Should such a potential disaster occur a pump (such as a Martin's transfusion pump) must be used and due attention paid to the dangers of hypocalcaemia, metabolic acidosis and hypothermia which may result from massive transfusion. Calcium gluconate 10%, sodium bicarbonate 8·4% and a blood warming apparatus should be kept ready to hand. However the prevention of overtransfusion is equally important, not only because the patients are anuric but also because they are more than usually likely to develop pulmonary oedema. They may not be dialysed until the third post-operative day, and in the absence of an immediate diuresis from the transplanted kidney, any accidental overload of the circulation cannot be corrected, other than by venesection, until dialysis takes place.

MONITORING

Most anaesthetists would argue that it is advisable to monitor central venous pressure in these difficult patients, especially if their pre-operative condition has not been fully stabilized by adequate dialysis. However we have not always found this possible because of the frequent shortage of

TABLE 2

Complication	Cause	Suggested treatment and/or prevention
Inhalation of vomit	Full stomach	Mist mag. trisil.
a At induction	Unprepared patient	Preoxygenation + Cricoid pressure
b On extubation	Unprepared patient	Positioning of patient in lateral head down posture for extubation
Prolonged apnoea a Depolarising relaxants	Low plasma pseudo-cholinesterase following haemodialysis	IPPV
b Non-depolarising relaxant	Potentiation by neomycin type antibiotics	IPPV (and/or dialysis)
Hypotension	i Haemorrhage	Transfusion
	ii Inferior vena caval obstruction	Surgical technique
	iii Antihypertensive therapy	Transfusion (?Metar-aminol)
	iv Bleeding from inadequate heparin reversal	Protamine sulphate
Hypertension	Vasopressor agents released from ischaemic kidney	Halothane in anaesthetic Hypotensive agents (e.g. hexamethonium or chlorpromazine)
Metabolic imbalance		
i Cardiac arrhythmia and arrest	Hyperkalaemia	Avoid repeated suxamethonium Calcium gluconate Avoid stimulation under light anaesthesia
ii Respiratory insufficiency	Metabolic acidosis	Give sodium bicarbonate
Pulmonary oedema	Uraemia	Adequate preoperative haemodialysis
	Overtransfusion	Accurate blood replacement Beware mannitol

superficial veins and the necessary time. Sphygmomanometry with a brachial cuff has proved adequate for monitoring the blood pressure and has the advantage of not interfering with peripheral arteries that may be needed for shunts.

For the electrocardiogram it is probably better to use plates rather than needle electrodes because of the danger of infection.

COMPLICATIONS

Table 2 lists some of the complications which have been reported in the literature with suggestions as to their cause and treatment.

RECOVERY

Patients on immunosuppressive therapy require careful barrier-nursing during their postoperative recovery. It is not practicable to return them to the general recovery room in a large hospital and special arrangements must be made for them in the transplant unit, where extreme care is taken in the provision of a clean environment.

REFERENCES

CALNE R.Y. (1969) Cadaveric kidneys for transplantation. *Br. Med. J.* ii, 555.

CHURCHILL-DAVIDSON H.C., WAY W.L. & DE JONG R.H. (1967) The muscle relaxants and renal excretion. *Anaesthesiology*, **28,** 540.

COHEN E.N., WINSLOW BREWER H. & SMITH D. (1967) The metabolism and elimination of d-tubocourarine H³. *Anaesthesiology*, **28,** 309.

DHUNER K.G., LUNKBERG H. & PETERHOFF V. (1968) Anaesthesia in renal transplantation. *Scand. J. Urol. & Nephrol.* **2,** 31.

EMERY E.R.J. (1963) Neuromuscular blocking properties of antibiotics as a cause of post-operative apnoea. *Anaesthesia,* **18,** 57.

FELDMAN S.A., COHEN E.N., GOLLING R.C. (1969) The excretion of gallamine in the dog. *Anaesthesiology*, **30,** 593.

LEVINE D.S. & VIRTUE R.W. (1964) Anaesthetic agents and techniques for renal homotransplants. *Canad. Anaesth. Soc. J.* **11,** 425.

LIST W.F. (1967) Serum potassium changes during induction of anaesthesia. *Br. J. Anaesth.* **39,** 480.

LÖFSTRÖM B. (1967) Anaesthetic problems in renal transplantation. *Scand. J. Urol. & Nephrol* **1,** 161.

PERKINS R.J. (1964) Apnoea with intramuscular colistin therapy. *J.A.M.A.* **190,** 421.

ROTH F. & WÜTHRICH H. (1969) The clinical importance of hyperkalaemia following suxamethonium administration. *Br. J. Anaesth.* **41,** 311.

SALAMAN J.R., CALNE R.Y., PENA J., SELLS R.A., WHITE H.J.O. & YOFFA D. (1969) Surgical aspects of clinical renal transplantation. *Br. J. Surg.* **56,** 413.

STRIKER T.D. & MORROW A.G. (1968) Effect of succinylcholine on the level of serum potassium in man. *Anaesthesiology,* **29,** 214.

STRUNIN L. (1966) Some aspects of anaesthesia for renal homotransplantation. *Br. J. Anaesth.* **38,** 812.

VANDAM L.D., HARRISON J.H., MURRAY J.E. & MERRILL J.P. (1962) Anaesthetic aspects of renal homotransplantation in man. *Anaesthesiology,* **23,** 783.

WYNANT G.W. (1967) The anaesthetist looks at tissue transplantation: three years experience with kidney transplants. *Canad. Anaesth. Soc. J.* **14,** 255.

CHAPTER 14

The Technique of Renal Transplantation

R.Y. Calne

This operation has now become standard practice in a large number of centres and for the most part is based on the extra-peritoneal approach, first used by Kuss *et al* in 1951. A discussion of the numerous minor variations would be out of place. I will describe instead our standard procedure. Although a supra-inguinal incision gives satisfactory exposure the upper end involves cutting the muscular fibres of the external oblique and this can lead to bleeding in the wound edge. I therefore prefer the J-shaped incision described by Alexandre in which there is no cutting of muscle, instead the fascia of the linear semilunaris and the anterior rectus sheath are incised (Fig. 1). The common and external iliac vessels are exposed in the extraperitoneal plane. The inferior epigastric vessels are carefully defined, ligated and divided as is the round ligament in the female. In the male the spermatic cord is controlled with a sling and freed from surrounding structures so that it will fit loosely across the lower pole of the transplanted kidney. The essentials are satisfactory continuity of the renal artery and vein to an artery and vein of the recipient, a safe domicile for the kidney and free ureteric drainage. The iliac vessels are carefully inspected for anatomical anomalies but more important is the likelihood of severe atherosclerotic disease at the origin of the internal iliac artery. If atherosclerotic plaques are found these can be removed by endarterectomy or alternatively the external iliac artery can be used with end-to-side anasto-

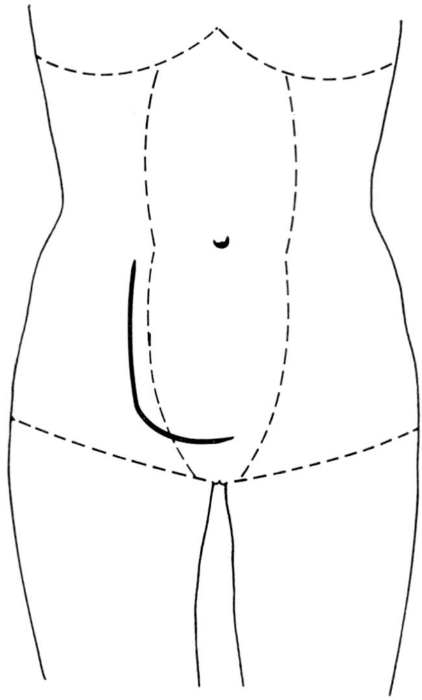

FIG. 1. J-shaped incision of Alexandre.

mosis. The choice of site for the operation is not of great importance, either kidney can be easily accommodated on the right or the left side, although there is slightly easier lie for the vessels if the internal iliac artery is being used, for the left kidney to be transplanted to the right iliac fossa, and vice versa; whereas when an end-to-side anastomosis to the iliac artery is being performed homolateral transplantation is preferable. If the patient has already had one transplant, the new graft is placed on the other side. If he has had multiple transplants then it may be safer to insert the new graft intra-peritoneally, anastomosing the renal vein to the common iliac vein or vena cava and the renal artery to the common iliac artery or terminal aorta. Having decided upon the details of the proposed anastomoses the appropriate iliac vessels are controlled and clamped. If the internal iliac artery is to be used this is ligated just proximal to its major division and the proximal part of the vessel is freed from surrounding tissues and turned forwards for convenience of handling. If the transplant is from a live donor, the details of the anatomy can be inspected *in situ* before the donor kidney is removed. We do not perfuse such transplants, which are simply immersed in a dish of iced saline and immediately grafted.

With cadaver donors, in our own institution the kidneys are carefully dissected from the cadaver before removal so that any abnormality of the anatomy is determined and noted beforehand. This saves wasting time during the grafting operation and it may prevent unnecessary dissection in the recipient. If the kidney is coming from another institution where the organ has been removed en masse with the cava and aorta without kidney dissection, additional time must be spent in clarifying the anatomy and planning the recipient operation. This is done when the kidney is removed from ice whilst it is still cold, but after the initial dissection has been performed on the recipient. Systemic heparin is not used.

The kidney is carefully orientated correctly so that the vessels and ureter lie in the right position relative to each other without any twisting or kinking. An appropriately sized anterior venotomy is performed, taking a minute portion of the wall of the external iliac vein by picking it up with forceps and cutting with curved scissors. It is helpful to control the kidney with a tape looped around it so that the assistant does not need to hold the kidney in his hand, getting in the way of the operation and warming the organ

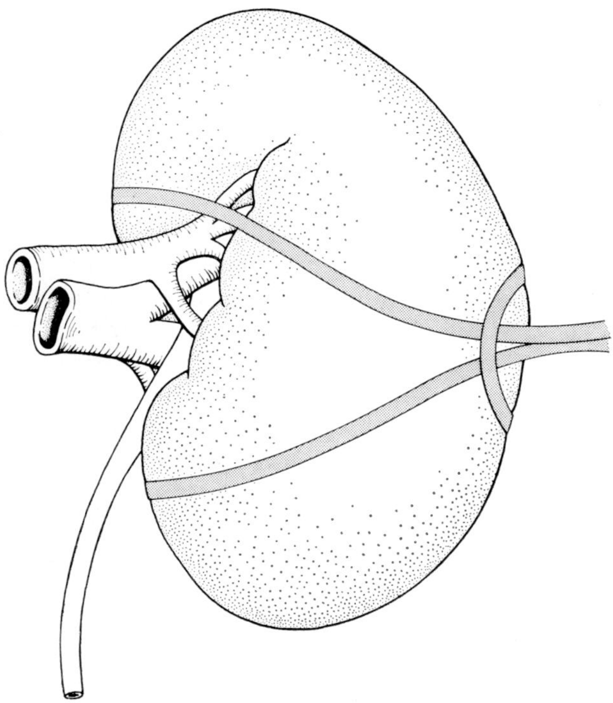

FIG. 2. Kidney controlled with a tape sling to facilitate handling and prevent warming of the organ.

(Fig. 2) (Merrill *et al* 1956). The venous anastomosis is usually performed with a running 5/0 atraumatic silk stitch with a needle at each end. The wall furthest away from the surgeon is sutured from inside the lumen and the nearer wall from outside. The area of the anastomosis is irrigated with heparinized saline during the procedure. If an end-to-end anastomosis is performed between the renal artery and the internal iliac, a 6/0 running stitch is usually used. If however the renal artery is to be implanted end-to-side to the external iliac artery with or without a Carrel patch, a 5/0 running stitch is used. The clamps are removed first from the iliac veins and then the artery. The kidney should rapidly take on a satisfactory salmon pink colour with normal tone. The tension rapidly increases if the renal vein is temporarily constricted between finger and thumb. If the kidney does not perfuse satisfactorily there are a variety of possibilities that need to be considered.

1 There is a gross technical fault in the performance of the anastomoses. Thus if the kidney is pale and soft there may be an error in the arterial anastomoses or the intima of the renal artery may have been fractured during removal of the kidney by excessive traction. This is a very unfortunate complication, difficult to rectify and often missed. The failure of the kidney may be attributed to hyperacute rejection, when in fact it is due to dissection of the intima of the renal artery. If there is an error in the venous anastomosis with a normal arterial inflow, the kidney will rapidly become extremely tense and cyanosed. Surgical errors require appropriate revision. It is usually best to reclamp the iliac vessels and work in a dry field bearing in mind that the additional time will add to the ischaemic damage of the kidney which by now will be warm.

2 The kidney has undergone hyperacute rejection. In this condition there is usually initial satisfactory perfusion of the kidney for a few minutes and then the kidney becomes flaccid. Constriction of the renal vein does not result in rapid increase in tone in the kidney, which becomes progressively more and more cyanosed. This complication is particularly likely in a patient who has had a previous transplant or multiple transfusions or pregnancies. There is no treatment that can help. The only satisfactory management is to remove the transplant immediately.

3 The kidney has undergone severe ischaemic damage from the time of the death of the donor to its transplantation. Such a kidney is usually paler than normal with diminished tone but to establish the diagnosis by inspection immediately after transplantation may be very difficult. The condition is also likely to be confused with the final complication—number 4. If in doubt, it is probably wisest to leave such a transplant *in situ* and await events.

4 Temporary reversible intravascular spasm is especially likely to occur in cadaver transplants where the donor has died violently with release of noradrenalin or has been given large doses of vasoconstrictor drugs, particularly noradrenalin and methedrine. Despite satisfactory anastomoses and no evidence of intimal tear, the kidney looks pale, feels soft and constricting the renal vein does not result in rapid increase in tone. The appearances are very similar to those described with ischaemic damage above. This condition may persist for some time and usually fills the operating team with despondency, but nevertheless it is consistent with excellent eventual renal function when the spasm wears off. The application of papavarine to the renal artery externally or injection of dilute procaine solution into the lumen of the venal artery may reverse the spasm, but sometimes does not. Eventually the spasm ceases spontaneously.

Once it has been decided that the vascular anastomoses are satisfactory, the capsule is incised from pole to pole along the maximum convexity. This allows for kidney swelling which is due to renal oedema, a result of ischaemic damage. Capsulotomy is not performed in live donor transplants.

URETERIC DRAINAGE

This is the most difficult and controversial part of the technique. I feel that for first kidney transplants there are advantages in implanting the ureter directly in the bladder and of course this is essential if the ureters of the recipient are grossly diseased and dilated. With a uretero-neocystostomy, if there is leakage from the ureter or stenosis due to poor technique, infection or rejection, the drainage can be revised using the recipient's own ureter. Moreover should the first transplant fail a second transplant can utilize the recipient's own ureter for anastomosis without dissecting around the bladder. Such dissection is likely to lead to infection in the perivesical spaces that result from previous fibrosis and it is better at second and subsequent transplants to avoid this area if possible. A variety of techniques have been used to implant the ureter. I now use a simple technique similar to that used in canine renal transplants, with some modifications described by Woodruff (1969). Without extensive dissection of the bladder the lateral wall is approached and a 2 cm incision is made in the muscle of the bladder until the mucosa pouts. A 0·5 cm incision is made at the lowermost point of this incision in the mucosa. A culture is taken from the inside of the bladder with a bacterial swab. The ureter is trimmed back so that there is no tension on it but also no long redundant loop and an incision is made

1 cm longitudinally in the end of the ureter so as to spatulate the end. If there is a brisk diuresis of urine at this time, the ureteric anastomosis is not splinted. If however, there is no diuresis, as is commonly experienced in many of our cadaveric transplants, a right-angled forceps is introduced into the bladder through the incision. It is passed across to the other side of the bladder on the vault, a stab incision is made at this point and a number 6 Tizzard catheter is pulled from the outside of the bladder through the

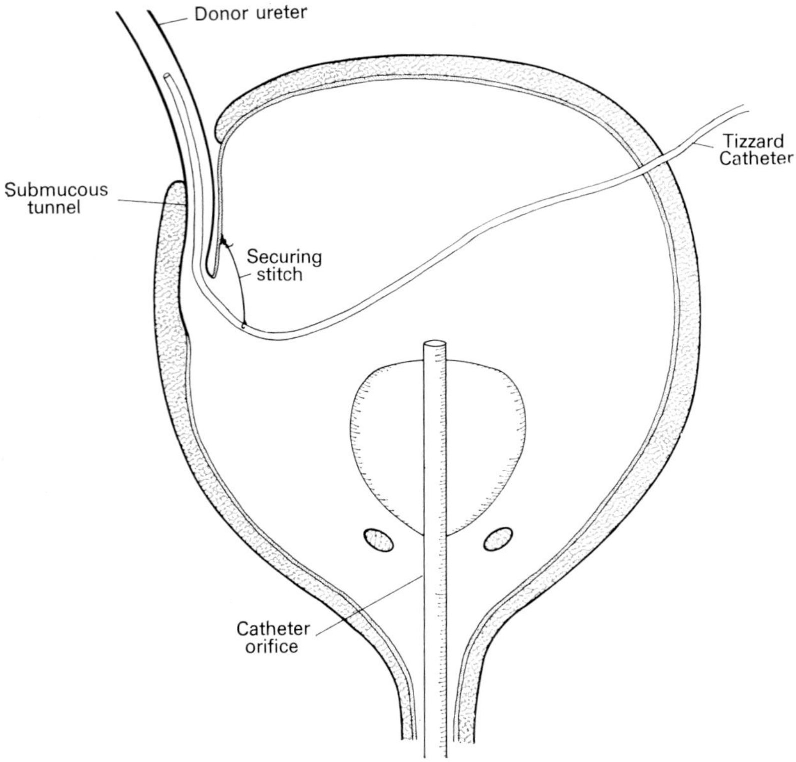

FIG. 3. Standard technique for ureter-to-bladder anastomosis over a Tizzard catheter.

lumen and is then passed up the ureter. This catheter is secured to the mucosa of the bladder adjacent to the anastomosis with a 4/0 chromic catgut stitch. A similar atraumatic running stitch is used for the anastomosis which is through all coats of the spatulated end of the ureter and through the mucosa of the bladder. Three or four interrupted catgut stitches are then used to approximate the muscle over the ureter where it lies adjacent to the mucosa, thus forming a sub-mucosal tunnel (Fig. 3). This technique is very simple and quick and seems to be in no way inferior to other more elaborate procedures. If a Tizzard catheter has been used to stent the ureteric anastomosis this is brought out through a stab incision medial to the main skin incision. The Tizzard catheter is left in for 4 days, when a retrograde pyrelogram is performed by injecting hypaque through the catheter and taking an X-ray. If the urinary drainage tract is satisfactory the catheter is removed. The catheter is small enough to allow urine to pass between it and the walls of the ureter. When the catheter is removed a passage is left for urine to pass, which might otherwise have filled with epithelial debris, fibrin or blood clot. For second and subsequent kidney transplants, where possible we have utilized the recipient's own ureter, anastomosing this to the pelvi-ureteric junction of the transplant. The end of the recipient ureter is spatulated by a 1 cm incision that matches up with an oblique cut at the pelvi-ureteric junction of the donor kidney. The anastomosis is performed with interrupted 4/0 atraumatic catgut stitches. Cushing clips have been used to mark the poles and maximum convexity of the kidney, as described by Hume *et al* (1963), but these are now no longer used since it was found that quite often the clips, although still adherent to the capsule of the kidney, became separated from the substance of the kidney as the capsule was stripped when the kidney enlarged.

A minute cortical biopsy is taken from the lower pole of the kidney at the end of the operation and haemostasis is secured with an atraumatic stitch. A careful search is then made for any bleeding points in the recipient and on the donor kidney. Sometimes small vessels in the hilum or the capsule of the kidney tend to bleed at the end of the operation. These are carefully ligated. A Silastic tube drain 1 cm in diameter is brought out from the upper extremity of the wound through a stab incision lateral to the main wound. Wound closure is with interrupted catgut for the fascia and interrupted silk for the skin. The sub-cutaneous tissues are sprinkled with penicillin and sulphonamide powder. A urinary catheter is inserted per urethra. We use a Foley catheter with an orifice to the lumen below the balloon as well as above. This ensures dependent drainage of the bladder neck region. The catheter is drained continuously into a sterile bag as is the Tizzard ureteric catheter if one has been used.

In an uncomplicated case the whole operating time should be between 1 and 2 h and blood loss should be minimal so that the operation is not shocking to the patient and the post-operative course is thereby made smooth.

Great care is taken to identify and anastomose all renal arteries of the graft, although a minute accessory polar vessel can be safely sacrificed, the small resulting infarct being of no consequence. There are multiple veno-venous communications in the kidney so it is not essential to anastomose more than one large renal vein. However if there are two veins of equal size that can be conveniently anastomosed this is the preferable procedure (Smith *et al* 1962).

REFERENCES

HUME D.M., MAGEE J.H., KAUFFMAN H.M. Jr., RITTENBURY M.S. & PROUT G.R. Jr. (1963) Renal homotransplantation in man in modified recipients. *Ann. Surg.* **158,** 608.

KUSS R., LEGRAIN M., CAMEY M., DESARMENIEN J., MATHE G., NEDEY R. & VORCH C. (1961) *Mem. Acad. Chir.* **87,** 183.

MERRILL J.P., MURRAY J.E., HARRISON H.H. & GUILD W.R. (1956) *J. Amer. med. Ass.* **160,** 277.

SMITH G.T., CALNE R.Y., MURRAY J.E. & DAMMIN G.J. (1962) *Surg. Gynec. Obstet.* **115,** 682.

WOODRUFF M.F.A., NOLAN B., ROBSON J.S. & MACDONALD M.K. (1969) Renal transplantation in man. Experience in 35 cases. *Lancet,* i, 6.

CHAPTER 15

Post-operative Management of Patients and Immunosuppression

D.B. Evans

Cadaveric renal transplantation with existing preservation methods has to be performed at any time of day or night and therefore always has an element of an emergency about it. Patients on haemodialysis programmes and awaiting transplantation should theoretically be well prepared, free from infection, their blood pressure controlled and in fluid and electrolyte balance. They are usually anaemic but because of the long and gradual development of the anaemia, they are usually well adapted to this state. However, they may have recently partaken of a meal or have had to travel for 1–2 h from home or work in order to reach the transplant unit, arriving only a short time before the beginning of the operation.

Pre-operative preparation may therefore have to be performed hurriedly e.g. shaving of the abdomen and emptying of the stomach by nasogastric suction, and in some cases, these procedures along with the setting up of intravenous infusion may have to be performed in the operating theatre ante-room. Ideally hospital blood banks should reserve crossmatched blood for prospective transplant recipients but if this is not practical the blood transfusion laboratory should be supplied with a weekly sample of serum from all prospective transplant candidates so that when a suitable donor is available, crossmatching can be commenced prior to the patient's arrival in hospital.

Opinions vary regarding the intensity of isolational nursing of the grafted patient and practices have changed even within single units over the course of time. Confinement in a sterile environment with sterilization of all equipment and food entering the area represents one extreme which was undoubtedly important in the era of total body irradiation. Other units observe minimal precautions amounting only to the wearing of masks and the cleaning of hands. The following account describes our practice in Cambridge during the past 4 years—it has proved fairly adequate and does not give the patient a feeling of complete imprisonment. The precautions taken to prevent the transfer of infections from other patients to the transplant recipient (reverse barrier conditions) seems to have been effective in that nearly all infections developing in our patients after transplantation could be traced to endogenous sources.

THE NURSING MANAGEMENT OF THE PATIENT AFTER TRANSPLANTATION

Accommodation

At the end of the transplantation operation, the patient is returned to a single bedded ward, the floors, walls and equipment of which have been cleaned with a suitable disinfecting agent e.g. sodium hypochlorite whilst the operation was under way. Sterilized bed linen was used initially but has later been exchanged for freshly laundered linen. All unnecessary personal effects are removed from the room but a television set is provided for the entertainment of the patient. After the patient returns to the room, the limited personnel entering the room to nurse, examine or visit the patient put on masks and gowns and hands are washed carefully before touching the patient. It has been found to be of great psychological advantage to allow visits by close relatives during the period of isolation. Staff and visitors with infections are excluded.

During the first 10 post-operative days when the patient has an indwelling bladder catheter, a healing abdominal wound and sometimes a drainage tube, all potential portals of entry for bacteria, these reverse barrier conditions are continued. At the end of this period he is allowed out of his room and if well enough and the weather reasonable, out for walks in the grounds. During the summer months patients are encouraged from the 3rd or 4th post-operative days to sit out on a balcony in the sunshine.

Observation of the patient

A minimum number of nurses are allowed into the room and usually one nurse per shift is made responsible for the patient. Routine temperature, pulse and B.P. readings are taken and recorded hourly during the first

12–24 h depending upon the patient's general condition and any significant changes in these signs are reported promptly to the resident medical staff. If no complications have arisen, the observations are thereafter recorded 2–4-hourly.

Careful attention is paid to the patient's fluid intake and output, all volumes are tabulated and a daily weight chart kept. A stool chart is kept to record the presence or absence of occult blood.

Attention to the patient's comfort is of paramount importance—frequent turning in order to protect pressure areas and frequent mouth care are practised. Passive movements of the limbs and breathing exercises are encouraged by the nurse and later intensified under the physiotherapist's supervision. Intravenous fluid therapy is given for the first 24–48 h but as bowel sounds return and flatus is passed, intravenous infusions are discontinued and oral fluids substituted. From the 3rd day a light diet is allowed and suppositories or enemata given if necessary to stimulate bowel action.

Catheters

Where indwelling bladder catheters are used, careful closed drainage is observed. If blood clots block the catheter, washouts are given with 1 : 1000 hibitane or 1% neomycin. Care must be taken in using the latter solution as absorption may occur from the bladder mucosa.

Where a ureteric catheter is used, small (2–5 ml) careful washouts of the same solution may also be given if obstruction is suspected. After a ureteric pyelogram on day 3 this catheter is usually removed.

Wounds

These are not inspected unless infection or haemorrhage are suspected. Sutures are usually removed between days 10 and 14 unless contra-indicated.

Ambulation

The patient is encouraged to sit out after the first 24 h and allowed to walk around the room a day or so later. Graduated exercises are thereafter encouraged, depending on the patient's condition, and after abdominal drains have been removed, patients are encouraged to put on their day clothes.

Drugs

Steroids, azathioprine and other immunosuppressive agents are administered parenterally during the first 24 h and thereafter by mouth if possible. Hypotensive drugs, antiemetics and analgesics may also have to be given by injection during the early post-operative period. Post-operative hyperkalaemia can be controlled by haemodialysis or retention enemata of ion exchange resins suspended in methyl cellulose. Other measures such as intravenous sodium bicarbonate, calcium gluconate or insulin and dextrose may have to be used.

Bacteriology

Routine nose, throat, shunt exit site swabs and midstream urine specimens are taken every 3–4 days and blood cultures daily. In the event of a post-operative fever, these investigations are made more frequently. If post-operative respiratory infection occurs, culture of the sputum is performed and chest X-rays taken. If any of these investigations reveal a significant infection, appropriate chemotherapy is prescribed.

Haemodialysis

Post-operative oliguria is common after cadaveric renal transplantation and repeated haemodialysis treatment has to be continued. We have to use the general dialysis room for this purpose, the patient being isolated as far as possible. Ideally, however, the patients should be dialysed in isolation. Regional heparinization is practised during the first 14 days after transplantation and special care is taken to maintain a steady blood pressure for fear of aggravating the ischaemic renal damage.

Subsequent progress

After barrier restrictions are lifted at 10 days the patient is allowed to mix with other non-infectious patients. Recording of temperature, pulse and B.P. are continued 4-hourly and the patients are encouraged to monitor and tabulate fluid intake and output. Daily adjustments in fluid intake and dietary allowances may have to be made until the patients have reached a steady state.

Psychological aspects

During what may be a protracted stay in hospital a close attachment grows between patients and the nursing staff and many of the former become emotionally very dependent upon the nurses. At the same time the nurses may become attached to certain of the patients and may react emotionally to adverse changes in their patients' conditions. Heavy emotional stresses may consequently result and many members of the nursing staff may not feel adequately equipped to deal with these situations. The presence of a stable ward sister can be a great advantage in running such a unit for she can, by gaining the confidence of her juniors, help them over these periods of stress.

MEDICAL MANAGEMENT

The patient after receiving a renal allograft is susceptible to the usual post-operative complications that might befall anyone who has been subjected to a comparable surgical operation. In addition to these 'usual hazards', his progress may be influenced by the following important factors:

1 The patient is usually significantly anaemic.
2 He had been suffering from terminal renal failure and pre-operative preparation may not have been ideal with resulting hypoproteinaemia, bleeding tendencies, hypertension, heart failure etc.
3 He was likely to be anephric prior to transplantation and may be very sensitive to alterations in blood and extracellular volumes.
4 He is being treated with steroids and azathioprine—drugs which increase the risk of post-operative infection, marrow depression and metabolic upsets.
5 The onset of renal function may be delayed.

If immediate renal function is established, provided fluid and electrolyte balance are maintained, the post-operative course of the patient may not pose too many problems—this set of circumstances usually follows live donor transplants and occasionally follows a cadaveric transplant. Far more commonly in our experience, post-operative oliguria or anuria prevails and the pre-operative renal failure regime has to be continued until allograft function returns.

It has been demonstrated by many workers that the highest morbidity and mortality to their allograft recipients occurs during the first 3 months after transplantation, and furthermore the risk to the patient and his graft may be related to the time taken for the recovery of graft function.

General management

The nursing procedures have already been outlined and it should be again emphasized that careful monitoring and tabulating of routine observations by the nurses is of vital importance and medical staff must be on the alert for alterations in pulse rate, blood pressure, temperature and urinary output. Failure to appreciate changes and to take appropriate steps early might endanger the survival of the graft or the patient.

All patients should be examined at least daily and notice should be taken of any new signs. Unusual symptoms described by the patient, no matter how neurotic he may be, should always be investigated. Careful routine search for infection is important as many of the well known cardinal signs may be missing in the presence of immunosuppressive drugs. Likewise gastrointestinal haemorrhage or perforation may develop insidiously and only by obsessional observation and monitoring will these be discovered. Blood pressure control is important for any marked rise or fall may endanger the function of the graft and appropriate measures should be promptly administered. If persistent and intractable hypertension develops, full investigation as to its cause should be undertaken (*vide infra*).

An efficiently run transplant ward should really function as an intensive care unit and any dilettante approach will sooner or later lead the participants into trouble. Daily combined ward rounds by physicians and surgeons should be performed so that a complete picture of all problems can be discussed and therapy decided. Routine blood and urine tests should be carried out during the first 2 months:

a	*Daily*	
	Haematology	Haemoglobin PCV
		Total leucocyte count
		Platelet count
	Biochemistry	Plasma urea, creatinine and electrolytes
		Creatinine clearance
		Urine urea, protein and sodium
	Bacteriology	Blood cultures (first 2 weeks)
b	*Twice weekly*	
	Bacteriology	Throat and nose swabs
		Sputum (if available)
		MSU for culture
	X-rays	Chest
c	*Once weekly*	SGPT (alanine transferase)
		Calcium, Phosphate and Alk. Phosphatase
		Plasma protein; fasting blood sugar

All these results are tabulated on a large monthly flow sheet chart and scrutinized on the daily ward round.

After the patient's discharge careful follow-up in the outpatient department is necessary as described later and a full blood count, urea, electrolytes and creatinine clearance are measured on each occasion.

Patients living outside the immediate range of the transplant unit are referred back to their parent hospital where they are usually followed up by the referring physician. He then undertakes their surveillance according to a prescribed regime. Any problems are naturally referred back to the unit, and if possible the patients are encouraged to visit the transplant unit for 6-monthly checks.

HAEMODIALYSIS TREATMENT OF THE PATIENT AFTER RENAL TRANSPLANTATION

Where ischaemic tubular necrosis of the cadaveric homograft has occurred a 2–3 week period of oliguria is expected. Where most cadaveric grafts are obtained from accident units dealing with road traffic accidents, long periods of warm ischaemia are expected, so that tubular necrosis is the rule rather than the exception. It is vital during this oliguric period to continue haemodialysis therapy on the same lines as preoperatively—making sure that regional heparinization is performed for the first 14 days. Dialysis is usually continued until there is evidence that the patient's blood urea or creatinine is showing a spontaneous fall. During the recovery phase, urine output seems to be dependent on the osmotic drive provided by a high blood urea and consequently oliguria usually follows on the day immediately after dialysis. Once diuresis is well established, however, little change in urinary output follows a period on haemodialysis.

Patients undergoing irreversible rejection will have to continue haemodialysis to cover the allograft nephrectomy and the subsequent period while they are awaiting a second transplant. An attempt should always be made when an elective operation is to be performed to do this approximately 24 h after the completion of the last haemodialysis period. In addition, after a major operation, it would seem sensible to wait for 48–72 h before performing the next dialysis for however skilled one is at regional heparinization, there is a slight risk of loss of control with resulting serious haemorrhage.

IMMUNOSUPPRESSION

Standard therapy

Steroids—hydrocortisone, prednisone or prednisolone

THE OLIGURIC PATIENT

An initial parenteral dose of 200 mg soluble hydrocortisone is given by the anaesthetist during the transplant operation. This is followed by 100 mg intramuscularly 8-hourly so that a total of 500 mg is given during the first 24 h. A further 500 mg is given in divided doses during the subsequent 24 h. Seventy-five milligrammes prednisolone orally is given daily in two divided doses from the second post-operative day until the patient's urine output is sufficient to lower the blood urea. The dose is then reduced to 50 mg/day for 30 days. The daily dose is thereafter reduced by 5 mg at monthly intervals so that 7 months after transplantation the patient is taking 20 mg/day. This dose is maintained until the end of the 1st year. During the 2nd year it is reduced gradually to 10 mg by the end of that year. Further small reductions may be possible subsequently.

Patients with immediate function

The regime during the first 3 days after operation is identical whether diuresis is delayed or immediate. Afterwards, the prednisolone is reduced to 50 mg/day for 30 days and thereafter reduced as outlined before.

Azathioprine

A loading dose of 5 mg/kg is given on the day of operation. If immediate diuresis occurs a dose of 2–2·5 mg/kg/day can then be given. If tubular necrosis of the allograft leads to oliguria, the dose of azathioprine should be kept at 1–1·5 mg/kg/day in order to prevent bone marrow depression. Provided regular haemodialysis is continued, most patients tolerate this dose quite well. As renal function improves, the dose can be increased gradually to a maximum maintenance dose of 2·5–3 mg/kg/day. During the first 2 months careful daily monitoring of the leucocyte and platelet counts is necessary in order to avoid overdosage. The dose of azathioprine is thereafter kept at the maximal tolerated dose indefinitely.

Anti-rejection therapy for established rejection

The dose of prednisolone is increased to 200 mg/day for 3 days and then reduced by 25 mg every other day down to 50 mg/day. Azathioprine is maintained at the maximum tolerated dose. In the absence of leucopenia or thrombocytopenia, Actinomycin C is given in a dose of 200 μg intravenously on each of 3 successive days. Most patients will tolerate two or three such anti-rejection regimes within the first 2 months but the advisability of repeating these doses will depend upon the histological appearance of the renal biopsy and to the response to previous courses.

Antilymphocytic serum preparations

These have been used in Cambridge as anti-rejection therapy in 7 patients with allograft rejection. In the first five patients 10 ml of antilymphocyte serum were given daily intramuscularly, the second three patients received

TABLE 1

	Basic Normal function	ATN	Rejection
Steroids	500 mg hydrocortisone: 2 days 75 mg prednisolone: 2 days 50 mg prednisolone: 30 days 45 mg prednisolone: 30 days etc.	500 mg hydrocortisone: 2 days 75 mg prednisolone: diuresis 50 mg prednisolone: 30 days 45 mg prednisolone: 30 days etc.	Prednisolone 200 mg: 3 days Prednisolone 175 mg: 2 days Prednisolone 150 mg: 2 days Prednisolone 125 mg: 2 days Prednisolone 100 mg: 2 days Prednisolone 75 mg: 2 days Prednisolone 50 mg: 30 days
Azathioprine	5 mg/kg b.w./day on 1st day 2–2·5 mg/kg b.w./day	5 mg/kg b.w./day on 1st day 1 mg/kg b.w./day: diuresis 1·5–2–2·5 mg/kg b.w./day	2·5 mg/kg b.w./day
Actinomycin C			200 μg i/v for 3 days

20 ml of antilymphocyte globulin in 200 ml 5% dextrose daily by intravenous infusion (Mee & Evans 1970). Most patients tolerated up to 10 daily injections but in almost all cases thrombocytopenia prevented further treatment. Benefit resulted in only three patients and in these the value of the antilymphocyte preparations was not proved.

Dipyridamole and anticoagulants

Mathew *et al* (1967), Mowbray (1969) and McMillan (1968) observed improvement in the function of kidneys undergoing rejection or tubular necrosis after the administration of anticoagulants and ADP antagonists. P. Kincaid-Smith (1969) reported absence of endothelial thickening and disruption of the internal elastic lamina of arterioles in renal allografts in patients treated with dipyridamole and anticoagulants. These substances may prove valuable as adjuvants to the basic immunosuppressive regimes described above, but as yet they have not been widely used, nor is their value proven.

SIDE EFFECTS OF IMMUNOSUPPRESSIVE THERAPY

X-rays	Bone marrow depression Infection Radiation sickness GI tract necrosis
Corticosteroids	Cushing's syndrome Delayed healing Infections GI tract ulceration Bone disease Cataracts Diabetes Mellitus Myopathies Psychoses Purpura Pancreatitis
Azathioprine	Bone marrow depression Alopecia Megaloblastic anaemia Liver dysfunction Wasting

Actinomycin C	Bone marrow depression
A.L.S.	Local skin reactions, urticaria Fever, tachycardia Arthralgia Serum sickness and anaphylaxis Leucopenia and thrombocytopenia

REFERENCES

KINCAID-SMITH P. (1969) Modification of the vascular lesions of rejection in cadaveric renal allografts by dipyridamole and anticoagulants. *Lancet*, ii, 920.

MATHEW T.H., KINCAID-SMITH P., MARSHALL V.C. & EREMIN J. (1967) Phenylbutazone in the treatment of acute rejection. *Ist. Int. Congress of Transpl. Soc. Paris* (*Abstract*), p. 256.

MCMILLAN R. (1968) Heparin in delayed transplant function. *Lancet*, i, 1178.

MEE A.D. & EVANS D.B. (1970) Antilymphocyte serum preparations in the treatment of renal allograft rejection. *Lancet* ii, 716.

MOWBRAY J.F. (1969) Platelet thrombi in rejection episodes. *Proc. R.S.M.* **62**, 597.

CHAPTER 16

Complications

D.B. Evans
W.A.B. Smellie

INTRODUCTION

Renal transplantation is fraught with many complications—medical, surgical and those resulting from immunosuppressive therapy. Morbidity and mortality are highest during the first 3 months after transplantation. These may be related to ischaemic damage to the allograft which commonly follows cadaveric transplantation.

The operation of renal transplantation is not an insignificant surgical procedure and for the patient to withstand such an operation adequate preparation by dialysis is essential (see Chapter 12). Few patients in terminal renal failure with hypertension, electrolyte inbalance and other complications will survive the immediate post-operative period whereas with good preparatory methods, the risk is hardly more than for a normal healthy individual. If immediate renal function does not return, continued dialysis treatment should be available so as to sustain life until the transplanted organ functions adequately.

Other pre-operative preparatory measures include the eradication of infections, the removal of infected kidneys and the treatment of peptic ulcers.

Tissue typing is currently performed on donors and recipients (see Chapter 3) so that bad matches are avoided thus reducing the risk of immunological rejection. Crossmatching of the recipient's serum against the donor's lymphocytes is routinely performed to avoid transplantation in those with circulating cytotoxic antibodies against the donor.

DISORDERED RENAL FUNCTION

In cadaveric renal transplantation programmes, donor kidneys are often obtained from patients dying of road traffic accidents, so that the time between death and admission to the hospital may be considerable. Even

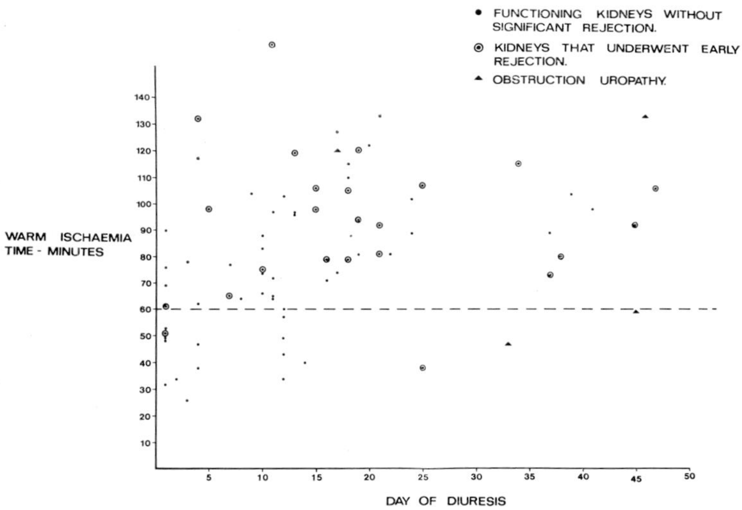

FIG. 1. Graph of warm ischaemia time (time from donor's death to cooling plus anastomosis time) in minutes plotted against the number of days taken by the allograft to excrete 1 l. of urine.

after admission and the certification of death, permission to remove kidneys has to be obtained from the coroner and if possible the relatives of the dead person. Often the time between death and the removal and perfusion of the kidneys is in excess of 1 h, resulting in almost all cases in significant ischaemic damage to the organ. The degree of damage to the kidney depends upon the warm ischaemia time and may range from tubular necrosis (ATN) which is usually reversible to cortical necrosis, which may be irreversible (Fig. 1).

With the exchange of kidneys between different hospital centres particularly between different towns, the total ischaemia periods for organs are becoming more and more prolonged.

If acute tubular necrosis has resulted from the period of ischaemia, this will be evident in the histology of the initial biopsy taken at the end of the operation. A period of oliguria is then to be expected which may extend for 7–28 days. During this time, the pre-operative dialysis régime has to be continued, care being taken to keep the patients' clotting times within safe limits. Because of the risk of bleeding, some units undertake peritoneal dialysis during the 2 weeks after transplantation, but the risk of infection must be weighed against that of haemorrhage.

Immediately after the removal of cadaveric kidneys for purposes of grafting, they are usually perfused with an ice cold multi-electrolyte solution. This manoeuvre serves (a) to cool the organ from the core thus slowing down its metabolic processes, (b) to wash out blood and (c) to give the surgeon an opportunity to assess whether the organ perfuses completely. The latter observation is important, for a badly perfused kidney, if transplanted, may subsequently show patchy areas of cortical necrosis, due to intrarenal vascular obstruction. Poorly perfused kidneys should therefore be discarded.

It takes a kidney with ATN up to 3–4 weeks to function adequately—this is a similar finding to that seen in ATN resulting from other causes such as haemolysis, multiple injuries etc. Providing the patient has been adequately dialysed the return of renal function will be gradual—with a slowly rising urinary output and glomerular filtration rate. Transient tubular defects such as glycosuria and potassium losing states may take several weeks or months to recover, and reversal of diurnal urinary rhythms usually recover during the course of several months. If the patient has not been dialysed, however, and if the blood urea is very high, the return of renal function may be heralded by a massive diuresis—requiring very careful fluid and electrolyte replacement.

During the oliguric period, when immunosuppressive drugs have to be given in attenuated doses, it is impossible clinically to know what is happening to the kidney and formal investigations short of a renal biopsy may be of little assistance.

Hyperacute rejection

Kissmeyer-Nielsen *et al* (1966) described immediate rejection in kidneys transplanted into pre-immunized multiparous women. Subsequent reports have appeared (Williams *et al* 1968; Starzl *et al* 1968; Myburgh *et al* 1969) all patients in these reports having been sensitized by previous transplants, pregnancies or by blood transfusions. Where immediate rejection occurs, the phenomenon can usually be witnessed on the operating table—the well perfused kidney suddenly becoming flabby and cyanosed within minutes of completing the vascular anastomosis. This phenomenon is well known to surgeons who have transplanted across major blood groups and in xenografting. A biopsy of this type of kidney usually shows the presence of interstitial haemorrhage, leucocytic infiltration and fibrinoid necrosis of the glomerular arterioles. Although treatment with heparin has been suggested (Starzl *et al* 1968) its value is not universally accepted. When hyperacute rejection of a graft occurs, there is little to be gained by leaving it *in situ* as it will undoubtedly have to be removed later.

If cytotoxicity testing is performed routinely prior to transplantation hyperacute rejection should theoretically not occur though reports of such events have appeared. However, as more and more patients are surviving one, two or more kidney grafts, the incidence of preformed antibodies is rising and the likelihood of finding suitable kidneys for these patients is diminishing.

Acute rejection

This occurs fairly commonly in the majority of kidney grafts. Many acute rejection crises are relatively mild, some may resolve spontaneously and others respond well to antirejection therapy, but in a few cases an intense reaction occurs which is resistant to treatment. In the functioning allograft the development of acute rejection is not usually difficult to diagnose and may manifest itself by the following features:

a a fall in urinary output and the development of oedema;
b a fall in glomerular filtration rate;
c a rise in blood urea and creatinine;
d a fall in urinary sodium excretion;
e an increase in proteinuria;
f the development of hypertension, tachycardia and fever;
g an enlargement and tenderness of the allograft;
h increased number of lymphocytes excreted in the urine;
i thrombocytopenia.

Not all these features reveal themselves simultaneously. The early detection of rejection can often only be made as a result of careful daily monitoring of a large number of parameters. A fall in urinary solute output coupled with a rise in proteinuria and the development of hypertension and tachycardia may preceed any measurable rise in blood urea or a fall in the creatinine clearance. The proteinuria usually becomes nonselective

(Braun *et al* 1967). Careful serial measurements of the thrombocyte count may also prove valuable (Mowbray 1969).

However, in the oliguric patient the clinical picture is much less clear cut and consequently, because of the paucity of clues, rejection episodes are undoubtedly missed and treatment delayed. In our experience enlargement and tenderness of the kidney may be unhelpful as they may occur in urinary or venous obstruction or may represent perirenal extravasation of blood, urine or lymph. Fever and tachycardia may be signs of infection and careful exclusion of this is necessary before attributing them to rejection. The development of hypertension is certainly an important sign, but renal artery stenosis or hypervolaemia due to sodium retention from other causes must be excluded.

A rapidly rising blood urea without a concomitant rise in blood creatinine should always make one suspicious of gastrointestinal haemorrhage.

It can therefore be appreciated that the diagnosis of acute rejection in the oliguric recipient is one of the most difficult problems in renal transplantation and it is therefore important that the whole clinical picture with as many as possible additional investigations be duly considered.

Additional investigations to determine the cause of oliguria or anuria

1 I_{131} *Renography*

This method using I_{131} labelled para-aminohippuran, may be of value in determining the viability of the kidney graft and in differentiating between vascular occlusions or obstruction to the outflow of urine from the allograft ureter. It is impossible to distinguish between oliguria due to tubular necrosis and rejection. Care must be taken in the interpretation of these renographic patterns as the 'normal curve' may be much flatter than that seen in a normally positioned kidney. This is probably due to the proximity of the graft to the bladder.

2 *Renal scintiscanning*

After the intravenous injection of Hg_{203} labelled chlormerodrin, scintiscanning over the allograft will give an indication of the viability of the graft and may indicate the presence of obstruction. Unfortunately, however, it gives little information as regards differentiation between tubular necrosis and rejection. Renal scanning after injection of I^{125} labelled fibrinogen may help make the distinction (Salaman 1970).

3 *Xenon washout studies*

Experimental work in dogs using Xe^{133} intrarenally indicated differential blood flow patterns in the cortex, the corticomedullary junction, the medulla and perirenal fat. Diminution in cortical blood flow heralded the onset of rejection (Truniger *et al* 1965). This method however is not practical for general use in human renal transplants.

4 *Arteriography*

The investigation of post-transplant hypertension by angiography has been reported by Smellie *et al* (1969). The development of a bruit over the transplanted organ is often associated with renal arterial narrowing and could be detected radiographically. In cases of rejection, diffuse narrowing of intrarenal arteries may be seen and in many cases absence of cortical filling and 'beading' of the intrarenal arterioles can be seen. O'Connor *et al* (1966) found no correlation between histological and angiographic findings in rejection. Since cortical biopsies may not include portions of arcuate or interlobular arteries, this lack of correlation does not seem surprising.

5 *Ultrasonics*

Sampson (1969) showed that by using an ultrasonic meter which depends upon the Doppler effect on blood passing through the renal artery, small changes in blood flow could be detected and he found close correlation between these changes and the development of other signs of rejection.

6 *Serum complement*

Levels of C′2 (second component of complement) have been shown to fall during the 3rd–10th days after the onset of rejection and to return to normal levels on its reversal. BlC globulin (C′3) has been shown to rise by 50% at the onset of rejection then to fall significantly and to return to normal levels when rejection was successfully reversed.

Because of the delayed fall in levels of these components of complement they are probably of little value in early rejection detection but serial measurements may be useful information from the point of view of subsequent management.

7 *Lymphocyte migration index (LMI)*

Eddelston *et al* (1969); Smith *et al* (1969) followed the LMI in patients who had undergone hepatic and renal transplantation and there appeared to be significant correlation between inhibition of migration with severity of graft rejection.

8 *Serum and urinary enzyme studies*

Renal tissue is rich in lactic dehydrogenase (LDH) and any condition resulting in tissue damage may be expected to be accompanied by an increased urinary concentration of the enzyme. Measurements of urine and serum LDH—isoenzymes however have been studied in relation to renal transplant rejection and characteristic patterns and levels have been described (Prout *et al* 1964), but most workers consider the serum LDH to be too insensitive a test. Some workers have felt that measurements of serum alkaline phosphatase was more valuable than LDH. Urinary lysozyme concentrations were found to rise after transplant ischaemia and a secondary peak occurred before rejection crises (Najarian *et al* 1965).

9 *Renal biopsy*

This has been the one investigation that has given us most information in regard to diagnosing the cause of delayed renal function (Millard *et al* 1970). Cortical biopsies according to the technique of P. Kincaid-Smith using a Vim Silverman or Trucut (Baxter) biopsy needle can be fairly easily obtained and if the usual precautions are taken regarding clotting and bleeding tendencies, the morbidity should be insignificant. Morphologically, evidence of rejection and ATN are diffusely distributed throughout the organ, so that the biopsy taken from one or other pole will, in general, be representative and allow for a fairly confident diagnosis.

During the early post-operative period biopsies can be helpful therefore in investigating the cause of delayed function and where rejection having been diagnosed on clinical grounds had not responded in the anticipated fashion to antirejection therapy (Millard *et al* 1970). Acute rejection may be the result of mononuclear cellular infiltration of the allograft with accompanying oedema of the interstitial spaces. Reversal of the rejection by high steroid doses is usually accompanied by diminution in the number of cells and degree of swelling. Where fibrinoid necrosis and severe vascular damage has occurred, however, reversal of this process is unlikely despite repeated antirejection treatment.

Chronic rejection

It has been suggested that histocompatibility matching of the donor and recipient plays little part in determining the initial outcome of a renal allograft but rather will influence the long term survival of the graft beyond 1 year. Where two or more antigenic incompatibilities have been present between the donor and recipient increasing histological damage represented by basement membrane thickening in the glomeruli and intimal thickening of the blood vessels have been demonstrated by Porter *et al* (1963).

Clinically, these changes may be reflected in gradually diminishing renal function with the development of a heavy nonselective proteinuria and hypertension. If treatment with high doses of steroids is given at this stage, some improvement in function may result presumably by reducing inflammatory responses in the kidney and by disaggregating platelets which might be attached to the damaged vascular endothelium.

Heavy proteinuria from the transplanted kidney may in some cases be the result of the development of glomerulonephritis. This phenomenon was first observed in grafts exchanged between identical twins where the recipient had previously suffered from glomerulonephritis. Characterization of the selectivity of the permeability of the glomerular basement membrane may be a useful guide, but electron microscopy of biopsy specimens and immunofluorescent studies are more likely to resolve the problem as to whether the condition is due to chronic rejection or glomerulonephritis. The presence of subepithelial lumps as seen on electron-microscopy of the glomerular basement membrane lends support to the possibility that glomerulonephritis is the cause. In addition it would seem unlikely that glomerulonephritis would affect the allograft in a patient who originally suffered from polycystic disease or pyelonephritis.

In some cases of chronic rejection improvement in function may result by increasing the dosage of steroids and by the use of anticoagulant drugs and Dipyridamole (McMillan 1968; Kincaid-Smith 1969).

The cardiovascular system

Failing renal function more often adversely affects the cardiovascular system than almost any other. Fluid and electrolyte inbalance may lead to hypertension, fluid retention and heart failure as well as changes in cardiac muscle function. Uraemic pericarditis may occur but its exact cause is unknown and the refractory anaemia associated with uraemia adds to the cardiac load. Patients with generalized vasculitis as a complication of a collagen disorder are usually excluded from dialysis and transplantation because of the high incidence of generalized vascular, arthritic and other possible complications which may occur. Cardiomyopathies have also been described (Bailey *et al* 1967).

Timely commencement of regular dialysis treatment usually forestalls many of these complications but if hypertension, heart failure or hyperkalaemia have become established, dialysis with ultrafiltration in association with hypotensive agents, exchange resins and sodium restriction will correct them. Strict adherence to a diet will ensure the maintenance of a reasonable electrolytic balance during the interdialysis period whereas indiscrete indulgement in foods containing excess sodium or potassium may result in pulmonary oedema or cardiac arrest.

Some hypertensive patients are refractory to hypotensive therapy, salt restriction and haemodialysis, and in such individuals high circulating renin levels may be found (Gleadle *et al* 1969). Bilateral nephrectomy usually facilitates the control of hypertension in those cases.

The control of blood pressure as measured by sphygmomanometric readings is a satisfying finding but more important is the serial observation of the electrocardiogram for disappearance of signs of left ventricular strain and also for the return to normal of the cardiac silhouette radiologically. The longer such patients are maintained by efficient haemodialysis, the better will they be able to withstand transplantation particularly if after surgery, oliguria persists. These patients are sensitive to significant alterations in blood volume and care should therefore be exercised with intravenous infusions and overenthusiastic measures to increase their haemoglobin levels by a 'topping up' bottle of blood should be strictly curbed. Inadvertent precipitation of acute left ventricular failure calls for emergency dialysis or phlebotomy.

Atheromatous changes in the arterial tree are particularly common even in young patients with longstanding hypertension and abnormalities in calcium metabolism may add to their problems by causing vascular calcification. Not only are the coronary arteries likely to be involved in this process but the cerebral and peripheral vessels also. Surgical anastomosis of a calcified internal iliac artery may be very difficult and often an endarterectomy has to be performed. Thus, patients with calcific vascular disease are not ideal candidates for transplantation and may be the victims of myocardial or cerebral infarctions in the postoperative period.

The development of peripheral ischaemia is rare in young adults but in one patient aged 20 years with longstanding renal failure, gangrenous changes occurred in his hand after the insertion of a Scribner shunt in the ulnar artery—the radial artery having previously been used. Another patient 2 years after successful renal transplantation developed ischaemic necrosis of the lateral side of the tip of his right index finger. His heart was in sinus rhythm, he had no other sign of vascular insufficiency and the proximal digital arteries to his finger pulsated normally. The iscahaemic area separated leaving a completely healed scar after 4 months. The finger is now painless and fully functional. This was probably the result of a localized digital artery thrombosis which may have been associated with the mild trauma of using a paint spray gun in his occupation as a coach repairer.

Renal artery stenosis

This complication which may affect the allograft artery has been described by many authors (Smellie *et al* 1969). Not only may stenosis occur at the line of anastomosis but also in the artery distal to the anastomosis. Such a complication may manifest itself by the development of severe hypertension in the absence of biopsy evidence of rejection and an audible bruit may develop over the allograft artery. The diagnosis may be confirmed by selective arteriography and prompt surgical correction should be performed.

Venous thrombosis in the legs has been seen in this unit in only six patients; these have not necessarily occurred on the same side as the transplanted kidney. In two further male patients multiple small pulmonary emboli were observed but no evidence of deep venous thromboses were found in the legs clinically—it seems possible that thrombosis in the pelvic veins may have been the source of the emboli, though had phlebograms been performed the site of thromboses might have been located. Under such conditions anticoagulant therapy has been given with benefit.

Increased capillary fragility is a recognized complication of steroid therapy but thrombocytopaenia may give a similar appearance of petechial haemorrhages, extensive ecchymoses and a positive Hess Test.

Venous occlusion

This is fortunately an unusual complication of renal transplantation. The venous drainage in the kidney has such good anastomotic connections that where multiple renal veins are present, all but the major vessels can be tied off with impunity. However, extravascular pressure by a haematoma may lead to venous obstruction. Allograft vein thrombosis may occur as a result of spread from pelvic vein or iliac vein thrombi. Sudden development of heavy proteinuria and swelling of the kidney should make one suspicious and pertrochanteric venography will usually confirm the diagnosis. Severe ischaemic damage to an allograft may lead to intrarenal venous thrombosis resulting in massive intrarenal haemorrhage with clinical enlargement.

Pulmonary

Patients with terminal renal failure are prone to pulmonary congestion and oedema due to water and sodium retention. Uraemic lung is a time honoured syndrome which closely resembles acute left ventricular failure but Gibson (1967) found low or normal right atrial and pulmonary artery pressures in a series of patients studied. He concluded that there is probably an increase in pulmonary capillary permeability in uraemic patients.

After transplantation, pulmonary oedema may again occur due to overloading the circulation and in the presence of immunosuppressive therapy, infections may supervene. Infection with bacteria, fungi, parasites and viruses can occur in the lungs in such patients.

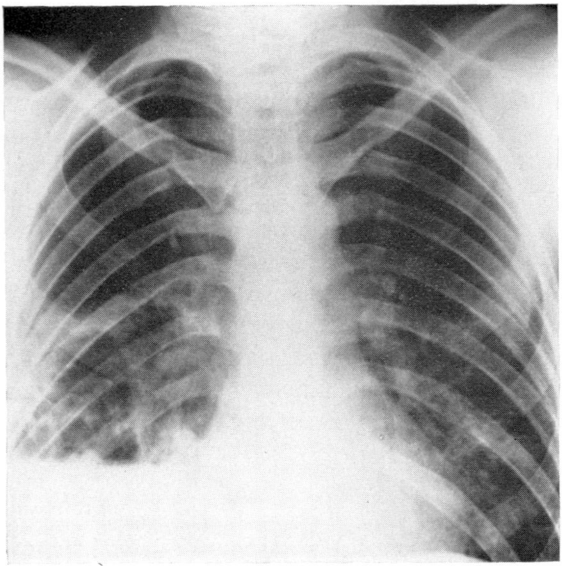

FIG. 2. Chest radiograph showing a large abscess in the right lower lobe following post-operative aspiration pneumonitis (patient N.M.).

Latent tuberculosis may be lit up and any patient with a previously suspected or known tuberculous infection should be covered by prophylactic antituberculous therapy during immunosuppression.

Bacterial pneumoniae may respond to prompt antibiotic therapy but occasionally cavitation with abscess formation may occur. Two of our patients developed lung abscesses—one following an inhalation pneumonia post-operatively and the other following a lobar pneumonia (Fig. 2). Both required drainage and developed bronchopleural fistulae (Fig. 3). Reduction in immunosuppressive drugs is important if healing is to occur even at the risk of losing the graft through rejection.

Pulmonary emboli may follow deep vein thrombosis in the legs. This condition has been found to be associated with erythraemia (Swales & Evans 1969) and usually responds to anticoagulant therapy. In two of our patients calcification of old pulmonary infarcts has occurred.

'Transplant pneumonitis' has been described (Slapak *et al* 1968) and is a condition thought to be due to cross reaction of antirenal antibodies with

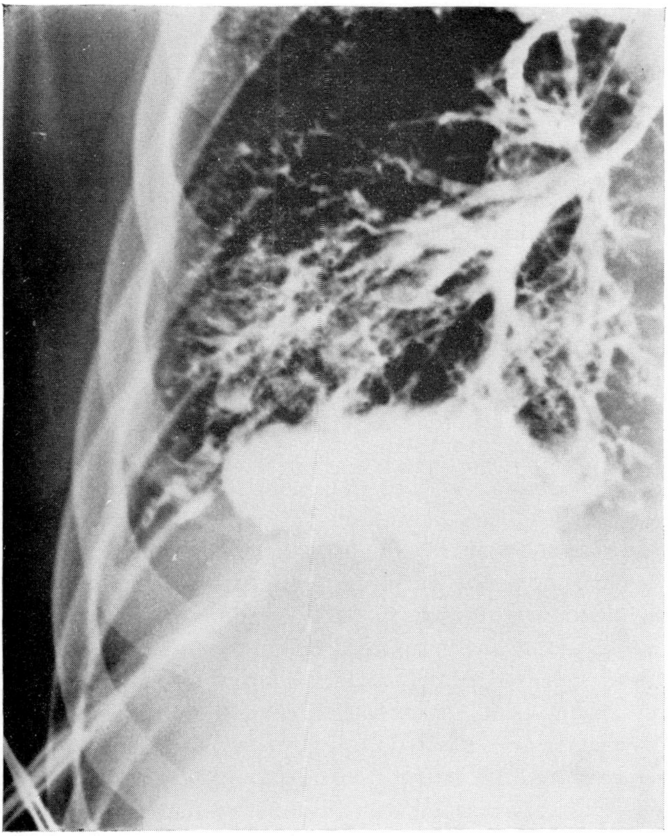

FIG. 3. Bronchogram of patient N.M. 1 year after rib resection and drainage of right lower lobe abscess. 1 month later, right lower partial lobectomy was successfully performed.

lung epithelium. Their patients were undergoing allograft rejection when they developed an alveolar capillary diffusion block and improvement occurred as a result of increasing the dose of steroids. The condition is characterized clinically by intense dyspnoea with minimal physical signs in the chest, a diffuse shadowing radiologically, often an intractable cough but no significant sputum. In some of our patients with similar clinical syndromes, viral and fungal causes for the diffusion defect were found and the condition worsened by increasing the dose of steroids.

Pneumothorax following lung abscesses or due to the rupture of emphysematous cysts or tuberculous cavities is an especially difficult complication to deal with in the suppressed patient. Drainage with suction must be performed and even then it is usually very difficult to stick the lung on to the chest wall because of the lack of an inflammatory response. An irritant such as colloidal kaolin has to be infused into the pleural cavity in order to stimulate a reaction but in the presence of steroids this may be unsuccessful.

Haematopoietic system

Uraemia impairs the immune response to a variable extent, but the white cell count and myeloid elements in the marrow are usually normal in appearance. Thrombocytes though present in normal numbers may not behave normally and have been shown to have diminished adhesiveness and other qualitative abnormalities resulting in a bleeding diathesis (Castali *et al* 1966).

The erythrocyte series is directly influenced by longstanding renal disease and chronic anaemia is an invariable accompaniment of this condition. It is unresponsive to the common haematinics—iron, folate and B12.

Erythropoietin is a hormone thought to be produced or activated by normal kidney tissue and in some cases of renal cysts and renal tumours, an excess of this hormone has been demonstrated. Excessive secretion is accompanied by overstimulation of the erythropoietic system resulting in erythaemia. In the normal individual the most potent stimulus to erythropoietin production is chronic anaemia. However, the anaemia of chronic renal failure is not usually accompanied by a high erythropoietin level, in fact activity may be even absent (Brown 1965). The removal of the patient's own kidneys and maintenance of life by intermittent haemodialysis has been shown to increase blood transfusion requirements suggesting that a source of erythropoietic stimulus may have been removed (van Ypersele de Strihou & Stragier 1969). It has also been shown by Crockett *et al* (1967) that efficient haemodialysis with maintenance of a low blood urea usually allows for spontaneous erythropoiesis suggesting that perhaps 'uraemia' *per se* may have a depressant effect on erythropoietin production or on its activity or even on the bone marrow itself. Certainly red cell life may be shortened significantly by chronic uraemia.

Successful renal allografting produces a dramatic effect on haemopoiesis and after discharge from hospital (where haemoglobin levels are kept at a low level by virtue of repeated phlebotomies) the patient's haemoglobin and haematocrit are usually back to normal levels within 2 months. Swales & Evans (1969) showed that in a few patients normal levels may be exceeded, and in this group of patients there was a high incidence of thrombotic phenomena—venous thrombosis, cardiac infarction and cerebral thrombosis. Phlebotomy or anticoagulation is probably indicated in such patients until haemoglobin and haematocrit levels return to normal as they almost invariably do. The aetiology of this phenomenon is uncertain; there may be excessive erythropoietin production, though in some instances haemoconcentration due to a low circulating plasma volume may be responsible.

Azathioprine, by its indiscriminate effect on rapidly dividing cells often depresses the level of circulating leucocytes—mainly of the granulocyte series. We have not observed any consistent depression of the lymphocytes in our patients. During the oliguric post-operative period, it has been already stressed that the dose of azathioprine should be kept low (1 mg/kg body weight/day), for if this dose is exceeded, leucopaenia often follows. If this state of affairs does occur, the drug will have to be witheld until the marrow recovers. An additional disadvantage of this is that during the period of no azathioprine therapy, the allograft may be left 'uncovered'. Once renal function is stable, a constant dose of azathioprine can usually be prescribed. We have sometimes seen thrombocytopaenia accompanying leucopaenia but as there are other possible causes such as immune rejection, bleeding etc., one cannot always be certain that azathioprine is responsible.

Depression of all bone marrow components can occur in any case with overwhelming septicaemia—this is not too uncommon an event in immunosuppressed patients.

Over the period of several months after successful renal transplantation, patients on azathioprine and steroids sometimes develop folic acid deficiency. Azathioprine is not a folic acid antagonist like methotrexate but acts by inhibiting the formation of nucleic acids. A possible mechanism of folate deficiency may be by interfering with the turnover of jejunal epithelium thus leading to a malabsorption of folate. Folate supplements parenterally will be curative.

Thrombocytopaenia may result from certain batches of antilymphocytic globulin and we have seen this complication several times (Mee & Evans 1970).

The liver

Reports have appeared from intermittent dialysis units throughout the world of epidemics of hepatitis (Jones *et al* 1967; Eastwood *et al* 1968). The virus is thought to be transmitted via blood products or non-disposable dialysers from patient to patient but in Sweden (Franksson 1969) an outbreak was reported in a transplantation unit using disposable dialysers. Patients and members of medical, nursing, technical laboratory and portering staff have been affected and several deaths have occurred. Transplantation surgeons are also at risk in this regard. The one common feature to units where hepatitis has developed has been the liberal use of blood transfusions in an attempt to maintain the patient's haematocrit level. The larger British dialysis units have now abandoned routine blood transfusions and by increased dialysis efficiency transfusions have become unnecessary. The transfer of patients from one dialysis unit to another e.g. whilst on holiday or for purposes of transplantation, may transmit hepatitis from one unit to another and therefore should be discouraged. Home dialysis seems to be the surest way of preventing hepatitis outbreaks provided, of course, blood transfusions are kept to an absolute minimum. In 1967 Blumberg *et al* found that 20% of cases of viral hepatitis possessed Australia antigen (Au). In 1969 he reported that Au antigen had been found in 58% of cases of post-transfusion hepatitis and in 38% of cases of infectious hepatitis. Turner & White (1969) found that as many as 80% of cases of viral hepatitis were positive to Au antigen during the early weeks of the disease. After this most patients were able to clear their blood of antigen and recover; but in cases of unresolved hepatitis 50% of patients had persistent Au antigen. It therefore would appear that in future screening of all blood donors for Australia antigen may be possible so that only blood from negative reactors will be used for transfusion purposes.

Precautions against hepatitis should be undertaken by all members of the dialysis and transplantation unit staff e.g. the wearing of gloves and protective clothing whenever blood or excreta or soiled materials have to be handled. We advise the use of gloves for 'blood letting' and similar procedures. Staff members should not be allowed to eat in the wards and disposable utensils should be used by the patients. The value of prophylactic γ-globulin in preventing or attenuating an attack of hepatitis is currently under review.

After renal transplantation, abnormalities of liver function may be found if looked for—raised alanine aminotransferase and alkaline phosphatase, often associated with slight tender hepatomegaly. In the majority of patients this is a self limiting condition but in a few cases liver failure may supervene. In such a group Evans *et al* (1969) found a varied histological pattern at necropsy amounting to portal fibrosis, liver cell necrosis and intracellular cytomegalic inclusions. Calne (1961) showed that azathioprine given to dogs with renal transplants developed a cholestatic jaundice with a rise in alkaline phosphatase. It is interesting that in clinical renal transplantation where azathioprine is given, liver cell damage (assessed by a rise in SGPT) is much commoner than cholestasis.

Pancreatic complications

a *Exocrine function*

Pancreatitis has been described as a complication of steroid therapy (Carone & Liebon 1957). In a comparison of autopsies performed on patients who had been on long-term steroid therapy and those who had not, the incidence of pancreatitis was eight times greater in the steroid treated group. Strumpf & Wilens (1955) had earlier reported pancreatic lesions in rabbits treated with cortisone. There has been no experimental evidence to suggest any relationship between pancreatitis and azathioprine therapy.

Johnson & Nabseth (1970) in a survey of 1321 renal transplants performed in many centres found 23 cases of pancreatitis with 12 deaths

The aetiology is not completely clear but an association has been found with hyperparathyroidism and it has been shown that high serum calcium levels may activate trypsinogen to produce trypsin (Haverback *et al* 1960). Tilney *et al* (1966) suggested an autoimmune basis as they described vasculitis in the pancreases of two of their patients undergoing renal allograft rejection.

Cytomegalovirus infection has also been a feature of some cases. Treatment consists of reducing the steroid dosage along with supportive measures and surgical drainage. Hyperparathyroidism if present should be corrected.

b *Endocrine function*

Diabetes mellitus may occur in patients given long-term steroid drugs (Starzl 1964). It seems probable that the steroids merely light up a latent condition though in the five cases seen by us, no family history of diabetes mellitus was found. It is usual to pick up the condition during the first 3 months after transplantation whilst the patients are on relatively high steroid doses, and insulin or oral hypoglycaemic agents may be necessary for adequate control. Recurrent antirejection therapy usually aggravates the condition. It is usually a mild condition and we have yet to see the development of diabetic retinopathy, nephropathy or neuropathy after transplantation.

Chronic renal failure per se, is sometimes accompanied by carbohydrate intolerance (Hampers *et al* 1966; Wright *et al* 1968) and several mechanisms have been postulated. However, haemodialysis is usually followed by improvement. After transplantation there is no good reason to believe that diabetes mellitus is a particular hazard in such patients.

Gonads

Depression of gonadal function is common in renal failure with loss of libido and amenorrhoea in the female and loss of potency in the male (Schreiner & Maher 1965). Oligozoospermia has been described in males with uraemia but improvement in libido, potency and fertility in men and return of menstruation in women have occurred with efficient dialysis treatment (Elstein *et al* 1969).

Renal transplantation invariably restores gonadal function and several of our male patients have fathered children after transplantation. Reports from the USA of women becoming pregnant and delivering normal babies after transplantation have been published but so far none of our own patients has become pregnant since renal transplantation.

Infectious complications

Patients treated with corticosteroids and antimetabolite drugs for malignant conditions as well as for renal transplantation are especially prone to infectious complications with bacterial, fungal, protozoal and viral agents (Rifkind *et al* 1964; Hutter & Collins 1962; Rifkind 1965; Rifkind *et al* 1967).

Host factors

1 DRUGS

Steroids and azathioprine are the most commonly used basic immunosuppressive drugs with local irradiation to the graft and actinomycin C as anti-rejection crisis agents. These drugs are nonspecific in their actions and diminish the resistance of patients to invasion by micro-organisms in addition to the suppression of the immune response.

Bone marrow depression frequently follows the indiscriminate use of azathioprine during periods of poor renal function. The resulting leukopaenia may increase the susceptibility of the patient to infections by depressing immunoglobulin synthesis and phagocytic activity. Furthermore, the rapidly dividing cells of the gastrointestinal tract may be inhibited with the result that ulceration occurs and enteric micro-organisms may gain entry into the blood stream.

The precise ways in which steroids alter the host's responses to infection are not completely understood. They are known to have anti-inflammatory properties and to interfere with healing processes but in addition they may depress phagocytosis and antibody synthesis. It is the experience of most workers that high steroid doses (as may be required in patients whose kidney grafts are undergoing rejection) are often accompanied by a high incidence of infection.

2 Functional and technical considerations

It is gratifying to observe the smooth progress of a recipient of an allograft where there are minimal immunological and no technical problems. However functional mishaps such as delayed function following ischaemic tubular necrosis and technical troubles e.g. urinary fistulate and local haemorrhage are often complicated by infection. In some cases, owing to the difficulty in making a definite diagnosis of rejection, antirejection therapy may have considerably increased the patient's susceptibility to infection.

3 Immunological factors

As already mentioned in respect of drug therapy, immunological rejection with the need for high steroid doses carries a correspondingly high risk of infection—often apparently harmless organisms proliferate unrestrained giving rise to bizarre and sometimes fatal syndromes.

4 Debility and inanition

Severely ill patients with terminal uraemia are bad risks for a transplantation operation unless adequately prepared. Bed ridden patients with such complications as metabolic bone disease and congestive cardiac failure need a prolonged course of haemodialysis and physiotherapy in order to transform them into subjects fit for surgery followed by immunosuppressive drugs.

5 Pre-existing infections

Eradication of pre-existing infection before starting the patient on immunosuppressive drugs is always indicated. In the majority of our patients who developed significant infections after transplantation the offending organisms could be traced to the host. Forty-five per cent of nasopharyngeal carriers of pyogenic staphylococci developed staphylococcal infections in their wounds or at the sites of arteriovenous shunts as opposed to 20% of negative carriers.

Chronic genito-urinary infection was the cause of terminal renal failure in approximately 20% of our cases and where pretransplant bilateral nephrectomy was not performed, recurrent infection of the urine occurred in 66% of cases whether previously infected or not. It is now our policy to remove the kidneys of all patients before transplantation as we have found post-transplantation urinary infections in patients who originally suffered from glomerulonephritis—the presence of nonfunctioning blind collecting systems acting as stagnant culture media.

Intra-abdominal sepsis following repeated peritoneal dialysis is another source of infection that can spread when the patient is immunosuppressed. It is best to avoid peritoneal dialysis but if it is necessary as a lifesaving procedure strict asepsis and the prompt treatment of infection by the appropriate antibiotic are important. In the presence of intraperitoneal infection, clinical signs may be minimal and in one recent case peritonitis developed as a result of the rupture of previously undiagnosed diverticulitis. Classical signs of peritonitis were absent.

Latent infections

Herpes simplex virus and herpes zoster—varicella virus not uncommonly develop in immunosuppressed patients and often the only course available is to withdraw immunosuppressive therapy. Inappropriate antibiotics may aggravate the situation. Systemic H. simplex has developed *de novo* in one of our patients 18 months after successful transplantation—this improved after infusions of plasma (presumably containing significant γ-globulin concentrations).

A previous history of tuberculosis is an indication for extensive search for activity. Should an active focus be found, intermittent haemodialysis with antituberculous chemotherapy should be the treatment of choice. The possibility of transplantation should be reviewed and considered when the process is healed. Thereafter, or in the case of old healed tuberculosis, transplantation and immunosuppression should be covered by appropriate chemotherapeutic drugs—care being taken to monitor blood levels in the presence of diminished renal function. Cytomegalovirus infections may be latent, but more often may be transmitted via fresh blood transfusions.

Cross infection

Cross infections are not usually a major problem provided reverse barrier conditions are observed during the period that the patient has unhealed wounds urinary catheters and drains *in situ* but in four of our cases infections transmitted via the donor organ have given rise to septicaemias and secondary haemorrhages. In each case the donor had been maintained on a respirator for periods of 48 h or more before death and the same organisms had been isolated from their bronchial secretions as were responsible for septicaemias in the recipients. Care should be taken therefore in avoiding the use of organs from infected donors for transplantation purposes.

The incidence of infection rises rapidly in a patient who undergoes repeated acute rejection episodes and requires high antirejection doses of steroids. Under those conditions one has to weigh the advantages of saving the suspect allograft against the disadvantage of precipitating irreversible infectious complications in the recipient. Our current policy tends to be conservative and if renal biopsy shows severe rejection with vascular changes, it is felt that repeated antirejection doses are unlikely to save the graft so that it is removed. Experience with the opposite viewpoint usually resulted in the death of the patient with multiple foci of sepsis, generalized intestinal ulceration and prolific fungal infection.

Bacterial infections

Gram-positive organisms, mainly *Staph. pyogenes*, are commonly present in the nasopharynx of hospitalized patients and may lead to shunt and wound sepsis. Septicaemias may result in the immunosuppressed patient. Treatment by drainage of wounds and appropriate antibiotics successfully eradicates the infection in most cases.

Gram-negative organisms are far more troublesome and usually stem from an autogenous source in the gastrointestinal or urinary tracts. Sometimes infected peritoneal cavities following repeated peritoneal dialysis may lead to dissemination of organisms, or to interference with intestinal function. Removal of infected kidneys before transplantation greatly reduces the risk of post-operative urinary tract infection and if leakage of urine occurs, of pelvic sepsis. Prostatitis and epididymo-orchitis may complicate prolonged bladder catheterization and a pseudomonas aeruginosa septicaemia followed such a sequence in one of our cases.

Pseudomonas aeruginosa and *proteus* spp. infections are particularly likely to affect patients who are emaciated, immobile and who have suffered considerable immunological reactions—in these cases the large steroid dosages undoubtedly contribute to the infection which is often fatal.

Two patients with lung abscesses following pneumonia both harboured multiple infecting organisms in their respiratory tracts—these included *Staph. pyogenes*, *ps. aeruginosa* and *candida albicans*. Improvement occurred in both following systemic and local therapy with appropriate antibiotics and antifungal agents coupled with drastic reduction in immuno-suppressive therapy.

Antibiotic therapy

Prophylactic antibiotics are rarely given in medical practice as they often lead to the emergence of bacteria resistant to the antibiotic agent used. They also alter the balance of normal bacterial flora in the nasopharyngeal, respiratory and gastrointestinal systems with the result that saprophytic organisms including fungi and protozoans are allowed to proliferate. Unusual syndromes may result from this saprophytic overgrowth against which our present therapy is often grossly inadequate.

When a significant bacterial infection develops following transplantation it is almost always necessary to treat it with the appropriate antibiotic, but in order to diminish the possibility of overgrowth with resistant strains of bacteria, a narrow spectrum antibiotic should be selected whenever possible. In addition, it is important to use doses which will give adequate serum levels against the specific organisms and if in the presence of disordered renal function the dose regime is uncertain, measurement of serum levels should be carried out in the laboratory. Therapy should not be prolonged beyond the time necessary to eliminate the infection.

Fungal and other infections

In spite of careful management and elimination of pre-operative infections and technical factors, the incidence of fungal, viral and protozoal infestations is very high in recipients of all organ grafts (Rifkind *et al* 1967; Brettschneider *et al* 1969). Immune rejection necessitating large steroid doses and the use of antibiotics to counter bacterial infections are undoubtedly the two most important predisposing factors. Diagnosis of these infections during life may be difficult and males tend to be affected more commonly than females (Rifkind *et al* 1967).

Fungi

Candida albicans and *Aspergillus* spp. are the two commonest infecting organisms. Both may be harboured in the respiratory and gastrointestinal tracts of normal individuals and aspergillus may in addition be found in the atmosphere. It is not surprising therefore that *aspergillus* infections mainly colonize lung tissue particularly abscess cavities and devitalized areas (Fig. 4). Rifkind *et al* (1967) found that *aspergillus* had a predisposition for brain tissue and when found either at craniotomy or autopsy, was often associated with haemorrhagic necrosis. Our experience is similar. Any unexplained personality or behavioural changes or the development of epilepsy after transplantation should be investigated with a view to excluding fungal invasion. One patient observed by us developed cerebellar ataxia, which was later found to be due to an aspergillus fumigatus abscess in a cerebellar hemisphere.

Candida albicans tends to invade the gastrointestinal tract—oral and oesophageal ulceration being fairly common. Wound and urinary tract

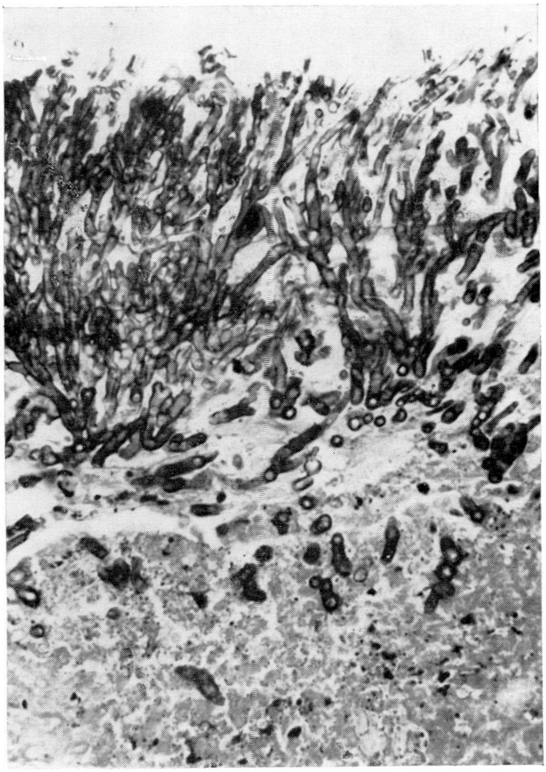

FIG. 4. *Aspergillus* sp. in necrotic lung tissue extending through the visceral pleura. Abscesses containing *Aspergillus* were also present in the allograft and the brain. H.E. ×600.

infections with candida have also been observed particularly when urinary fistulae have occurred.

Oral candidiasis is amenable to topical therapy with gentian violet, nystatin or fungilin (Amphotericin B), but oesophageal ulceration will only respond to systemic amphotericin B therapy. Amphotericin B is nephrotoxic and therefore careful observation of renal function is necessary. We have found that small doses e.g. 0·2 mg/kg body weight/day are usually adequate.

Histoplasmosis, nocardosis and coccidioidomycosis have been described as complications of renal transplantation, causing granulomatous lesions in skin, lungs and central nervous system (Park *et al* 1967).

Regular measurement of fungal antibodies in the patient's serum may be of value in the detection of significant fungal infections—a rising titre may accompany clinical infection or represent occult infection. In immunosuppressed patients however it must be remembered that antibody development may be depressed and therefore of little diagnostic aid.

Mortality is high amongst patients developing significant fungal infection; in the main this is undoubtedly due to the difficulty in making a diagnosis during life, but the possibility of improved and safer antifungal agents gives hope that such infections will one day be amenable to treatment.

Viruses

Herpes simplex and Herpes zoster—varicella viruses are common organisms in the general population and are frequently reactivated in patients with malignant diseases and in those receiving immunosuppressive therapy.

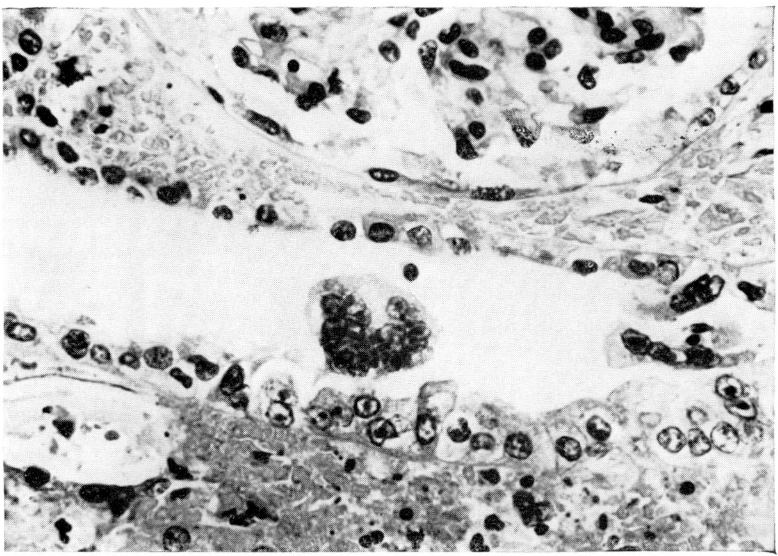

FIG. 5. Renal allograft of patient dying from fulminating varicella. Intranuclear inclusion bodies in epithelial cells lining a tubule and in a multinucleate cell in the lumen. H.E. ×600.

Many of our patients have suffered from herpes simplex mouth ulceration and one patient developed severe dendritic corneal ulcers. These local lesions usually respond to local idoxyuridine. Generalized Herpes simplex infections following lung infection however are usually fatal.

Herpes zoster has, in our patients, been a relatively benigh condition—complete resolution occurring in the course of a month. One patient who developed haemorrhagic varicella on the other hand, had a fulminating and fatal course and at autopsy, the varicella virus had invaded most of the patient's tissues (Fig. 5).

Cytomegalovirus infection complicating immunosuppressive therapy is widely recognized and intranuclear inclusion bodies may be widespread in necropsy material (Fig. 6). Examination of the urinary deposit of renal

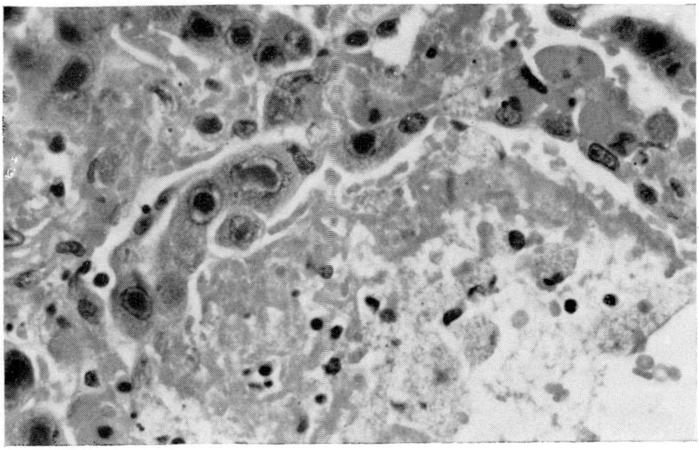

FIG. 6. Lung. Cells in alveoli containing intranuclear inclusions in cytomegalovirus infection. H.E. × 500.

transplant recipients will reveal a high incidence of cytomegalic inclusions even in the absence of any other sign of infection. Liver dysfunction may occasionally be attributed to this virus but again the picture is clouded by the possibility of azathioprine toxicity and viral hepatitis (Evans *et al* 1969).

If eradication of infection can be ensured pre-operatively and by good tissue matching technique, significant histocompatibility mismatches avoided, post-operative rejection crises and infections may be kept to a minimum. The use of antibiotics to combat bacterial infections following rejection is the commonest factor in allowing the proliferation of fungi and viruses. To accept the inevitable loss of a graft that has some residual function is one of the hardest problems facing a transplant team but in the face of severe rejection complicated by infection, it is often the only solution at present.

Neurological complications

In longstanding chronic renal failure the nervous system is frequently involved. Muscle twitching with flapping tremor, drowsiness and nocturnal insomnia, major epileptiform convulsions and eventual coma were a common sequence of events before the advent of intermittent haemodialysis. With prolongation of life by dieting and haemodialysis, however, another complication has emerged—peripheral neuropathy (Tenckoff *et al* 1965; Heron *et al* 1965). This is a progressive condition involving initially the lower limbs, and affecting both sensory and motor fibres. By nerve conduction studies, it can be detected before clinical signs appear and by early and efficient haemodialysis it can be arrested or even improved. Its aetiology is as yet uncertain but the restoration of normal renal function by transplantation results in its complete resolution.

Disturbances of calcium metabolism are often associated with changes in neuromuscular function and tetanic cramps and muscle weakness may result. Myopathies may also occur in association with calcium disturbances.

Malignant hypertension if untreated may result in hypertensive encephalopathy and cerebral irritation and sometimes epilepsy may occur during haemodialysis in the presence of high levels of blood urea.

There is an association between polycystic disease of the kidneys and aneurysms on the Circle of Willis and subarachnoid haemorrhage may occur.

Following transplantation most of these neurological complications resolve naturally. However several complications may result either from the direct effect of the drugs or as the result of immunosuppression.

Post-operative hypertensive crises with major epilepsy can occur in the previously unprepared patient but the steroids themselves may be directly responsible in some cases. If no other good reason for hypertension can be found an underlying allograft artery stenosis should be looked for. The relentless development of chronic rejection often accompanied by hypertension needs careful observation and treatment for fear of cerebrovascular damage.

Cerebrovascular calcification may predispose to cerebral infarction in the post-operative period and mycotic aneurysms from bacteraemic vegetations on heart valves may occasionally be seen.

Hereditary nephritis with deafness constitutes a well known syndrome but most cases of deafness and vestibular disturbances seen by us either before or after transplantation could usually be attributed to toxic antibiotics which had been administered carelessly—Gentamycin, Streptomycin, Kanamycin, Colomycin and Neomycin are usually responsible and it must always be remembered that toxic blood levels may be achieved even from topical applications or local instillations of these antibiotics. Careful monitoring of blood levels cannot be overemphasized if these drugs must be used.

Thrombocytopaenia due to any cause may result in cerebral or subdural haemorrhages. The only way to avoid this is by careful daily platelet counts and titration of immunosuppressive therapy accordingly.

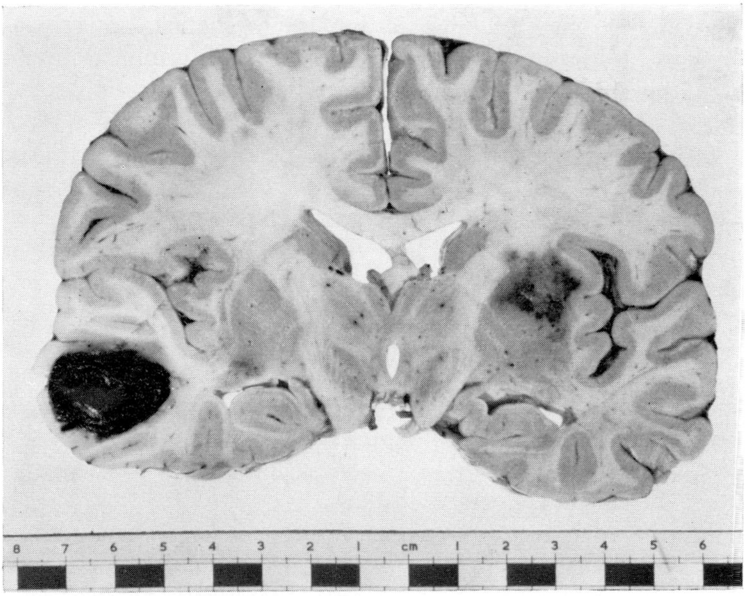

FIG. 7. Coronal section of brain. Haematoma of left temporal lobe. The area of 'softening' in the right basal ganglia consisted of a group of micro-abscesses containing Aspergillus spp. The patient died 117 days after transplantation and similar fungus was present in lesions in the lungs. ×0·9.

Infections of the central nervous system tend to follow the patterns seen in other systems—one should be aware of their possibility and any change in personality, behaviour or the development of localizing signs should be investigated by lumbar puncture and brain scans. The infections are usually secondary to septicaemias, lung or sinus infections and may be caused by bacteria, fungi or viruses. Fungi may also be secondary invaders of brain infarcts probably transported by the bloodstream from the intestines or respiratory tree (Fig. 7).

Bone and joint complications

The bony complications of chronic renal disease have been reviewed by Stanbury (1967). A combination of osteomalacia and secondary hyperparathyroidism are seen most commonly but osteoporosis and osteosclerosis have been described. In children with renal failure changes of rickets and slipped femoral epiphyses may occur (Darryl Shea & Mankin 1966). The exact mechanisms of these multiple abnormalities are not fully understood but diminished intestinal calcium absorption resulting in a negative calcium balance undoubtedly is an important factor. Large doses of vitamin D usually improves calcium balance but its administration is not without its hazards. With advancing renal failure, inorganic phosphorus accumulates in the body and if the $(Ca^{++}) \times (PO_4'')$ product reaches a critical level, there is danger of metastatic deposition of calcium phosphate in para-articular tissues and elsewhere. Para-articular deposition leads often to painful joints which may become swollen and red. This has been dubbed 'pseudo-gout' because of its similarity to gout. The pain in the joints is probably due to calcium phosphate crystals being shed into the synovial fluid. Reduction in plasma phosphate levels either by using a phosphate binding substance such as aluminium hydroxide or by effective

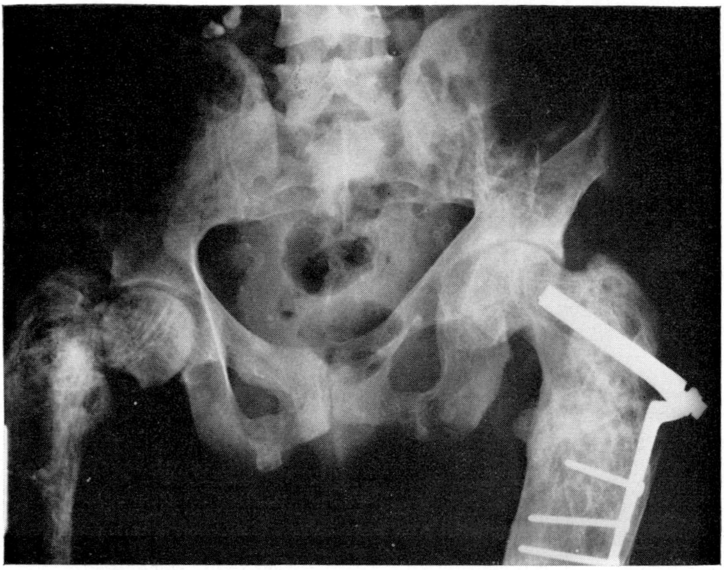

FIG. 8. X-ray of the pelvis of a patient with primary hyperparathyroidism showing extensive osteitis fibrosa cystica with pathological fractures of both hips and distortion of the pelvic brim.

haemodialysis may give clinical remission and the deposit can be seen to resolve radiologically.

Primary hyperparathyroidism may lead to renal calcification, urinary lithiasis and ultimately renal failure. It is usually accompanied by changes of osteitis fibrosa in the bones, with Looser's zones and spontaneous fractures (Fig. 8). Distortion of the pelvis may occur giving the classical triradiate shape of the pelvic brim in the more severe cases.

In secondary hyperparathyroidism, bone changes certainly occur but they are not usually as severe and extensive as in the primary variety (Figs. 9 and 10). This metabolic abnormality occurs as a result of renal failure and by timely commencement of haemodialysis with careful control of the dialysate

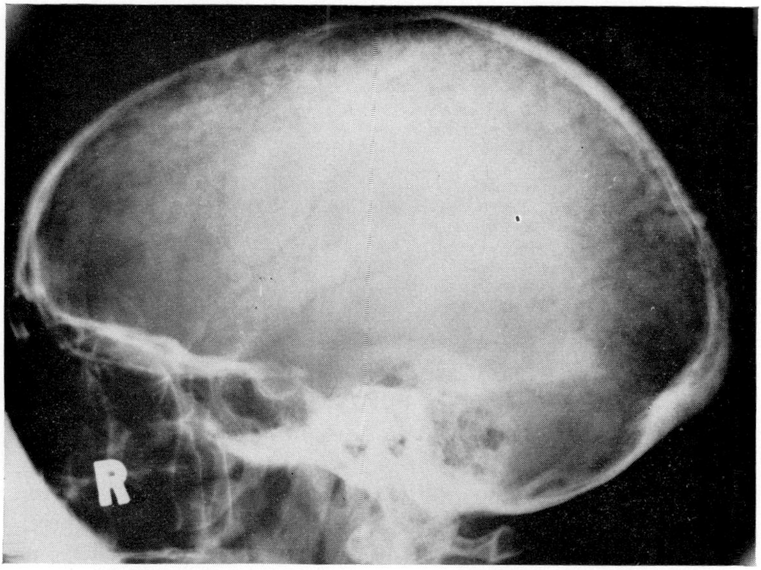

FIG. 9. Secondary hyperparathyroid changes in the skull of a patient with renal failure.

calcium concentration radiological resolution of the bony manifestations usually occurs (Wing 1968). Successful renal transplantation has a similar effect. The management of fractures is often conservative as adequate internal fixation cannot be guaranteed.

Where there is persistence or even deterioration of biochemical and radiological evidence of hyperparathyroidism, the possibility of parathyroid autonomy has to be considered. Under these conditions parathyroidectomy should be performed (McPhaul *et al* 1964) (Wilson *et al* 1965).

Although renal transplantation relieves many of the orthopaedic problems in renal failure, complications may arise as a result of immunosuppressive therapy.

Osteoporosis

This manifests itself by compression fractures and wedging of vertebrae (Figs. 11a and 11b), spontaneous sternal fractures, march fractures of the

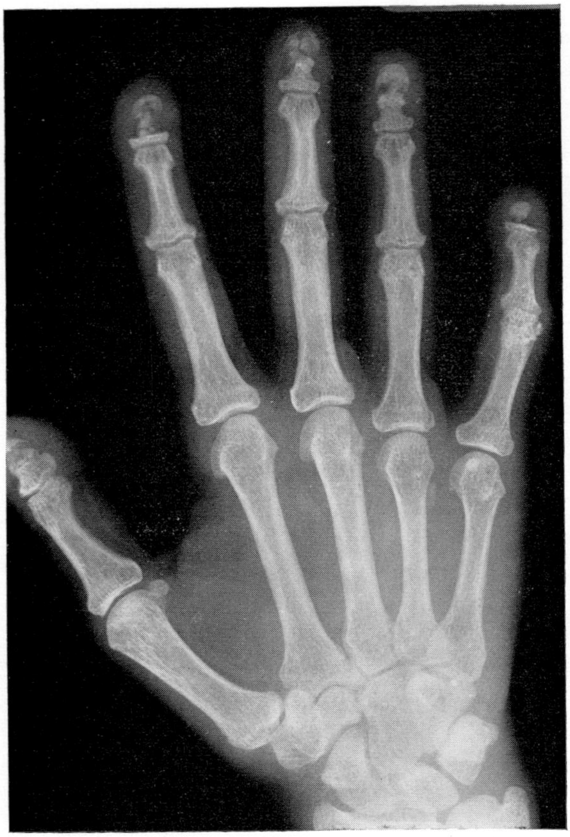

FIG. 10. X-ray of hand of patient with secondary hyperparathyroidism showing destruction of the distal phalanges and subperiosteal erosions in the intermediate phalanges.

metatarsal bones etc. The basic defect is probably in the bone matrix and is usually ascribed to the steroid therapy. Improvement usually results from reducing the dose of steroids, high protein feeding, and calcium supplements. Anabolic steroids may be of some use.

Avascular necrosis

This condition may occur in any of the major joints but is most prevalent in the hips and knee joints. The incidence varies in reported series but as many as 37% of 6-month survivors reported by Creuss *et al* (1968) have had joint involvement. This complication has been much less frequent in our cases. The onset is often within the first 3 months after transplantation

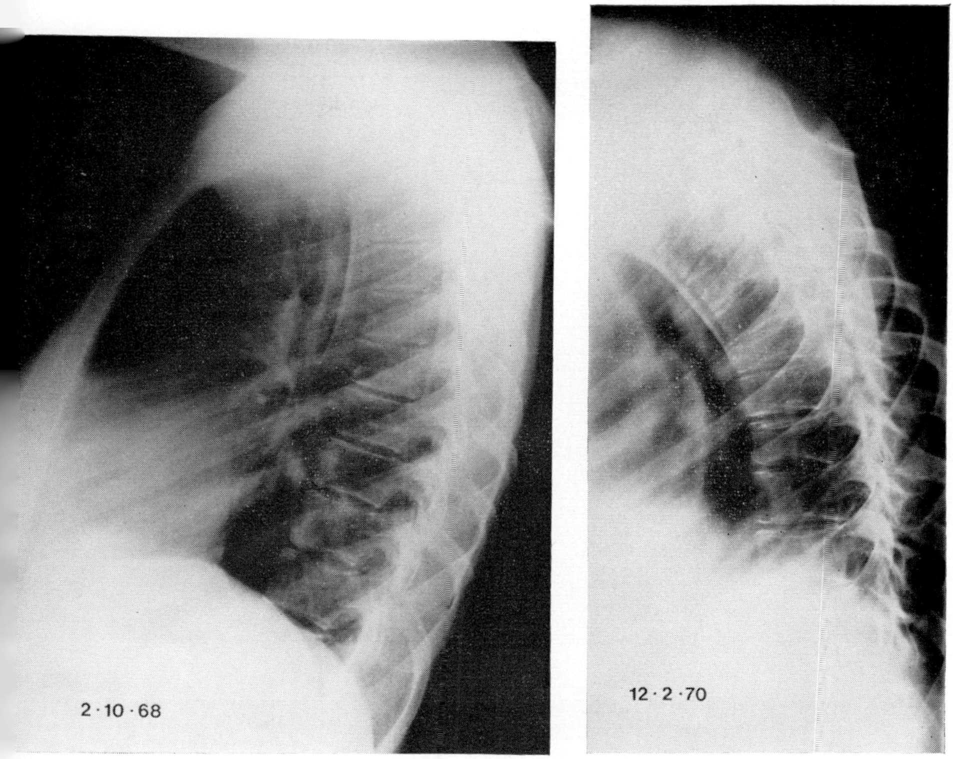

(a) (b)

FIGS. 11a and 11b. Two X-rays of the spine of a 20-year-old girl before and 4 months after renal transplantation. Kyphosis due to wedging of the thoracic vertebrae is shown—probably a complication of steroids.

with pain related to the relevant joint made worse by weight bearing. Symptoms precede radiological changes often by several weeks although critical examination of radiographs will usually reveal early changes in many cases. The radiographic changes are subchondral bone demineralization followed later by collapse due to fracture of the bone trabeculae. In time, complete distortion of the joint may occur reminiscent of the Charcot type of joints (Figs. 12a and 12b). The aetiology is unknown but it would appear that the secondary radiological changes are due to bone infarction. Steroid therapy in rheumatoid arthritis patients produces the same type of radiological change. Fat embolism and infection have also been incriminated. Experimental work with azathioprine in animals has not produced these joint changes.

Treatment involves the prevention of bony collapse of the joint surfaces

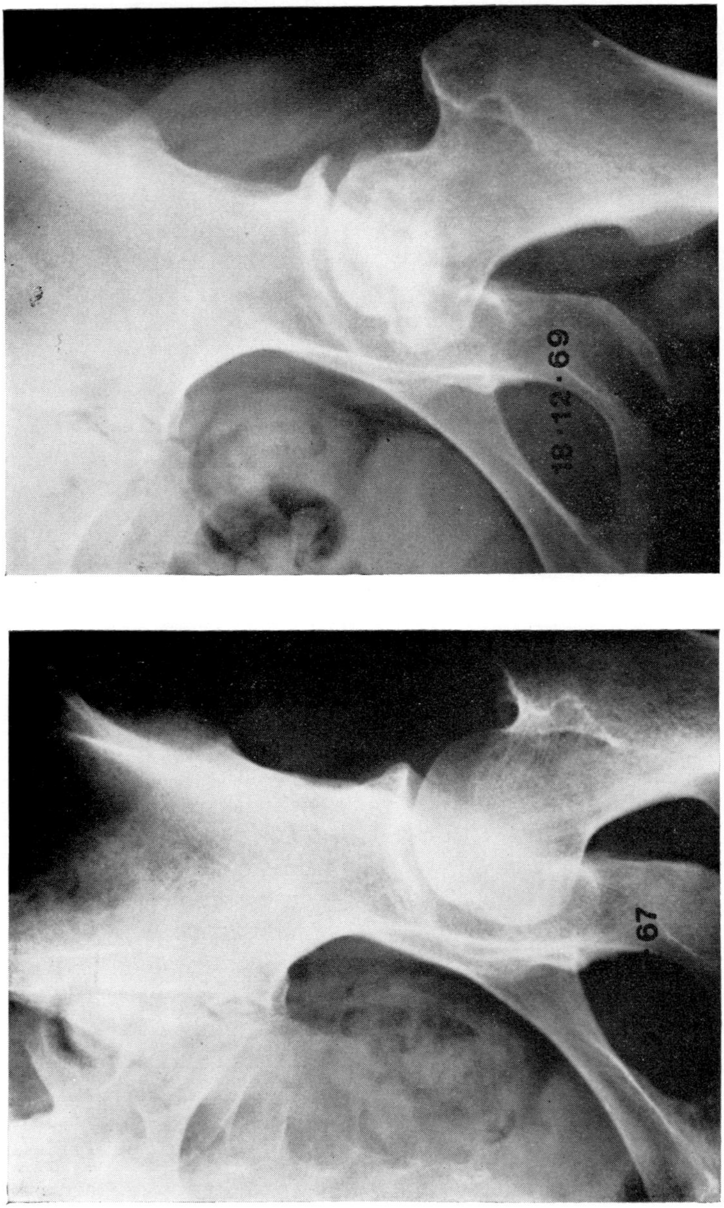

(b)

(a)

FIGS. 12a and 12b. X-rays of the femoral head of a patient 2 months after renal transplantation showing normal appearance with a follow-up film 26 months later showing changes due to avascular necrosis.

by avoiding load bearing and joint replacement if symptoms warrant it in the advanced case.

Osteomyelitis

Osteomyelitis of the lower end of the tibia developed in one of our patients as a complication of staphylococcal septicaemia from a carbuncle on the shoulder. This caused a small osteolytic area in the bone with an associated cellulitis of the overlying skin. He responded well to appropriate antibiotic therapy which in such cases should be over a prolonged period.

Various other musculoskeletal symptoms have been observed in renal transplant patients. These amount to non-specific aches and pains in muscles and joints but if these patients are followed up for long periods definitive clinical and radiological signs may develop. In some cases however, no cause is found, though in a proportion of these, serological tests for rheumatoid factor are positive suggesting that there may be an underlying autoimmune process (Irby & Hume 1968).

Skin complications

One of the striking features of patients with severe renal failure is their pale, muddy complexions. This is due to a combination of anaemia and the retention and deposition of chromogens and sometimes iron pigment in the dermis. There seems to be a predilection for exposed surfaces and scar tissue, the intensity of the pigmentation tending to be directly related to the duration of impaired renal function. Enforced protein restriction in addition may reduce the connective tissue of the skin which tends to lose its elasticity and texture. Often a dry flaking appearance of the skin may be observed and more rarely 'urea frost'—a hoary deposit on the face thought to be due to crystallization of urea in the sweat. Irritation of the skin may be a troublesome symptom—the causative factor is unknown but an association has been suggested between it and disordered calcium metabolism particularly secondary hyperparathyroidism (Hampers *et al* 1968). Alleviation of symptoms may follow parathyroidectomy. Chronic eczematous changes, due to persistent irritation is occasionally seen but the precise relationship with renal failure is uncertain. Efficient haemodialysis is said to cure all these symptoms but skin pigmentation usually remains unchanged until restoration of normal renal function has been achieved by transplantation.

The direct effects of immunosuppressive drug therapy on the skin are basically those observed in patients suffering from Cushing's syndrome. The moon face, hirsutism particularly on the forehead and back, striae and purpura are well known and are particularly prone to develop when the dose level of steroids is high, a gradual improvement in the general appearance occurs as the steroid dose is reduced. Azathioprine tends to produce a diffuse thinning of the scalp hair particularly in women but provided the dose of 2–2·5 mg/kg body weight/day is not exceeded, total alopecia is unlikely to occur. Petechiae and purpura are common where thrombotyopenia occurs, but may occur without platelet deficiency probably due to the steroid effect on capillary fragility. Under these circumstances a positive Hess test is easily elicited. By their effect on sebaceous gland secretion, steroids often cause papular or pustular acneiform lesions on the face, neck and shoulders. Even though the pustules are sterile if cultured, improvement follows a long-term course of small doses of tetracycline. Lowering the dose of steroid will of course also help in this respect.

The immunosuppressive drugs alter the natural defence mechanisms of the host and this applies to the skin as well as other systems. Microorganisms which are normally quiescent on the skin may find conditions conducive to proliferation such as the virus of warts and herpes simplex.

Brownish scaly patches with slight erythema are commonly seen especially on the upper trunks of these patients and are due to a condition known as pityriasis versicolor. This condition is due to an increase in the numbers of and to a change to the mycelial form of a normal commensal yeast—pityrosporum orbiculare. Examination of these under a Wood's lamp reveals yellow fluorescence and direct microscopy of skin scrapings shows numerous yeasts and filaments.

Patients carrying *candida albicans* in large numbers on the intertriginous skin often harbour candida in the respiratory tract and gut. Dermatophyte infections in our experience have not been a problem but they may well develop in steroid treated patients. Pre-existing dermatoses such as chronic eczema and psoriasis may be chronic sources of infection—an important consideration when arteriovenous shunts and other skin wounds have to be inflicted. Attempts to clear them up should be made though often after a successful transplant remission occurs possibly as a result of immunosuppression. Systemic infections may present with skin manifestations—we have seen erysipeloid lesions due to bacterial emboli in a case of *ps. aeruginosa*, septicaemia and disseminated fungal and virus infections may produce diffuse erythematous or vesicular eruptions e.g. varicella-Zoster and disseminated histoplasmosis (Park *et al* 1967).

The careful examination of the skin of the whole body of any immumosuppressed patient is important and may often give useful clues as to the diagnosis in any baffling infection of unknown aetiology e.g. a skin biopsy in a case of a disseminated erythematous rash revealed clusters of acid fast bacilli in the dermal cells making a diagnosis of lepromatous leprosy.

Eyes

Severe untreated hypertension accompanying renal failure may present with deteriorating vision due to hypertensive retinopathy which may lead to retinal detachment. We have also seen spontaneous retro-orbital haemorrhages resulting in transient amblyopia. Adequate treatment with hypotensive agents and haemodialysis results in marked improvement in the retinopathy.

When disordered calcium metabolism complicates renal failure deposition of calcium in the conjunctiva may lead to 'red eyes' as described by Berlyne & Shaw (1967). This is distinct from band keratopathy and is often associated with a high plasma phosphate concentration. Improvement will occur by efficient haemodialysis and lowering of the phosphate/calcium product.

Successful renal transplantation usually reverses these conditions but in the event of rejection leading to diminishing renal function they may reappear. The ocular effects of topical and systemic corticosteroids has been well reviewed by David & Berkowitz (1969). They found raised intraocular pressure in about 30% of patients on systemic steroids. Posterior subcapsular cataracts occur in 11–38% of patients on long-term systemic steroids and exophthalmos, chemosis and external ocular myopathies may occur more rarely. Subconjunctival haemorrhages are not uncommon.

Acute increases in steroid dosages in our patients have been occasionally accompanied by marked conjunctival oedema, usually associated with other evidence of fluid detention. This usually subsides as the dose of steroids is reduced.

Long-term steroid therapy has produced central posterior lenticular cataracts in 4% of our cases but we have not looked particularly for increased intraocular pressure. Infection with herpes simplex virus may produce dendritic ulcers which if neglected may produce iridocyclitis and infections of the anterior chamber. Corneal opacification may be the end result. Herpes zoster if it involves the first segment of the trigeminal nerve may likewise result in conjunctival and corneal ulceration. Involvement of the lachrimal glands may lead to a kerato-conjunctivitis sicca—the aetiology of this is not known.

Steroid induced diabetes mellitus in our experience has been mild and quite easy to control by dieting and oral hypoglycaemic agents. Occasionally insulin has had to be prescribed during the period when the patient is on high steroid doses. It is theoretically possible for diabetic retinopathy to develop in longerm survivors of transplantation, though its incidence in Cushing's disease has been reported as being very low (Sprague *et al* 1956).

Psychological aspects

Prolonged dialysis therapy whether it be peritoneal or haemodialysis can impose considerable emotional strain on the patients, their families and staff of dialysis units (De-Nour & Czaczkes 1968; Cramond *et al* 1968; Menzies & Stewart 1968). The increasing debility consequent upon the advance of renal failure often leads to severe depression in any patient of moderate intelligence. Many who fail to gain a place in a dialysis or transplantation programme because of medical or other contra-indications are fortunately spared the final realization that death is imminent by the clouding of the sensorium which accompanies azotaemia or by some terminal catastrophe. The assessment of a patient's eligibility for dialysis or transplantation may be extremely difficult when they have reached the terminal stages of the disease and if selection has to be made one often has to depend upon the evidence of acquaintances, the family doctor, employer etc. and on the patient's previous co-operation during the period of conservative therapy.

In the cases of those who are offered dialysis or transplantation, the chance of a new lease of life may not always result in a feeling of relief and elation. In some cases a feeling of guilt may be aroused—the patient may become more depressed and in one such case we have witnessed a suicidal attempt when the patient succeeded in tearing apart his arteriovenous shunt.

Another patient became paranoid and refused to accept that she was in dire need of dialysis treatment. She improved remarkably as a result of electroconvulsive treatment and has remained perfectly stable for 9 months despite losing an allograft through rejection.

Once the concept of regular dialysis treatment has been accepted, the monotony of twice or thrice weekly visits to a hospital centre may in some patients develop into a phobia, particularly if the dialysis techniques of the particular unit do not encourage patient participation. They may resent their dependence on nursing and medical staff leading to a chronically irritating relationship. Such patients would be far better treated in their own homes. The challenge of responsibility for their equipment and therefore their own lives and well being provides a worthwhile stimulus.

The indiscriminate use of some drugs either singly or in combination may cause abnormal emotional reactions, resulting in depression, drowsiness, catatonic states, mutism etc. Care should be exercised in prescribing psychotropic, hypotensive and other drugs to subjects with gross impairment of renal function.

Successful renal transplantation usually restores a patient to a normal physical and psychological state. However, in the early post-operative phase the obsessional attention by the staff to alterations in renal function is nearly always transmitted to the patient, so that one can often assess a patient's fluid balance merely by looking at the anxious expression on his face—a deficit of as little as 100 ml of urine is often enough to plunge him into the depths of despair. This fear of rejection or other complication is naturally a depressive influence on the majority of intelligent patients but analogous situations can be encountered in other branches of medicine.

Steroid drugs frequently stimulate a sense of euphoria but in some susceptible subjects a state of excitability may be engendered. We have seen patients who have become hysterical and others psychotic under the influence of antirejection doses of steroids—in all cases improvement followed a reduction in the dosage and by the judicious use of sedative or tranquillizing drugs.

The incidence of serious psychiatric disorders in our series of 98 renal transplant patients is nevertheless fairly low. Despite the close relationships with other patients on the unit and the inevitable sense of comradeship that results, the urge for self survival is strong and the ability of many patients to dissociate their medical progress from that of their companions serves to keep up the general morale of the community.

URINARY TRACT COMPLICATIONS

A careful pre-transplant urological assessment of each potential kidney recipient is necessary. Failure to observe this rule greatly increases the incidence of post-operative urinary tract complications. Thus, bladder neck obstruction and foci of infection such as mega-ureters and diverticula must be excluded. As described in an earlier section, in the majority of instances the recipient's own kidneys are removed before transplant. The pre-operative urological work-up will include urine cultures, and if the history is suggestive of pyelonephritis, cystograms and cystoscopy to check for ureteric reflux and bladder neck obstruction respectively.

The fact that there is such a wide variety of described manoeuvres available for re-establishing continuity of the urinary tract after renal transplant (Leading article 1966) suggests that complications following this part of the operation are not uncommon. This is to be expected on general grounds when considering that the recipient is previously debilitated, often anaemic, and is now immunosuppressed. However, each of the many methods described seems to be relatively safe in the hands of those who regularly employ it. The method of this unit is to implant the ureter by a relatively simple technique with a short sub-mucosal tunnel. More elaborate procedures, such as the Leadbetter-Politano operation (Politano *et al* (1958); Hume (1968)) involve the retention of a greater length of donor ureter, with the increased hazard of ischaemia at the distal tip, and also the making of a large anterior cystotomy, a potential source of serious disruption. Retention of the recipient ureter and anastomosis of it to the pelvis of the transplanted kidney is often suitable, but is contra-indicated in the presence of previous sepsis, with or without ureteric reflux. In centres where cadaveric transplants are performed with long periods of ischaemia, tubular necrosis is the rule rather than the exception, and this is the case in our own unit. Problems of early urinary leakage are therefore uncommon. Of much more frequent early concern to us is the question of obstruction of the transplanted ureter. An obstructive renogram pattern may support this diagnosis, but the only certain method of confirmation of exclusion is retrograde ureteric catheterization, which may be technically difficult to perform.

Urinary leaks may be manifested in several ways. If they occur early, while the drains are still *in situ*, a frank vesicocutaneous fistula develops. More commonly, the anastomotic breakdown is not total, and a small volume only of urine is extravasated. This sort of leak is probably fairly common and only gives rise to serious trouble if infection is superimposed. A significant urinary leak usually requires reimplantation of the ureter, with or without a temporary nephrostomy (Hume *et al* 1963).

In the post-operative period urinary production may be suppressed by the accumulation of fluid in the tight space around the kidney. This is usually a haematoma, and return of renal function may be expected after its evacuation. Sometimes this collection is not of altered blood but of lymph, presumably produced from recipient and or donor renal lymphatics cut at the time of operation. This collection may require multiple aspirations, but disappears eventually. Secondary infection introduced from without is the obvious danger.

Spontaneous rupture of the kidney is a frightening complication seen in two of our patients, and now reported with increasing frequency from other centres (Murray *et al* 1968). This usually presents between 5 and 14 days after operation with intense pain around the transplant, associated with urinary suppression and an increasing haematoma. The patient may become shocked from a combination of blood loss and pain. At exploration a swollen kidney is encountered with a split of varying depth in the substance of the cortex. If at all possible the kidney should not be removed, and the bleeding controlled by judicious underrunning with atraumatic chromic catgut and the use of topical clotting agents. Both our patients recovered completely with these measures and achieved good renal function. Biopsies showed an intensely oedematous kidney with a moderate mononuclear infiltrate only. Anti-rejection therapy, comprising large doses of prednisone, was used on each occasion to cover the possibility that this change was immunological in origin. The aetiology of the condition remains obscure, but what is certain is that capsulotomy at the time of transplant, which we perform routinely, does not, necessarily, prevent it.

The majority of patients with transplanted kidneys, whether from related living or cadaveric donors, sometime during their post-operative course demonstrate a significant bacteruria. Analysis of the series from the Medical College of Virginia suggests that 75% are so affected, Prout *et al* (1967). The two most commonly found organisms are *B.-coli* and *strepto-coccus faecalis*, but many others have been encountered. The vast majority of these infected urines become sterile after the appropriate antibiotic treatment. Failure to render urine sterile after effective treatment should raise the possibility of an underlying anatomical reason, and an IVP is performed. This may show some stenosis of the uretero-vesical anastomosis with some proximal hydro-ureter and hydronephrosis. On occasion a retained remnant of the patient's own ureter has been demonstrated to be the cause of continuing urinary infection and has required removal in order to render the urine permanently sterile.

Some degree of hydronephrosis is commonly seen but is usually not significant. A well defined lesion that we and others have encountered is ureteric obstruction some 3–6 cm below the pelvi-ureteric junction, and well above the uretero-cystotomy. The cause of this lesion is not known, but it may be the result of pressure from an oedematous kidney; indeed little is known of the dynamics of the upper urinary tract after renal transplantation. Reflux up the transplanted ureter is very rarely encountered but is not specifically excluded in most series because of the danger of introducing infection at the time of performing a micturating cystogram.

Renal stones have developed in the pelvis of the transplant, (Hume *et al* 1963), and if encountered should always raise the possibility of hyper-parathyroidism.

GASTROINTESTINAL COMPLICATIONS

1 *Constipation*

Constipation in the early days post transplant is extremely common. Prolonged bed rest and dietary restrictions are the most likely causes, but alteration of the normal bowel alignment by the presence of a retroperitoneal mass behind the caecum may contribute to the problem. The condition responds to traditional remedies.

2 *Appendicitis*

Appendicitis may occur at any time, and high steroid levels may modify the presentation considerably. If the graft is in the right iliac fossa acute rejection with perirenal tenderness must be excluded and this may at times be extremely difficult. Some Centres routinely perform appendicectomy at the time of recipient nephrectomy to avoid this problem (Hume 1968). However, appendicectomy in the uraemic patient is not without risk, particularly if steroid therapy is to be added in the near future, and we prefer to accept the slight hazard of later disease except when the appendix is obviously abnormal at laparotomy.

3 *Diverticulitis*

This condition may also be hard to diagnose in the presence of high levels of prednisone. We have had a patient who succumbed to septicaemia from an unsuspected paracolic abscess secondary to diverticulitis, in whom there was no past history of colonic disorder. Other Centres have encountered diverticulitis more frequently than we have and the morbidity has been high (Penn *et al* 1970).

4 *Gastrointestinal haemorrhage*

Peptic ulceration is a not uncommon complication of transplantation and carries a high mortality. A distinction must be made between an established penetrating peptic ulcer and the multiple superficial stress ulcers of steroid therapy. All patients accepted for a transplant programme should have a pre-operative barium meal, and in cases where there is a definite past history of ulcer, or where the X-ray shows abnormality, corrective surgery should be undertaken at the time of recipient nephrectomy. On most occasions the chronic ulcer arises in the duodenum and here vagotomy with a drainage procedure is the treatment of choice. Prophylactic vagotomy has been advocated by some workers for all potential recipients (Penn *et al* 1968), but there is no convincing evidence in man that vagotomy protects against stress ulcers, and these are the lesions most commonly encountered.

If a transplanted patient presents with a significant gastrointestinal bleed it is essential to secure a first class barium or gastrografin study at the earliest opportunity. If a local lesion is demonstrated, surgery is performed forthwith.

At operation considerable judgment is required, and if as is likely, the ulcer arises in the duodenum, the merits of a relatively straightforward vagotomy and underruning of the ulcer with pyloroplasty have to be weighed against the operation of Polya partial grastrectomy, with its slightly increased hazards, but more certain control of the haemorrhage. If no ulcer is demonstrated with barium studies a tentative diagnosis of superficial erosions may be made. In advanced uraemia or if the platelet count is depressed these erosions may be found not only in the stomach but also throughout the upper small intestine. We have had a patient in whom the 'gastritis' extended to the gastric epithelium in a large Meckel's diverticulum. Where erosions are suspected a traditional conservative management is initially employed. This consists of blood replacement, gastric lavage with bicarbonate and antacids by mouth, and the avoidance of other oral drug therapy. Imuran administration is stopped, and if the situation is not too critical, the steroid dosage may be gradually decreased; if an acute situation has arisen, however, a steroid boost may be indicated. Conservative management should not be persevered with in the face of prolonged or severe haemorrhage, even where erosions have been diagnosed with some confidence. At operation a Polya-type gastrectomy with or without vagotomy is usually indicated. Most units that have had success in their management of severe gastrointestinal haemorrhage in transplanted patients advocate early surgery whatever the suspected source of the bleeding.

REFERENCES

BAILEY G.L., HAMPERS C.L. & MERRIL J.P. (1967) Reversible cardiomyopathy in uraemia. *Trans. Am. Soc. Artif. Int. Org.* **13**, 263.

BERLYNE G.M. & SHAW A.B. (1967) Red eyes in renal failure. *Lancet*, i, 4.

BLUMBERG B.S., GERSTLEY B.T.S., HUNGERFORD D.A., LONDON W.T. & GUTRICK A.I. (1967) A serum antigen (Australia antigen) in Down's syndrome, leukaemia and hepatitis. *Ann. Int. Med.* **66**, 924.

BRAUN W.E. & MERRILL J.P. (1967) Urine protein selectivity in renal transplant patients. *Proc. 1st Int. Congr. Transpl. Soc.* (*Abstract*), 252.

BRETTSCHNEIDER L., TONG J.L., BOOSE D.S., DALOZE P.M., SMITH G.V., HUGUET C., BLANCHARD H., GROTH C.G. & STARZL T.E. (1968) Specific bacteriologic problems after orthotopic liver transplantation in dogs and pigs. *Arch. Surg.* **97**, 313.

BROWN R. (1965) Plasma erythropoietin in chronic uraemia. *Br. Med. J.* ii, 1036.

CALNE R.Y. (1961) Inhibition of the rejection of renal homografts in dogs by purine analogues. *Trans. Bull.* **28**, 445.

CARONE F.A. & LIEBON A.A. (1957) Acute pancreatic lesions in patients treated with ACTH and adrenal steroids. *New Engl. J. Med.* **275**, 690.

CASTALI P.A., ROZENBERG M.C. & STEWART J.H. (1966) The bleeding disorder of uraemia. *Lancet*, ii, 66.

Cramond W.A., Knight P.R., Lawrence J.R., Higgins B.A., Court J.H., MacNamara F.M., Clarkson A.R. & Miller C.D.J. (1968) Psychological aspects of the management of chronic renal failure. *Br. Med J* i, 539

Cruess R.G., Blenner Lassett J., Macdonald F.R., Maclean L.D. & Dossetor J. (1968) Aseptic necrosis following renal transplantation. *J. Bone & Jt. Surg.* **50**-A, 1577.

Crockett R.E., Abillod R.A., Lee B.N., Moorhead J.F., Stevenson C.M., Varghese Z. & Shaldon S. (1967) Maintenance of 50 patients on intermittent haemodialysis without blood transfusion. *Proc. E.D.T.A.* **4**, 17.

Darryl Shea & Mankin H.J. (1966) Slipped capital epiphysis in renal rickets. *J. Bone & Joint Surg.* **48A**, 349.

David D.S. & Berkowitz J.S. (1969) The ocular effects of topical and systemic corticosteroids. *Lancet*, ii, 149.

de-Nour A.K. & Czaczkes J.W. (1968) Emotional problems and reactions of the medical team in a chronic haemodialysis unit. *Lancet*, ii, 987.

Eastwood J.B., Curtis J.R., Wing A.J. & de Wardener H.E. (1968) Hepatitis in a maintenance haemodialysis unit. *Ann. Int. Med.* **69**, 59.

Eddelston A.L.W.F., Williams R., Calne R.Y. (1969) Cellular immune response during rejection of a liver transplant in man. *Nature, Lond.* **223**, 674.

Elstein M., Smith E.K.M. & Curtis J.R. (1969) Reproductive potential of patients treated by maintenance haemodialysis. *Br. med. J.* ii, 734.

Evans D.B., Millard P.R. & Herbertson B.M. (1969) Hepatic dysfunction associated with renal transplantation. *Lancet*, ii, 929.

Franksson C. (1969) Hepatitis and liver damage among patients and staff in a transplantation unit. *Transpl. Proc.* **1**, 209.

Gleadle R.I., Brown J.J., Curtis J.R., Fraser R., Lawson D.H., Lever A.F., Linton A.L., McVeigh S., Robertson J.I.S., de Wardener H.E. & Wing A.J. (1969) Plasma renin concentration and the control of blood pressure in patients with chronic renal failure: the effect of haemodialysis. *Proc. E.D.T.A.* **VI**, 131.

Gibson D.G. (1967) Haemodynamic factors in development of acute pulmonary oedema in renal failure. *Lancet*, ii, 1217.

Hampers C.L., Sobidner J.S., Doak P.B. & Merrill J.P. (1966) The effect of chronic renal failure and haemodialysis on carbohydrate metabolism. *J. Clin. Invest.* **45**, 1719.

Hampers C.L., Soeldner J.A., Gleason R.E., Bailey G.L., Diamond J.A. & Merrill J.P. (1968) Insulin glucose relationships in uraemia. *Am. J. Clin. Nutrition*, **21**, 414.

Haverback B.J., Dyce B., Bundy H. & Edmondson H.A. (1960) Trypsin, trypsinogen and trypsin inhibitor in human pancreatic juice: mechanism for pancreatitis associated with hyperparathyroidism. *Am. J. Med.* **29**, 424.

Heron J.R., Konotey-Ahulu F.I.D., Shaldon S. & Thomas P.K. (1965) Nerve conduction in chronic renal failure treated by dialysis. *Proc. E.D.T.A.* **II**, 138.

Hume D.M. (1968) In *Human Transplantation*, ed. Rapaport & Dausset, pp. 114, 117.

Hume D.M., Magee J.H., Kaufman H.J. Jr., Rittenbury M.S. & Prout G.R. (1963) Renal homotransplantation in man in modified recipients. *Ann. Surg.* **158**, 608.

Hutter R.V.P. & Collins H.S. (1962) The occurrence of opportunistic fungus infection in a cancer hospital. *Lab. Invest.* **11**, 1035.

IRBY R. & HUME D.M. (1968) Joint changes observed following renal transplants. *Clin. Orthopaedics & Related Research*, **57**, 101.

JOHNSON W.C. & NABSETH D.C. (1970) Pancreatitis in renal transplantation. *Ann. Surg.* **171**, 309.

JONES P.O., GOLDSMITH H.J., WRIGHT F.K., ROBERTS C. & WATSON D.C. (1967) Viral hepatitis: a staff hazard in dialysis units. *Lancet*, i, 835.

KINCAID-SMITH P. (1969) Modification of the vascular lesions of rejection in cadaveric renal allografts by dypiridamole and antigens. *Lancet*, ii, 920.

KISSMEYER-NIELSEN F., OLSEN S., POSBERG PETERSEN V. & FJELDBORG O. (1966) Hyperacute rejection of kidney allografts associated with pre-existing humoral antibodies against donor cells. *Lancet*, ii, 662.

LEADING ARTICLE (1966) Ureter in renal transplantation. *Br. med. J.* ii, 1343.

MATTHEW T.H., KINCAID-SMITH P., EREMIN J. & MARSHALL V.C. (1968) Percutaneous needle biopsy of renal homografts. *Med. J. Aust.* **1**, 6.

McMILLAN R. (1968) Heparin in delayed transplant function. *Lancet*, i, 1178.

McPHAUL J.J., McINTOSH D.A., HAMMOND W.S. & PARK O.K. (1964) Autonomous secondary (renal) parathyroid hyperplasia. *New Engl. J. Med.* **26**, 1342.

MEE A.D. & EVANS D.B. (1970) Antilymphocyte serum preparations in the treatment of renal allograft rejection. In press.

MENZIES I.C. & STEWART W.K. (1968) Psychiatric observations on patients receiving regular dialysis treatment. *Br. med. J.* i, 544.

MILLARD P.R., HERBERTSON B M & EVANS D.B. (1970) Renal biopsy in clinical management of renal transplantation. A light-microscopy study. *Lancet*, i, 113.

MOWBRAY J. (1969) Platelet thrombi in rejection episodes. *Proc. R.S.M.* **62**, 597.

MURRAY J.E., WILSON R.E., TILNEY N.L., MERRILL J.P., COOPER W.C., BIRTCH A.G., CARPENTER C.B., HAGER E.B., DAMMIN G.J., HARTWELL HARRISON J. (1968) Five years experience in renal transplantation with immuno-suppressive drugs. *Ann. Surg.* **11**, 425.

MYBURGH J.A., COHEN I., GECELTER L., MEYERS A.M., ABRAHAMS C., FURMEN K.I., GOLDBERG B. & VAN BLERK P.J.P. (1969) Hyperacute rejection in human kidney allografts. Schwartzman or Arthus. *New Engl. J. Med.* **281**, 131.

NAJARIAN J.S., NOBLE R., BRABY P. & BRAINER H.D. (1965) Lysozyme determination as a measure of rejection of kidney homotransplantation. *Surg. Forum*, **16**, 258.

O'CONNOR J.F., COUCH N.P., LINDQUIST R., DAMMIN G.J. & MURRAY J.E. (1966) A correlation of arteriography, histology and clinical course in kidney transplantation. *Ann. N.Y. Acad. Sci.* **129**, 637.

PARK R.K., GOLTZ R.W. & CAREY T.B. (1967) Unusual cutaneous infections associated with immunosuppression. *Arch. Derm.* **95**, 345.

PENN I., BRETTSCHNEIDER L., SIMPSON T., MARTIN A., STARZL T.E. (1970) Major colonic problems in human homotransplant recipients. *Arch. Surg.* **100**, 61.

PENN I., GROTH C., BRETTSCHNEIDER L., MARTIN A.J., MARCHIORO T.L. & STARZL T.E. (1968) Surgically correctable intra-abdominal complications before and after renal homotransplantation. *Ann. of Surg.* **168**, 865.

POLITANO V.A. & LEADBETTER W.F. (1958) An operative technique for correction of vesico-ureteral reflux. *J. Urol.* **79**, 932.

PORTER K.A., THOMSON W.B., OWEN K., KENYON J.R., MOWBRAY J.F. & PEART W.S. (1963) Obliterative vascular changes in four human kidney homotransplants. *Br. med. J.* **2**, 639.

PROUT G.R., HUME D.M., LEE H.M., WILLIAMS G.M. (1967) Some urological aspects of 93 consecutive renal homotransplants in modified recipients. *J. Urol.* **97,** 416.

PROUT G.R. Jr., MACLAG E.V. Jr. & HUME D.M. (1964) Serum and urinary lactic dehydrogenase in patients with renal homotransplants. *Surgery,* **56,** 283.

RIFKIND D., MARCHIORO T.L., WADDELL W.R. & STARZL T.E. (1964) Infectious diseases associated with renal homotransplantation. *J.A.M.A.* **189,** 397.

RIFKIND D. (1965) Cytomegalovirus infection after renal transplanation. *Arch. Intern. Med.* **116,** 554.

RIFKIND D., MARCHIORO T.L. SCHNECK S.A. & HILL R.B. Jr. (1967) Systemic fungal infections complicating renal transplantation and immunosuppressive therapy. Clinical, microbiologic, neurologic and pathologic features. *Am. J. Med.* **43,** 28.

SALAMAN J.R. (1970) *Brit. Med. J.* **2,** 517.

SAMPSON D. (1969) Ultrasonic method for detecting rejection of human renal allotransplants. *Lancet,* ii, 976.

SCHREINER G.E. & MAHER J.F. (1965) Haemodialysis for chronic renal failure. *Ann. Int. Med.* **62,** 551.

SMELLIE W.A.B., VINIK M. & HUME D.M. (1969) Angiographic investigation of hypertension complicating human renal transplantation. *Surg. Gynec. Obst.* **128,** 963.

SMITH M.G.M., DOMINGUEZ J.A., EVANS D.B., BEWICK M., WILLIAMS R. (1969) Changes in leucocyte migration after renal transplantation. *Br. med. J.* **4,** 275.

SPRAGUE R.G., RANDALL R.V., SALOSSA R.M., SCHOLZ D.A., PRIESTLY J.T., WALTERS W. & BULBULIAN A.H. (1956) Cushings syndrome: progressive and often fatal disease. *Arch. Int. Med.* **98,** 389.

STANBURY S.W. (1967) Bony Complications of Renal Disease. In *Renal Disease,* Second edition, ed. BLACK D.A.K. Oxford: Blackwell.

STARZL T.E. (1964) In *Experience in Renal Transplantation.* W.B.Saunders.

STARZL T.E., LERNER R.A., DIXON F.J., GROTH C.G., BRETTSCHNEIDER L. & TERASAKI P.I. (1968) Schwartzman reaction after human renal homotransplantation. *New Engl. J. Med.* **278,** 642.

STRUMPF H.H. & WILENS S.L. (1955) Pancreatic lesions and peripancreatic fat necrosis in cortisone treated rabbits. *Amer. J. Path.* **31,** 563.

SWALES J.D. & EVANS D.B (1969) Erythraemia in renal transplantation *Br. med. J.* ii, 80.

TENCKOFF H.A., BOEN F.S.T., JEBSEN R.H. & SPIEGLER J.H. (1965) Polyneuropathy in chronic renal insufficiency. *J.A.M.A.* **192,** 91.

TILNEY N.L., COLLINS J.J., Jr. & WILSON R.E. (1966) Haemorrhagic pancreatitis —a fatal complication of renal transplantation. *New Eng. J. Med.* **274,** 1051.

TRUNIGER B., ROSEN S.M., KRIEK H., MERRILL J.P. & MURRAY J.E. (1965) Intrarenal distribution of blood flow in the rejecting homotransplanted dog kidney. *Surg. Forum,* **16,** 254.

TURNER G.C. & BRUCE WHITE G.B. (1969) S.H. antigen in haemodialysis associated hepatitis. *Lancet* ii, 121.

VAN YPERSELE DE STRIHOU C. & STRAGIER A. (1969) Effect of bilateral nephrectomy on transfusion requirements of patients undergoing chronic dialysis. *Lancet,* ii, 705.

WILLIAMS G.M., HUME D.M., HUDSON R.P., MORRIS P.J., KANO K. & MILGROM F. (1968) Hyperacute renal homograft rejection in man. *New Engl. J. Med.* **279,** 611.

WILSON R.E., BERNSTEIN D.S., MURRAY J.E. & MOORE F.D. (1965) Effects of parathyroidectomy and kidney transplantation on renal osteodystrophy. *Am. J. Surg.* **110,** 380.

WING A.J. (1968) Optimum calcium concentration of dialysis fluid for maintnenance haemodialysis. *Br. med. J.* **4,** 145.

WRIGHT A.D., LOWY C., RUSSELL FRAZER T., SPITZ I.M., RUBENSTEIN A.H. & BERSOHN I. (1968) Serum growth hormone and glucose intolerance in renal failure. *Lancet,* ii, 798.

ACKNOWLEDGEMENTS

We should like to thank Dr S.O.B. Roberts for dermatological advice; Mr D. Rosborough for orthopaedic advice; the Department of Medical Photography and Illustration (Addenbrooke's Hospital); Mrs J. Small for typing the chapter and Miss A. Trelogan for checking our proofs.

CHAPTER 17

The Pathology of Renal Transplants

B.M. Herbertson
P.R. Millard

1. INTRODUCTION

One of the most impressive aspects of the pathology of human renal transplantation is the wide range of factors which may affect the behaviour of the grafted kidney and the wellbeing of the recipient. Although the genetic relationship between the donor and the recipient and the consequent antigenic similarities and differences are undoubtedly of great significance, the structure and function of a renal transplant also depends on many other features. These include the quality of the donated kidney, the adequacy of the anastamoses, the possible development of infection, and the nature of the patient's original renal disorder. It is not surprising, therefore, that the morphological changes developing in a renal transplant may be rather complex and difficult to interpret. Fortunately the pathologist is greatly aided by experience gained from experimental studies. In such investigations an analysis of the factors affecting transplanted tissues can be systematically examined and the effect of varying individual conditions demonstrated. Indeed few developments in medical practice provide a better illustration of the importance of adequate interplay between the various scientific disciplines and between experimental and clinical studies.

In this section the factors affecting human renal allografts are considered and the structural changes described. The account is primarily based on a study of transplanted cadaver kidneys and for descriptive convenience the renal allograft is considered from the viewpoint of its natural history, namely, (1) the donor phase (life span in the donor), (2) the transplantation phase (the period between death of donor and revascularization in the new host), and (3) the recipient phase (life span in the recipient). (Herbertson 1970.)

The pathology of human renal isografts and renal xenografts transplanted to man is not discussed in this section. The interested reader is referred to a review by Porter (1966a).

A Donor phase

The investigations performed before transplanting a kidney are discussed elsewhere. However, despite thorough investigations there is always the possibility of transplanting an abnormal kidney. Moreover, there are usually age differences between the recipient and donor and variable degrees of ischaemic damage to the graft resulting from the mode of death.

1 *Transmission of disease*

Bacterial, viral and fungal infection transmitted from donor to recipient has been reported (Evans 1969; Hume 1966; Hood *et al* 1965) and the occurrence of malignant tumours in the recipient similar to those in the donor has also been described (MacLean *et al* 1965; Martin *et al* 1965). The use of a diseased kidney is avoidable if there are accompanying macroscopic changes. However, this may not always be the case. Porter *et al* (1963) used a kidney from a donor with malignant hypertension and in another centre a kidney with diabetic glomerulosclerotic lesions and a second with sarcoid granulomas were inadvertently used (Millard *et al* 1970).

2 *Age changes*

Although the average age of cadaver kidney donors is probably about 45 years (Calne *et al* 1968), kidneys have been used from donors of all age groups, including stillborn infants (Martin *et al* 1969) and septuagenarians (Woodruff *et al* 1969). In all series donor and recipient ages have rarely been matched but, because of the frequency of ageing changes in older donors, most centres avoid using kidneys from the aged. However, the significance of age disparity is not at present clear. While White *et al* (1968) reported that age difference was unimportant, Reeve *et al* (1969) found that kidneys transplanted from older patients functioned less satisfactorily than those from younger donors.

3 *Mode of dying*

The patient who dies suddenly, and whose kidneys are quickly removed and subjected to satisfactory preservation techniques may be a better donor than one who dies slowly. In the latter patient renal blood flow may have been reduced for an ill-defined period prior to death. Moreover, treatment with anti-hypotensive drugs, although maintaining blood pressure, may further reduce blood flow through the kidneys (Goodman & Gilman 1965) and increase the degree of ischaemic damage. Such a patient may also have received potentially nephrotoxic drugs. Terminal invasion of the bloodstream by bacteria is a further additional hazard in patients dying slowly.

B **Transplantation phase: interval between death of donor (or removal of kidney from live donor) and revascularization in recipient**

The factors affecting the morphology of the transplanted kidney during this phase are considered in the section on Organ Preservation (Chapter 3).

C **Recipient phase**

After the surgeon releases the vascular clamps the revascularized but denervated kidney is subjected to the physiological demands of the new host, a wide range of therapeutic agents and an immune reaction of varying intensity. With time, during which the single kidney will have to adapt itself to provide the function formerly supplied by two kidneys, the effects of infection, hypertension and primary renal disease may also play their part in modifying both its present function and morphology. Thus, in assessing any morphologic change in any or all of the individual components of the transplanted kidney attention must also be given to these factors as well as to those discussed in the preceding phases. Unquestionably, however, the host's immune reaction is the most important of these considerations. A brief presentation of these various aetiological factors will be given before describing the morphological consequences of renal transplantation.

1 *Immune rejection*

a Immediate rejection in a sensitized recipient

Morphologically, immune rejection is manifested in two distinct forms. One form, first documented by Kissmeyer-Nielsen *et al* (1966), occurs within minutes of completing the transplant operation, while the other much commoner type occurs at variable intervals after the transplantation procedure. Kissmeyer-Nielsen *et al* (1966) associated rapid or immediate rejection with pre-existing cytotoxic antibodies in two recipients who were both multiparous women and who had both received numerous blood and plasma transfusions. The glomerular capillaries in the kidneys of both patients were engorged and contained fibrin-platelet deposits while the other structures appeared essentially normal. Immediate rejection may also occur in some cases of major ABO incompatibility (Porter 1967) and in both instances humoral antibodies are probably a major factor contributing to the rejection process. Thus from these initial experiences it has now become apparent that in transplantation the recipient should not be given a kidney from a donor with red cells containing A or B antigens that the recipient does not possess. Blood transfusions should be kept at a minimum in prospective candidates and all such patients should be tested for cytotoxic antibodies before receiving a kidney graft.

b REJECTION DUE TO SENSITIZATION BY THE TRANSPLANTED KIDNEY

Allograft rejection in the normal experimental animal is a continuous, relentless process culminating fairly rapidly in a functionless necrotic graft. In the majority of immunosuppressed human recipients the rejection process appears to be essentially similar although pursuing a more protracted course, possibly partly due to the uraemic state (Dammin *et al* 1957). With close donor-recipient tissue matching the graft may even function effectively for years but with major antigenic differences the kidney may be very rapidly destroyed. This rapid destruction can occur despite increased immunosuppression and in some patients may follow sensitization by previous renal allografts (Gifford *et al* 1967). Successful transplantation of second and even third renal allografts has, however, been performed (Hume *et al* 1966), even with the initial rejected kidney still *in situ* (Boak *et al* 1969).

The effect of the rejection process is primarily on the vascular endothelium and is probably mediated by the infiltrating mononuclear cells (Gowans 1965). However, the demonstration of deposits of immunoglobulins in some of these vascular lesions (Porter 1967), suggests that humoral antibodies are also involved. The damaged endothelium is then a potential site for platelet deposition with thrombus formation and partial or complete occlusion of the vessels involved (Kincaid-Smith 1967). If the rejection episode subsides or is modified these lesions may heal and secondary effects from ischaemia develop in nephrons and interstitial tissue. In more aggressive rejection episodes, often associated with major degrees of histocompatibility antigen mismatches, the vascular damage is more profound and fibrinoid necrosis of arteries and arterioles is a dominant feature.

With all types of rejection an important feature is the apparently random distribution of the lesions. Rarely are all structures equally involved and even the mononuclear cell infiltrate is commonly focal in nature. Thus in allografts in which several rejection episodes have occurred lesions of clearly different ages and in varying stages of healing are seen. At present there is no adequate explanation for this patchy distribution, but it is probably due to several factors, including the siting of the initial ischaemic damage during the pretransplantation period as well as alterations in renal blood flow and distribution during rejection episodes (Retik *et al* 1967).

2 *Other factors*

a Regeneration and compensatory enlargement

The removal of a kidney from one host and transfer to another host necessarily involves severing the lymphatic, nervous and blood vascular supply as well as the ureteric drainage. Of these parameters the surgeon will only attempt to reconstruct the blood vascular supply and ureteric drainage thus leaving the kidney in the new host free of nervous and lymphatic connections. Further the recipient's own kidneys have often been removed, and in any event the host is in functional renal insufficiency. After unilateral nephrectomy compensatory enlargement of the remaining kidney is an accepted phenomenon, and in man may occur in all age groups, including people in their seventies. The enlargement is uniform involving glomeruli, tubules, blood vessels, calyces, pelvis and ureter (Hodson 1967). Almost all transplanted kidneys have dimensions and weights beyond those accepted as normal. This change in size and weight is partly contributed to by oedema fluid and increase in total cell content (Williams *et al* 1964), as well as any hypertrophy and hyperplasia. Microscopically, many glomeruli and some tubules with their lining cells appear enlarged and similar observations apply to the thickness of vessel walls. However, no accurate measurements of vessel wall thickness have been made and many other factors may contribute to this increase.

The endothelium of the vascular anastomoses reforms over these sites and it is likely, though as yet undemonstrated that lymphatic regeneration follows a similar but slower pattern. The regeneration of nerves has been shown to be beginning by 4 weeks after transplantation (Dammin 1968). Associated with the anoxia at the time of transplantation degeneration and necrosis of tubular cells occur and it is therefore common to see evidence of regeneration in the tubules in almost all early allograft biopsies. Thus in spite of being transplanted to an anatomically abnormal site and into a new host the transplanted kidney, like the single kidney, undergoes similar processes of enlargement with coincident regeneration of any damaged parts.

b Drugs and other therapeutic agents

Milne (1967), in a succinct summary of the interaction of drugs and kidney function, emphasized the importance of normal renal function, liver function and protein metabolism for the effective removal of such agents from the body. When any or all of these functions are altered the normal detoxication pathways for an individual drug will be affected and potentially harmful levels of drugs may occur in body tissues. The recipient of a cadaver kidney is in renal failure and will probably remain so for a variable period after receiving the graft. This patient will of necessity be given immunosuppressive agents and antibiotics which besides possibly being nephrotoxic may also injure the liver and bone marrow.

While nephrotoxicity of individual agents is often recognized the interaction of many or all of these agents is seldom understood and extreme caution is necessary before attributing an effect on the patient or the transplanted kidney to any particular therapeutic agent. Fortunately the potentially toxic role of many drugs, both direct and indirect, is probably minimized by the use of dialysis during the early post-operative stages.

However, to the morphologist the drugs azathioprine and amphoteracin B are of particular interest. The role of azathioprine is difficult to assess. Sheil *et al* (1968) in dogs found that discontinuing this drug, even after having been administered for some years, resulted in a considerable increase in size in the allografted kidney suggesting that compensatory enlargement of the graft, and possibly regeneration, were formerly inhibited, The bizarre tubular appearances seen in cadaver human transplants are described below and attention is also drawn to the fact that with time when lower drug dosages are given these abnormal appearances decrease and a more normal tubular epithelium appears. It is highly possible that azathioprine and other immunosuppressant drugs affect regeneration of tubular epithelium as well as having some effect on the degree of tubular cell hypertrophy. The proven hepatotoxicity of azathioprine in normal dogs (Starzl & Putnam 1969) is also pertinent in human organ transplantation.

Amphoteracin B, a fungicide, is recognized as a nephrotoxic agent causing tubular damage and occasionally followed by renal calcification (Garrod & O'Grady 1968). Many patients receiving grafts have been given amphoteracin B and calcification does sometimes occur in tubules and vessels of the graft. Although renal failure, and associated hyperparathyroidism may be responsible for such calcium deposition the possible role of amphoteracin B must also be considered.

c Infection

The association between organ transplantation, immunosuppression, and bacterial, viral and fungal infections is now widely documented (Hill *et al* 1967; Evans 1969). While many of these infections affect the lungs and brain it is not uncommon for the renal allograft also to be involved. Pyelonephritis therefore may be found in allografts at any period post-operatively but is especially likely to occur in patients developing either a urinary fistula or any form of ureteric obstruction.

Fungal infection may be superadded to this bacterial infection but more commonly is confined to the allograft ureter and particularly to those ureters in which a fistula is present. Thus in any patient with a urinary fistula the possibility of fungus gaining entry at this site should constantly be borne in mind. While bacterial and fungal infection can clearly be detrimental to the function of the transplant and cause morphological changes it is more difficult to assess the role of viruses. Virus infection may be associated with kidney dysfunction either as the prime mediator or alternatively by encouraging secondary bacterial infection (Jensen 1967). Many patients receiving renal allografts experience viral infections, particularly by the herpes group (Evans 1969) and in a few of these patients viral hepatitis develops. Herpes simplex and zoster seem to have no detrimental effect on renal function and rarely do patients die from these diseases. In a patient dying from generalized haemorrhagic varicella the evidence of direct harm to the kidney by the varicella virus was more convincing. The grafted kidney was functioning satisfactorily until the patient contracted chicken-pox. She rapidly developed renal failure and numerous intranuclear inclusion bodies were present in all parts of the kidney. Many patients receiving renal allografts show evidence of cytomegalovirus infection either by the presence of rising antibody titres or by culture of the virus from the urine (Craighead *et al* 1967). Also the typical intranuclear inclusion bodies are not infrequently seen in cells lining tubules, blood vessels and within glomeruli in both biopsy and allograft nephrectomy specimens. Their presence may be coincident with impaired renal function but there are generally other factors more commonly recognized as causing renal failure *per se*. Viral hepatitis may be a lethal complication in renal transplantation (Evans *et al* 1968) but again there is no evidence of direct injury to the transplanted kidney.

d Hypertension

The renal lesions and the mechanisms involved in hypertension have been extensively reviewed by Heptinstall (1966) and Peart (1967). Many patients with renal failure are hypertensive but with regular dialysis, hypotensive drugs, and in some cases bilateral nephrectomy, the hypertension may be controlled. Following the introduction of a functioning allograft the blood pressure may be maintained at normal levels. However, should a rejection episode occur it is not uncommon for there to be a coincident rise in blood pressure and in patients with long-term grafts a more gradual rise in blood pressure often develops. While this latter observation may be due to sustained subclinical rejection it may also be associated with stenosis at the arterial anastomosis (Papadimitriou *et al* 1969) or along the length of the donor renal artery (Smellie *et al* 1969).

e Anastomoses

Of the three anastomoses performed by the surgeon the venous anastomosis is the least prone to complications, of which thrombosis is the commonest (Clarke *et al* 1970). In contrast, thrombus formation, haemorrhage (sometimes due to infection), and stenosis may all occur at the arterial anastomosis. The relationship between renal artery stenosis and profound atrophy of proximal convoluted tubules and hypertension is well recognized (Heptinstall 1966) and may contribute to the diverse changes seen in renal allografts. In addition, if there are multiple renal arteries, technical or other complications may result in infarction of part of the kidney.

Whether ureteric drainage is achieved by direct implantation into the bladder or by anastomosis to the patient's ureter, a fistula may develop. Once this occurs bacterial and fungus infection may follow and later involve the graft (see above). Graft infection, associated with hydronephrosis, may also theoretically complicate stenosis of the ureteric anastomosis or kinking of the ureter during its course to the bladder. In practice, however, this has been uncommon even in the presence of considerable angulation of the ureter. Calculus formation equally might be expected but has personally been found at autopsy only once.

f Original renal disorder

Most recipients of renal allografts are suffering from glomerulonephritis, pyelonephritis or congenital polycystic disease of 'adult' type. A minority are suffering from a wide range of renal disorders including primary renal hypertension, amyloidosis and other connective tissue disorders (Table 1).

TABLE 1. Causes of renal failure in 63 recipients of renal transplants in Cambridge series 1966–1970. (Based on morphological features of kidney specimens)

Chronic glomerulonephritis	29
Chronic pyelonephritis	17
Congenital polycystic disease of 'adult' type	7
Malignant hypertension	2
Renal artery stenosis	2
Amyloidosis	1
Uraemic medullary cystic disease	1
Renal hamartomata associated with tuberous sclerosis	1
Original disorder not identified	3

Potentially many of these disorders, particularly systemic ones, may occur in the transplanted kidney. However, with glomerulonephritis it is far more difficult to be sure that transmission of the disease has occurred. From experience with identical twins receiving their twin's kidney it is known that glomerulonephritis may be transmitted to the new kidney (Glassock *et al* 1968). However, morphological appearances similar to those of glomerulonephritis may appear in rejected grafted canine kidneys (Sheil *et al* 1968). While Dixon *et al* (1969) have demonstrated glomerulonephritis in renal allografts, a precise interpretation of glomerular changes is difficult and at present often impossible (Porter *et al* 1967).

II. MORPHOLOGY

A Macroscopic features

1 *Appearances of hyperacute rejection in a sensitized recipient*

Unlike the features described below these appearances can be evident before the completion of the transplant operation (Starzl *et al* 1968) and have been graphically described by Kissmeyer-Nielsen *et al* (1966). The kidney loses its normal tone and colour within minutes of completing the vascular anastomoses, becoming flabby and cyanotic: this change is generally uniform and the vascular anastomoses are patent. If the graft is not removed immediately it becomes necrotic and when subsequently examined, is soft, grey-pink and not enlarged. Alternatively the cortex may be more affected than the rest of the parenchyma, having a dark red appearance. Blood clot fills the main and intrarenal blood vessels. The lining of the pelvis and ureter is a dark purple and they may contain altered blood clot and debris. The appearances are similar to those of a kidney in an advanced stage of autolysis.

2 *Appearances of rejection following sensitization by the renal allograft*

In these circumstances the macroscopic appearance of the allograft varies greatly but three principal forms are found. Superimposed on any of these basic patterns there may be infarcts, infection, and deformities arising from ureteric obstruction.

a LARGE HAEMORRHAGIC KIDNEY

The kidney is enlarged, on occasion to 485 g (14·0 × 8·5 × 4·0 cm), firm yet friable, with a smooth dark purple surface to which the capsule is not significantly adherent (Fig. 1). Scattered throughout the substance of the organ are recent and older haemorrhages of variable size. In the cortex these are often arranged in a linear fashion and the cortico-medullary junction may appear as an ill-defined dark purple band. The cortex is generally widened. The medullary pyramids are engorged and there are

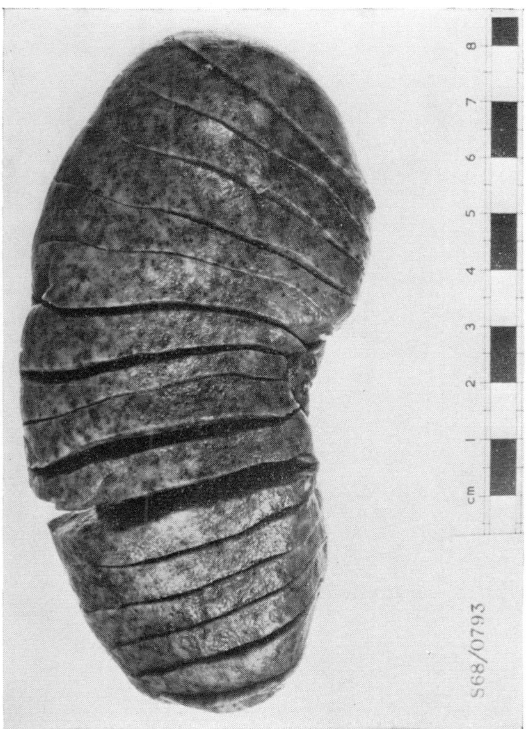

FIG. 1. Kidney 39 days after transplantation. A large haemorrhagic renal allograft (300 g). ×0·75.

haemorrhages in the pericalyceal fat. The lining of the major calyces, pelvis and allograft portion of the ureter is reddish purple, often ending abruptly at the donor-recipient junction. The pelvis and ureter often contain blood clot and debris. On the cut surface of the kidney arteries of all sizes tend to be unduly conspicuous, and may be filled with thrombus and, in some cases, their walls are thickened and include yellow material.

b Large pale kidney

The appearance is exactly similar to the 'large pale kidney' found in some renal disorders (Fig. 2). The kidney is enlarged in all its components, strikingly pale, with a firm rubbery consistency and smooth outer surface. Clear colourless fluid oozes from the cut surface and there is oedema of the pale calyceal, pelvic and ureteric linings. In most cases the intrarenal vessels are not unduly conspicuous and main vessels are patent.

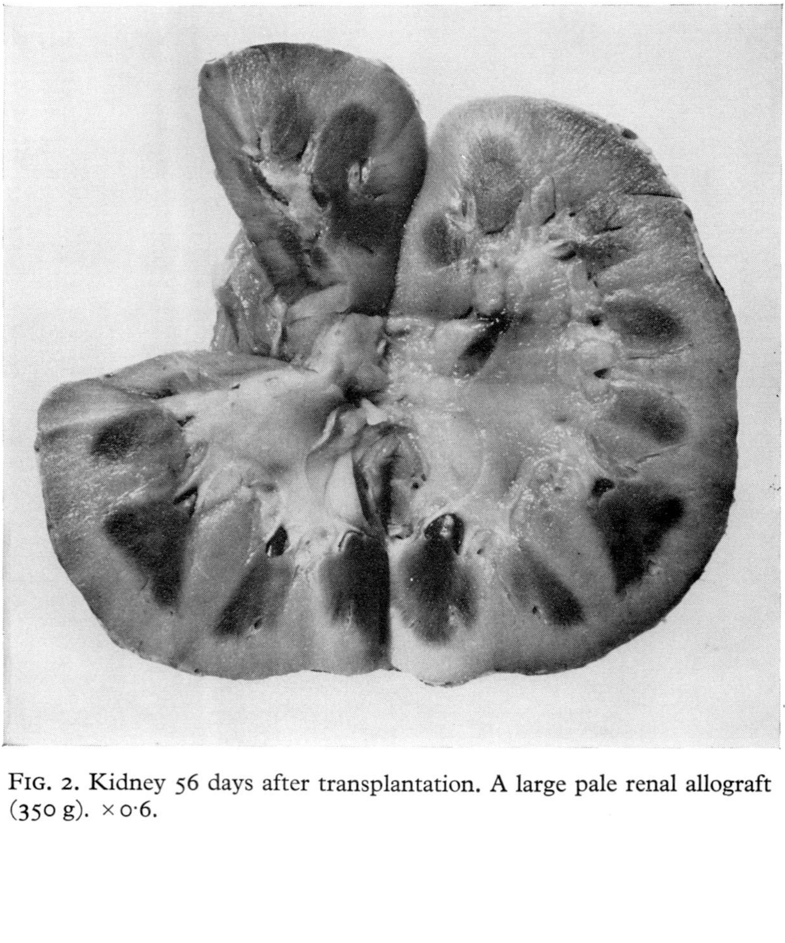

FIG. 2. Kidney 56 days after transplantation. A large pale renal allograft (350 g). ×0·6.

This type of kidney, together with some of the miscellaneous features enumerated below has been the commonest macroscopic appearance observed. Twenty of these kidneys had an average weight of 301 g, the heaviest being 650 g. These features have been present within 1 month of transplantation but may develop after much longer periods. The factors contributing towards the renal enlargement are oedema, the mononuclear cell infiltration, compensatory hypertrophy and hyperplasia and increase in interstitial connective tissue.

c SMALL SCARRED KIDNEY

The kidney is small with a thickened firmly adherent capsule. The surface is pale with deep and shallow scars (Fig. 3). Some of these may be coincident with calyceal deformities, while others overlie areas of grossly narrowed cortex (Fig. 4). The entire parenchyma is pale, firm and extremely tough

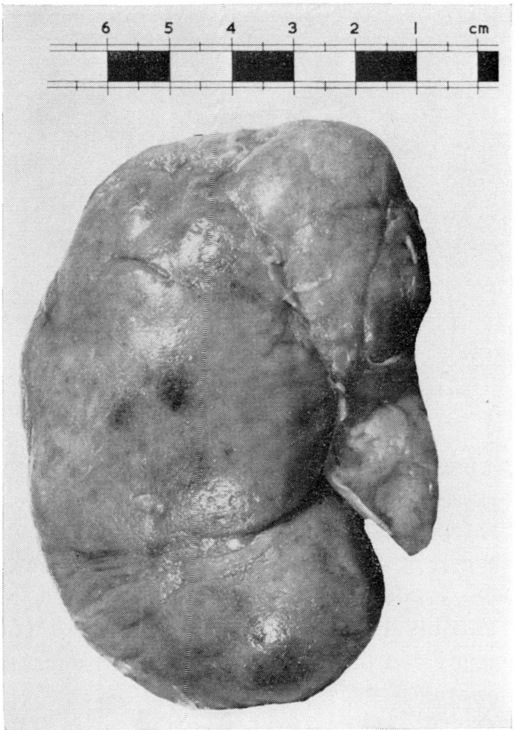

FIG. 3. Kidney 760 days after transplantation. A small scarred kidney (110 g) ×0·8.

with blurring or total loss of the corticomedullary boundary. The pelvis and calyces may be deformed and the ureteric wall thinned; the mucosal linings are pale and smooth. The lumen of the ureter may be narrowed due to stenosis at the anastomotic site or due to fibrous bands and adhesions. Vessels are clearly visible and their walls thickened. In some instances there may be stenosis of the renal artery, either at the anastomosis or along its length; alternatively this vessel may be kinked.

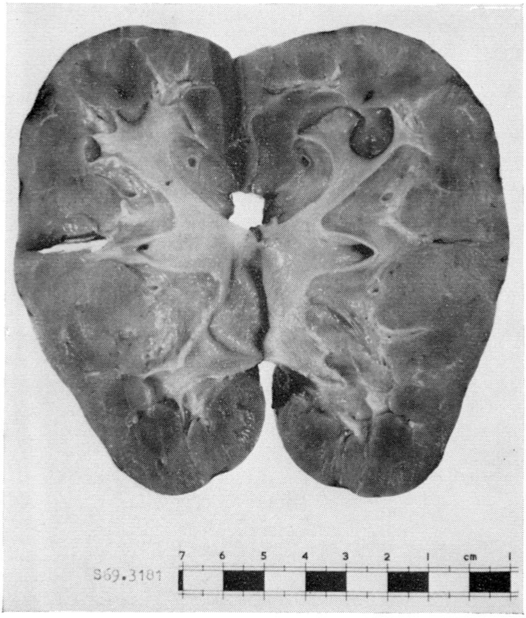

FIG. 4. Kidney 388 days after transplantation. A small scarred kidney (99 g). ×0·55.

The classification of the macroscopic features as presented above is based upon a personal study of 55 renal allografts. Microscopically these grafts have presented a wide range of features involving all components of the renal substance. The various factors contributing towards these lesions have already been considered and the overall importance of immune rejection stressed. Probably because of the variable and episodic nature of immune rejection, no constant pattern of lesions has occurred with any of these macroscopic appearances. Thus a detailed account of the microscopic features of each type of kidney would be inappropriate. Further, while this classification is probably helpful it is not all embracing and few allografts fit neatly into any one of the groups described. However, in spite of these reservations some broad generalizations about associated macroscopic and microscopic features can be made which may be of help to the clinician.

The flabby, cyanotic kidney is characterized by fibrin-platelet deposits in glomeruli and arterioles. The main features of the large haemorrhagic kidney are interstitial haemorrhage and patchy arteriolar and glomerular fibrinoid necrosis but other vascular, interstitial, and tubular changes are also frequently present. The large pale kidney often shows considerable mononuclear cell infiltration, interstitial oedema and an increase in connective tissue. Arterial lesions, particularly severe intimal narrowing, also occur but only if the kidney has been transplanted more than a few weeks. The small scarred kidney usually represents the cumulative effects of chronic arterial and glomerular lesions and interstitial tissue changes. As with some forms of glomerulonephritis it seems likely that many renal allografts progress through a phase of a 'large pale kidney' before becoming small and scarred.

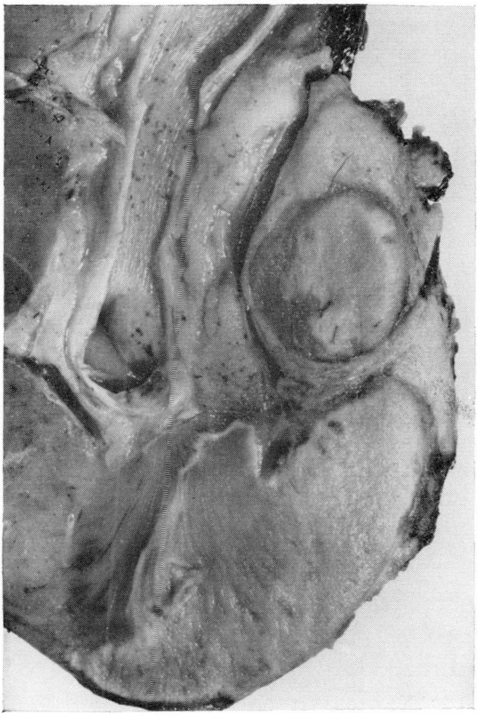

FIG. 5. Kidney 41 days after transplantation. An infarct of the lower pole of a large pale allograft. The artery to this region was almost entirely occluded by recent intimal thickening. × 1·2.

3 *Miscellaneous appearances*

Infarcts have the classical appearances and may be large or small. The larger infarcts are often associated with the presence of multiple renal arteries and hence often polar in distribution (Fig. 5). The smaller infarcts, often confined to the cortex, are probably evidence of severe rejection episodes (Fig. 6). They are of varying ages, widely distributed and may

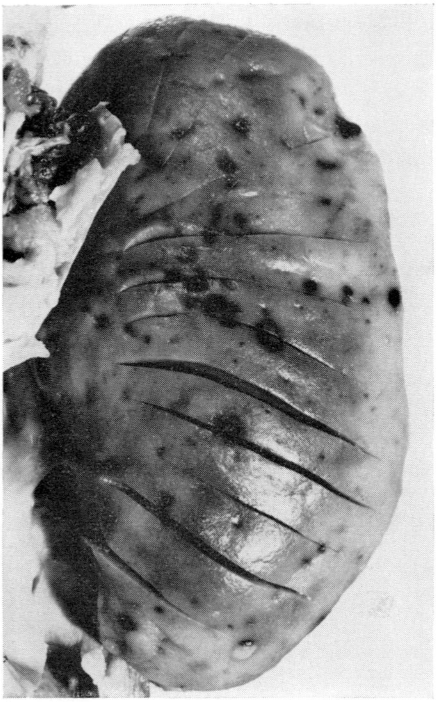

FIG. 6. Kidney 84 days after transplantation. A large pale kidney (250 g) with multiple small infarcts, many with haemorrhagic borders ×0·6.

occur in all parts of the renal parenchyma. In other instances the peripheral part of the entire cortex may become necrotic, appearing as a yellowish white band around the kidney (Fig. 7). Retik *et al* (1967), have shown in dogs that during a rejection episode the cortical blood flow is reduced due to redistribution of blood within the kidney. It is likely that similar alterations in renal blood flow occur in human renal allografts during rejection crises.

Bacterial, fungal and viral infections of the allograft occur, either as a part of a systemic infection or associated with an ascending infection from a ureteric fistula or the bladder. Bacterial infection is localized in scattered foci throughout the renal substance. These foci have a pale yellow colour, giving a granular appearance to the surface of the organ. If infection persists the area becomes scarred and the overlying capsule firmly adherent.

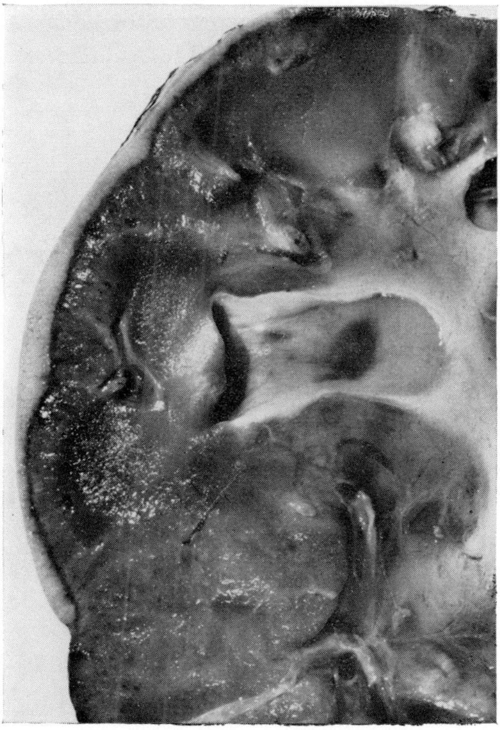

FIG. 7. Kidney 77 days after transplantation. Necrosis of peripheral part of cortex. The walls of the intrarenal arteries are thickened and the calyces dilated. × 1·15.

Fungal infection produces a similar macroscopic appearance. Cytomegalovirus infection *per se* does not appear to cause any alteration in the gross morphology of the kidney, but is more often found in the large haemorrhagic type of allograft than the other types. A patient with fulminating haemorrhagic varicella had an enlarged kidney with scattered petechial haemorrhages and extensive haemorrhage into the pericalyceal fat, the lining of calyces, pelvis and ureter.

B Microscopic features

1 *Interstitial tissue*

The earliest change that may be seen is the presence of oedema fluid. This may occur in moderate amounts in biopsies taken after revascularization and is probably a reflection of the total ischaemia time and the degree of handling. Later, however, the oedema is usually due to immune rejection (Kountz *et al* 1963) and accounts, in part, for the increased size of the renal allograft (Williams *et al* 1964). Concurrent with oedema there is a variable infiltrate of mononuclear cells (Fig. 8). This cellular infiltrate may occur

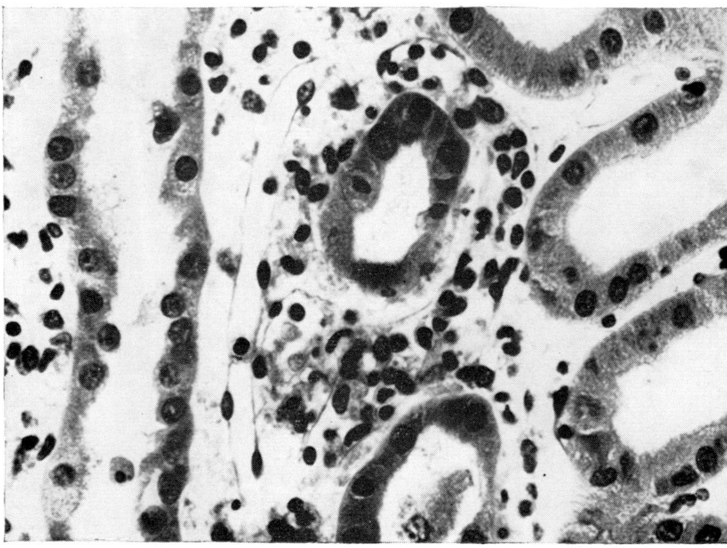

FIG. 8. Allograft biopsy 14 days after transplantation. Mononuclear cells in intertubular capillary on right and in oedematous interstitial tissue. H.E. ×440.

within 5 days of transplantation and at any subsequent time. The fine structure of the cells involved has been described by Porter (1967), and is similar to that of the cells involved in rejection of other tissues (Wiener *et al* 1964; Porter 1966b). Porter (1967) recognized three types of cells; lymphoid cells, plasma cells and macrophages. The lymphoid cells are divisible into large cells (immunoblasts), and smaller cells (immunocytes), both rich in ribose nucleic acids. Many of these cells are pyroninophilic and dividing cells are seen. Eosinophil polymorphs may also form part of the infiltrate in a few individuals. In the early stages of a rejection episode lymphoid cells are commonest, plasma cells appearing later. The cells first appear in intertubular capillaries (Fig. 8), later migrating through and damaging the endothelium of these capillaries to appear in the interstitial tissue (Kountz *et al* 1963; Porter 1967). As the cellular infiltrate increases the cells are particularly conspicuous around the intrarenal veins, frequently infiltrating their walls, and in the interstitial tissue around glomeruli and between tubules. These appearances are common in biopsy specimens during the early post-operative period and do not always provide a definite indication of the future function of the graft.

If the rejection process persists the mononuclear cell infiltrate increases involving much of the renal parenchyma. The cells also infiltrate walls of arteries, appearing first beneath the endothelium and later in the media and adventitia. With increased immunosuppressive therapy the cellular infiltrate in the interstitial tissue may subside although the vascular changes initiated may continue to progress.

A characteristic of any severe rejection episode is extensive, but often patchy, interstitial haemorrhage. This may be due to the capillary damage described by Porter (1965) but hypertension and thrombocytopenia may also contribute. Extensive interstitial haemorrhage is reported as commoner in renal allografts treated with X-irradiation (Porter 1966b).

Fibroblastic proliferation with the development of increasing amounts of interstitial fibrous connective tissue invariably follows these changes and eventually results in contraction and scarring of the kidney. This is seen in its most pronounced form in the longstanding allograft where the severe arterial changes described below are also an important contributory factor. Like these arterial changes and the mononuclear cell infiltrate the interstitial fibrosis is both patchy in distribution and variable in amount.

2 *Arteries*

A wide range of changes involving arterioles and arteries of all sizes develops and these are often responsible for the ultimate fate of the graft. Generally the smaller vessels are more involved in kidneys surviving for a shorter time, the larger vessels only becoming affected in the longer term kidneys (Darmady *et al* 1964). Further, many of these lesions develop at points of bifurcation. A most important change and the only one of immediate prognostic importance in kidneys personally studied has been fibrinoid necrosis (Fig. 9). Unlike other reported series (Starzl 1964) this change has not been found to be reversible with increased immunosuppressive therapy and kidney function has never significantly improved with such treatment.

Fibrinoid necrosis principally affects afferent and efferent glomerular arterioles (Fig. 10). However, these vessels are never equally involved and many remain normal. The lesions may be focal or affect the entire length and circumference of the vessels. There is generally a slight neutrophil polymorph infiltrate in the necrotic vessel wall and there may be accompanying haemorrhage spreading into the surrounding tissues. In many of these arterioles thrombosis occurs and may totally occlude the lumen. Fibrinoid necrosis, usually with thrombosis, often extends into glomerular tufts and frequently also involves interlobular arteries (Fig. 9). Arcuate

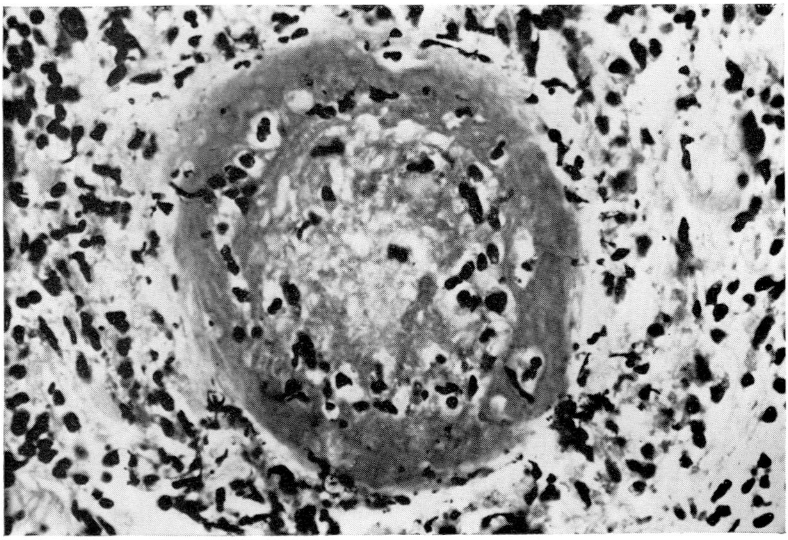

FIG. 9. Interlobular artery 39 days after transplantation. Fibrinoid necrosis with mononuclear cells and neutrophil polymorphs in artery wall and surrounding tissue. H.E. ×380.

arteries can be affected but this occurs less frequently. This change represents a severe immune reaction and may be seen not only within the first few weeks after transplantation but also after a year or more of good renal function.

Other arterial changes that occur include a mononuclear cell infiltrate and a variety of other lesions in the intima and media. The mononuclear cell infiltrate generally accompanies a substantial cell infiltrate in the interstitial tissue, the cells being similar, and first appearing beneath the endothelium. In some instances mononuclear cells infiltrate the media and if the rejection episode is particularly severe occasional neutrophil polymorphs may also appear. With this type of reaction the endothelial cells are swollen and Porter *et al* (1968) have demonstrated granular intimal deposits. Sometimes macrophages distended with lipid are also present, the lipid possibly being derived from the breakdown of platelets (Figs 11 and 12). The damage to the intima encourages the formation of thrombus which may complicate any of the above changes. Should the rejection

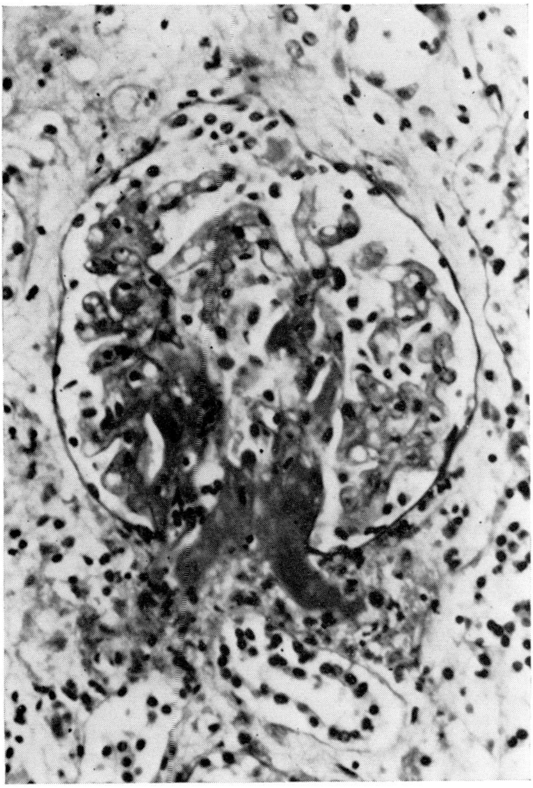

FIG. 10. Glomerulus 39 days after transplantation. Fibrinoid necrosis of afferent and efferent glomerular arterioles with extension into glomerular tuft. P.A.S. ×250.

episode be modified by therapy or be of a more insidious nature a different type of arterial lesion occurs. The lumen of the vessel in the early stages is narrowed, and in some cases totally occluded by loose, very cellular tissue. This is generally arranged evenly around the lumen but does occasionally occur eccentrically. There is a slight or moderate mononuclear infiltrate

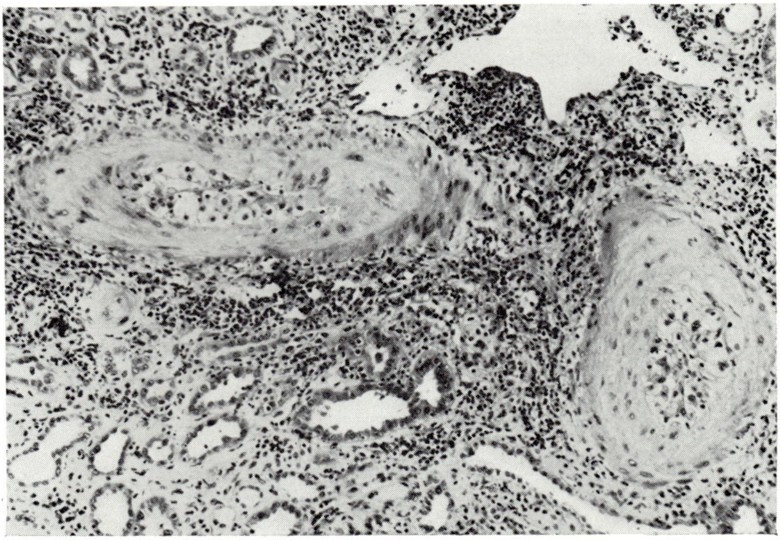

FIG. 11. Arcuate arteries 26 days after transplantation. Macrophages distended with fat narrowing the lumen of two arcuate arteries. A substantial infiltrate of mononuclear cells in the interstitial tissue and in the wall of the arcuate vein which is patent. H.E. ×110.

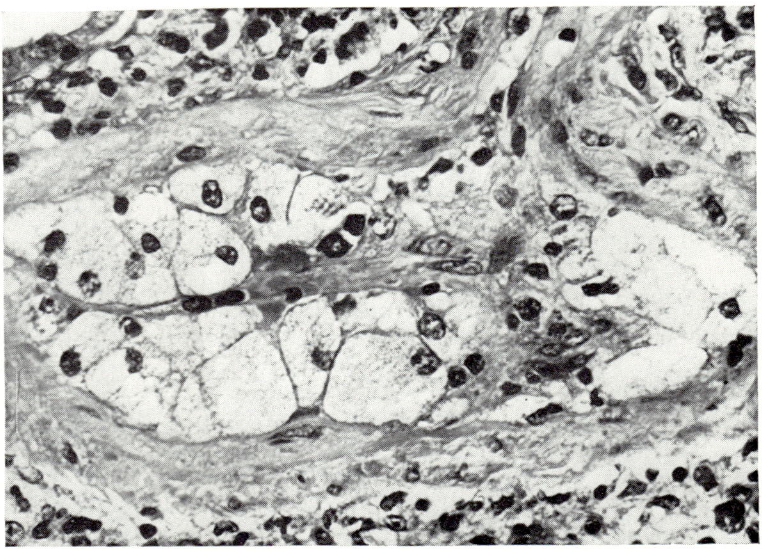

FIG. 12. Arcuate artery 26 days after transplantation. Higher-power of artery similar to Fig. 11. H.E. ×380.

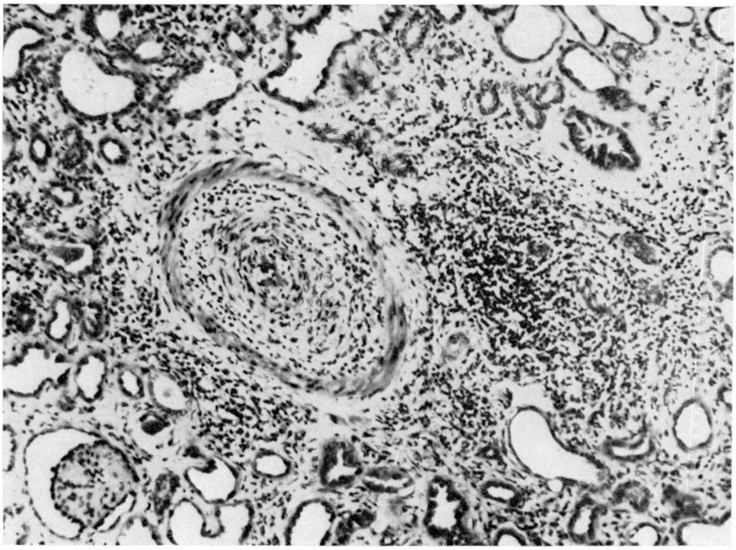

FIG. 13. Interlobular artery 57 days after transplantation. Profound intimal thickening with cellular connective tissue and a moderate mononuclear cell infiltrate in intima and surrounding tissue H E. × 120.

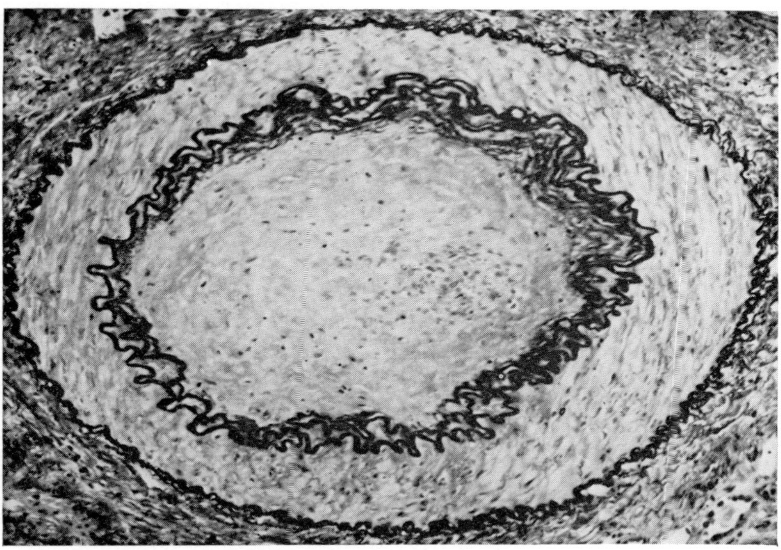

FIG. 14. Arcuate artery 117 days after transplantation. Total occlusion of lumen by fibrous connective tissue. The internal elastic lamina is intact. E.P.S. × 100.

within the thickened intima (Fig. 13). Later, the cellular intimal thickening is replaced by dense fibrous tissue, the lumen of the vessels becoming narrower or even occluded (Fig. 14). Accompanying the intimal thickening fragmentation or wide breaks in the internal elastic lamina can occur (Fig. 15). However, sometimes wide breaks in the internal elastic lamina may be seen without gross changes in the intima, although this is unusual (Fig. 16). Where changes in the intima and internal elastic lamina are present varying degrees of atrophy and fibrosis of the media are seen. Thus the final effect is a grossly narrowed vessel, possibly with breaks in the internal elastic lamina, and a scarred media. The external elastic lamina generally seems to be unaffected but there may be increased connective tissue in the adventitia. Most reports describe these changes in long-standing allografts but they may occur within 3 or 4 weeks of transplantation. Kincaid-Smith (1969) has claimed a reduction in their incidence with the use of anticoagulants. If her experience is confirmed it strongly supports the idea that the thickened tissue is partly due to organization of mural thrombus associated with immune damage.

The role of immune reaction in causing vascular lesions in renal allografts is supported by the work of Porter *et al* (1968) and McKenzie & Whittingham (1968) who have shown deposits containing immunoglobulins, complement components and fibrin in vessel walls at varying times after transplantation with new deposits occurring during rejection crises.

3 *Veins*

The commonest abnormality in veins is an infiltrate of mononuclear cells in their walls (Fig. 11). This change may be seen at any time during a rejection episode and the cells involved are similar to those in the interstitial tissue. Porter *et al* (1964) drew attention to venous thrombosis in canine renal allografts where they found a 5% incidence. Intra-renal venous thrombosis is not uncommon in human renal allografts, occurring in 22 of a series of 47 transplanted kidneys (Fig. 17). This higher incidence of venous thrombosis in human allografts may be due to many factors including immune rejection. This change has been seen as early as 10 days after transplantation but may equally occur at any stage and veins of all sizes may be involved. Generally the thrombus is small and does not completely occlude the lumen of the vessels. Due to the many potential intrarenal venous shunts these lesions are probably of little importance to the viability of the graft. However, they may well account for the substantial fibrous intimal thickening seen in veins in some long-term grafts. Occasionally this change may develop early after transplantation. For example, a

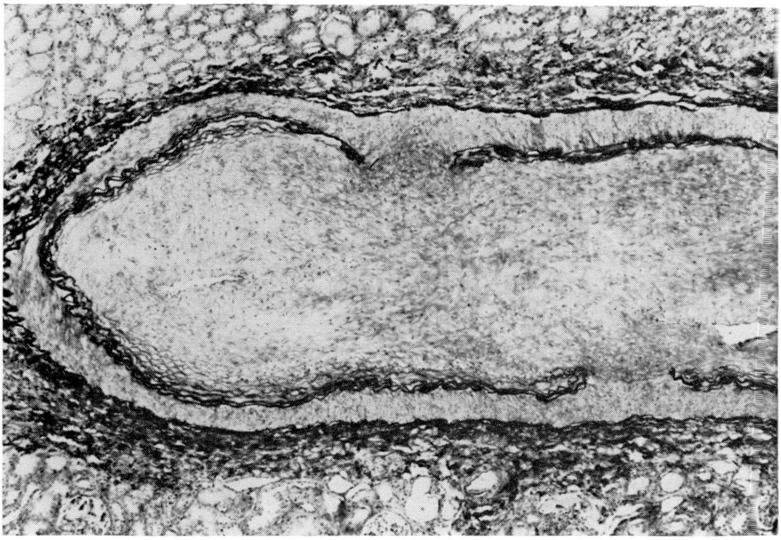

FIG. 15. Lobar artery 117 days after transplantation. Profound fibrous connective tissue thickening of intima with almost complete occlusion of lumen. Large breaks in internal elastic lamina. E.P.S. ×40.

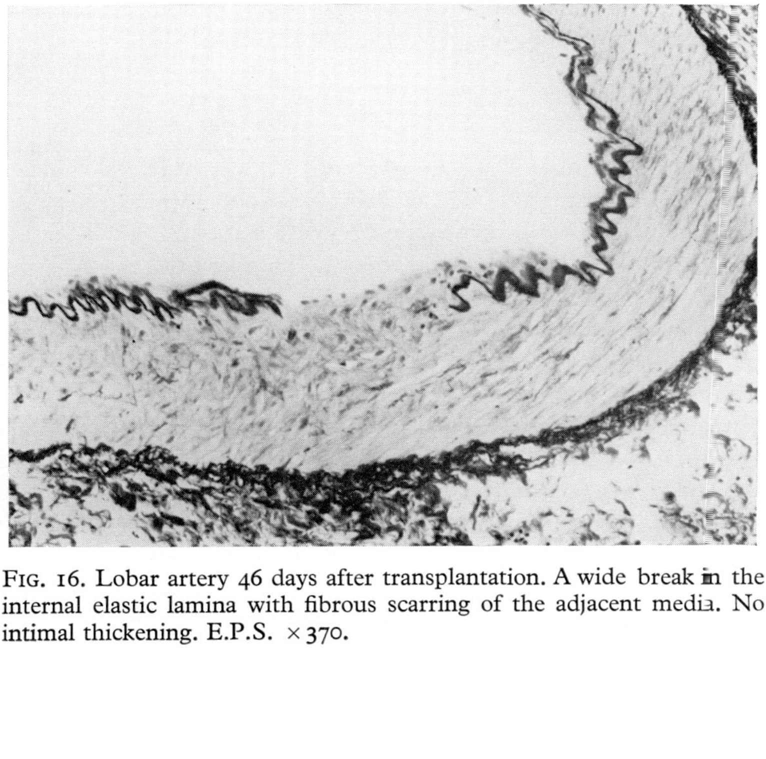

FIG. 16. Lobar artery 46 days after transplantation. A wide break in the internal elastic lamina with fibrous scarring of the adjacent media. No intimal thickening. E.P.S. ×370.

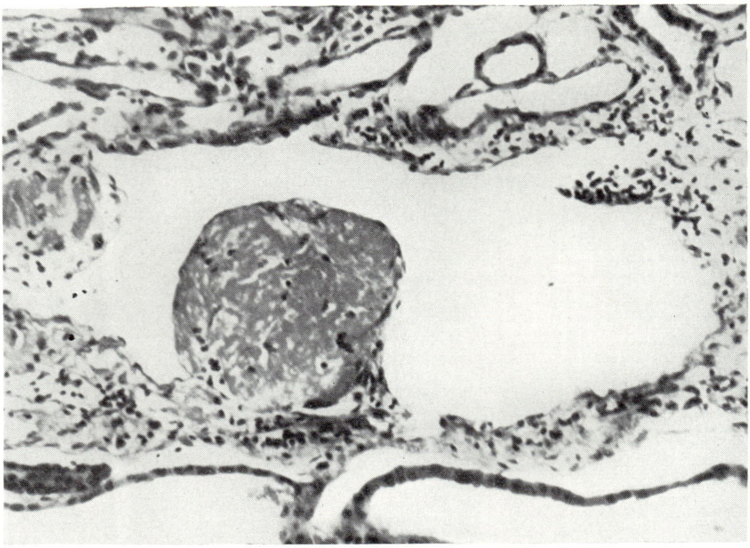

FIG. 17. Interlobular vein 54 days after transplantation. Organizing mural thrombus. Slight mononuclear cell infiltration of vein wall. H.E. ×200.

kidney removed 43 days following transplantation showed considerable fibrous intimal thickening in veins.

4 *Glomeruli*

A range of lesions may occur in glomeruli at any stage following transplantation. The interpretation of these changes and further understanding of their pathogenesis will only come by using a wide range of techniques including electron microscopy and immunofluorescence.

Immediate rejection can result in engorgement and deposits of amorphous eosinophilic material in glomerular tufts within minutes of revascularization of the graft (Kissmeyer-Nielsen *et al* 1966). This material contains fibrin and probably consists of platelet-fibrin aggregates. Similar deposits occur in glomerular arterioles. Accompanying these changes is an infiltrate of neutrophil polymorphs in glomerular tufts but mononuclear cells are conspicuously absent. This type of lesion develops in some recipients previously sensitized by multiple pregnancies or blood transfusion or when there are ABO blood group incompatibilities (Starzl 1964).

In other forms of immune rejection a variety of glomerular changes may develop. One type of lesion is occlusion of glomerular capillaries by aggregates of platelets and fibrin (Porter 1966b). This change is commonly associated with fibrinoid necrosis and thrombosis of arterioles and may result in necrosis of part or the whole tuft. In the region of the basement membranes of such lesions Porter *et al* (1968) have demonstrated IgM and components of complement. However, this change does not affect all glomeruli and some appear normal.

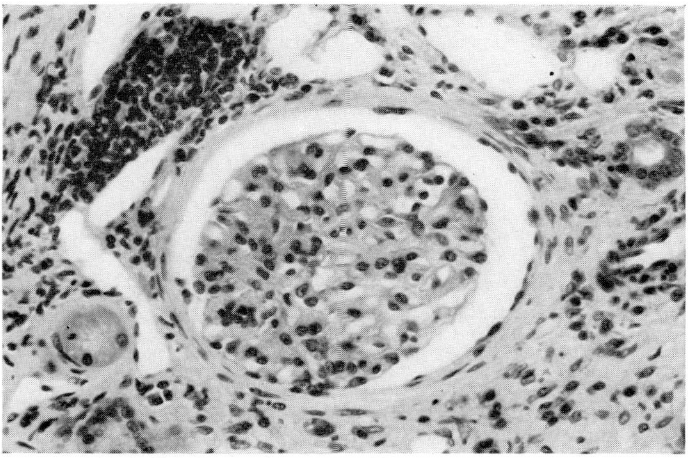

(a)

FIG. 18

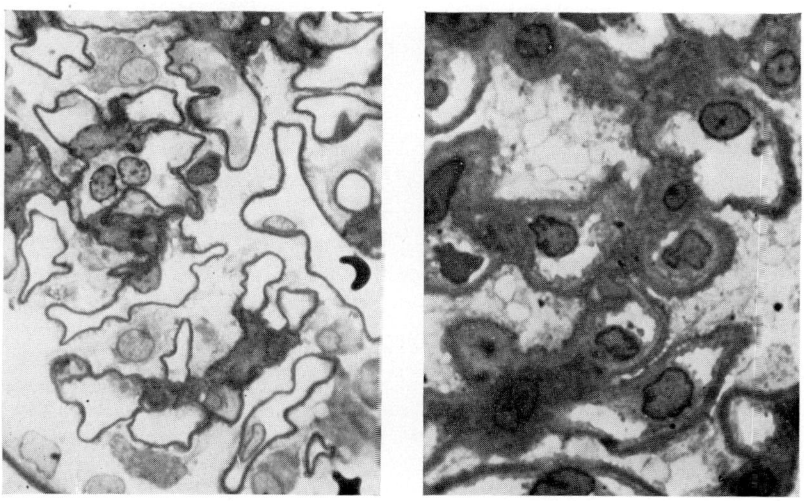

(b)

FIG. 18

In long-term renal allografts alterations may develop in glomerular basement membranes and in the mesangial regions (Figs. 18, 19 and 20). These appearances may be associated with proteinuria and the nephrotic syndrome (Harlan *et al* 1967). Conventional light microscopy reveals a thickening in these regions which resembles the appearances seen in either membranous glomerulonephritis, or lobular glomerulonephritis. However, the glomerular changes in any one graft are rarely uniform. Electron microscopy studies by Porter *et al* (1968) have revealed two types of lesions involving the basement membrane. In one group subendothelial deposits of amorphous material containing IgM and complement components were the significant features, while in another group there were large 'lumpy-bumpy' subepithelial deposits of electron-dense material containing IgM, IgG and complement components. Both types of lesion were associated with hypertrophied endothelial and epithelial cells, and hyperplasia of mesangial cells.

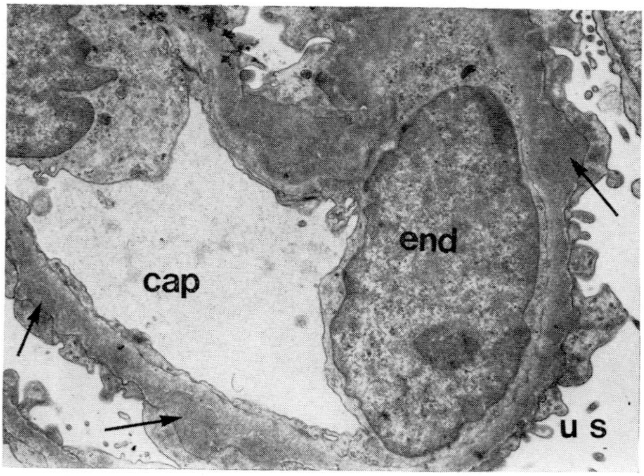

(c)

FIG. 18. Biopsy of a kidney 777 days after transplantation. A patient with chronic idiopathic membranous glomerulonephritis received a transplant. After 2 years of satisfactory renal function he developed severe proteinuria (up to 23 g/day). (a) Thickened basement membranes in a glomerulus with slight periglomerular fibrosis. H.E. ×235. (b) *Right:* Irregular thickening of basement membranes in a further glomerulus from the same biopsy. *Left:* Part of a normal glomerulus from a different kidney. Epon: Azure II ×650. (c) Electron micrograph of part of a capillary loop from the abnormal glomerulus in Fig. 18b. Subepithelial deposits (arrows). cap = capillary lumen. end = endothelial cell. u s = urinary space. Epon: lead citrate ×5000.

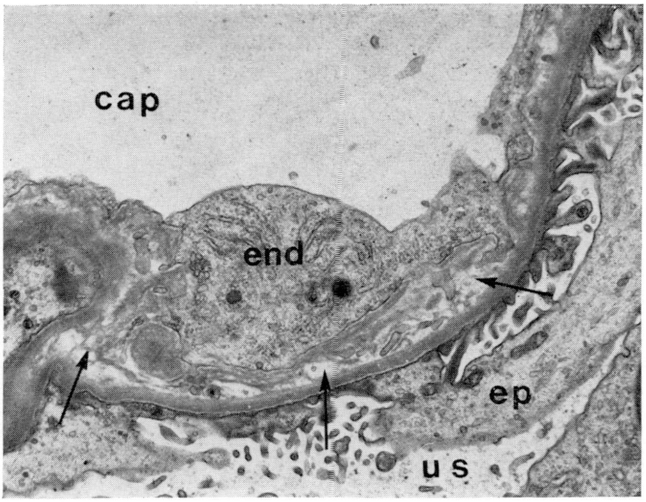

FIG. 19. Glomerulus in a biopsy 40 days after transplantation. Biopsy of the third allograft in a patient whose original renal disorder was chronic pyelonephritis. Cytotoxic antibodies were present prior to the third graft. An electron micrograph showing subendothelial deposits (arrows) of varying density. Abbreviations as for Fig. 18c. Epon: lead citrate ×4250.

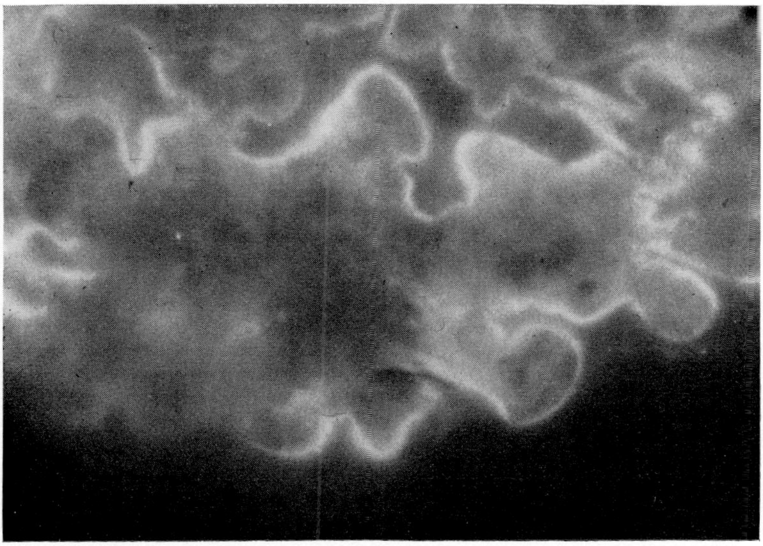

FIG. 20. Glomerulus in an allograft 120 days after transplantation. Linear deposits C3 in glomerular basement membrane. Immunofluorescence.

The lesions seen in the first group are similar to those produced by antibodies against glomerular basement membranes. The 'lumpy-bumpy' subepithelial deposits may occur in the presence of circulating antigen-antibody complexes (Dixon 1968). These glomerular lesions in the grafted kidney could represent glomerulonephritis, a state that may well have occurred in kidney grafts between identical twins (Glassock *et al* 1968). However, exact identity between twins, as discussed by Maynard-Smith & Penrose (1955), has not always been established. Similar glomerular lesions have also occurred in allografts in patients who were not suffering from glomerulonephritis as their original renal disease (Porter *et al* 1968). Further, similar light microscopy appearances have been seen in canine renal transplants (Sheil *et al* 1968). It therefore seems probable that in part these lesions reflect a continuing immune process as a result of the antigenic disparity between the graft and the host. At present the cause of these two changes remains unclear and deserves further study.

Associated with these main changes a wide variety of nonspecific appearances may occur at any interval after transplantation. Various factors including ischaemia due to profound narrowing of arteries may affect glomeruli. Thus atrophy of glomeruli and adhesions of tufts, periglomerular fibrosis and epithelial cell proliferation even to crescent formation can occur. Porter (1966b) has reported hyperplasia of the juxtaglomerular apparatus in 31 out of 33 renal allografts.

5 *Tubules*

In the transplanted kidney a number of factors including immune rejection, ischaemia, ureteric obstruction, infection and drugs can injure the tubular cells and so affect renal structure and function. Biopsy material from cadaveric renal allografts taken soon after revascularization invariably shows degenerative changes and necrosis of a proportion of cells lining proximal tubules. Distal tubules and collecting tubules show similar changes only when many proximal tubular cells are necrotic. The extent of necrosis is directly related to the length of the ischaemia times. MacGillivray & Calne (1966), in a small number of patients, found a relationship between the degree of mitochondrial swelling, the period of ischaemia and the subsequent immediate post-operative function of the transplant.

Although the tubular cells have considerable capacity for regeneration, the transplanted patient is receiving cytotoxic drugs which may affect tubular cell proliferation and account in part for the pleomorphism seen in the earlier stages after transplantation. After a few days it may be difficult to distinguish proximal and distal tubules, most being lined by a similar epithelium. These lining cells are often strikingly pleomorphic with nuclei

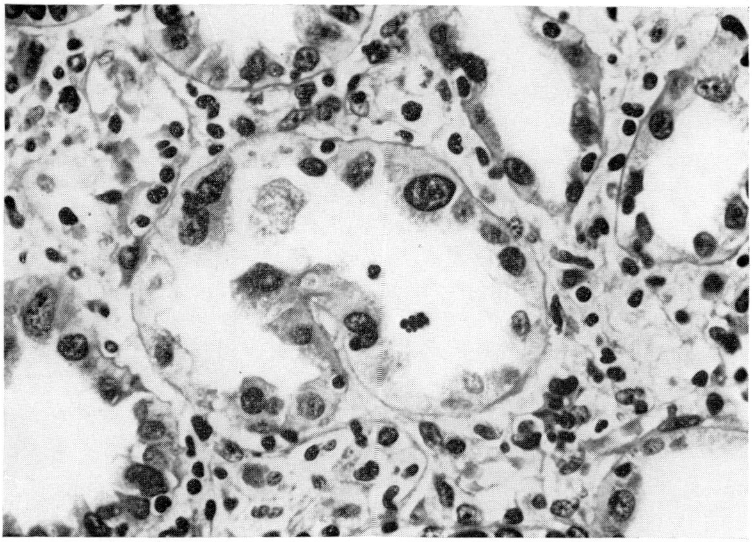

(a)

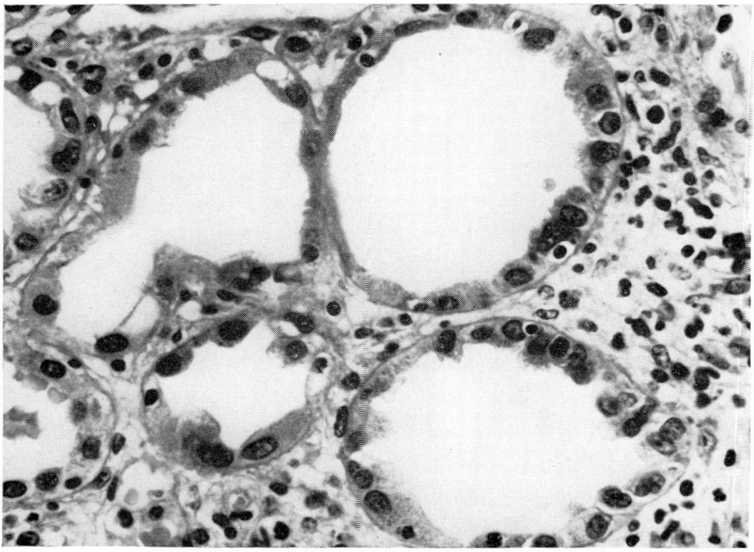

(b)

FIG. 21a, b. Tubules 39 days after transplantation. Cellular and nuclear pleomorphism of tubular cells. The types of the tubules are difficult to identify. Mononuclear cell infiltration in interstitial tissue. H.E. ×395.

of variable shape and size (Fig. 21). Many cells are flattened, while others are large and bulge into the lumen of the tubule. Some of these cells are undergoing apparently normal mitosis. At this stage most tubules are patent but some may contain desquamated epithelial cells, necrotic debris, and occasional birefringent oxalate crystals. These appearances persist until good renal function is achieved. At this stage the tubules may appear normal.

Once the transplant is established different appearances may be seen in tubules, probably reflecting the concurrent processes of cell destruction and regeneration. Many tubules become atrophic, particularly in the cortex, giving a false impression of an increase in the number of glomeruli present. This change is similar to that seen in renal artery stenosis, but without the good preservation of the tubular epithelium. Other tubules may be dilated and their contents may be similar to those described above but can also include neutrophil polymorphs and eosinophilic material resembling thyroid colloid. The pathogenesis of these tubular changes is usually difficult to determine. In some instances ischaemia is probably responsible but in others the injury may be caused by the action of sensitized cells or cytotoxic antibodies.

Ridson *et al* (1968) have drawn attention to the relationship between the extent of tubular damage and renal function in glomerulonephritis. They found that the greater the tubular changes the more advanced the degree of renal failure. This observation is probably also applicable to renal allografts.

6 *Pelvis and ureter*

Generally the morphological appearances of rejection of the pelvis and donor ureter are similar to those seen in the kidney. In both structures a mononuclear infiltrate, oedema, interstitial haemorrhage, and arterial and venous changes occur and their intensity and type are similar to those in the grafted kidney. In addition, associated with severe rejection episodes, the epithelium of both pelvis and ureter may be partly absent or even the full thickness of the wall necrotic. Also in the ureter of long-term renal allografts there is often an increase of fibrous connective tissue and atrophy of smooth muscle; ultimately this portion of the ureter may be represented as a fibrous tube with a flattened and thinned epithelium. The development of ureteric fistula and dilatation and infection of the transplanted ureter and pelvis have already been discussed.

7 *Vascular anastomoses*

Although the intrarenal vessels are often severely affected by immune rejection, the major recipient artery and vein contributing to the vascular anastomoses rarely show similar features. The changes seen are a combination of the effects of surgical trauma and repair processes, superimposed upon features present in these vessels prior to transplantation. Thus in the venous anastomoses shortly after transplantation necrosis of the media at the anastomotic juncture and loss of the intima at this site associated with an inflammatory cell infiltrate occur. With time, the damaged media is replaced by fibrous tissue and the endothelium reforms. Thrombus formation at the anastomotic site is an uncommon complication.

Similar appearances are seen at the arterial anastomoses, and are superimposed upon any pre-existing fibroelastic intimal thickening and medial fibrosis. Atherosclerosis of either donor or recipient arteries may be present prior to transplantation. The absence of endothelium, medial necrosis and an inflammatory cell response are again early features. At this stage whether infection is present or not rupture of this anastomosis may occur (Calne *et al* 1968) but again thrombus formation is unusual. With time the intima overlying the anastomotic junctions is usually represented by thickened fibrous tissue, the internal elastic lamina fragments and disappears, and the media is replaced by a thin band of fibrous tissue; suture material persists. Fibrous intimal thickening and slight medial fibrosis commonly develop in the donor and recipient arteries immediately adjacent to the anastomosis. On occasions this thickening may be sufficient to cause significant stenosis to the arterial supply of the graft (Kincaid-Smith 1969).

C Allograft biopsy

The renal allograft is often biopsied after the completion of the transplantation procedure (initial biopsy) and biopsies may also be taken at later intervals. The latter procedure is either a percutaneous needle biopsy or a biopsy performed as part of an open operation. In either case, if sufficient tissue is available, this should be divided into three portions for light microscopy, electron microscopy and immunofluorescence. This approach is particularly important in examining tissue from long-term kidneys since these biopsies may include glomerular lesions which are difficult to interpret (see above). Also the tissue for light microscopy studies from all biopsy specimens must always be serially sectioned since due to the patchy nature of the rejection process lesions may only be present in parts of the specimen. Without serial sectioning such lesions may easily be missed. Suitable techniques for preparing tissue for light microscopy are basically modifications of routine histology laboratory procedures and are outlined by Disbrey (1971).

The initial biopsy provides an invaluable base line of the transplanted kidney for both pathologist and clinician. The tissue will show the effect of the ischaemic damage prior to revascularization and so give a broad indication of the likely post-operative anuric interval. Also, even though the kidney is macroscopically normal this biopsy can reveal significant renal disorders as well as the severity of age changes. In a few patients the biopsy will show features of immediate rejection associated with cytotoxic antibodies (see above) and no function can be anticipated from such a kidney.

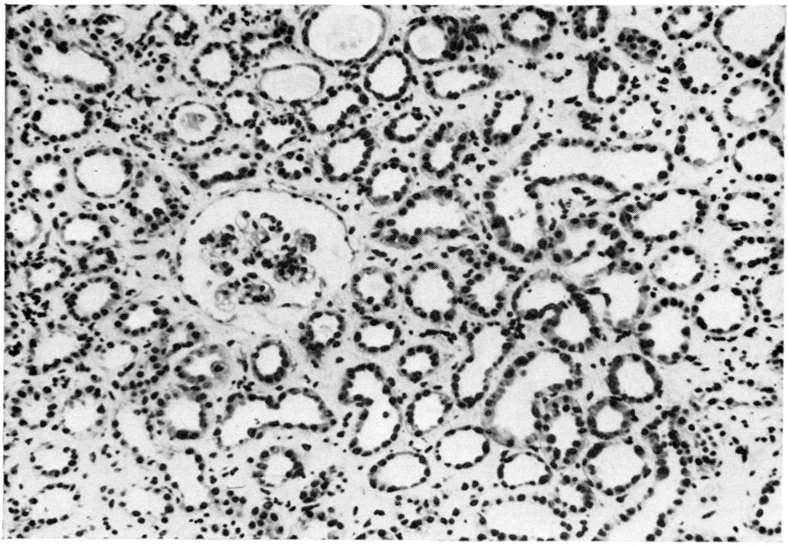

FIG. 22. Allograft biopsy 45 days after transplantation. The cadaver kidney failed to function. At laparotomy after 45 days a ureteric obstruction was discovered. This was relieved and adequate renal function developed. Patent tubules lined by rather flattened epithelium. Oedema and slight increase in interstitial connective tissue. Only occasional mononuclear cells present. A biopsy at 15 days showed similar features. H.E. × 130.

The clinical indications for biopsying the renal allograft post-operatively are discussed elsewhere. The biopsy in all instances is a part of the investigation of impaired renal function and should always be interpreted in conjunction with information gained from other sources. But, while a diversity of circumstances may be responsible for absent or poor function of the graft, immune rejection is obviously a very likely cause and, at present, morphologic appearances provide the only exact criteria for this diagnosis.

The most valuable contribution of the later biopsy is therefore the recognition of immune rejection and any of the microscopic features described above can be seen in these biopsy specimens. The diagnosis may however be missed if the specimen is not serially sectioned or if the process principally affects the larger vessels near the hilum of the kidney. Further, since rejection may advance rapidly or be irreversible it is most helpful to the clinician if the biopsy is processed and examined as soon as possible. The clinician then may be given an idea of the condition of the graft at that time. If there is no evidence of immune rejection in the biopsy, other causes of poor renal function should be more fully investigated. Of these tubular necrosis and ureteric obstruction are of particular importance during the early post-operative period. Tubular necrosis, morphologically, is easily recognized. In biopsy specimens the diagnosis of ureteric obstruction can only be presumptive and is reached by excluding other causes of anuria, particularly immune rejection (Fig. 22). In the longer-term allografts immune rejection may still be the cause of deficient function but infection and glomerular disorders also occur. The recognition of any of these conditions in biopsy specimens at any post-operative interval is helpful since this enables the clinician to avoid the dangers of increased immunosuppression.

III. CONCLUSIONS

An attempt has been made in this chapter to stress the wide range of factors that affect an individual renal allograft. There are probably few human disorders in which a greater variety of factors is involved. Even so, the structural changes in the grafted kidney are not unique and in many respects are similar to those seen in some naturally occurring diseases affecting the kidney, for example polyarteritis nodosa. This is not surprising since injury of living tissue, however caused, can provoke only a limited range of cellular respones. Thus, in spontaneous renal disorders the number of basic patterns of reaction is relatively small and few of the resulting lesions are specific. Identification of a particular renal disease is therefore often difficult. In the grafted kidney the problem of interpretation tends to be more complex and identifying the causes of individual lesions is at present frequently impossible. The continuing contribution of experimental work towards solving these problems and the importance of uniting laboratory and clinical studies has already been mentioned. However, direct analogy between laboratory experiments and clinical observations is not always appropriate and many challenging problems about the morphology of renal allografts remain.

REFERENCES

BOAK J.L., GOODWIN T.J., HULME B., KENYON J.R., OWEN K., PEART W.S. PORTER K.A. & THOMPSON A.E. (1969) Transplantation of second cadaver donor kidneys. *Br. J. Surg.* **56,** 622.

CALNE R.Y., EVANS D.B., HERBERTSON B.M., JOYSEY V., MCMILLAN R., MAGINN R.R., MILLARD P.R., PENA J.R., SALAMAN J.R., WHITE H.J.O., WITHYCOMBE J.F.R. & YOFFA D.E. (1968) Survival after renal transplantation in man: an interim report on 54 consecutive transplants. *Br. med. J.* ii, 404.

CLARKE S.D., KENNEDY J.A., HEWITT J.C., MCEVOY J., MCGEOWN M.G. & NELSON S.D. (1970) Successful removal of thrombus from renal vein after renal transplantation. *Br. med. J.* i, 154.

CRAIGHEAD J.E., HANSHAW J.B. & CARPENTER C.B. (1967) Cytomegalovirus infection after renal allotransplantation. *J.A.M.A.* **201,** 727.

DAMMIN G.J. (1968) The Pathology of Human Renal Transplantation. In *Human Transplantation,* ed. RAPAPORT F.T. & DAUSSET J., p. 170. New York and London: Grune & Stratton.

DAMMIN G.J., COUCH N.P. & MURRAY J.E. (1957) Prolonged survival of skin homografts in uraemic patients. *Ann. N.Y. Acad. Sci.* **64,** 967.

DARMADY E.M., OFFER J.M. & STRANACK F. (1964) Study of renal vessels by microdissection in human transplantation. *Br. med. J.* ii, 976.

DISBREY B.D. (1971) In *Histopathology: Select Topics,* ed. COOK H.C. London: Ward Lock.

DIXON F.J. (1968) The pathogenesis of glomerulonephritis. *Am. J. Med.* **44,** 493.

DIXON F.J., MCPHAUL J.J. & LERNER R.A. (1969) The contribution of kidney transplantation to the study of glomerulonephritis: the recurrence of glomerulonephritis in renal transplants. *Transplantation Proc.* **1,** 194.

EVANS D.B. (1969) Infectious complications of transplantation surgery. *Proc. roy. Soc. Med.* **62,** 597.

EVANS D.B., MILLARD P.R. & HERBERTSON B.M. (1968) Hepatic dysfunction associated with renal transplantation. *Lancet,* ii, 929.

GARROD L.P. & O'GRADY F. (1968) *Antibiotic and Chemotherapy.* (2nd edition). Edinburgh and London: Livingstone.

GIFFORD R.W., DEODHAR S.D., STEWART B.H., NAKAMOTO S., SHIBAGAKI M. & KOLFF W.J. (1967) Retransplantation after failure of first renal homografts: studies in 19 patients. *J.A.M.A.* **199,** 135.

GLASSOCK R.J., FELDMAN D., DAMMIN G.J., REYNOLDS E.S. & MERRILL J.P. (1968) Recurrent glomerulonephritis in human renal isotransplants: a clinicopathologic study. *Proc. 1st International Congress. Transp. Soc.,* p. 361.

GOODMAN L.S. & GILMAN A. (1965) *The Pharmacological Basis of Therapeutics* (3rd edition) Chapter 24. New York: Macmillan Co.

GOWANS J.L. (1965) The role of lymphocytes in the destruction of homografts. *Br. Med. Bull.* **21,** 106.

HARLAN W.R., HOLDEN K.R., WILLIAMS E.M. & HUME D.M. (1967) Proteinuria and nephrotic syndrome associated with chronic rejection of kidney transplants. *New Engl. J. Med.* **277,** 769.

HEPTINSTALL R.H. (1966) Hypertension. I. Essential Hypertension. II. Secondary Forms of Hypertension. In *Pathology of the Kidney* by HEPTINSTALL R.H., p. 119 and 151. Boston: Little, Brown & Co.

HERBERTSON B.M. (1970) The pathology of renal transplantation. *Proc. IVth Int. Congress Nephrol.* (In press.)

HILL R.B., ROWLANDS D.T. & RIFKIND D. (1967) Death after transplantation: an analysis of 60 cases. *Am. J. Med.* **42,** 327.

HODSON C.J. (1967) Radiology of the Kidney. In *Renal Disease* (2nd edition), ed. BLACK D.A.K., p. 136. Oxford and Edinburgh: Blackwell.

HOOD A.B., INGLIS F.G., LOWENSTEIN L., DOSSETOR J.B. & MACLEAN L.D. (1965) Histoplasmosis and thrombocytopenic purpura: transmission by renal transplanatation. *Canad. Med. Ass. J.* **93,** 587.

HUME D.M. (1966) Renal Homotransplantation in Man: Studies in 63 cases. In *The Kidney.*, ed. MOSTOFI F.K. & SMITH D.E., p. 409. Baltimore: Williams & Wilkins.

HUME D.M., LEE H.M., WILLIAMS G.M., WHITE H.J.O., FERRÉ J., WOLF J.S., PROUT G.R., SLAPAK M., O'BRIEN J., KILPATRICK S.J., KAUFFMAN H.M. & CLEVELAND R.J. (1966) Comparative results of cadaver and related donor renal homografts in man, and immunologic implications of the outcome of second and paired transplants. *Ann. Surg.* **164,** 352.

JENSEN M.M. (1967) Viruses and kidney disease. *Am. J. Med.* **43,** 897.

KINCAID-SMITH P. (1967) Histological diagnosis of rejection of renal homografts in man. *Lancet,* ii, 849.

KINCAID-SMITH P. (1969) Modification of the vascular lesions of rejection in cadaveric renal allografts by Dipyridamole and anticoagulants. *Lancet,* i, 920.

KISSMEYER-NIELSEN F., OLSEN S., PETERSEN V.P. & FJELDBORG O. (1966) Hyperacute rejection of kidney allografts, associated with pre-existing humoral antibodies against donor cells. *Lancet,* ii, 662.

KOUNTZ S.L. WILLIAMS M.A., WILLIAMS P.L., KAPROS C. & DEMPSTER W.J. (1963) Mechanism of rejection of homotransplanted kidneys. *Nature, Lond.* **199,** 257.

MACGILLIVRAY J.B. & CALNE R.Y. (1966) The effects of ischaemia in cadaveric renal transplants. *Br. J. Urology,* **38,** 121.

MACLEAN L.D., DOSSETOR J.B., GAULT M.H., OLIVER J.A., INGLIS F.G. & MACKINNON K.J. (1965) Renal homotransplantation using cadaver donors. *Arch. Surg.* **91,** 288.

MCKENZIE I.F.C. & WHITTINGHAM S. (1968) Deposits of immunoglobulin and fibrin in human allografted kidneys. *Lancet,* ii, 1313.

MARTIN L.W., GONZALEZ L.L., WEST C.D., SWARTZ R.A. & SUTORIUS D.J. (1969) Homotransplantation of both kidneys from an anencephalic monster to a 17 pound boy with Eagle-Barrett syndrome. *Surgery,* **66,** 603.

MARTIN D.C., RUBINI M. & ROSEN V.J. (1965) Tumour transplant (Letter to the Editor). *New Engl. J. Med.* **272,** 435.

MAYNARD-SMITH S. & PENROSE L.S. (1955) Monozygotic and dizygotic twin diagnosis. *Ann. Hum. Genet.* **19,** 273.

MILLARD P.R., HERBERTSON B.M. & EVANS D.B. (1970) Renal biopsy in clinical management of renal transplantation: a light microscopy study. *Lancet* i, 113.

MILNE M.D. (1967) Drugs, Poisons and the Kidney. In *Renal Disease* (2nd edition), ed. BLACK D.A.K., p. 546. Oxford and Edinburgh: Blackwell.

PAPADIMITRIOU M., CHISHOLM G.D. & SHACKMAN R. (1969) Hypertension in patients on regular haemodialysis and after renal transplantation. *Lancet,* i, 902.

PEART W.S. (1967) Hypertension and the Kidney. In *Renal Disease* (2nd edition), ed. BLACK D.A.K, p. 638. Oxford and Edinburgh: Blackwell.

PORTER K.A. (1965) Morphological aspects of renal homograft rejection. *Br. Med. Bull.* **21,** 171.

PORTER K.A. (1966a) Renal Transplantation. In *Pathology of the Kidney*. HEPTINSTALL R.H., p. 601. Boston: Little, Brown & Co.

PORTER K.A. (1966b) Tissue Transplantation. In *Recent Advances in Pathology* (8th edition), ed. HARRISON C.V., p. 242. London: Churchill.

PORTER K.A. (1967) Rejection in Treated Renal Allografts. In *Tissue and Organ Transplantation*, ed. PORTER K.A. *J. clin. Path* **20,** 518.

PORTER K.A., ANDRES G.A., CALDER M.W., DOSSETOR J.B., HSU K.C., RENDALL J.M., SEEGAL B.C. & STARZL T.E. (1968) Human renal transplants. II. Immunofluorescent and immunoferritin studies. *Lab. Invest.* **18,** 159.

PORTER K.A., CALNE R.Y. & ZUKOSKI C.F. (1964) Vascular and other changes in 200 canine renal homotransplants treated with immunosuppressive drugs. *Lab. Invest.* **13,** 809.

PORTER K.A., DOSSETOR J.B., MARCHIORO T.L., PEART W.S., RENDALL J.M., STARZL T.E. & TERASAKI P.I. (1967) Human renal transplants. I. Glomerular changes. *Lab. Invest.* **16,** 153.

PORTER K.A. THOMSON W.B., OWEN K., KENYON J.R., MOWBRAY J.F. & PEART W.S. (1963) Obliterative vascular changes in four human kidney homotransplants. *Br. med. J.* ii, 639.

REEVE C.E., MARTIN D.C., GONICK H.C., KAUFMAN J.J., RUBINI M.E., MIMMS M.M., GOODWIN W.E., KOPPEL M.H., KOPPEL J.D. & GOLDMAN R. (1969). Kidney transplantation: a comparison of results using cadaver and related living donors. *Am. J. Med.* **47,** 410.

RETIK A.B., HOLLENBERG N.K., ROSEN S.M., MERRILL J.P. & MURRAY J.E. (1967) Cortical ischaemia in renal allograft rejection. *Surg. Gynec. Obstet.* **124,** 989.

RISDON R.A., SLOPER J.C. & DE WARDNER H.E. (1968) Relationship between renal function and histological changes found in renal biopsy specimens from patients with persistent glomerularnephritis. *Lancet*, ii, 363.

SHEIL A.G.R., DAMMIN G.J., MITCHELL R.M., MOSELEY R.V. & MURRAY J.E. (1968) The management, function and histology of long functioning renal allografts in dogs on immunosuppressive drug therapy. *Ann. Surg.* **167,** 467.

SMELLIE W.A.B., VINIK M. & HUME D.M. (1969) Angiographic investigation of hypertension complicating human renal transplantation. *Surg. Gynec. Obstet.* **128,** 963.

STARZL T.E. (1964) *Experience in Renal Transplantation*. Philadelphia: Saunders.

STARZL T.E., LERNER R.A., DIXON F.J., GROTH C.G., BRETTSCHNEIDER L. & TERASAKI P.I. (1968) Schwartzman reaction after human renal homotransplantation. *New Engl. J. Med.* **278,** 642.

STARZL T.E & PUTNAM C.W. (1969) Efforts to Mitigate or Prevent Rejection. In *Experience in Hepatic Transplantation*, ed. STARZL T.E. & PUTNAM C.W., p. 193. Philadelphia: W.B.Saunders.

WHITE H.J.O., EVANS D.B. & CALNE R.Y. (1968) Function of cadaver renal homografts in relation to age of donor, cause of death, and ischaemia time. *Br. med. J.* **4,** 739.

WIENER J., SPIRO D. & RUSSELL P.S. (1964) An electron-microscopic study of the homograft reaction. *Amer. J. Path.* **44,** 319.

WILLIAMS M.A., MORTON M., TYLER H.M. & DEMPSTER W.J. (1964) A biochemical approach to the study of rejection of canine renal homotransplants. II. Chemical analysis of kidney homogenates. *Br. J. exp. Path.* **65,** 235.

WOODRUFF M.F.A., NOLAN B., ROBSON J.S. & MACDONALD M.K. (1969) Renal transplantation in man: experience in 35 cases. *Lancet*, i, 6.

ACKNOWLEDGEMENTS

We wish to thank Dr P.J.Lachmann for Fig. 20 and Miss J.Metherell for help in preparing Figs. 18 and 19. We are grateful to Mr L.Beard, Miss J.Fendick and Mr S.W.Patman for their help with illustrations.

CHAPTER 18

Long-term Care and Follow-up

W.A.B. Smellie

Long-term care of a transplanted patient begins the day that he leaves hospital. This moment is at a very variable time after the transplant operation. In some units it is the deliberate policy to keep patients within the centre for 120 days post-transplant (Hume 1970), partly for the purposes of study. The vast majority of units, however, keep their patients only until they have reached a satisfactory equilibrium of renal function. Under optimal circumstances this may be as little as 3 weeks, but on average is between 4 and 6 weeks after operation.

The precise method of subsequent supervision differs in various regions, largely depending on the distance between the transplanting centre and the patient's home. Those who live within a reasonable distance of our unit are followed-up by us, according to a protocol to be described later. Those who are referred from afar are usually followed at their local hospital by a renal physician who retains contact with our unit and discusses problems as they arise. The family practitioner is early incorporated into the programme of care and is told of the particular signs and symptoms to expect in case of trouble.

Weekly follow-up is the rule for the first 3 months after discharge, fortnightly for the next 9 months, and every 3 weeks between the 1st and 2nd year. Thereafter patients are followed up monthly.

At each follow-up a complete physical examination is undertaken with special reference to the blood pressure. The urine is cultured, the patient brings with him a collection of his previous 24 hours' urine production, and the creatinine clearance is estimated. Routine blood work is performed, including differential white cell and platelet counts and routine serum chemistry. Serum calcium and phosphates and liver function tests are estimated on alternate visits.

Routine radiology is not undertaken, apart from a chest X-ray at 6-monthly intervals. An IVP is performed on all patients at the time of their discharge, and is not repeated unless an especial indication arises. Routine renal biopsies have not been our practice, although in some centres they have been of considerable help (Kincaid-Smith 1969). Our policy is to biopsy the kidney only if the situation deteriorates and further information is required for the management of the patient.

Immunosuppressive drugs are continued indefinitely with minor adjustments in dose. Signs of intolerance include changes in blood count, hepatitis, and all the complications of long-term steroid therapy. Whenever possible, the daily maintenance dose of Imuran is between 2–2·5 mg/kg body weight, and of Prednisone between 10–12 mg/day. Patients with poorly tolerated kidneys, however, may require larger steroid dosage.

If at any time during the follow-up period there is a suspicion that a rejection episode is occurring, the patient is admitted for further investigations and anti-rejection treatment if necessary. As previously mentioned, rejection crises diminish in frequency with time, and after the 2nd year are rarely encountered. More common in those patients into their 3rd year who are not tolerating their kidneys well is a slow deterioration of renal function, occurring over many months and often associated with the development of hypertension. This is the process of chronic rejection, which responds poorly to all the methods of immunosuppression currently available. Although a course of anti-rejection management may be employed, a satisfactory response is unusual. It has been tempting in the management of several patients in this and many other units where well matched kidneys have had an essentially benign post-operative course, to consider reduction of immunosuppression to below the maintenance levels previously described. No unit, however, has a statistically significant group of long-term survivors and at the present it would seem unwise to alter a régime which has produced in some series dependable results in patients now in their 8th year post-transplantation.

If the transplanted patient suffers from an intercurrent illness he is managed from the point of view of prednisolone as is any other patient on a maintenance dose of steroids. His daily dose is immediately doubled and is brought back to the previous level as rapidly as possible after the acute episode is over. Major surgical operations will require a pre-operative boost of steroids, which may need to be continued into the post-operative period for a few days. The Imuran dosage during the time of acute crisis need not be altered unless concern is caused by deteriorating white blood or platelet counts. The only other situations where continuing Imuran dosage may be dangerous is in the presence of oliguria, or in patients with gradual deterioration of renal function and creatinine clearances of less than 20 ml/min.

Patients may ask advice of the managing physicians about pregnancies. In transplanted women there are several potential hazards. The transplanted kidney may have to compete with a rapidly expanding uterus for space within the pelvis, and obstruction of the transplanted ureter may be expected to occur. Of rather more serious import than purely mechanical considerations are the theoretical possibilities of foetal abnormality produced by long-term Imuran therapy (Murray *et al* 1964), or in some units where local irradiation to the graft is undertaken, by the accidental irradiation of the ovary. The advice of most units to their female patients is not to start a pregnancy, but this advice has on occasion been ignored. There are two patients in the Medical College of Virginia series who have produced normal infants at term (Hume 1968) and who did not suffer significant deterioration of renal function during pregnancy. There are many instances of male transplanted patients on long-term immunosuppression having fathered children (Hume *et al* 1963) and there has been no report of foetal abnormality.

The development of neoplasia in transplanted immunosuppressed patients has long been feared on theoretical grounds (Swanson & Schwarz 1967) and this fear has now been confirmed (Doak *et al* 1968), although happily trouble is infrequent. This whole problem is considered in detail in Chapter 8.

We advise our patients not to undergo immunization procedures using live or attenuated viruses or organisms, though this has not been a universal practice in other units. There is no doubt that relatively benign conditions can behave in atypical fashion in immunosuppressed patients; we have witnessed a rapid death from chickenpox of a recipient who developed the disease within a few days of a completely satisfactory transplant from her father, and in whom the course of the illness was fulminating and relentless.

In spite of rigid follow-up and the above listed restrictions a patient with a successful transplant can lead a relatively normal existence. There is no occupation which is specifically contra-indicted. The rapid return to physical and mental health of a patient often previously chronically sick and protein starved for many years is one of the most satisfying sights to witness in medicine today.

REFERENCES

DOAK P.B., MONTGOMERIE J.Z., NORTH J.D.K. & SMITH M., (1968) Reticular cell sarcoma after renal homotransplantation and azathioprine and prednisone therapy. *Br. med. J.* ii, 746.

HUME D.M. (1968) In *Human Transplantation*, by RAPAPORT & DAUSSET, p. 131.

HUME D.M. (1970). Personal communication.

HUME D.M., MAGEE J.H., KAUFMAN H.J. Jr., RITTENBURY M.S. & PROUT G.R., Jr. (1963) Renal homotransplantation in man in modified recipients. *Ann. Surg.* **158,** 608.

KINCAID-SMITH P. (1969) Modification of the vascular lesions of rejection in cadaveric renal allografts by dyperidanole and antigens. *Lancet,* ii, 920.

MURRAY J. E., SHIEL A.G.R., MOSELEY R., KNIGHT P., MEGAVIC J.D., & DAMMIN G.J., (1964) Analysis of mechanism of immunosuppressive drugs in renal homotransplantation. *Ann. Surg.* **160,** 449.

SWANSON M.A. & SCHWARZ R.S. (1967) Immunosuppressive therapy. *New Engl. J. Med.* **277,** 163.

CHAPTER 19

Results

W.A.B. Smellie

The majority of human kidney transplants performed are reported to the Human Kidney Transplant Registry in Boston, where data is extracted for central processing and analysis. This Registry, founded in 1963, produces an annual report. At the time of its last report (Human Transplant Registry, 1970) 3645 cases were available for study. The overall results are given in Table 1.

TABLE 1.

3645 Transplants analysed			
	Identical twin (1%) %	Related living donors (43%) %	Cadaveric donors (56%) %
1 year functional survival	89	78	52
2 year functional survival	87	75	41

From the eighth report of the human kidney registry (1970)

A similar service for kidney transplant operations performed in Europe is provided by the Renal Research Unit and Department of Urology at Leeds, who also produce an annual report. 1239 patients are available for analysis

TABLE 2.

1239 patients considered	Living donors		Cadaveric
	Parental %	Sibling %	donors %
1 year functional survival	60	75	42
2 year functional survival	59	66	40

From the annual report on renal transplantation in Europe 1969

in their most recent study (Parsons *et all* 1969), of whom 442 were transplanted during the year 1 April 1968, to 1 April 1969. The overall results from this analysis are given in Table 2.

The conclusion to be drawn from comparison of these two reports is that the results at two years of cadaveric transplantation are very similar in different parts of the world. However, it would appear that the results of related living donor transplantation are worse in Europe than elsewhere.

In Europe at present cadaveric donors outnumber related living donors by about three to one; in our unit from a series of 142 transplants, related living donors have been used on seven occasions only. In the USA this trend is reversed, with the result that in the overall analysis (see Table 1) related living donors and cadaveric donors each supply roughly half the total numbers used.

The reasons for the disparity in results between cadaveric and related living donor transplants are both immunological and mechanical. Clearly, related living donors must have a better chance of genetic similarity with the recipient than randomly selected cadaveric donors, and siblings are more likely to be genetically similar than are parents. There is no problem in coinciding the operation of kidney removal and insertion when performing a transplant using a living donor. When a cadaveric donor is used, however, ischaemia, organ perfusion and storage, and the logistics of transport all present their particular problems. The end result is that cadaveric donor kidneys have longer warm and total ischaemia times, and are much less likely to be well matched with the recipient unless very special precautions are undertaken. A central organization for typing cadaveric donors and selecting the optimal match from a large pool of recipients, often in hospitals widely separated, is in operation in many areas, including the United Kingdom, the Benelux countries, Scandinavia, France and the west coast of America. By this means it is hoped that cadaveric donor transplant figures will improve, although the programmes are not yet sufficiently advanced for any definite conclusion to be reached. There is no doubt at present that a good match is often procured at the expense of a very considerable prolongation of cold ischaemia time, and the advantages of the former in the face of the latter may not be as significant as was at first hoped. However, it does seem quite certain that in the future better systems of organ procurement and preservation, and a more profound understanding of the immunological background of various tissue types will all contribute to a general improvement in results.

An emerging unit can improve on the average results previously described if it rigidly uses cadaveric kidneys with short warm ischaemia times of less than 60 min. Centres where the supply of donor kidneys is plentiful, and where the local feeling allows the use of donor kidneys from respirator cases, are well placed to produce minimally ischaemic organs. However, policy has to be declared at the beginning of a proposed programme of renal transplantation and it is the philosophy of many, including our own unit, since we are attempting to provide treatment for the community, to perform the maximum number of transplants possible, rather than to restrict the procedure to the few cases in which technical success can be almost guaranteed. Accurate figures are hard to obtain but it is probable that at present in the United Kingdom only between six and seven hundred patients are maintained on chronic home dialysis (Dunworth 1969) whereas more than 2000 young patients die annually from renal failure (Annual Statistical Report for England and Wales), who might have benefitted from either transplantation or chronic dialysis. An ideally supported unit for the management of terminal renal failure should have facilities for both chronic dialysis and transplantation, as some patients are better treated by one method than by the other.

In general our policy is to accept for transplantation kidneys from cadaveric sources with up to 90 min of warm and 12 h of cold ischaemia and it is hoped that improvement in perfusing solutions and methods will in future prolong the acceptable time of cold ischaemia still further. Prospective tissue typing has been undertaken since May 1968, and each case is judged on its individual merits.

The results using this policy in the 87 cadaveric first kidney transplants performed in our unit more than 1 year ago are given in Table 3.

TABLE 3.

	% Functional Survival
1 year functional survival	53
2 year functional survival	49

Cambridge results from cadaveric donors: first kidney transplants 1 January 1971

In view of the above discussion direct comparison of the results of cadaveric renal transplantation may be difficult, since some centres remove kidneys from cases of *coma depassé*, which from the point of view of ischaemia, are the same as kidneys from living donors, while others pursue a policy similar to ours.

MULTIPLE TRANSPLANTATION

The problem of management of patients who have a failed renal transplant is becoming increasingly difficult. If the first graft failed for technical reasons the prospects for a further graft are often favourable. However, if the graft failed because of rejection, particularly if function was maintained for some considerable time, the situation may be more complex. This is largely because cytotoxic antibodies may have developed in the patient's serum. If a further transplant is performed in a patient with preformed cytotoxic antibodies to the second graft, the phenomenon of hyperacute rejection and immediate kidney destruction may be witnessed (Kissmayer-Nielson *et al* 1966; Williams *et al* 1968). This phenomenon is seen with increasing frequency by all transplant units of experience. It is in this group of patients that the correct use of typing facilities is so vital, as it should be possible before operation to detect cytotoxic antibodies to the proposed donor's cells. No form of therapy yet devised can alter the titre of circulating cytotoxic antibodies, which however does tend to diminish with time and may indeed fluctuate. These antibodies are produced initially by the mismatched antigens of the original transplant, blood transfusion or pregnancies and provided that a further donor can be found who does not carry these same mismatched antigens, hyperacute rejection on theoretical grounds can be avoided. An analysis of multiple transplants must in each case take into account the history of the previous transplant and also the mode of immunosuppression of the patient during the period of failure of his previous graft. A sharp reduction in immunosuppression therapy at this stage, though tempting on general terms, may allow immunization to occur and may preclude a further satisfactory transplant.

Of the 23 patients transplanted for a second time at the Medical College of Virginia, (Hume & Lee 1970), only eight are still functioning on their second kidney, although two of these are now more than 5 years post-operation. Of the 15 patients with a failed second transplant six have been transplanted for a third time, and of these one is functioning satisfactorily at 56 months. Of the five whose third transplant failed, two were transplanted on a fourth occasion and of these one is living at 26 months. Thus, even in the most experienced hands, multiple transplants have produced disappointing results.

In our unit 19 patients have been transplanted for a second time and two for a third. Four of these 19 patients lost their first kidney from technical reasons, and 16 because of rejection. Three of the four in the first group were transplanted successfully on the second occasion and have functioning grafts 2 years later. Of the 16 who lost their first kidney for immunological reasons 11 were successfully transplanted on a second occasion. Those five who had unsuccessful second grafts lost them from either hyperacute rejection or rejection within the first few months. One patient transplanted a third time lost this graft from fulminating early rejection without it ever achieving function. This was particularly disappointing in view of the fact that there were no cytotoxic antibodies to this third donor demonstratable before operation, and there was no major mismatch between donor and recipient. The other patient received her third kidney recently. It is at present functioning well; the donor and recipient were HL-A identical.

REFERENCES

DUNWORTH J. (1969) Parliamentary question time. *Lancet*, ii, 1311.

HUME D.M. & LEE H.M., (1970) personal communication.

KISSMEYER-NIELSON F., OLSEN S., PETERSON V.P. & FJILDBORG O. (1966). 'Hyperacute rejection of kidney allografts associated with pre-existing humoral antibodies against donor cells. *Lancet*, ii, 662.

PARSONS F.M., CLARK P.B. (1969). *Annual Report on Renal Transplantation in Europe*.

REGISTRAR GENERAL'S ANNUAL STATISTICAL REPORT FOR ENGLAND AND WALES (1962). Published 1964.

8TH REPORT OF THE HUMAN TRANSPLANT REGISTRY (1970).

WILLIAMS G.M., HUME D.M., HUDSON R.P., MORRIS P.J., KANO K. & MILGROM F. (1968). Hyperacute renal homograft rejection in man. *New Engl. J. Med.*, **279**, 611.

ACKNOWLEDGEMENTS

I am grateful to Dr David Hume and Dr H.M.Lee for providing data from the Medical College of Virginia transplantation programme.

Part 3
Liver Transplantation

CHAPTER 20

Indications for Liver Transplantation and Assessment of Recipient

Roger Williams

Published reports on the prognosis of certain forms of liver disease which theoretically would be suitable for transplantation, make gloomy reading. Primary hepatomas are in general highly malignant tumours and most patients are dead within 4 to 6 months of diagnosis (Lawrence *et al* 1966; Nelson *et al* 1966). Although carcinomas arising from the bifurcation of the hepatic duct grow more slowly and tend to metastasize late they are because of their site in the hilum of the liver rarely resectable. In some patients a tube can be passed through the growth with relief of jaundice and with worthwhile survival for several years but the average survivals in the two largest series reported were 15·5 and 14·6 months (Klatskin *et al* 1965; Whelton *et al* 1969). In only a quarter of the children born with extrahepatic biliary atresia is it possible to correct the anatomical defect (Cameron & Bunton 1960), the others usually dying before the age of 3 years.

It is more difficult to generalize about the prognosis of cirrhosis for statistics from different countries vary because of geographical differences in the type of cirrhosis found and those from special units are fallacious because of selection by patient referral. However, Stone *et al* (1968) analysed the course of 155 patients admitted with cirrhosis to a busy general hospital in Birmingham during the years 1959 to 1964. The calculated 5 year survival was only 14·3% showing that cirrhosis has an outlook worse than that of many forms of cancer. The onset of ascites is an ominous sign and only 28·6% survive more than 8 months. In another series from two busy general hospitals the mortality of the first episode of bleeding from varices was 54% (Hislop *et al* 1966).

Acute hepatic necrosis whether due to fulminant hepatitis or to drug toxicity carries an appalling mortality. In the latest account from the Fulminant Hepatic Failure Surveillance Study (Trey *et al* 1970), the mortality of the 284 patients who went into coma was 82%, with a figure of 96% for those with a halothane induced hepatic necrosis. Although it has been said that, the liver can regenerate in these patients this seems very doubtful when one looks at the histological appearance at autopsy with almost complete destruction of the liver cells and only a few surviving bile ducts. This is a disease which strikes at all ages and the patients have usually been in good health prior to its onset. It is possible that the transplanted liver would also be attacked by the hepatitis virus. Although the patient should have developed an immune reaction by that time, this might be depressed by the immunosuppressive treatment. It would be prudent to give γ-globulin both to the recipient and to those involved in the transplant surgery and after care.

TABLE 1. Recorded deaths in England and Wales during 1964 (from Terblanche & Riddell 1967)

	0–60 years
Primary hepatoma	145
Primary biliary tract carcinoma	195
Cirrhosis	490
Acute hepatitis/yellow atrophy	160
Total	990

The number of patients who died of these conditions in England and Wales during 1964 is shown in Table 1, which gives data abstracted by Terblanche & Riddell (1967) from the Registrar General's Statistical Review for that year. Not all of these patients would have been suitable for transplantation. About a third of those with a primary hepatoma will already have metastases by the time of diagnosis. In others where the growth is localized to one lobe, partial hepatectomy is the preferred method of treatment. The figures for primary biliary tract carcinoma include those arising from the gallbladder and those at the lower end of the common bile duct for which transplantation would not be considered. Similarly, the deaths from cirrhosis include those with alocholic cirrhosis (probably a third of the total) and many of these patients would be unsuitable candidates for transplantation because of their psychological disability. A very approximate estimate of the total number that might be treated by liver transplantation per year in this country is of the order of 500 patients.

Each of these conditions has particular problems with respect to transplantation. In a primary hepatoma, the large size of the liver and the frequent vascular adhesions make the recipient hepatectomy technically difficult. Previous operations particularly when they have involved the porta hepatis as in cases of hepatic duct carcinoma, add to the surgical difficulties—pre-operative infection being the most serious hazard. In cirrhosis, bleeding is the main problem due both to the portal hypertension and to the haemorrhagic diathesis. The frequently associated metabolic disturbances and renal failure are further hazards. Hepatic coma is not a contra-indication and a previous portacaval anastomosis with lowering of the portal pressure can facilitate the surgery. In extrahepatic biliary atresia difficulties arise from the small size of the vessels and the frequently associated congenital anomalies.

TABLE 2. The diagnosis and number of patients treated by orthotopic transplantation (January 1971)

	No. patients
Primary hepatoma	6
Carcinoma of hepatic duct	5
Cirrhosis with liver failure	9
Secondary deposits	2
Extrahepatic biliary atresia	1
Total	23

Our selection of patients (given in Table 2), has been rather different from that of Starzl (1969). Of his first 25 patients, who were operated on between 1 March 1963 and 11 February 1969, 12 had extrahepatic biliary atresia and six primary hepatoma without underlying cirrhosis.

In assessing recipients for transplantation particular attention must be paid to screening for metastases and to the detection and treatment of systemic or local infections. We have taken 60 years as an upper age limit and a stable pre-illness personality is essential. One important pre-operative investigation is hepatic arteriography done via a catheter inserted percutaneously into the femoral artery. In the recipient whose arteriogram is illustrated in Fig. 1, the right hepatic artery rose from the superior mesenteric artery and the left from the coeliac axis. Knowledge of such anatomical variation is of help to the surgeon. It is not yet clear whether metastic

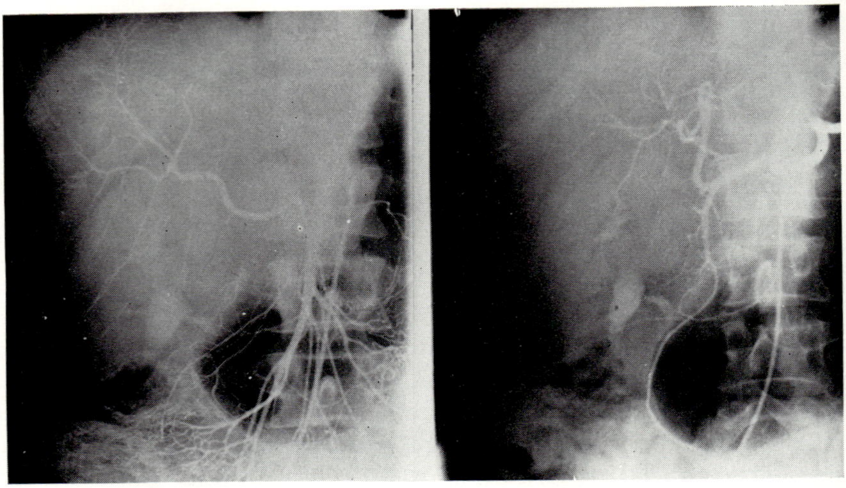

FIG. 1. Illustrating anatomical variation in hepatic arterial supply of a patient SG who had an adenocarcinoma arising at the hepatic duct bifurcation (from Williams 1970).

growth apparently confined to the liver will be an indication for liver allografting.

HETEROTOPIC VERSUS ORTHOTOPIC TRANSPLANTATION

The advantages of a heterotopic approach are that the residual function of the donor liver is retained, at least initially, and the difficulties of the recipient hepatectomy are avoided. However, it is difficult to find room for an extra liver in the abdomen. Moreover the auxillary organ appears to compete with the recipients own liver for some essential metabolite in the portal venous blood. It has been shown in dogs and rats after auxillary transplantation that the organ which has first access to the portal blood flow retains its functional and morphological integrity whereas the other organ undergoes atrophy (Marchioro *et al* 1967; Lee & Edgington 1968). In man the function of the recipient's own liver will already be severely impaired by episodes of rejection. Evidence of graft atrophy was observed in a patient of Starzl's who survived for 34 days after heterotopic transplantation (Starzl 1969). It is, of course, only applicable to non-malignant conditions and in cirrhosis, which would be the largest potential group, there is a significant risk of a hepatoma developing—18·4% in the Birmingham series (Stone *et al* 1968). For these and other reasons we do not favour heterotopic grafts.

ASSESSMENT OF DONOR

Unfortunately the liver is extremely sensitive to warm ischaemia and if left at body temperature without a blood supply for more than 15 min serious damage will occur. If such a liver is transplanted the recipient almost inevitably develops within a few hours a severe haemorrhagic diathesis resistant to all forms of therapy.

The most suitable donors are those with irreversible brain damage who are on ventilators and in whom the decision has been made by Consultant Staff independant of the transplant team to cease resusciation. Only when respiration and heart beat have stopped does the operation on the donor start, the aim being to cool the liver as soon as possible by perfusion of a chilled fluid through a catheter placed in the superior mesenteric vein, details of which are given later. In assessing the suitability of a donor particular attention should be paid to occurrence of periods of hypotension, for these will have the same effect on the donor liver as prolonged warm ischaemia after death. Systemic infection of the donor, carcinoma or previous hepato-biliary disease are also absolute bars. On general grounds organs from donors less than 50-years-old are preferred though liver function is relatively little affected by age (Thompson & Williams 1965), and Peters from Starzl's group who examined 30 patients dying after the age of 50 found that the hepatic artery was completely spared of atheroma in 80% (Starzl 1969).

REFERENCES

CAMERON R. & BUNTON G.L. (1960) Congenital biliary atresia. *Br. med. J* ii, 1253.

HISLOP I.G., WATERS T.E., KELLOCK T.D. & SWYNNERTON B. (1966) The natural history of haemorrhage from oesophageal varices. *Lancet*, i, 945.

KLATSKIN G. (1965) Adenocarcinoma of the hepatic duct at its bifurcation within the porta hepatis. *Am. J. Med.* **38**, 241.

LAWRENCE G.H., GRAUMAN D., LASERSOHN J. & BAKER J.W. (1966) Primary carcinoma of the liver. *Am. J. Surg.* **112**, 200.

LEE S. & EDGINGTON T.S. (1968) Heterotopic liver transplantation utilizing inbred rat strains. *Am. J. Path.* **52**, 649.

MARCHIORO T.L., PORTER K.A., BROWN B.I., OTTE J.B. & STARZL T.E. (1967) The effect of partial portacaval transposition on the canine liver. *Surgery*, **61**, 723.

NELSON R.S., ELIZALDE R.DE & HOWE C.D. (1966) Clinical aspects of primary carcinoma of the liver. *Cancer, Philadelphia*, **19**, 533.

STARZL T.E. (1969) *Experience in Hepatic Transplantation.* Philadelphia, London, Toronto: W.B.Saunders.

STONE W.D., ISLAM N.R.K. & PATON A. (1968) The natural history of cirrhosis. *Quart. J. Med.* **37,** 119.

TERBLANCHE J. & RIDDELL A.G. (1967) The strategy of liver transplantation. In *The Liver,* ed. READ A.E. London: Butterworth.

THOMPSON E.N. & WILLIAMS R. (1965) The effect of age on liver function with particular reference to bromsulphalein excretion. *Gut,* **6,** 266.

TREY C., LIPWORTH L. & DAVIDSON C.S. (1970) Parameters influencing survival in the first 318 patients reported to the fulminant hepatic failure surveillance study. *Gastroenterology,* **58,** 306.

WHELTON M.L., PETRELLI M., GEORGE P., YOUNG W.B. & SHERLOCK S. (1968) Carcinoma of the junction of the main hepatic duct. *Quart. J. Med.* N.S. **38,** 211.

ACKNOWLEDGEMENTS

The authors of Chapters 20, 25, 26 and 27 are grateful to the research fellows and clinical staff of the Liver Unit at King's College Hospital, as well as Mr John Winch and Mr John Dawson of the Department of Surgery, who have helped at one time or another in the care of these patients. Members of the Department of Chemical Pathology have also been of invaluable assistance in the post-operative management. We are also indebted to Dr M.G.M.Smith for his considerable assistance with the immunological studies and to Dr M.O.Rake for his work on the haematological changes. Various aspects of the research have been generously supported by grants from the Wellcome Trust and the Wates Foundation.

CHAPTER 21

Selection of Donors for Liver Transplantation

V.C. Marshall

Selection of donors for liver transplantation, although possessing broad similarities to those required for cadaver kidney procurement, demands more stringent criteria. This is because cooling of the liver must begin within 15 min of death if severe agonal damage is to be prevented. Consent of the relatives for organ removal, and suitable blood and tissue matching between donor and recipient should therefore preferably be obtained before death. Patients who are dead on arrival at the casualty department or who die suddenly and unexpectedly within the hospital are usually unsuitable.

The most suitable donor is therefore a young person with severe and irreversible brain damage from injury or neurologic disease, in whom the diagnosis of permanent loss of brain function can be made while temporary resuscitation by artificial ventilation is being carried out, and in whom circulatory status is not showing rapid deterioration.

The involvement of the transplant team does not begin until the diagnosis of brain death is confirmed by the clinicians in charge. Notification of the transplant team and continuation of resuscitation allows time to confirm the suitability of the donor, and to negotiate consent from relatives and coroner. Absence of previous liver disease should be confirmed and standard liver function tests shown to be normal.

Other factors are sought which will determine the patient's suitability or otherwise.

a Age is probably of relatively minor importance as a determinant of donor suitability. Atherosclerosis seems certainly no more common in the coeliac artery branches than in other vessels, and may be less so. An upper age limit of 45 years has however been suggested (Starzl & Putnam 1969). Anencephalic neonates have been used as donors for accessory grafts in children with biliary atresia. Orthotopic transplantation of an adult liver into a child with gross size discrepancy is impossible, but the reverse procedure can provide liver grafts with entirely adequate function, providing technical problems of vascular anastomosis can be met.

b Infection is so lethal a complication of organ transplantation that exclusion of transmissible infection in the donor is probably the most important factor other than exclusion of liver disease itself. Patients on respirators with tracheostomies for prolonged periods are particularly prone to bronochopulmonary infection, and isolation of pathogenic organisms from the stoma or bronchial secretions along with chest signs and systemic effects of fever and leucocytosis would be strong indications against the procedure. Positive bacteraemia should be an absolute contraindication.

Urinary tract infection from prolonged bladder drainage is another potential hazard. Intraabdominal infection, actual or potential, from recent surgery will also be a contraindication.

c Malignant neoplasm other than primary intracerebral ones are absolute contraindications to grafting.

d Inadequate perfusion of the liver during a protracted agonal phase may be very difficult to assess. A systolic blood pressure below 90 mmHg at normothermia for more than a few hours is potentially harmful. Some aid may be given by urine output, in that sustained renal function until death may be taken to infer adequate hepatic perfusion along with the kidneys, although this may be a dangerous assumption.

Prolonged and extensive resuscitation requiring cardiac massage and inadequate peripheral perfusion will be clear contraindications, especially as direct hepatic injury can occur from over-vigorous cardiac massage. Prolonged use of vasopressor drugs such as norepinephrine to maintain systolic blood pressure is also potentially deleterious.

Once brain death has been diagnosed, the time until final certification of death by the clinicians-in-charge may be utilized in assessment of the suitability of the patient as a donor, and in prevention of further agonal damage. Some of the potentially valuable measures are systemic hypothermia, which may have been instituted in neurosurgical patients, although it is probable that standard methods of hypothermia have minor effectiveness in prolonging hepatic tolerance to ischaemia. Hypotension is better treated by fluid and electrolyte infusions and by isoproterenol than by vasopressors. Other more specific agents which may prevent hepatic agonal damage are chlorpromazine, phenoxybenzamine and steroids.

Use of brain death as the criterion of donor death, and liver removal with an intact circulation, will make agonal damage least likely. Starzl, who has adopted this course in recent grafts, has stated . . . 'Initially the fear that the quality of terminal care provided for the donor might be thereby lessened caused us to speak out against the pronouncement of death in the presence of a heart beat. Our later experience has convinced us that such anxieties were unfounded'. (Starzl & Putnam 1969.)

In Cambridge, conventional criteria of death have been observed, and the state of British law, and of public and medical opinion, make the use of organs from patients with brain death alone unlikely in the near future.

The care of the patient serving as a donor must obviously rest with his clinician until the moment of death, but it is also apparent that adequate assessment of the suitability of a particular patient as a liver donor must usually involve fore-knowledge by the transplant team for a period of several hours before death. Without understanding and co-operation between members of the medical community, the procurement of suitable organs will therefore not be possible.

REFERENCES

STARZL T.E. & PUTNAM C.W. (1969) In *Experience in Hepatic Transplantation.* Philadelphia: W.B.Saunders.

CHAPTER 22

Anaesthesia for Liver Transplantation

J.V. Farman
S.A. Mason

INTRODUCTION

Although the term 'liver transplantation' suggests a single, uniform procedure it covers two distinct operations. The first is the insertion of an accessory liver, usually in place of the spleen. The second is the total replacement of the patient's liver by one from a recently deceased donor; this operation is fully described in the next section.

ORTHOTOPIC TRANSPLANTATION

Total replacement of the liver poses particular problems for the anaesthetist. This is not simply because it is a long operation, often accompanied by considerable blood loss. Nor is it because the operation must always be arranged at very short notice, because the patient is usually in hospital waiting for the operation, and some hours warning is usually given. An anaesthetic team of considerable skill and experience is needed, firstly, because the operation involves clamping and division of the inferior vena cava and portal vein, severely curtailing the venous return to the heart. Secondly, the insertion of the new liver produces profound metabolic and electrolytic disturbances which are not seen in any other operation. In particular the levels of potassium, hydrogen ions and glucose may become sufficiently abnormal to hazard the life of the patient. Lastly, the anaesthetist must take into account the possibility that the agents and techniques used may themselves damage the new liver.

Many of the complications mentioned above apply equally to the insertion of an accessory liver. In either case the operation is likely to last many hours, while the loss of blood may involve more than total replacement of the blood volume. Although most of the patients are conscious and mobile before operation, many have some disturbance of liver function, sufficient to reduce their ability to break down anaesthetic drugs or, by impairing the clotting mechanism, to increase the danger of surgery. While the importance of these factors should not be minimized, they are not peculiar to liver transplantation. They are discussed later, while the theoretical considerations and anaesthetic management of liver transplantation have been reviewed by Aldrete (1969[1], 1969[2]).

CIRCULATORY EFFECTS OF LIVER REPLACEMENT

The recipient operation begins with the process of 'skeletonizing' the liver. This consists of a careful removal of all ligamentous attachments, division of the common bile duct and exposure of the supra- and infra-hepatic portions of the inferior vena cava, the portal vein and the hepatic artery. In patients with cirrhosis who have portal hypertension this may entail considerable bleeding from engorged anastomotic vessels (Aldrete 1969[1]). These patients are also likely to suffer from abnormalities of the coagulation mechanisms. Patients with hepatic malignancies may also bleed profusely during skeletonization, while the dissection required to eliminate local spread may be quite extensive and time consuming.

As the diseased liver is removed the major vessels are clamped and then divided. This completely obstructs the venous return flow from the mesenteric region and the lower half of the body. Only in some patients with cirrhosis who have well developed anastomoses, is the venous return to the heart likely to be maintained. The normal hepatic blood flow is of the order of 1·2 l./min via the portal vein and 0·3 l./min via the hepatic artery. The flow in the infrahepatic inferior vena cava is normally about 1·5 l./min, making a total of 3 l./min. If the resting cardiac output is 5 l./min, the venous return to the heart will be reduced by more than half when the clamps are applied.

Starling's work (Patterson & Starling 1916) showed the clear cut dependence of cardiac output on venous return flow. The reduction in output caused by inferior vena caval obstruction is normally accompanied by an increase in peripheral resistance and a rise in heart rate, while arterial pressure is maintained at least temporarily (Scott 1968). While deep anaesthesia interferes with these respones, light anaesthesia with nitrous oxide and a relaxant permits them to remain at least in part. The technique of anaesthesia described turns this concept to account in the belief that the best possible distribution of cardiac output is likely to result.

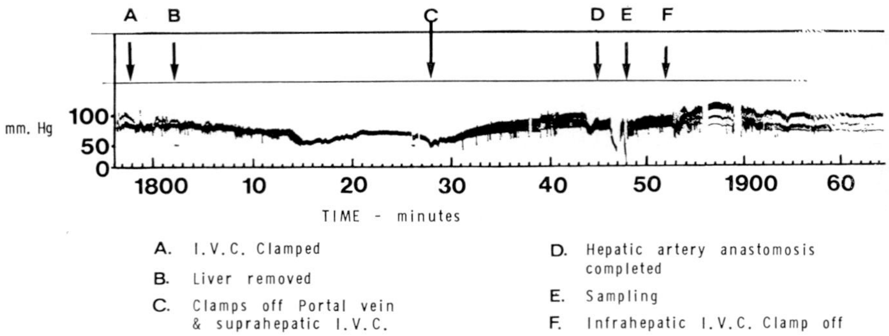

Fig. 1.

Figure 1 shows the effect on the arterial pressure of clamping the vessels supplying the liver in a patient with a cholangio-carcinoma (case 19). At the beginning of the tracing the pressure was 120/75 mmHg, but it fell immediately 100/80 mmHg when the inferior vena cava was clamped. The pulse pressure remained constant at 15–20 mmHg for the next 16 min, but the mean arterial pressure declined steadily during this time to about 90/75 mmHg. At 18·14 there was a further fall to 60/50 mmHg. The speed of transfusion was increased and the patient given 1 g of calcium gluconate and 10 mEq of sodium bicarbonate, after which the pressure rose again. The pulse pressure did not increase again until the clamps were removed from the portal vein and the suprahepatic vena cava. There was an initial further fall followed by a progressive recovery of both mean arterial and pulse pressures over the next 10 min. When the hepatic artery anastomosis was completed and the clamp removed there was a fall in pressure. At 18·53 the infrahepatic caval clamp was removed and the arterial pressure rose at first to 140/90 mmHg but settled within a few minutes to 120/80 mmHg. When the vessels were clamped the heart rate rose at first from 80 to 140 beats/min and the venous pressure fell to −1 cm H_2O. This is shown in Fig. 2, in which the arterial pressure has been replotted to the same time scale. The heart rate later fell and the venous pressure rose to atmospheric.

Although this case is typical, not all patients showed an exactly similar

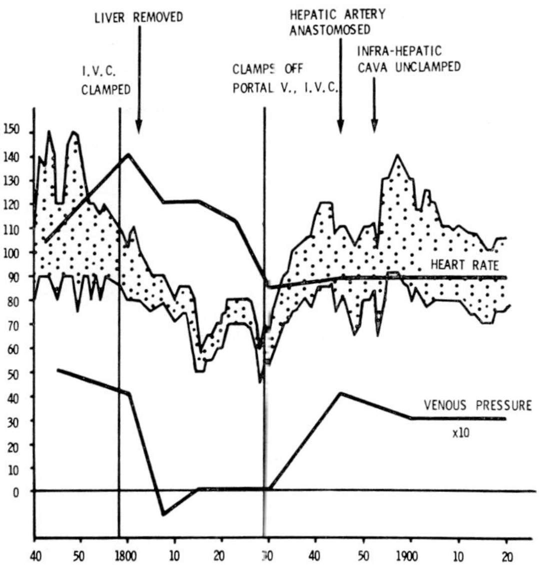

Fig. 2.

pattern. The rises in heart rate and falls in arterial pressure occurred in every case, but venous pressures have been variable, sometimes falling and sometimes remaining elevated. Aldrete *et al* (1969[2]) have made a similar observation. Two possible causes are variation in the position of the tip of the measuring catheter and the effect of artificial respiration. An elevated venous pressure during the anhepatic period will not therefore be a guarantee of an adequate right atrial pressure, but a fall will be a definite indication to increase the speed of transfusion. Observations of arterial pressure made by Aldrete almost exactly match those that we have made. In interpreting them it should be remembered that a fall in cardiac output will be followed by a fall in arterial pressure or an increase in peripheral resistance, or by a combination of the two. Increased resistance does not necessarily depend on sympathetic activity but may be due to elastic closure of arterioles.

The blood loss accompanying the operation is usually heaviest while the diseased liver is being removed. Occasionally it proved impossible to secure all bleeding vessels until after removal. In patients with clotting defects (see Chapter 24) blood loss may be extremely heavy, amounting to 20 l. in one case. Table 1 shows the measured loss in each patient; the mean was 6·5 l. (calculated for all cases). The mean loss in the four small children was 1 l. and was in each case approximately equal to the blood volume

TABLE I

Case	Age years	Weight kg	Diagnosis	Duration h	Measured blood loss ml	Anhepatic time min
1	48	71	Cirrhosis	$5\frac{1}{2}$*	8,500	—
2	47	52	Cholangiocarcinoma	$6\frac{1}{2}$	6,500	50
3	10/12	7·7	Biliary Atresia	$4\frac{3}{4}$	1,036	20
4	41	60	Hepatoma	$8\frac{3}{4}$	14,500	32
5	46	59	Cholangiocarcinoma	$5\frac{1}{2}$	3,960	34
6	57	40	Biliary cirrhosis	$5\frac{1}{2}$	2,900	25
7	43	50	Hepatoma	$6\frac{1}{4}$	17,000	32
8	17	50	Hepatitis	8	9,670	40
9	57	61	Cholangiocarcinoma	6	3,700	37
10	44	38	Hepatoma	$5\frac{1}{2}$	9,000	50
11	2 10/12	18·7	Biliary Atresia	$4\frac{1}{2}$*	1,140	—
12	56	74	Hepatoma, cirrhosis	8	7,000	45
13	37	70	Cholangiocarcinoma	8	12,500	70
14	58	45	Cirrhosis	7 (died)	18,000	28
15	53	44	Cholangiocarcinoma	$7\frac{1}{4}$	2,700	37
16	65	95	Hepatitis	$3\frac{1}{2}$ (died)	7,200	70
17	54	—	Cirrhosis	6	8,355	30
18	2 1/12	9·6	Biliary Atresia	$6\frac{1}{2}$*	1,315	—
19	51	51	Cholangiocarcinoma	$6\frac{1}{2}$	3,000	32
20	46	50	? Hepatitis	6	6,492	50
21	2 10/12	11	Biliary Atresia	4*	940	—
22	31	67	Hepatic tumour	$5\frac{1}{2}$	2,700	40
23	28	63	Hepatoma	6	3,200	35
n	19 adults			23	23 4 children	19
Mean	44			$6\frac{1}{4}$	6500 1108	40

* Heterotopic transplant.

calculated from the body weight. The losses in the adults were on the whole greater than their calculated blood volumes. The amount of blood lost does not appear to be closely related to the diagnosis. In particular, patients with cirrhosis do not always bleed the most.

For transfusion we use the largest possible disposable plastic cannula, preferably the No. 14 Medicut (Argyle). This has a smooth internal shape and laboratory tests show that it is capable of passing more blood than any other type (Farman & Powell 1969). This is linked to a standard blood giving set via a warming coil which lies in a thermostat-controlled warming bath (Grant Instruments Limited). It is essential to warm the blood to body temperature, not only because of the danger of hypothermia developing in the patient, but because refrigerated blood has a viscosity three times greater than that of blood at 37°C. The use of a warming coil will therefore actually increase the maximum rate of flow which can be achieved. With this arrangement 500 ml of blood can be infused in under 5 min without the use of a pump.

METABOLIC EFFECTS OF LIVER REPLACEMENT

Acid-base disturbances

Any operation accompanied by heavy blood loss and rapid transfusion is likely to be accompanied by some degree of metabolic acidosis (Bunker 1966[1]). Although an attempt was made to use as much fresh blood as possible, including blood from the liver donor, the bulk of that used is bank blood stored for varying periods in Acid-Citrate-Dextrose solution. This contains 2 g of dextrose (glucose) and 3 g of monohydric disodium citrate in 120 ml, to which is added 420 ml of blood. The resulting mixture has a pH of 7·1 when first drawn, falling to 6·8 within 24 h (Mollison 1961). By the time it is 3 weeks old the pH has fallen to 6·3 or 6·4 due to release of lactic acid. This represents a base deficit of approximately 500 mEq/l. The initial effect of transfusion is a fall in plasma bicarbonate which buffers the acid. In normal patients the citric and lactic acids are metabolized, forming new bicarbonate and leading to the development of a metabolic alkalosis.

Very rapid transfusion may lower the pH even in normal patients (Bunker 1966) and may be accompanied by citrate intoxication and hyperkalaemia. In patients with impaired liver function the excess citric and lactic acids are metabolized very slowly. During the anhepatic period these dangers are inevitably increased. High levels of citrate in the plasma cause hypotension, low pulse pressure, low cardiac output and ECG changes (Q-T prolongation). These effects are due to a lowering of the serum ionized calcium level and can be reversed by giving calcium. The metabolic effects of blood transfusion, at any rate before the new liver is perfused, are therefore a combination of citrate intoxication, a lowering of pH and sometimes hyperkalaemia.

The fall in cardiac output which accompanies clamping of the inferior vena cava results in reduced tissue perfusion, particularly in the lower half of the body, the venous return from which is blocked. In spite of the sub-basal metabolic rate of anaesthetized patients, this factor alone is likely to cause anaerobic metabolism with production of organic acids which will be distributed throughout the body, causing a generalized metabolic acidosis.

The last and possibly most important factor responsible for the development of a metabolic acidosis concerns the donor liver. The technique and conditions of preservation of the liver are described elsewhere. The perfusate is a poorly buffered approximation to extra-cellular fluid. As the liver is cooled, hydrogen ions, potassium and glucose leak from the cells into the perfusate. Similar changes are to be expected in the portal blood after the portal vein is clamped. In two of our patients (cases 16 and 19) the pH of the effluent coming from the liver at revascularization was 6·85. This is equivalent to a hydrogen ion concentration of 120 nEq/l., three times the normal level. This was associated with P_{CO_2} of 70 mmHg and a base deficit of 25 mEq/l. A normal human liver weighing 1·5–2 kg would be expected to have an extracellular fluid volume of 500–600 ml. Hydrogen ions diffuse freely throughout the extra cellular fluid volume, so it can be assumed that even if the liver shrinks during storage, approximately 10–15 mEq of free acid will be released when it is revascularized. This is enough to produce a base deficit of 2 mEq/l. when distributed through the blood volume. This level will fall as the acid subsequently diffuses from the bloodstream into the whole extracellular fluid space. Experimental work on pig livers performed by Marshall (1970) supports this view and suggests that even after revascularization the liver may continue to release hydrogen ions for some hours. In view of these observations it is advisable to run to waste, via the infra-hepatic vena cava, the first portion of the effluent, up

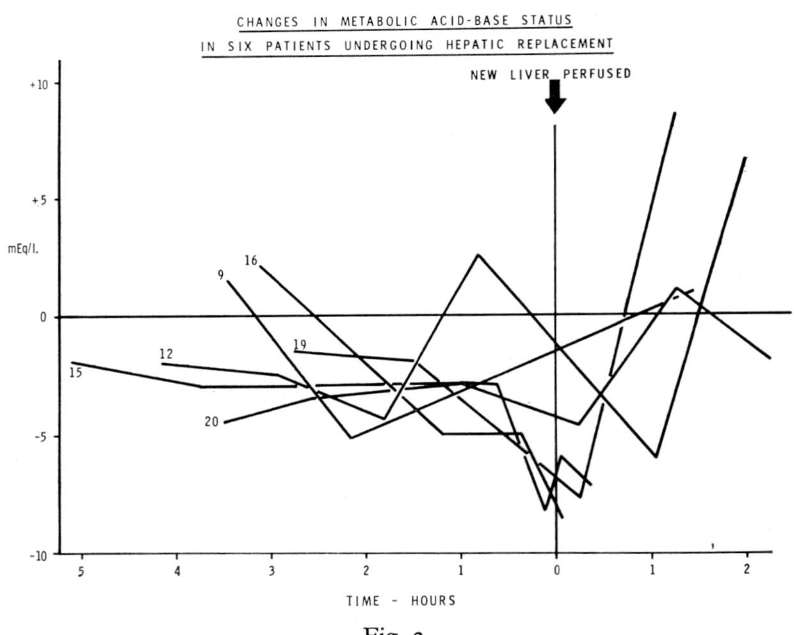

Fig. 3.

to 100 ml containing the highest concentration of hydrogen ions and potassium.

To reverse the metabolic acidosis which develops sodium bicarbonate is used. THAM buffer is contra-indicated as it causes a marked elevation of serum potassium (Moore *et al* 1962) and possible liver damage (Goldenberg *et al* 1968). It is neither possible nor desirable to neutralize each bottle of stored blood. We originally gave a small quantity, 10 mEq of sodium bicarbonate with each unit of blood, to prevent any large or rapid deterioration of acid-base state. Figure 3 shows the base excess/deficit in six patients. There was a general downward trend in all the patients before the liver was removed. (Case 12 showed a base excess of 2·5 mEq/l. after the infusion of 100 mEq of sodium bicarbonate). Samples taken immediately after revascularization of the new liver usually revealed further falls, due to the sudden release of acid mentioned above. Most patients needed further large doses of alkali (ranging from 80 to 200 mEq of $NaHCO_3$) to restore acid-base balance to normal. However this resulted in the development of metabolic alkalosis after revascularization of the new liver, due to breakdown of citrate and lactic acid. In view of this we now give 20 mEq with each unit of blood. This reduces the need for larger doses later in the operation.

Changes in plasma potassium

Not only does the donor liver release hydrogen ions into the perfusate, but potassium leaks out in considerable quantities. Experimental work by Ashby & Lines (1969) showed that when pig livers were perfused continuously, the potassium concentration in the perfusate rose for some hours (e.g. from 5·7 to 10 mEq/l.). In two of our cases (19 and 20) the potassium concentration in the perfusate at the time of revascularization was 17 and 25 mEq/l. respectively. In two cases in which the bulk of the perfusate was allowed to enter the general circulation (cases 5 and 7) gross electrocardiographic abnormalities were seen immediately after the suprahepatic caval clamp was removed. These took the form of prolongation of the Q-T interval and large T waves. This was probably the combined effect of a high serum potassium and a low serum ionized calcium.

Figure 4 shows changes in plasma potassium during four hepatic replacements. In three cases the level rose during the early part of the operation, possibly as a result of blood transfusion (21-day-old stored blood has a potassium concentration of between 15 and 30 mEq/l.). Three samples taken immediately after restoration of the hepatic circulation showed peak concentrations in each case. In one patient (case 16), in whom the concentration was already high, a concentration of nearly 7 mEq/l. was

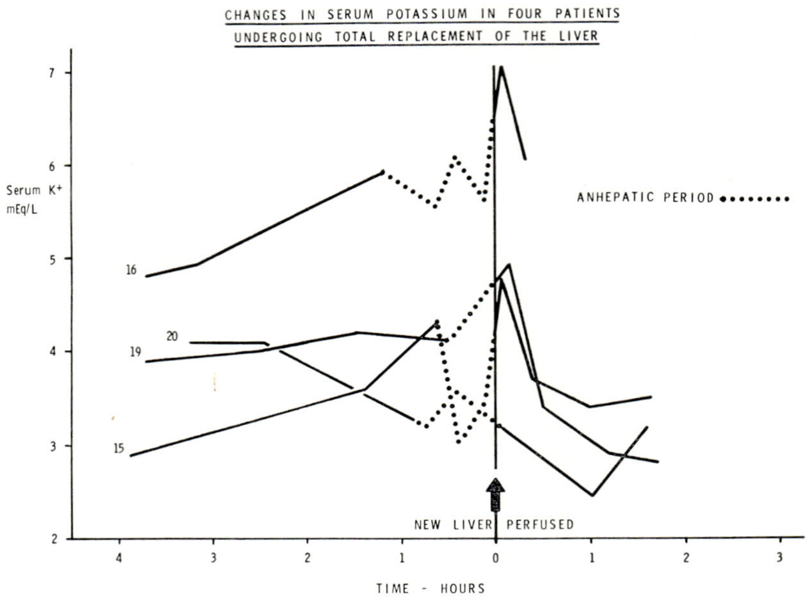

Fig. 4.

measured. This was accompanied by electrocardiographic abnormalities of the type described, followed by ventricular fibrillation. At the same time there was torrential haemorrhage from the supra-hepatic anastomosis which could not be controlled. This patient was given only a small dose (100 mg) of calcium chloride during the anhepatic period. Calcium ions have a protective effect against dysrhythmias resulting from high serum levels of potassium. It is important to give a dose of the order of 1 g of calcium chloride before the circulation is restored to the new liver.

We have found that, particularly in those patients in whom the initial hepatic perfusate was run to waste, the serum potassium level fell rather rapidly as the new liver was perfused. This is presumably because the liver starts to function once again and takes up potassium from the serum. Ashby and Lines and Marshall's observations in pigs support the idea that most of the potassium liberated from the donor liver is reabsorbed once the liver is revascularized. In four patients it was necessary to give supplementary potassium towards the end of the operation. There is no doubt that this is preferable to the risk of precipitating cardiac arrhythmias by flooding the circulation with a large quantity of potassium when the liver is revascularized.

Ashby & Lines also observed that if the serum potassium in pigs receiving liver transplants failed to fall after revascularization, or after some hours again rose, the animal usually died, revealing histological evidence of liver damage. Two patients who died shortly after operation showed high potassium levels. The first (case 17) had a cardiac arrest some hours post-operatively. A child (case 21) who had an accessory transplant showed a progressive rise before dying on the third post-operative day and was found at post-mortem examination to have severe ischaemic damage to the liver. Another child (case 3) died suddenly about 3 hours after the end of the operation. No acid-base or electrolyte estimations had been made. Autopsy shows no obvious cause of death but it is possible that it was due to acidosis and hyperkalaemia.

Blood glucose changes

Liver glycogen is the principle carbohydrate store. It has been thought for many years that hepatectomized animals develop a rapid and fatal hypoglycaemia which can be prevented by the infusion of glucose. It has therefore been assumed (Aldrete 1969) that patients undergoing liver replacement will become hypoglycaemic during the anhepatic period. Aldrete therefore gave his patients 25% glucose solution at 0·5 g/kg/h in order to maintain the serum concentration at between 150 and 350 mg/100 ml. After revascularization of the liver the dose was reduced to 0·2 g/kg/h. Severe hypoglycaemia nevertheless occurred in two patients in the post-operative period with convulsions, unconsciousness, hypotension and respiratory arrest (Aldrete 1969[2]). Treatment with 50% glucose was given successfully. Intravenous glucose infusion was needed for hours or days after operation.

Ashby & Lines' observations on pig liver transplants showed that perfused livers lose glucose. After revascularisation the serum glucose level fell, suggesting either that glucose is reabsorbed by the liver or that the freshly anastomosed liver is unable to secrete enough glucose to maintain a normal level in the recipient.

Blood glucose levels in four patients are shown in Fig. 5. None of them was given large doses of glucose during the early part of the operation. One (case 15) was given 25 g of glucose 80 min after the removal of her liver and 45 min after the new liver was revascularized. Her blood sugar level was already 300 mg/100 ml before the dose was given, but this was not known at the time. All these patients showed a general increase in the blood sugar level during the operation, with little or no fall during the anhepatic period. This finding was unexpected. Determinations of blood glucose in other cases suggest that this pattern is not unusual. All patients were given varying quantities of Acid-Citrate-Dextrose blood, containing

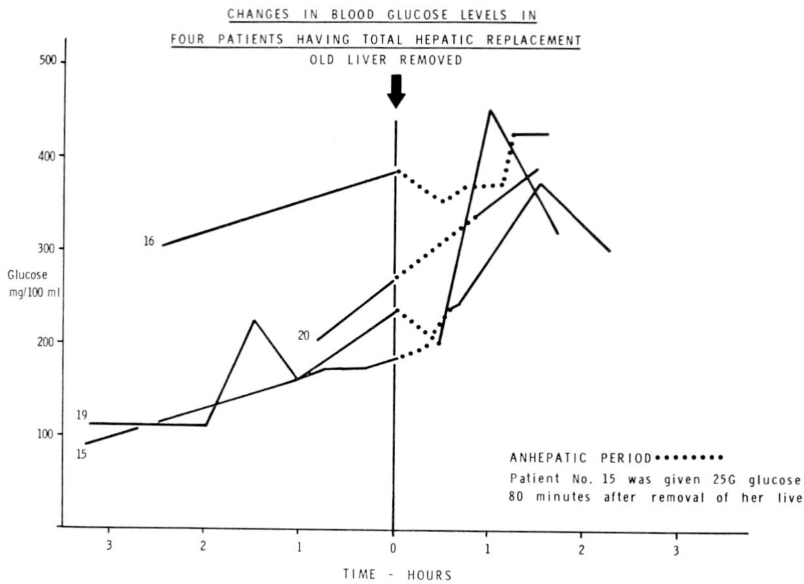

Fig. 5.

3 g glucose/unit, with glucose levels around 500 mg/100 ml. (Measurements of glucose levels in ten bottles of 21-day-old blood showed a mean of 516 mg/100 ml). Some of these patients were given infusions of glucose; case 15 received 100 ml of 4% glucose, case 20 received about 1 l. of 4% glucose via the arterial and central venous pressure catheters and cases 16 and 19 were each given about 250 ml of 4% glucose by the same route. An additional factor is the low metabolic rate in anaesthetized patients. Although this was not measured, Nunn & Matthews (1959) estimated that patients anaesthetized with relaxants have metabolic rates in the region of 80% of basal. The consumption of glucose would therefore be particularly low because of reduced muscle activity. There is no other available source of glucose in the body: muscle glycogen can only be used to satisfy the energetic demands of the muscles themselves.

A logical approach to this problem is to measure the blood glucose level shortly before the liver is removed and to give additional glucose if the level is below about 150 mg/100 ml. Crawley & Seager (1970) recommend the use of 'Dextrostix' reagent strips (Ames Co.) which are sufficiently accurate for clinical purposes although they are unable to discriminate between values in excess of 200 mg/100 ml. In view of Aldrete's experience and evidence from animal work (Ashby & Lines) it would seem that the greatest risk of hypoglycaemia is not during the anhepatic period but post-operatively. Glucose-containing fluid must therefore be infused during this period. The blood glucose level should be estimated at the end of the operation and the estimation repeated frequently during the first 48 h.

Temperature changes

A slowly progressive fall of temperature is commonly seen in long operations but one of the features of hepatic transplantation is that the donor liver is ice-cold at the time of insertion. It is essential that it be kept cold as

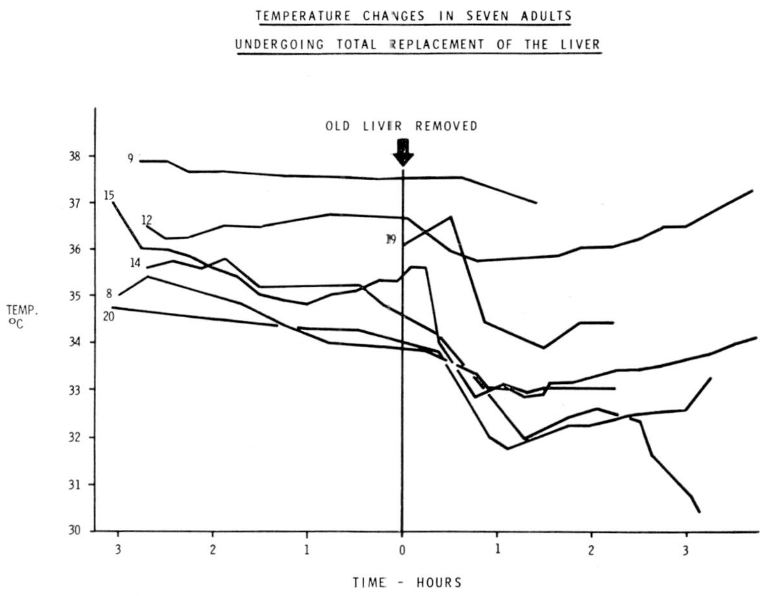

Fig. 6.

long as it is not perfused and that revascularization should precede re-warming. As an adult liver weights 1·5–2·0 kg it will require approximately 35 × 1·5 to 2·0 = 50–70 Kcal to raise its temperature to that of the patient. This heat must come from the recipient's body. In a patient weighing 50 kg this would be expected to lead to an overall fall in temperature of 1–1·5°C. Figure 6 shows temperature changes in seven patients, five of whom showed falls of about 2°C within 30 min. Two patients who had temperatures in the normal range (cases 9 and 12) showed little fall after insertion of the new liver suggesting that they had unusually high rates of metabolism. There was a tendency for the temperature to start to rise again after about

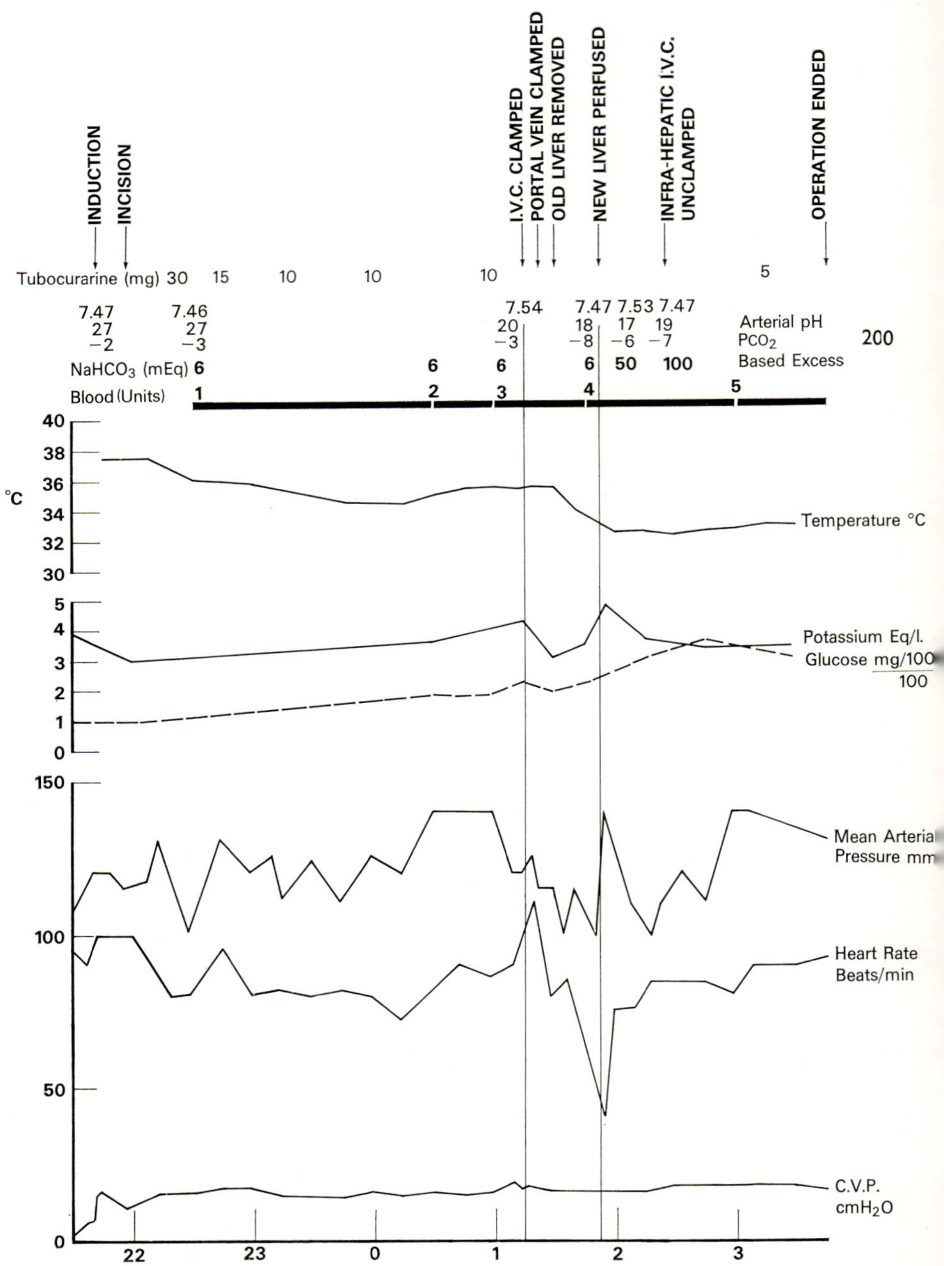
INDUCTION
INCISION
I.V.C. CLAMPED
PORTAL VEIN CLAMPED
OLD LIVER REMOVED
NEW LIVER PERFUSED
INFRA-HEPATIC I.V.C. UNCLAMPED
OPERATION ENDED
Tubocurarine (mg) 30 15 10 10 10 5
7.47 27 −2
7.46 27 −3
7.54 20 −3
7.47 18 −8
7.53 17 −6
7.47 19 −7
Arterial pH
PCO2
Based Excess
200
NaHCO3 (mEq) 6 6 6 6 50 100
Blood (Units) 1 2 3 4 5
°C
Temperature °C
Potassium Eq/l.
Glucose mg/100
100
Mean Arterial Pressure mm
Heart Rate Beats/min
C.V.P. cmH2O
22 23 0 1 2 3

Fig. 7.

1 h. Case 14 was exceptional; this patient bled profusely throughout the operation and the final drop of temperature proved to be terminal.

Although the temperature fall is self-limiting it is undoubtedly an advantage to employ some external means of warming the patient. The four children were placed on a warm water blanket and it proved possible to maintain their temperatures within 1 °C of normal.

Figure 7 shows the record of case 15, a 44-year-old woman. The relationship between the haemodynamic, temperature and biochemical changes and events during the operation is well demonstrated.

ANAESTHETIC TECHNIQUES FOR LIVER TRANSPLANTATION

The choice of drugs

Greene (1968) has discussed in some detail the role the liver plays in the degradation of anaesthetic drugs. Barbiturates and opioids are broken down in whole or in part by liver microsomal enzymes, as is the local anaesthetic lignocaine. Muscle relaxants are on the whole excreted unchanged, although d-tubeocurarine is partially degraded at any unknown site in the body. Suxamethonium is the only common exception, being hydrolyzed rapidly by serum cholinesterase. Although there is now evidence the most inhalational agents undergo biotransformation in the body, the main route of excretion is through the lungs. As these degradations take place mainly in the liver and as they delay rather than accelerate excretion, the effect of poor liver function will be to increase the rate of excretion, rather than the reverse.

Little & Whetstone (1964) have reviewed the effects of anaesthetic agents on the liver. They emphasized that the choice of drugs should not be at the expense of all other considerations. They also said that 'the skill with which the anaesthesia is administered is of considerably more importance than the anaesthetic itself'. In other words, the total effect of an anaesthetic sequence may be apparently unrelated to the known effects of the individual drugs on the liver. The factors important in protecting the liver in the anaesthetized patient are the pre-operative preparation, including restoration of clotting factors and serum protein (important for plasma-bound drugs such as d-tubocurarine), maintenance of adequate oxygen flux (i.e., avoiding hypoxia and hypotension), rapid and accurate replacement of lost blood and meticulous attention to the details of anaesthetic administration. Our experience would suggest that conventional relaxant-nitrous oxide techniques (Gray 1965) are satisfactory, and that the anaesthetist would do best to concentrate on the other points described in this chapter, with which he is probably less familiar. For inhalational supplements the choice of drugs should take into account both direct hepatic toxicity and effects on splanchnic blood flow. The most potent agents generally have the most profound effects on the liver. Although many inhalational anaesthetics are similar to chloroform in their effects, halothane has proved relatively harmless in patients (Bunker *et al* 1966). It has been used almost exclusively for pig liver transplant operations in Cambridge and no evidence of hepatic toxicity has been encountered (Calne, personal communication). Coultas *et al* (1969) published results of isolated dog liver perfusion. They showed that 2% halothane administered for 60 min produced depression of bile secretion and oxygen consumption. 1% methoxyflurane given for 60 min depressed BSP clearance and bile secretion; there was a rise in aspartate amino transferase (GOT) in the perfusate, with loss of potassium and often a loss of glucose, suggesting that this agent is hepatotoxic. Trifluoroethylvinyl ether is considered by Aldrete (1969[1]) to be the least toxic agent. It is not explosive in concentrations below 4% in oxygen. Cyclopropane is generally thought to be free of hepatotoxicity.

There is however, a marked difference between the effect of an agent on isolated liver slices or on an artificially perfused liver and its effect on the liver *in vivo*. This is because of the effects of anaesthetics on splanchnic and particularly hepatic blood flow. Zauder, Baez & Orkin (1964) showed in the dog that light diethyl ether anaesthesia increased hepatic oxygen tension, while trifluoroethylvinyl ether, cyclopropane, chloroform and halothane all reduced it. Only methoxyflurane consistently increased oxygen tension, at all levels of anaesthesia. On the other hand Price *et al* (1966) showed in human volunteers that, although splanchnic blood flow was reduced by cyclopropane and halothane, hepatic oxygen consumption did not suffer, although there was an increase in lactate/pyruvate ratio in hepatic venous blood after cyclopropane anaesthesia. Bunker *et al* (1966[2]) in the National Halothane Study, showed that the use of cyclopropane was followed by an appreciable incidence of jaundice. Splanchnic vasoconstriction is caused by hypoxia, hypercarbia, oligaemia and as a result of giving vasoconstrictor drugs. Induction of hypotension will reduce splanchnic blood flow. No inhalational agent is totally harmless to the liver.

Lastly, there is the occurrence of delayed sensitivity—this has been invoked as the cause of jaundice after halothane anaesthesia. In some patients repeated halothane anaesthetics may sensitise the liver (Klatskin 1968). In this case the first administration will have no untoward effects, but on subsequent occasions the patient may show post-operative fever and even jaundice. This is an extremely rare occurrence. Nevertheless it would seem wise to avoid the use of halothane in liver transplant patients who have received halothane previously, if at all possible.

Of the intravenously injected drugs, normal doses of barbiturates are unlikely to have any effect on the liver. Such doses depend for their duration of action on redistribution into other tissues rather than on metabolic degradation. Provided that repeated doses of such drugs are not used there should be no accumulation even if degradation does not take place.

The use of non-depolarizing relaxants is unlikely to pose a problem. Patients with liver disease may require larger than normal doses of d-tubocurarine. One explanation is that the low serum cholinesterase level reduces the rate of hydrolysis of acetylcholine, so that the patient needs larger doses of the d-tubocurarine in order to produce muscle relaxation (Dundee & Gray 1953). Our experience does not support this view; cases 7 and 13 had pre-operative cholinesterase levels of 16 and 21 units (normal level 65–120 units) but their d-tubocurarine requirements were only 0·24 and 0·25 mg/kg/h respectively (see Table 2). Aladjemoff, Dikstein & Shafir (1958) showed that in patients with high levels of γ-globulin d-tubocurarine is bound by the protein, thus hindering its extravascular diffusion and its access to the motor endplates. Baraka & Gabali (1968) have confirmed the correlation between γ-globulin levels and tubocurarine requirement in clinical practice. Our patients characteristically had normal or raised total serum protein levels with high globulin levels and reversal of the albumen : globulin ratio. Levels are given in Table 2. The doses of d-tubocurarine in 14 of the cases varied from 0·09 to 0·5 mg/kg/h. Adjuvant drugs were used in three of the children and one adult (phenoperidine, halothane, methoxyflurane) but did not appear to reduce relaxant requirements. Aldrete (1969) regarded gallamine, because of its renal excretion, as the agent of choice. On the other hand Kennedy & Farman (1968) showed that this drug increases cardiac output and is associated with heavier blood losses than with d-tubocurarine (Casale & Farman 1970). We have used this drug on two occasions (cases 1 and 11), but neither patient had an unusually great operative blood loss. Pancuronium does not appear to be affected by the level of hepatic function and is perhaps to be regarded as the agent of choice, on account of its lack of hypotensive effect.

The action of suxamethonium is likely to be prolonged in the presence of a low serum cholinesterase. Pre-operative enzyme levels in patients are given in Table 2; the mean pre-operative level in 11 cases was 41 units (normal 65–120 Warburg units). Suxamethonium (mean dose 70 mg) was given in nine patients, but prolonged apnoea was not encountered, even in those patients whose levels were low (cases 15 and 19).

TABLE 2

Case	Induction	Total relaxant dose	Relaxant mg/kg/h	Serum Globulin	Serum Total protein	Cholinesterase (normal 65-120 units)
1	—	Gallamine 240 mg	0·62	Raised	4·7	—
2	N_2O, Cyclopropane	Dtc. 75 mg	0·22	Raised	7·4	34 units (post-op)
3	N_2O, Cyclopropane	Dtc. 16·5 mg	0·43	—	—	—
4	N_2O, Cyclopropane Suxameth. 50 mg	Dtc. 210 mg	0·40	4·5	8·6	—
5	Methohexitone 50 mg Suxameth. 100 mg	Dtc. 130 mg	0·39	5·0	7·9	—
6	Methohexitone 100 mg	Dtc. 110 mg	0·5	5·6	8·6	—
7	Thiop. 175 mg	Dtc. 75 mg	0·24	Raised	7·2	16 units
8	Methohexitone 15 mg Suxameth. 50 mg	Dtc. 45 mg	0·14	4·5	6·8	—
9	Methohexitone 100 mg Suxameth. 100 mg	Dtc. 105 mg	0·29	3·8	6·2	—
10	Thiop. 200 mg	Dtc. 95 mg	0·45	—	7·0	—
11	N_2O, Halothane	Gallamine 60 mg	0·07	Raised	5·3	24 units

12	Thiop. 300 mg Suxameth. 100 mg	Dtc. 180 mg	0·3	2·8	6·5	—
13	N_2O, Dtc. 45 mg	Dtc. 120 mg	0·25	3·2	6·0	21 units
14	Thiop. 250 mg Pancuronium 8 mg	Pancuronium 10 mg	0·031	3·9	6·2	—
15	Thiop. 200 mg Suxameth. 50 mg	Dtc. 80 mg	0·25	—	—	49 units
16	Thiop. 100 mg Dtc. 30 mg	Dtc. 30 mg	0·09	Raised	5·0	28 units
17	Thiop. 150 mg	Dtc. 190 mg	—	3·8	7·1	—
18	N_2O, Halothane	Pancuronium 5·5 mg	0·087	Normal	6·9	25 units (post-op)
19	Thiop. 250 mg Suxameth 30 mg	Pancuronium 6 mg	0·018	—	—	42 units
20	N_2O, Halothane Pancuronium 8 mg	Pancuronium 16 mg	0·053	2·4	5·0	—
21	N_2O, Halothane	Dtc. 19 mg	0·43	—	—	47 units
22	Thiop. 400 mg Suxameth. 100 mg	Pancuronium 16 mg	0·044	Low	7·3	70 units
23	Thiop. 350 mg Suxameth. 50 mg	Pancuronium 20 mg	0·053	Raised	8·1	94 units

The production of cholinesterase by the normal liver is enough to raise the level by about 10 Warburg units/day (Lehmann, personal communication). The level of this enzyme is a very sensitive indication of hepatic function. A patient who is totally depleted of this enzyme by an organo-phosporus anti-cholinesterase will take approximately 2 weeks to regain the normal level once the drug has been stopped. Changes in the cholinesterase level during operation, as reported by Aldrete (1969) are therefore due entirely to enzyme present in transfused blood, rather than to production of new enzyme by the donor liver. We have observed that the cholinesterase level may reach a peak immediately after operation for this reason.

Monitoring

A cannula (usually No. 15 Jelco) is inserted under local anaesthesia into one radial artery. This has a three-way tap for sampling and is flushed with 4% glucose in 0·18% saline containing 10,000 units of heparin/l. All blood samples are drawn from this tap other than those taken for estimating clotting factors (which are taken from the SVC catheter). We have used either a dial-type pressure gauge (Tycos) or a pressure transducer (Consolidated Electrodynamics) and pen recorder (Devices M.2). In addition a cuff and clinical stethescope (Diasyst) are placed on one arm. In children a cuff and oscillometer are used.

A large venous catheter (No. 16 E-Z Cath) is inserted under local anaesthesia into the median cubital (24 in) or external jugular (12 in) vein and advance until its tip is in a central vein. This is connected to a proprietary venous pressure set, using 4% glucose in 0·18% saline. The tip position is checked by observing oscillations in the fluid column in time with the heart beat and respiration.

The electrocardiograph is taken from standard limb or precordial leads and displayed on an oscillascope or the pen recorder. A probe is inserted via one nostril into the pharynx for measurement of temperature. A urinary catheter is inserted and connected to a graduated collection bag.

Blood loss is measured by swab weighing, assuming that all swabs used are dry and of standard weight, and by measurement of suction bottle contents.

Samples should be taken hourly in adult patients for estimation of acid-base state (pH, $P\text{CO}_2$ Standard Bicarbonate and Base Excess), $P\text{O}_2$ and potassium, sodium and glucose levels. Dextrostix estimations of glucose level should also be done immediately before and during the anhepatic phase. Samples should be taken for acid-base and electrolyte estimations within 5 min after revascularization of the donor liver and hourly thereafter.

Anaesthesia in adult patients

In order to reduce the total time spent under general anaesthesia it is worth inserting the venous and arterial cannulae under local anaesthesia. The ECG electrode plates are also applied. This is normally done while the donor liver is being removed. It is advisable to offer the patient some sedation during this period and we have used diazepam, either by mouth (20 mg 2 hours beforehand) or intramuscularly (10 mg 1 hour beforehand) when time has allowed. Atropine may either be given by intramuscular injection at the same time, or intravenously at the time of induction. If it appears that the donor liver is likely to be removed earlier than expected, general anaesthesia is induced and the patient intubated. This enables the vascular cannulae to be inserted very rapidly.

The actual method of induction will vary according to the practice of the individual. We have used thiopentone in eight patients, methohexitone in four and inhalational agents (nitrous oxide, with or without cyclopropane or halothane) in the remainder. Endotracheal intubation is then performed, usually with the aid of a relaxant: suxamethonium (nine cases), pancuronium (two cases) or d-tubocurarine and topical lignocaine. Some patients were allowed to breathe spontaneously while drips were set up, while others were immediately given a long-acting muscle relaxant.

Artificial ventilation was performed in all cases, using a nitrous oxide-oxygen mixture. It is our practice to moderately hyperventilate these patients, both to ensure adequate oxygenation and in order to maintain a normal pH in the presence of a base deficit. The P_{CO_2} was maintained between 20 and 35 mmHg. Very low levels which may cause splanchnic vasoconstriction are avoided. Reversal at the end was usually with atropine and neostigmine. The patient who had received 4 mg phenoperidine during the course of the operation could not be de-curarized even though given 5 mg neostigmine and had to be ventilated for 10 h. Two patients (cases 8 and 9) needed no neostigmine but all the others were given neostigmine without waiting to see if they would breathe spontaneously. Case 13 was ventilated for 1 h after the end of the operation before spontaneous respiration was established. Case 7 suffered heavy and prolonged postoperative blood loss accompanied by metabolic acidosis: he was ventilated artificially after the operation until his death 27 h later. In neither of these cases was their inability to breathe spontaneously thought to be due to failure to reverse the relaxants.

Anaesthesia in children

Children present difficulties because of their small size and poor temperature-regulating ability while under anaesthesia. Monitoring of pressures may be difficult and it is usually necessary to cut down on to a vein in order to introduce a central venous catheter. We have not attempted to introduce arterial cannulae in these patients. Blood samples may be difficult to obtain and the volume removed may become quite large by the end of the operation. The volume of all samples should be recorded. The electrocardiogram is taken from adhesive chest electrodes which can also be used for impedance spirometry (Farman & Juett 1967). Access to the patient may be limited and an illuminated screen to fit on the operating table over the child's head is desirable. The child is always placed on a temperature control blanket.

We have used only inhalational anaesthetic agents in children. Induction is with nitrous oxide and cyclopropane or halothane, followed by endotracheal intubation. Anaesthesia is maintained with nitrous oxide and usually an inhalational agent (halothane or methoxyflurane) to permit the use of 50% oxygen without fear of the patient waking. Relaxants were used in all four children; d-tubocurarine in two (cases 3 and 21), gallamine in case 11 and pancuronium in case 18. The doses of curare and gallamine were within the expected range, but case 18, who also received methoxyflurane, required a very large amount of pancuronium (0·087 mg/kg/h).

Very strict attention must be paid to the replacement of lost blood. It is only too easy to go wrong when counting a large number of burette readings on a paediatric giving set. All relevant factors (measured loss, arterial pressure and venous pressure) should be taken into account when replacing lost blood. Serial determinations of haematocrit can prove invaluable under these conditions (Aldrete 1969).

OTHER TREATMENT DURING OPERATION

Mannitol 20 g (as 10% or 20%) solution is given early in the operation in order to promote diuresis and in an attempt to reduce ischaemic damage in the donor liver by virtue of its osmotic effect. All patients were given hydrocortisone hemisuccinate 200 mg at the time of revascularization of the donor liver, but other immunosuppressives were withheld until the post-operative period. Antibiotics were given intravenously during operation to protect the donor liver from infection.

POST-OPERATIVE CARE

Special attention should be paid to the patient in the early post-operative period. The arterial and venous catheters are left in place for 24–48 h both for pressure measurements and for taking samples. The patient should be nursed in an intensive care unit where a nurse and a doctor should remain in constant attendance. If possible it is preferable to continue automatic arterial pressure measurement than to disturb the patient by repeatedly inflating an arm cuff. Further loss of blood from the wound should be watched for and replaced.

The rate and volume of respiration should be recorded. Equipment for artificial respiration (including laryngoscope, tubes and self-inflating bag) should remain by the bedside until the patient has fully recovered. Four of our patients required artificial respiration either because of difficulty in establishing normal respiration at the end of the anaesthetic (cases 4, 7 and 13) or because they become apnoeic (case 20). Two of the children who had heterotopic transplants developed severe post-operative chest infections (cases 11 and 18). Estimation of the blood glucose level should be performed 2-hourly, using Dextrostix, for the first 8 h and extra glucose given if the level falls below 150 mg/100 ml. Serum potassium should be estimated at similar intervals and extra potassium given, as potassium chloride, if the level falls below 4 mEq/l. Hourly temperature measurements should be made and the patient warmed if necessary.

ACKNOWLEDGEMENTS

We would like to acknowledge the valuable help and advice we have received from Professor H.Lehmand, Dr M.P.Walsh and Dr J.G.Lines of the John Bonnett Clinical Laboratories, University of Cambridge; from Mr B.S.Ashby and Mr V.C.Marshall, working in the Department of Surgery, University of Cambridge and from the many anaethetists who have contributed to the care of these patients, particularly Dr J.R.Samuel.

REFERENCES

ALDRETE A.J. (1969)[1] *Anaesthesia and Intra-operative Care*. In *Experience in Liver Transplantation*, ed. STARZL T.E. Philadelphia: Saunders.

ALDRETE A.J., LE VINE D.S. & GINGRICH T.F. (1969)[2] Experience in anaesthesia for liver transplantation. *Anesth. Analg. Curr. Res.* **48,** 802.

ALADJEMOFF L., DIKSTEIN– SHAFRIR E. (1958) Binding of tubocurarine chloride to plasma proteins. *J. Pharmacol. Exper. Therap.* **123,** 43.

ASHBY B.S. & LINES J.G. (1969) Unpublished observations.

BARAKA A. & GABALI F. (1968) Correlation between tubocurarine requirements and plasma protein pattern. *Br. J. Anaeth.* **40,** 89.

BUNKER J.P. (1966)[1] Metabolic effects of blood transfusion. *Anesthesiol.* **27**, 446.

BUNKER J.P. (1966)[2] Chairman, *Et alii*. Summary of the National Halothane Study. *J. Amer. Med. Assoc.* **197**, 775.

CASALE F.F. & FARMAN J.V. (1970) Blood loss during Hysterectomy associated with the use of tubocurarine or gallamine. *Br. J. Anaesth.* **42**, 65.

COULTAS R.J., STRUNIN L., WALKER W.D., STRUNIN J.M., REYNARD A. & SIMPSON B.R. (1969) A comparison of the effects of Halothane and Methoxyflurane on the isolated perfused canine liver. *Br. J. Anaesth.* **41**, 790.

CRAWLEY B.E. & SEAGER R. (1970) Monitoring the blood sugar during surgery. *Anaesthesia* **25**, 73.

DUNDEE J.W. & GRAY T.C. (1953) Resistance to d-tubocurarine chloride in the presence of liver damage. *Lancet*, ii, 16.

FARMAN J.V. & JUETT D.A. (1967) Impedance spirometry in clinical monitoring. *Br. Med. J.* iv, 27.

FARMAN J.V. & POWELL D. (1969) Performance of disposable venous catheters, needles and cannulae. *Br. J. Hosp. Med. Equipment Supplement* 37.

GOLDENBERG V.E., WIEGENSTEIN L. & HOPKINS G.B. (1968) Hepatic injury associated with Tromethamine. *J. Amer. Med. Assoc.* **205**, 81.

GRAY T.C. (1965) Relaxants Used in Anaesthesia. In *General Anaesthesia*, 2, eds. EVANS F.T. & GRAY T.C., p. 149. London: Butterworths.

GREENE N.M. (1968) The metabolism of drugs employed in Anaesthesia. *Anesthesiology*, **29**, 127.

KENNEDY B.R. & FARMAN J.V. (1968) Cardiovascular effects of gallamine triethiodine in man. *Br. J. Anaesth.* **40**, 773.

KLATSKIN G. (1968) Mechanisms of Toxic and Drug Induced Hepatic Injury. In *Toxicity of Anaesthetics*, ed. FINK B.R. Baltimore: Williams & Wilkins.

LITTLE D.M. & WHETSTONE H.J. (1964) Anaesthesia and the liver. *Anaesthesiol.* **25**, 815.

MARSHALL V.C. (1970) Unpublished observations.

MOLLISON P.L. (1961) *Blood Transfusion in Clinical Medicine*. Oxford and Edinburgh: Blackwell.

MOORE D., BERNHARD W. & KEVY S. (1962) The efficacy of 2-amino-2-hydroxymethyl-1, 3-propanediol in the restoration of heparinized blood. *Clin. Res.* **10**, 203.

NUNN J.F. & MATTHEWS R.L. (1959) Gaseous exchange during halothane anaesthesia. *Br. J. Anaesth.* **31**, 330.

PATTERSON S.W. & STARLING E.H. (1914) On the mechanical factors which determine the output of the ventricles. *J. Physiol.* **48**, 357.

PRICE H.L., DEUTSCH S., DAVIDSON I.A., CLEMENT A.J., BEHAR M.G. & EPSTEIN R.M. (1966) Can general anaesthetics produce splanchnic visceral hypoxia by reducing regional blood flow? *Anaesthesiol.* **27**, 24.

SCOTT D.B. (1968) Inferior vena caval occlusion in late pregnancy and its importance in anaesthesia. *Br. J. Anaesth.* **40**, 120.

ZAUDER H.L., BAEZ S., ORKIN L.R. (1964) Tissue Perfusion During Anaesthesia. In *Anesthesia and the Circulation*, ed. FABIAN L.W. Oxford and Edinburgh: Blackwell.

CHAPTER 23

The Technique of Liver Transplantation

R.Y. Calne

The liver may be transplanted to the normal position after hepatectomy (orthotopic) or an additional liver may be inserted leaving the patient's own liver intact (accessory, auxiliary, or heterotopic). For malignant disease of the liver preliminary hepatectomy is obviously essential, but even for non malignant parenchymatous liver disease, the advantages of the orthotopic position are considerable. There is room to accommodate the transplant, which can be supported by anastomosis of the suprahepatic inferior vena cava to that of the recipient. The stitches include adventitia, which in this situation merges with the diaphragm and is relatively tough. The other anastomoses lie in correct relationship to each other. The advantages of an accessory liver are that preliminary hepatectomy, which may be a difficult operation, is omitted and any residual function of the patient's own liver may help tide him through the operation and immediately afterwards if the grafted liver does not function well. There are, however, serious disadvantages. The extra liver may not be easily accommodated within the abdomen and siting of the anastomoses to achieve satisfactory inflow of portal and systemic arterial blood to the liver, free drainage of venous blood from the liver, and biliary drainage may be difficult. Even if the anastomoses are satisfactory at the time of surgery they can become compromized when the patient regains an upright posture. We have performed four heterotopic liver transplants inserting the new liver in the splenic site. Although function was demonstrated in a neonatal liver transplanted into a child with biliary atresia using this technique, the operation is considered to be unsatisfactory and the technique will not be described here.

ORTHOTOPIC LIVER TRANSPLANTATION

This operation is complicated and time-consuming. At certain stages careful co-ordination is required so as not to subject the liver to excessive ischarmic damage. After removal of the recipient's own liver the surgeon has reached a point of no return and this adds to the tension of the operation. Although there can be difficulties with some of the technical procedures, the most important objective is to avoid any error in each individual manoeuvre, since the margin between technical disaster and a good functioning transplant is extremely narrow.

The operation can be considered to be in three parts—(1) donor hepatectomy, (2) recipient hepatectomy, (3) insertion of the graft (Calne 1969).

Donor hepatectomy

A liver for transplantation should be the same size or smaller than that of the recipient, but never larger, since a liver that is too large cannot be accommodated satisfactorily even in the orthotopic position. The liver is very sensitive to ischaemic damage and if left in a corpse without perfusion for more than 15 min at 37°C irreversible autolysis occurs and attempts to transplant such a liver will result in disaster. The procedure of liver transplantation is complicated and requires a large number of medical and nursing personnel continuously on call. Since time is required to prepare for surgery, some form of warning is necessary. It is obvious that the best chances of success are in cases where resuscitation has been attempted and where, for decisions unconcerned with the desirability of transplantation, it has been decided to terminate resuscitation. It is then possible to give the transplant team sufficient notice. Cold perfusion of the corpse with a heart-lung machine has been used to gain time by Marchioro *et al* (1963), but we have no experience of this technique in man.

Immediately after death of the donor has been confirmed by doctors independent of the transplant team, the abdomen is opened by a bilateral subcostal incision, a Bardic cannula is inserted into the superior mesenteric vein and heparinized Hartmann's solution (Heparin 2000 i.u./l.) at 4°C is infused under gravity from a drip stand into the portal vein (Fig. 1). The inferior vena cava is cannulated below the renal veins and blood is collected from the donor to prevent a rise in venous pressure. The blood can be used for transfusion into the recipient if the ABO groups are the same. Although the liver from a Group O donor can be used for any recipient, the Group O serum may haemolyse red cells of another group. Additional cannulation and cold perfusion of the abdominal aorta has been used in some cases.

Once the liver has started to cool it is removed as quickly as possible, the structures in the free border of the lesser omentum are separated from each other, and the common bile-duct is divided just above the duodenum, after careful identification and preservation of the junction of the cystic

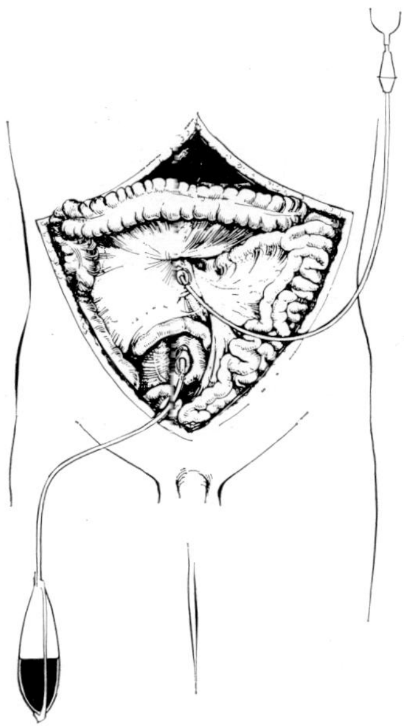

FIG. 1. Cooling of donor liver via superior mesenterid vein. Drainage of blood and perfusate from the inferior vena cava below the renal veins.

(By courtesy of the *British Journal of Surgery*.)

to the common duct. The cystic duct may descend behind the common duct and pass to below the first part of the duodenum before it joins the common duct at the sphincter of Oddi. It is extremely important to determine if this anomaly is present otherwise subsequent biliary drainage may be impossible. (Starzl 1969). The portal vein and hepatic artery are individually controlled with slings and a search is made for an additional hepatic artery, which usually passes behind the portal vein and arises from the superior mesenteric, an anomaly that occurs in approximately 15% of people. Ligation and division of the gastroduodenal artery help in this dissection. The right adrenal vein is ligated and divided and a sling is passed around the infrahepatic inferior vena cava (IVC). The peritoneal attachments of the liver to the diaphragm are divided, the diaphragm is incised and the suprahepatic IVC is divided in the chest close to the right atrium. The incision in the diaphragm is continued around the IVC to leave a short cuff of the diaphragmatic tendon. The right, left and posterior phrenic veins are individually ligated and divided. This is a very important step since failure to secure the veins will result in serious haemorrhage and the danger of air embolism after transplantation. The remaining connective tissue attachments of the liver are divided and attention is now directed to the most difficult part of the dissection, namely the hepatic artery. The spleen is mobilized and is gently pulled towards the right of the abdomen. bringing with it the tail of the pancreas and body of the stomach. The abdominal aorta is now identified and followed from the level of the renal arteries up to the diaphragm. The origins of the coeliac and superior mesenteric arteries are now defined. Since the arteries are not pulsating and are pale and collapsed, the dissection may be time-consuming. This was clearly recognized by the anatomist, Charles Bell, who in 1798 wrote: 'In dissecting the root of the coeliac artery and the aorta, betwixt it and the superior mesenteric artery much confusion arises, from the meshes of the semilunar ganglion'.

I have found it helpful to control the hepatic artery near the liver with a rubber sling and then to apply gentle traction to the spleen, follow the splenic artery to where it joins the coeliac, and then to secure the left gastric artery and splenic artery which are ligated and divided. If an hepatic artery arises from the superior mesenteric vessel the origin of the superior mesenteric artery is preserved, together with the coeliac, and both are removed in one large Carrel patch of aorta. If the entire hepatic arterial supply comes from the coeliac artery, this alone is included in a Carrel patch of aorta.

The liver is now ready to be removed for the body; the dissection usually takes between 50 and 60 min. The Hartmann's infusion solution is now changed to a plasma/bicarbonate/dextrose solution (preservation fluid containing 400 ml reconsituted human plasma, 10 ml 2% procaine, 80 ml 5% glucose, and 20 ml 1·4% sodium bicarbonate (Schalm 1969). Between 200 and 300 ml of this solution are infused and the cannula is then removed from the portal vein.

Similar perfusion of the coeliac artery with Hartmann's solution followed by plasma/bicarbonate/dextrose solution is then performed, approximately 100 cc of each solution is used. The liver is then removed and placed in a sterile plastic bag containing cold saline; this is inserted into another similar bag which is then surrounded by an ice-and-water mixture.

Recipient hepatectomy

The coagulation profile should be determined on the patient before surgery; if clotting defects are present fresh frozen plasma is given. Blood-loss during surgery may be considerable and it is not likely to cease until good liver function has been re-established in the patient. If there is a shortage of blood I think it is best to use ordinary stored blood during the operation and, if possible, fresh blood at the end of the operation. Two intravenous infusions are inserted into veins draining into the superior vena cava and the central venous pressure is monitored by one of these. A bilateral subcostal incision is made under light anaesthesia (Fig. 2). If the liver is

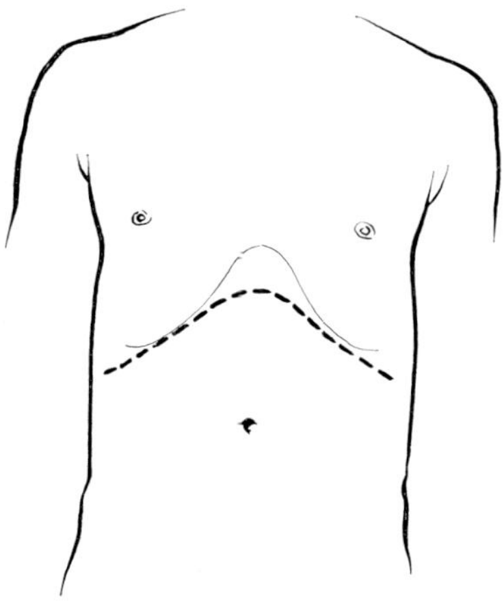

FIG. 2. Bilateral subcostal incision for both donor and recipient operations.
(By courtesy of the *British Journal of Surgery*.)

shrunk and cirrhotic, hepatectomy may be straightforward. A large liver, particularly if involved with adhesions from previous surgery, may be difficult to remove. Portal hypertension results in oedema of the tissues around the liver and excessive vascularity; these will slow the dissection. It is very important to secure and ligate all bleeding points, however small. The structures in the free edge of the lesser omentum are separated from each other and controlled with slings. A sling is passed around the infrahepatic IVC and the peritoneal attachments of the liver are divided. The chest is not opened. Freed from the parieties, the liver can be dislocated anteriorly, putting the right adrenal vein on stretch so that it can be ligated and divided. A sling is passed around the suprahepatic IVC below the diaphragm. At the completion of this stage of the operation the liver is attached only by its vascular connections and common bile-duct. The

TABLE I

Procedure A			Procedure B		
Donor	Min	Recipient	Donor	Min	Recipient
	0	Induction of anaesthesia	Resuscitation abandoned	0	Induction of anaesthesia
			Heart stopped	30	
			Cooling commences	40	
	60	Anaesthesia completed Surgery begins	Liver satisfactory	60	Anaesthesia completed Surgery begins
			Hepactectomy completed	90	
Resuscitation abandoned	160	Liver skeletonized	Liver out of ice	160	Recipient Hepatectomy completed
Heart stopped	190			190	Liver perfused with portal blood
Cooling commenced	205				
Hepatectomy completed	250				
	280	Liver perfused with portal blood			
Advantages	1	Minimal cold ischaemia time	Advantages	1	Operation not begun on recipient until it is known that the donor liver is satisfactory
	2	Hepatectomy not rushed		2	Less haemorrhage at critical period of surgery
				3	90 min shorter total operative time
Disadvantages	1	Operation begins on recipient before it is known that the donor organ is satisfactory	Disadvantages	1	70 min longer cold ischaemia time
	2	90 min in which the recipient may bleed and become shocked		2	Recipient hepatectomy must not be delayed

skeletonizing of the liver may well take up to 2 h. If the recipient operation is begun immediately after the death of the donor, a simple method of preservation by cold infusion will protect the donor liver from serious ischaemic damage for 3–4 h. The period of cold ischaemia can be shortened by continuing resuscitation of the donor until the recipient liver has been skeletonized. The exact timing of the recipient operation in relation to the death of the donor has varied in our experience. Table 1 shows the pros and cons of two approaches we have used. If skeletonization of the recipient's liver is completed before resuscitation on the donor is stopped the transplant has a minimal cold ischaemia time and hepatectomy on the recipient is not rushed. However the operation commences on the recipient before it is known that the donor organ is satisfactory and the recipient is anaesthetized for an extra 90 min during which period considerable bleeding may occur leading to shock. If the operation is not begun on the recipient until it is known that the donor liver is satisfactory there is less haemorrhage at the critical period of surgery before the new liver is inserted and the operation is 90 min shorter. However there may be up to 70 min longer cold ischaemia time for the graft and the recipient hepatectomy has to be performed quickly. We have decided to compromise and to start anaesthetizing the recipient and set up the various observational monitors and then at this point resuscitation of the donor ceases. The circulation in the donor may cease immediately or continue for 30 min or more. During this period of waiting the recipient is towelled up and the instrucments prepared. Immediately the circulation ceases the operation on the donor begins and as soon as it is apparent that the liver is anatomically normal the operation on the recipient begins. In Starzl's Unit, *coma depassé* or brain death is accepted as a diagnosis of death as far as the donor is concerned, and the liver is removed with the heart still beating and the circulation intact. This has obvious advantages as far as ischaemic damage to the donor liver is concerned, since skeletonization of the graft can be completed with an intact circulation (Starzl 1969). The ethical aspects of this procedure I have discussed in Chapter 10 but it should be pointed out that despite the disadvantages, utilizing traditional criteria of death, it is possible to get excellent initial function from a transplanted liver.

When it is known that the donor liver is satisfactory on anatomical grounds and has been preserved and cooled correctly, the recipient's liver is removed. The common bile-duct is divided above the duodenum, the hepartic artery is clamped with two bulldog clips and divided distal to the clips. The portal vein is similarly clamped and the infrahepatic IVC is occluded with a Crafford clamp; a Brock's atrial calmp is used to occlude the suprahepatic IVC. Occlusion of the portal vein and inferior vena cava will result in congestion of the intestinal tract and diminished venous return

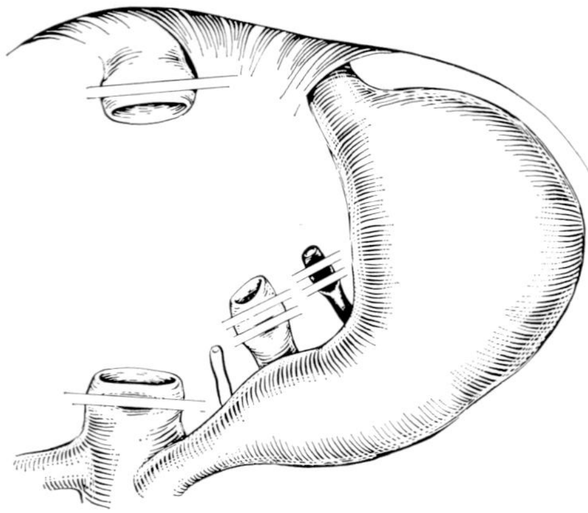

FIG. 3. Removal of liver from recipient with a section of vena cava. The portal vein and hepatic artery are clamped. The common duct is left open.

(By courtesy of the *British Journal of Surgery*.)

to the heart. A transient fall in blood-pressure commonly occurs and it may be necessary to infuse blood rather quickly into the superior caval system. The liver is usually removed with a portion of vena cava from the hepatic veins to the right adrenal vein (Fig. 3). On two occasions a child's liver was grafted into an adult, the ages of the children being $4\frac{1}{2}$ and 5 years respectively. In these cases the child's vena cava was considered to be too small for anastomosis to the recipient's IVC and therefore the liver was filleted

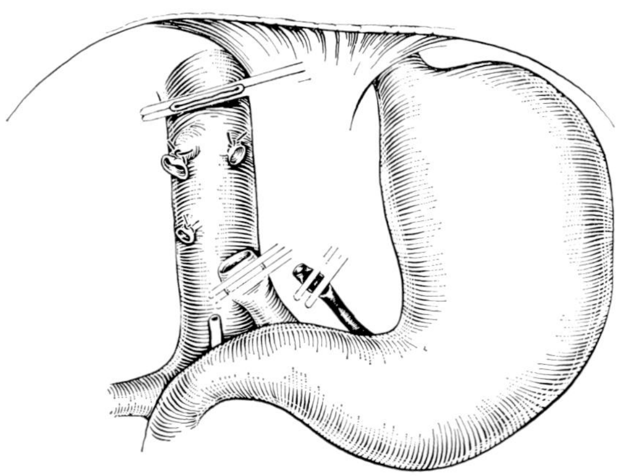

FIG. 4. Removal of recipient liver leaving vena cava intact. Accessory hepatic veins are ligated. Main hepatic vein is clamped.

(By courtesy of the *British Journal of Surgery*.)

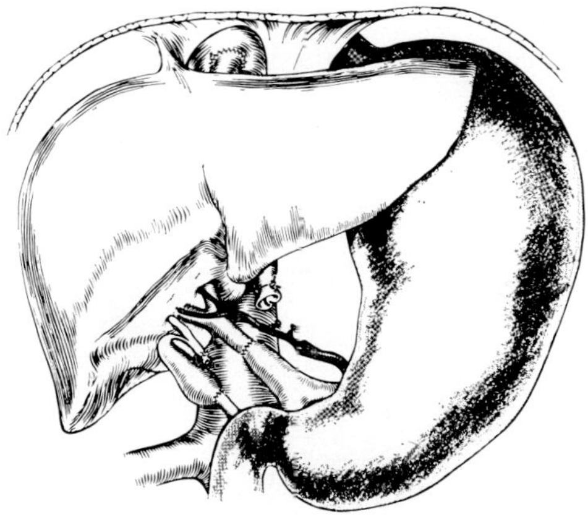

FIG. 5. Transplantation of liver from small donor into large recipient. The vena cava below the liver is ligated and that above the liver is anastomozed to the hepatic veins of the recipient. The coeliac artery is anastomosed end to end to the portal vein. The donor common duct is ligated and the gall-bladder joined to the recipient common duct.

(By courtesy of the *British Medical Journal*.)

off the IVC after it had been clamped above and below the liver and the inflow to the liver had been occluded. Thus it was possible in a dry field to oversew the adventitious hepatic veins and leave the main hepatic veins for anastomosis to the donor organ's suprahepatic IVC, the infrahepatic IVC of the donor being ligated (Fig. 4 and 5). In one case a previous end to side porto-caval shunt had cured portal hypertension facilitating recipient hehatectomy. Dissection of the anastomosis did not present great difficulties.

Insertion of the transplant

The objective here is to provide the new liver with satisfactory vascular inflow and outflow before it has time to become warm and undergo further warm ischaemic damage. The liver must be orientated so that the anastomoses will not become kinked or otherwise obstructed and so that bile drainage is free. Slight variations in technique have been used in the 23 clinical orthotopic liver transplants that we have performed. With the exception of the two child-to-adult cases, the suprahepatic IVC was anastomozed to that of the recipient with a running stitch of silk or mersilene, the posterior layer being sutured from within the lumen sometimes with two rows, if this was felt desirable on the grounds of security. The anterior layer was sewn from outside. In all cases the portal vein has been anastomozed end-to-end with a similar running silk suture. The infrahepatic IVC anastomoses were also end-to-end sutured in the same way as the portal-venous anastomosis except in the two child donors where the infra-hepatic IVC was ligated. No complication has developed to date in any of the venous anastomoses.

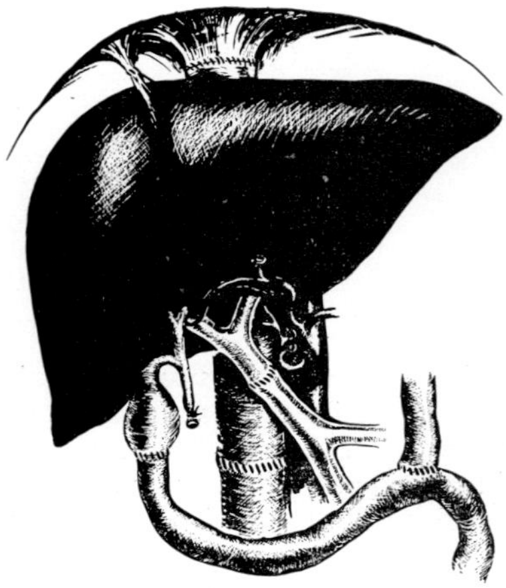

FIG. 6. Diagram of transplantation in which the main hepatic artery with coeliac and a patch of aorta is anastomozed to the aorta. The accessory hepatic artery from the superior mesenteric is anastomozed to the recipient hepatic artery. The gall-bladder is here anastomozed to a Roux loop of jejunum.

(By courtesy of the *British Journal of Surgery*.)

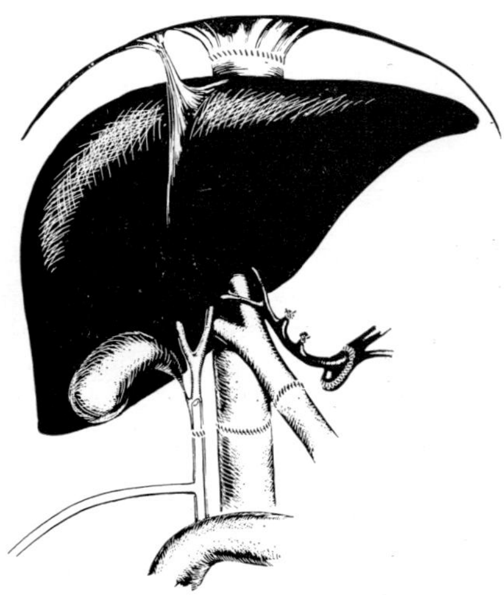

FIG. 7. Diagram of orthotopic liver transplantation with drainage of bile via a choledochodochostomy over a T-tube.

(By courtesy of the *British Journal of Surgery*).

In one case, a child recipient, the coeliac artery with a cuff of aorta was anastomozed end-to-side to the abdominal aorta (Fig. 6). In the other cases the coeliac artery was anastomozed to the hepatic artery of the recipient end-to-end or end-to-side (Fig. 7). There were three cases with additional hepatic arteries arising from the superior mesenteric artery. The main trunk of the superior mesenteric was anastomozed end-to-end to the hepatic artery in two cases (Fig. 6) and to the donor splenic artery in one. In one case the donor coeliac artery was occluded by atherosclerotic thrombus. A free graft of renal artery was used to join the recipient to the

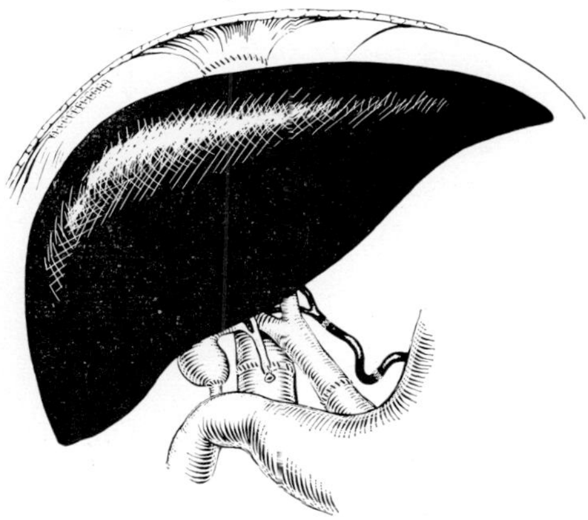

FIG. 8. The procedure in a case where the donor coeliac artery was occluded by atherosclerosis. Free graft of renal artery bridges the gap between the donor and recipient hepatic arteries.

(By courtesy of the *British Journal of Surgery*.)

donor hepatic artery (Fig. 8). There was only one arterial complication in this series, in a patient who developed multiple septic infarcts in the liver. At autopsy a mural clot was found where the hepatic artery had been clamped (Calne & Williams 1968; Calne, Williams *et al* 1968).

Biliary drainage

The best method of biliary drainage in clinical liver transplantation has not yet been clarified. On theoretical grounds it is desirable to retain the patient's sphincter of Oddi to prevent ascending infection, which is particularly likely to occur in patients given immunosuppression. In the pig it has proved to be satisfactory to anastomose the common bile duct end-to-end without any tube drainage. The common bile duct in the pig is of relatively large diameter and has a good blood supply. The blood supply of the human common bile duct is far more precarious in a liver transplantation operation. Nevertheless end-to-end anastomosis has been performed with a T-tube splinting the anastomosis, the long limb of the T-tube being brought out through the recipient common bile duct (Starzl 1969) (Fig. 7).

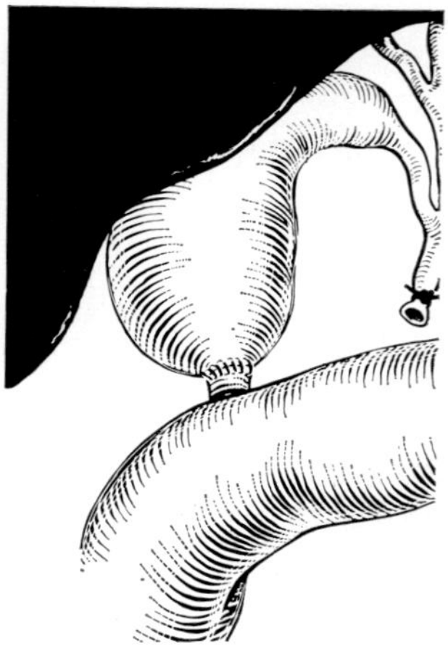

FIG. 9. Detail of cholecystcholedochostomy. Running 0000 chromic catgut suture through all layers.

(By courtesy of the *British Journal of Surgery*.)

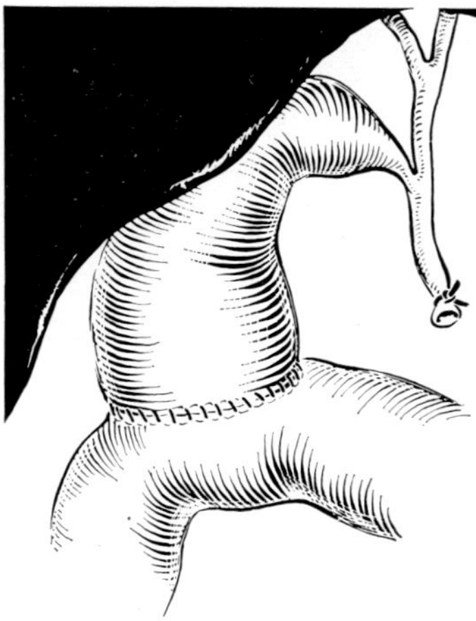

FIG. 10. Section layer of cholecystcholedochostomy. The seromuscular layer of the gall-bladder is sutured to the pancreas behind and the seromuscular layer of the duodenum in front.

(By courtesy of the *British Journal of Surgery*.)

Complications have arisen from cholangitis and ischaemic necrosis at the site of the anastomosis. Probably this form of T-tube drainage is unsatisfactory. Alternative modifications of end-to-end common bile duct anastomosis may be used in the future, since all other methods of bile drainage have disadvantages. Thus to tie the common bile duct below the entrance of the cystic duct and utilize the gall bladder for drainage has a weak link in the cystic duct, which is narrow and likely to be obstructed by biliary sludge and concretions and the danger of a long cystic duct being incorporated in the common bile duct ligature has already been mentioned. We have, however, utilized gall bladder to common bile duct drainage with satisfactory results (Figs. 8, 9 and 10). This technique does preseve the sphincter of Oddi and lessens the danger of cholangitis. Starzl, however, has had very little trouble with cholangitis after draining the gall bladder directly into the duodenum. This is certainly the most easy and straightforward technique. Alternatively the gall bladder may be joined to a Roux loop of jejunum (Fig. 6).

In all cases the falciform ligament of the donor liver was sutured to that of the recipient to help support the liver and prevent rotation (Starzl *et al* 1968). An external shunt of portal or IVC blood to the superior caval system is not necessary in humans, although it is an essential part of the technique of the operation in dogs (Starzl *et al* 1968).

The order of anastomoses has been suprahepatic vena cava followed by portal vein. As soon as the portal venous anastomosis is completed, blood is allowed to perfuse the liver. The initial effluent from the inferior vena cava is discarded, approximately 100 ml are allowed to flow freely out of the liver. This fluid is cold, ascidic, contains very high potassium levels and probably other dangerous metabolites as the result of ischaemic-damage of the liver and portal venous clamping on the splanchnic circulation. The infrahepatic IVC is then clamped and the clamps are taken off the suprahepatic IVC so that the liver receives its portal blood supply which drains into the inferior vena cava. The next anastomosis has been the arterial which is unclamped as soon as it is finished, then the infrahepatic caval and, finally, the biliary anastomosis. Starzl (1969) has performed second orthotopic liver grafts in two patients. He points out that in order to obtain enough suprahepatic vena cava for safe anastomosis it is necessary to retain a portion of the allograft vena cava inferior to the original anactomosis.

Ampicillin solution containing 2 g in 20 ml of saline is irrigated around the anastomoses and under the diaphragm, and the abdomen is drained with a 1 cm diameter Silastic drain brought out through a stab incision below the right extremity of the main wound which is closed with monofilamentous nylon, interrupted catgut and interrupted silk skin stitches.

No systemic heparin is given but, in addition to blood replacement, all patients are given intravenous infusions of bicarbonate, dextrose, and human fibrinogen. Most patients receive fresh frozen plasma, some in addition are given epsilon-aminocaproic acid (EACA) and aminomethyl cyclohexane carboxylic acid (AMCA), although these agents were throught not to have influenced the course of events to an important extent. Antibiotics are given systemically when infection has been suspected or demonstrated.

It is quite clear from the results reported by Starzl and others (1969) and from our own experience of 23 orthotopic liver transplant operations in man, that clinical transplantation of the liver can be surgically satisfactory. It is unlikely that one would be able to improve the condition of a liver by *in vitro* perfusion, so that the methods described above in the surgically successful cases will probably not be improved upon as far as initial function and morphological preservation of the liver are concerned. Nevertheless, a perfusion system that would allow 8 h or more of permissible ischaemic time, without severe continuing damage, would make the logistics of the operation far easier than at the present time. Encouraging results with an hyperbaric cold perfusion system have been reported (Brettschneider *et al* 1968).

It is of paramount importance that the transplanted liver is adequately perfused with portal and systemic arterial blood as soon as possible. If the patient is hypotensive when the anastomoses are completed, the grafted liver remains pale and assumes a bluish tinge. This is a disastrous situation and results in the same uncontrollable haemorrhagic state that occurs when a liver damaged severely by ischaemia is transplanted. The objective should be to over-correct blood-loss in the early stages of the operation. Operative haemorrhage can be massive and rapid in patients with portal hypertension and poor liver function. Adhesions from previous surgery may bleed profusely despite the utmost care taken to secure all bleeding points. Dilated thin walled venules under high pressure can bleed after minimal surgical trauma. Hypotension at the time of graft revascularization has resulted in the death of two of our patients. Uncontrollable capillary haemorrhage of up to 1 l. every 15 min occurred from multiple sites, where no large vessel had been left bleeding. In cases where this sequence can be anticipated, it is preferable to remove the donor liver before commencing to operate on the recipient. This prevents delay during which bleeding can take place, in the period following skeletonization of the liver whilst the donor hepatectomy is in progress. Removal of the patient's liver proceeds as rapidly as possible, with massive blood replacement continuing until the transplantation is completed. Satisfactory perfusion of the graft would be expected to halt the haemorrhage by reducing the portal pressure and enabling the liver to produce clot-promoting factors. This can tip the scales in favour of the patient's survival and prevents the hopeless transfusion of litres of blood in an irreversible situation. The vascular anastomoses which have been used appear to be satisfactory, but biliary drainage is still a problem. In patients with parenchymatous disease of the liver with a haemorrhagic diathesis there can be multiple deficiencies of coagulation factors. The continued uncontrollable haemorrhage that occurs if a poorly preserved liver is transplanted, or if the patient is shocked at the time of revascularization of the liver, has been mentioned and no matter what haematological advice is given, bleeding will not stop. Per contra, even though a patient may have been bleeding massively during the recipient hepatectomy, provided he is not shocked and the transplant has been well preserved initially, satisfactory perfusion of the liver graft is followed often within 20 min by a dramatic cessation of capillary haemorrhage: surely one of the most satisfying observations that can occur during surgery.

REFERENCES

BRETTSCHNEIDER L., DALOZE P.N., HUGUET C., PORTER K.A., GROTH C.G., KASHIWAGI N., HUTCHISON D. & STARZL T.E. (1968) The use of combined preservation techniques for extended storage of orthotopic liver homografts. *Surgery, Gynec. Obstet.* **126,** 263.

CALNE R.Y. & WILLIAMS R. (1968) Liver transplantation. I. Observations on technique and organisation in five cases. *Brit. med. J.* iv, 535.

CALNE R.Y., WILLAIMS R., DAWSON J.L., ANSELL I.D., EVANS D.B., FLUTE P.T., HERBERTSON P.M., JOYSEY V., KEATES G.H.W., KNILL-JONES R.P., MASON S.A., MILLARD P.R., PENA J.R., PENTLOW B.M., SALAMAN J.R., SELLS R.A. & CULLUM P.A. (1968) Liver transplantation in man. II. A report of two orthotopic liver transplants in adult recipients. *Br. med. J.* iv, 451.

CALNE R.Y. (1969) Surgical aspects of clinical liver transplantation in 14 cases. *Br. J. Surg.* **56,** 729.

MARCHIORO T.L., HUNTLEY R.T., WADDELL W.R. and STARZL T.E. (1963) Extracorporeal perfusion for obtaining postmortem homografts. *Surgery,* **54,** 900.

SCHALM S.W. (1969) A simple method for short-term preservation of a liver homograft. *Transplantation,* **8,** 877.

STARZL T.E. (1969) *Experience in Hepatic Transplantation.* London: W.B.Saunders.

STARZL T.E., GROTH C.G., BRETTSCHNEIDER L., PENN I., FULGINITI V.A., MOON J.B., BLAMCHARD H., MARTIN A.J. Jr. & PORTER K.A. (1968) Orthotopic homotransplantation of the human liver. *Ann. Surg.* **168,** 392.

CHAPTER 24

Haematological Management

P.T. Flute

The haematologist will be called upon to monitor marrow function during immunosuppressive therapy. This will require frequent estimations of haemoglobin and counts of white cells and platelets. He must also give advice regarding the considerable problems of haemostasis and thrombosis. The platelets may be reduced by depressed marrow production or by increased consumption, either due to sequestration in perisinusoidal spaces within the liver graft (Hutchison *et al* 1968) or by a process of disseminated intravascular coagulation (McKay 1968). Decreased synthesis or increased consumption of coagulation and fibrinolytic factors is also found in liver disease (Rake *et al* 1970a).

COAGULATION AND FIBRINOLYSIS

General principles

Stimulation of coagulation and fibrinolysis is the expected response to tissue damage, however it is caused. Although the precise stimulus has yet to be defined the common denominator is exposure of the blood to damaged cells (Fig. 1). The action of thrombin and plasmin is largely confined to the actual sites of stimulation by an excess of inhibitors in the blood and by the action of the reticulo-endothelial cells of the liver, lungs, and elsewhere.

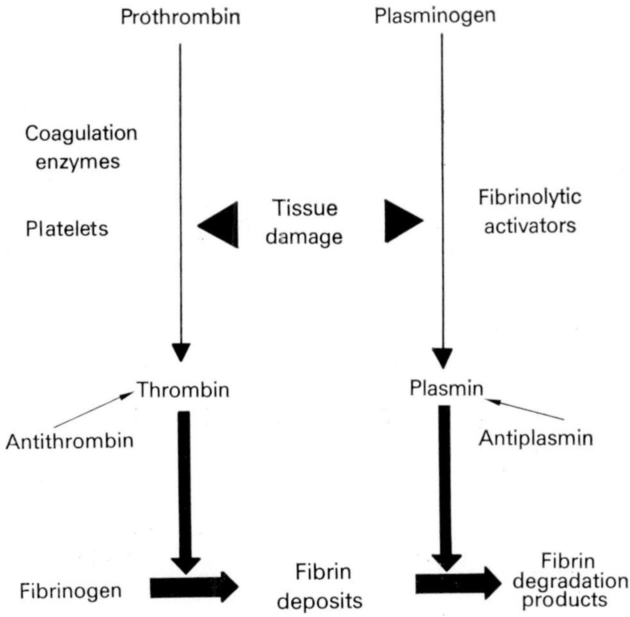

FIG. 1.

These rapidly and selectively clear the blood reaching them of active enzymes and of the end products of both systems, soluble fibrin monomer complexes and fibrin degradation products.

The local effect of stimulation will be the formation of haemostatic plugs. General effects which may be observed are the presence of the active intermediates and end products and, if the process is sufficiently intense, a falling blood concentration of platelets, coagulation factors, and plasminogen, as they are consumed faster than they can be replaced.

Complications which may arise are of three types. Firstly, if the stimulus is extreme the reduction of factors, supplemented by the presence of end products, particularly fibrin degradation products which have a complex antihaemostatic effect, may cause severe bleeding at the time of operation. Secondly, while active intermediates are circulating massive thrombosis may occur in areas of stasis within veins, producing a risk of pulmonary embolism. Thirdly, microthrombi may form, in capillaries and small vessels of different organs; if not rapidly dissolved by the fibrinolytic enzymes they may lead to tissue necrosis. The site of microthrombus formation is probably determined by variations in blood flow; typical examples would be necrotic lesions of the gut mucosa, or bilateral renal cortical necrosis with lesions in the glomeruli.

Operative changes

Transplantation of the liver in animals and man (Von Kaulla *et al* 1966; Flute *et al* 1969; Groth *et al* 1969) is regularly associated with an immediate fall in platelets, all the coagulation factors, and plasminogen, and with the appearance of active intermediates, soluble fibrin complexes, fibrinolytic activator, and fibrin degradation products (FDP). These changes of acute intravascular coagulation with secondary fibrinolysis are often no greater than those seen in other major surgical procedures, particularly those on the heart and lung in association with bypass procedures (Fig. 2), and are usually well tolerated. Complications may arise when they are accentuated by certain features peculiar to liver transplantation.

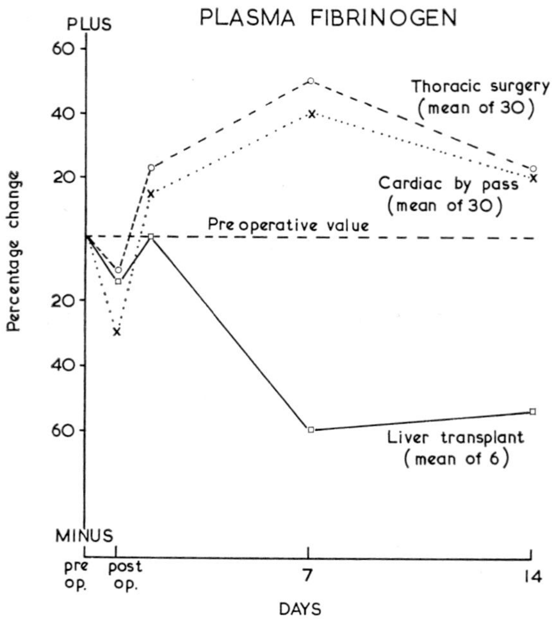

FIG. 2. Plasma fibrinogen after operation.

Multiple abnormalities may already be present due to pre-existing disease or its treatment. The donor organ can act as an intense stimulus to coagulation if it has been damaged by ischaemia. In early operations the foreign surfaces of artificial bypasses for decompression of the caval system would have contributed to the stimulus, but these are no longer in use. Diversion of blood flow from the liver may allow a temporary accumulation of active products due to interference with normal clearance mechanisms. Severe haemorrhage acts as a stimulus to coagulation and lysis and if hypovolaemia occurs a vicious circle may develop; it is particularly difficult to ensure prompt and adequate blood replacement during dissection of multiple porto-systemic collaterals. Acidosis may be a further contributory stimulus.

Post-operative changes

The fall of platelets, coagulation factors, and plasminogen, at operation are soon followed by a rise in their concentration due to increased production. Factor VIII reaches particularly high levels, but platelet increase may be delayed for a few days. These changes are again common to all major operations and suggest that liver synthesis is progressing normally.

However, the changes are modified after the 1st week, possibly by the immune response, perhaps sometimes due to the immunosuppresive therapy or to the continuing effects of ischaemic damage to the grafted organ. Platelets, fibrinogen, and plasminogen concentrations are normal or slightly reduced, at a time when certainly platelets and fibrinogen would be expected to be increased. Factor VIII is characteristically high and fibrin degradation products can be detected in the serum. The turnover of ^{125}I-labelled fibrinogen is increased, often for several months but with a gradual return to normal (Fig. 3). These are the changes of chronic intra-

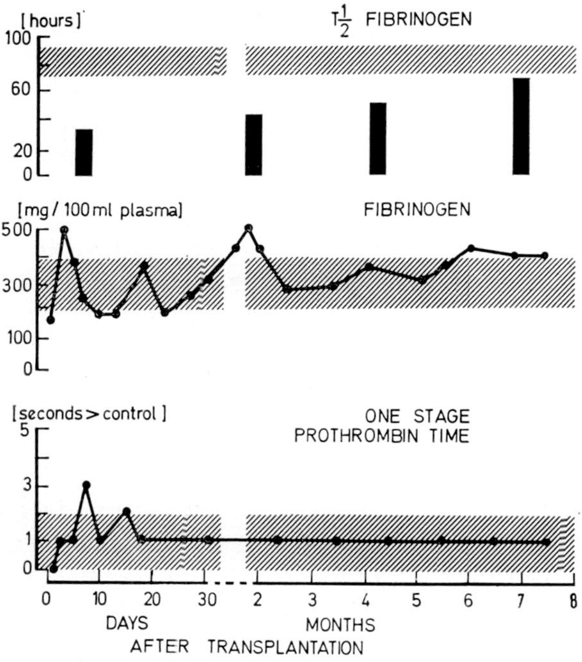

FIG. 3. Fibrinogen and prothrombin time after orthotopic liver transplantation in a single patient (the normal range is shaded).

vascular coagulation and suggest that active intermediates of coagulation may still be circulating, with a risk of thrombosis in areas of impaired blood flow. Fibrinogen synthesis is normal (Rake *et al* 1970b).

With poor function of the homograft, defective synthesis and increased consumption provoked by the stimulus of the damaged liver cells combine to prevent the expected increase of platelets and coagulation factors; the increased consumption makes it virtually impossible to replace them by transfusion. Similar blood changes, not necessarily associated with obvious bleeding, may be seen when acute rejection occurs or when the blood supply to the graft is impaired.

Laboratory assessment

The blood concentration of all the coagulation factors is best followed by simple tests, frequently repeated. One stage prothrombin and partial thromboplastin times will give an indication of all except factor XIII. Prolongation of these tests suggests decreased synthesis or increased consumption of the coagulation factors. Short times due to an increased synthesis of coagulation factors are more likely to be detected with the partial thromboplastin time. Assay of individual factors is possible but seldom of practical value except for fibrinogen. The synthesis of fibrinogen continues in all but the most severe hepatic failure and its measurement is, therefore, a useful guide to the presence of increased consumption of coagulation factors, especially when related to a fall in the platelet count, raised serum FDP, and an increase of factor VIII. The best method for confirming increased consumption is the measurement of fibrinogen turnover with ^{125}I-labelled human fibrinogen.

Circulating activator of fibrinolysis can be measured if the euglobulin fraction of plasma is tested on fibrin plates. This method is to be preferred to clot lysis times which depend on the patient's own plasminogen and fibrinogen because these may vary independently. However, an increase of circulating activator is not an inevitable accompaniment of fibrinolysis and frequently the levels are decreased after operation when decreased plasminogen and increased fibrin degradation products show that fibrinolysis is active. A rapid guide to the level of FDP is given by the thrombin clotting time. This may be prolonged in three ways: by severe fibrinogen deficiency; by heparin, when it will be corrected by protamine added in amounts up to 2 mg/100 ml; and by fibrin or fibrinogen degradation products, when it will be returned to normal by the addition of much larger amounts of protamine, of the order of 20 to 40 mg/100 ml.

Intravascular coagulation may also be indicated by haemolytic anaemia of microangiopathic type showing a falling haemoglobin not related to bleeding, increased reticulocytes, and fragmented red cells. It should be emphasized that an increased turnover of fibrinogen has been found in the absence of these changes.

PRACTICAL MANAGEMENT

Pre-operative

Existing abnormalities should be corrected as far as possible. Vitamin K may be required and can be supplemented with transfusions of fresh frozen plasma. In the presence of severe hepatic necrosis these measures are often ineffective because of the increased consumption. Removal of the damaged liver brings the stimulus to massive consumption to an end and the operation can be successful if transfusion with fresh blood is continued until this stage of the operation is passed.

Operative

Laboratory tests are of little help in predicting the onset of severe bleeding. Since many of the cases who bleed excessively do so because of an accentuation of the tendency to disseminated intravascular coagulation it is important to minimize the possible stimuli. Blood loss must be replaced promptly and adequately; the use of fresh blood will minimize the tendency to a fall in platelets as well as coagulation factors. Five units or more of fresh blood can usually be obtained from the donor of the liver graft and then can be transfused into the recipient provided it is compatible. Hypoxia, hypothermia, acidosis, and hypocalcaemia, must be controlled. If the graft itself is damaged by ischaemia these methods are unlikely to be successful. If bleeding becomes a problem the immediate rapid transfusion of 1 l. of fresh frozen plasma and 4 g of fibrinogen will supply coagulation factors though not platelets.

Anticoagulants and fibrinolytic inhibitors are usually unnecessary. In experimental animals subjected to severe haemorrhage, or the infusion of tissue materials, heparin blocks the changes in both coagulation and fibrinolysis. Therefore, if bleeding fails to respond to transfusion, 10,000 units of heparin may be given in an attempt to reduce the stimulus to coagulation; its action can be rapidly reversed with protamine if no response is obtained. Acidosis may prevent its effect. Fibrinolytic inhibitors are less useful, they block the stimulation of fibrinolysis but allow the coagulation changes and, therefore, the risk of thrombosis in the microcirculation to continue unchecked. In two patients with severe hepatic necrosis and multiple deficiencies which could not be corrected by transfusion, 1 g of the fibrinolytic inhibitor tranexamic acid was given intravenously 1 h before operation and again just before removal of the recipient's liver; no untoward effects were observed (Flute *et al* 1969).

Post-operative

There is no certain laboratory test to predict the occurrence of thrombosis. However, the increased fibrinogen turnover suggests that a tendency to thrombosis continues for long periods and continuous heparinization during the first few weeks merits consideration and is indicated for the treatment of a clinically obvious episode. Bleeding from the gastrointestinal tract may be a manifestation of local necrosis due to microthrombosis and may then respond to heparin. Often it occurs at a time when the blood urea is rising and substitution of renal function by dialysis may stop the bleeding.

SUMMARY

The operation is dominated by the stimulation of coagulation and an increase of fibrinolysis now regarded as secondary to the coagulation. Evidence of less intense stimulation continues after the operation for many weeks. Further experience is needed to show when replacement of missing factors by transfusion, of fresh blood, fresh frozen plasma, or fibrinogen concentrates, should be supplemented by heparin.

REFERENCES

FLUTE P.T., RAKE M.O., WILLIAMS R., SEAMAN M.J. & CALNE R.Y. (1969) Liver transplantation in man. IV Haemorrhage and thrombosis. *Br. med. J.* iii, 20.

GROTH C.G., PECHET L. & STARZL T.E. (1969) Coagulation during and after orthotopic transplantation of the human liver. *Arch. Surg.* **98**, 31.

HUTCHISON D.E., GENTON E., PORTER K.A., DALOZE P.M., HUGUET C., BRETTSCHNEIDER L., GROTH C.G. & STARZL T.E. (1968) Platelet changes following clinical and experimental hepatic homotransplantation. *Arch. Surg.* **97**, 27.

MCKAY D.G. (1968) Disseminated intravascular coagulation. *Proc. Roy. Soc. Med.* **61**, 1129.

RAKE M.O., FLUTE P.T., PANNELL G. & WILLIAMS R. (1970a) Intravascular coagulation in acute hepatic necrosis. *Lancet*, i, 533.

RAKE M.O., MCFARLANE A.S. & WILLIAMS R. (1970b) Protein synthesis after transplantation of the liver, in preparation.

VON KAULLA K.N., KAYE H., VON KAULLA E., MARCHIORO T.L. & STARZL T.E. (1966) Changes in blood coagulation before and after hepatectomy or liver transplantation in dogs and man. *Arch. Surg.* **92**, 71.

CHAPTER 25

Post-operative Care

Roger Williams

During the first 24 h after transplantation the patient needs constant surveillance. Excluding complications directly related to surgery, such as post-operative haemorrhage, many other problems can arise. Our own experience has provided instances of a respiratory arrest due to retained secretions, hyperkalaemia with a cardiac arrest, other cardiac arrhythmias and of hypokalaemia (see the section on Anaesthesia). Cardiac monitoring with an oscilloscope and ratemeter is essential and the serum electrolytes should be estimated at least 4-hourly. The blood gases also need to be checked regularly and assisted respiration may be needed during the 1st post-operative day. Particular problems related to the haematological changes and coagulation disturbances will be dealt with separately. Physiotherapy is essential both for the chest and to prevent venous thrombosis in the legs.

Once the first 24 h are over the patient's general condition usually begins to improve. Encouraging indications of an adequately functioning liver are a fall in serum bilirubin and improvement in tests of coagulation. Intravenous feeding can usually be discontinued by the 4th to 5th day and in the uncomplicated case the patient will be out of bed at the end of the 1st week and walking by the third.

Details of immunosuppressive therapy and antibiotic cover during this period will be given separately. Other therapy that may be needed includes infusions of salt-poor human serum albumin particularly during the 2nd and 3rd weeks. In our experience the serum albumin tends to fall at this time and the patient may develop oedema. Certain of the liver function tests namely serum bilirubin, alkaline phosphatase and serum transaminase are estimated daily during the first 10 days, the serum proteins less frequently. The subsequent routine varies accordingly to the progress and whether rejection or other complications develop. Serial scintiscanning is also a considerable help in assessing the function of the graft.

IMMEDIATE RESULTS

The immediate results of an orthotopic transplantation can be most encouraging. This is well shown by the improvement in liver function tests of a 40-year-old woman (Case EC) with complete biliary obstruction

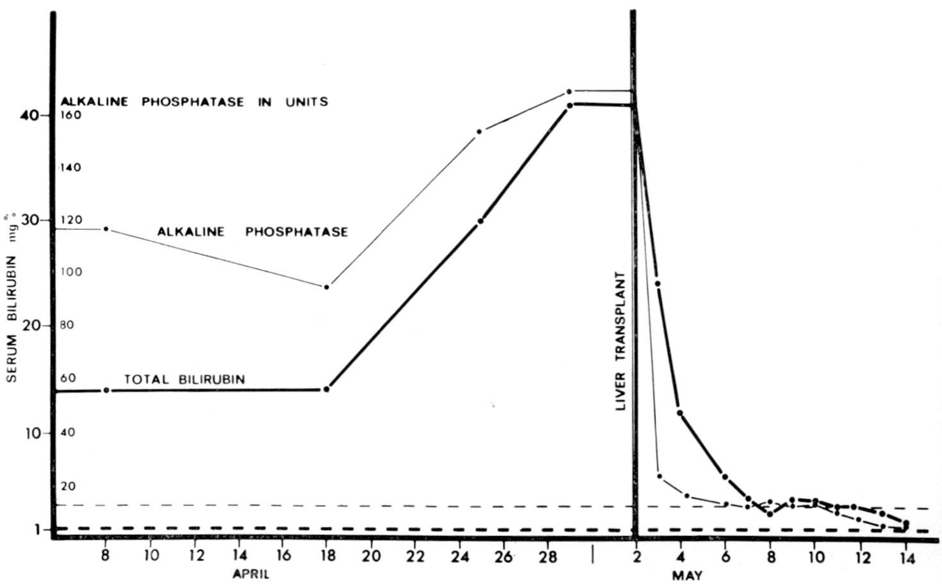

FIG. 1. The liver function tests of a patient with a carcinoma of hepatic ducts before and after transplantation (from Calne & Williams 1968).

due to a carcinoma of the hepatic duct (Fig. 1). Prior to transplantation her serum bilirubin had risen to 42 mg/100 ml, and the serum alkaline phosphatase to 150 KA u/100 ml. Within a week of transplantation both values had fallen to near normal limits.

EFFECT ON ACUTE AND CHRONIC HEPATIC ENCEPHALOPATHY

One of our patients, was in deep hepatic coma with non-reactive pupils at the time of transplantation. Corresponding with this is the EEG recording which showed high voltage slow waves of delta frequency many having the slow and sharp wave form ('biphasic') which is characteristic of severe hepatic coma (Fig. 2). The latter is regarded as of serious prognostic import, and none of the other patients with acute hepatic failure and this type of EEG abnormality that we have seen during the past two years have

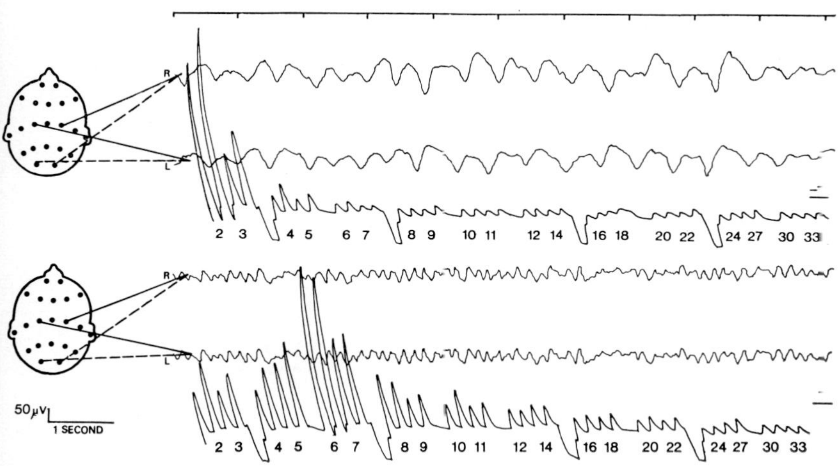

FIG. 2. EEG readings in a patient with acute hepatic coma before and 18 h after orthotopic transplantation. Below the EEG records is the automatic printout of the electronic waveform analyser giving the summated voltage at each individual frequency (from Parkes *et al* 1970).

survived. However, on the day following transplantation the recording showed considerable improvement with some normal alpha activity present. He regained consciousness on the first post-operative day and was talking on the second.

Conventional EEG recordings are difficult to quantitate and assessment of changes from serial recordings is particularly difficult. However, using an electronic waveform analyser it is possible to determine the summated voltage at each individual frequency of 2–33 c/s over a 10 s recording period. This is automatically printed below the EEG tracings as shown in Fig. 2, the first deflection representing activity of the right hemisphere, the second that from the left. The height of the deflection is directly proportional to the summated voltage. It can be seen that in this patient before transplantation most of the activity was at 2–3 c/s but on the day following, peak activity had already shifted to 6–7 c/s (Parkes *et al* 1970).

From this automatic analysis print-out it is also possible to calculate a single figure—the mean dominant frequency—which gives an estimate of mean frequency in that recording. It is particularly useful in illustrating changes over a period of time and in Fig. 3 it has been used to show the

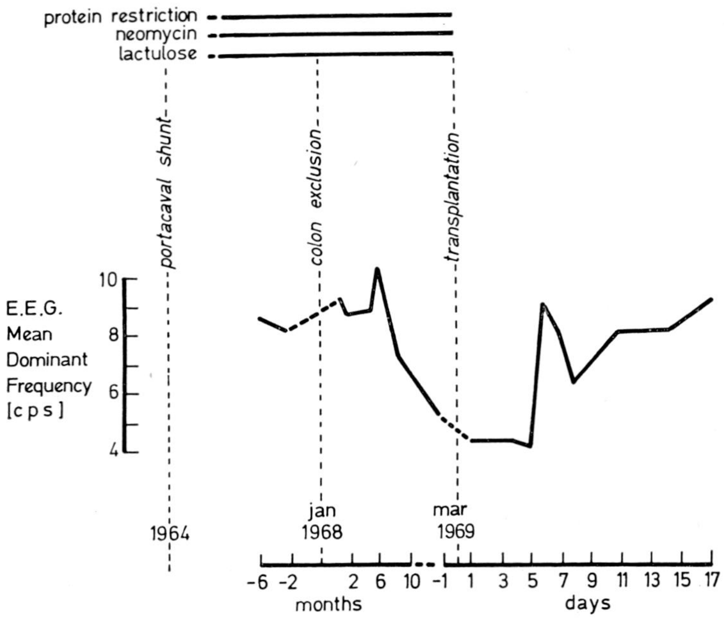

FIG. 3. Illustrating changes in mean dominant frequency in patient GK with chronic encephalopathy before and after transplantation (from Williams 1970).

effect of transplantation in a patient G.K. with chronic encephalopathy. This patient had cirrhosis and had a portacaval anastomosis done in 1964, because of bleeding from varices. Subsequently he developed hepatic encephalopathy and despite a low-protein diet, neomycin and lactulose his clinical condition and EEG steadily deteriorated. In 1968 a colonic exclusion with a caeco-rectal anastomosis was performed. Following this he improved clinically and the mean dominant frequency rose to normal and remained so for 8 months. Then his condition deteriorated again, the mean dominant frequency dropping to 5 c/s. Following transplantation there was a rapid rise on the 5th post-operative day to a near normal level. On the 8th day there was slight deterioration which corresponded to the onset of a minor episode of rejection with transient confusion and rise in serum enzymes but no change in serum bilirubin. By the 17th day he had a normal EEG recording (Parkes *et al* 1970). During these first 2 weeks there was a correspondingly rapid improvement in his mental state, his writing became clearer and the hepatic flap disappeared. We were surprised at the rapidity and extent of recovery of a patient with such severe and chronic encephalopathy in whom one might have expected that some at least of the brain damage was irreversible.

Other effects

Other manifestations of cirrhosis are also reversed. Figure 4 shows the fall in titre of the serum mitochondrial antibody in a patient with primary biliary cirrhosis. The significance of this antibody in the pathogenesis of

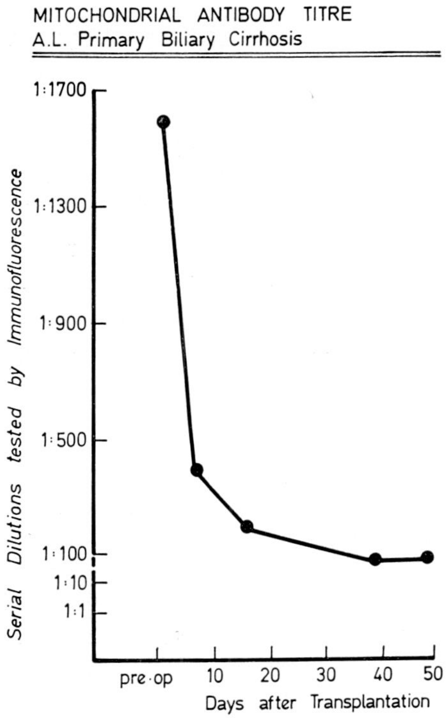

FIG. 4. Changes in serum mitochondrial antibody titre in a patient with primary biliary cirrhosis treated by an orthotopic transplantation (by courtesy of Dr Deborah Doniach and from Williams 1970).

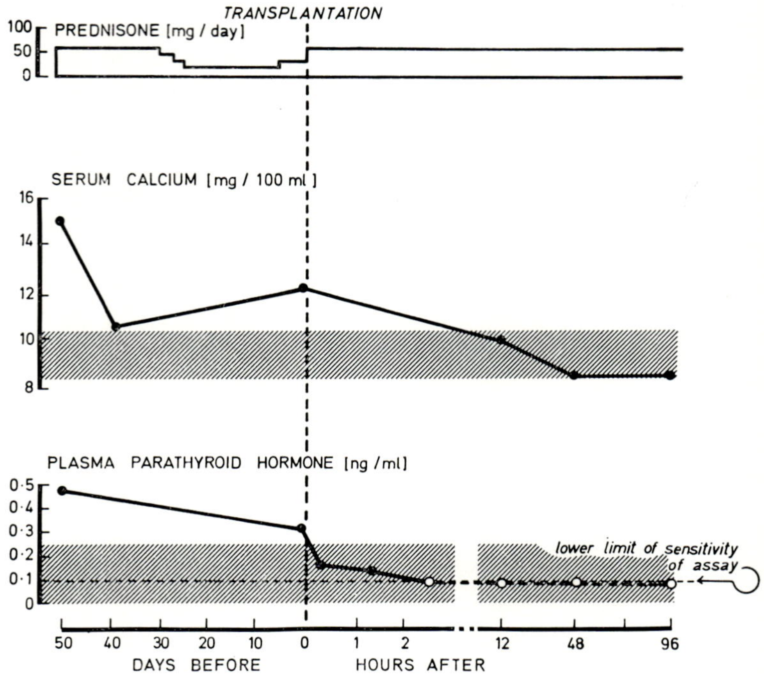

FIG. 5. Showing effect of transplantation on the hypercalcaemia and increased plasma parathyroid hormone level of a patient with a primary hepatoma producing parathyroid hormone (from Knill-Jones *et al* 1970).

primary biliary cirrhosis, of which it is so characteristic, is uncertain, but the fall in titre following removal of the diseased liver is of some interest. Patients with primary biliary cirrhosis who have been treated with prednisone or azathioprine have not shown a similar fall in titre. However, there was a fall in rubella antibody titre in our patient and the further studies of serum antibodies following transplantation are needed.

In a 57-year-old man with a primary hepatoma unequivocal production of parathyroid hormone by the tumour was demonstrated. The serum calcium was considerably elevated at 17·6 mg/100 ml and the serum phosphate was low at 1·4 mg/100 ml. Increased levels of parathyroid hormone in the plasma were demonstrated by an immunoassay technique. Following transplantation both the serum calcium and the raised parathyroid hormone level fell to normal (Fig. 5). At the time of surgery there was a higher concentration of parathyroid hormone in the hepatic vein (0·54 ng/ml) than in either the portal vein or hepatic artery (0·20 and 0·39 ng/ml respectively) and an extraction of the tumour but not of the normal liver tissue showed significant parathyroid hormone activity (Knill-Jones *et al* 1970).

REFERENCES

CALNE R.Y. & WILLIAMS R. (1968) Liver transplantation in man. I. Observations on technique and organization in liver cases. *Br. med. J.* iv, 535.

KNILL-JONES R.P., BUCKLE R.M., PARSONS V., CALNE R.Y. & WILLIAMS R. (1970) Hypercalcaemia and increased parathyroid hormone activity in a primary hepatome: Studies before and after transplantation. *New Engl. J. Med.* **282,** 704.

PARKES J.D., MURRAY-LYON I.M. & WILLIAMS R. (1970) Neuropsychiatric and electroencephalographic changes before and after transplantation of the liver for hepatoma or cirrhosis. *Quart. J. Med.* N.S. **39,** 1515.

WILLIAMS R. (1970) Liver transplantation in man. *Br. med. J.* i, 585.

CHAPTER 26

The Occurrence and Patterns of Rejection

Roger Williams

EARLY REJECTION

Early episodes of jaundice starting about the 6th–8th post-operative day have been observed in a number of our patients, and have also been described by Starzl (1969). One such episode is illustrated in Fig. 1. Liver function tests on 5th, 6th and 7th days were virtually normal. On the 8th day the serum bilirubin rose to 2·2 mg/100 ml and there was also a slight rise in the serum transaminase. Over the next week the serum bilirubin continued to rise with accompanying moderate increases in serum transaminase and alkaline phosphatase levels. The possibility of a toxic reaction to azathioprine was considered and this was stopped on the 10th day, but there was no improvement, and A.L.G. which had been discontinued after the first week owing to lack of supplies was restarted. From the 4th day the dose of prednisone was increased to 200 mg daily. Subsequently, there was a rapid fall in serum bilirubin and transaminase and by the beginning of the fourth week liver function tests were much improved.

In this patient A.L.G. had been stopped before deterioration in liver function, but in other cases similar rises in serum bilirubin and transaminase were observed though A.L.G. continued to be given daily. In this patient it appeared to be the increased dose of prednisone which lead to control of the jaundice, but in some of Starzl's patients similar episodes of jaundice attributable to rejection improved spontaneously without any change in immunosuppressive therapy and this has also been observed in the dog.

Percutaneous liver biopsies done at this time have shown histological appearances consistent with rejection as will be described later.

Other characteristic features of these early rejection episodes are a rise in white cell count and E.S.R. and a fall in the platelet count. Fever may be present depending on the dose of steroids. The patient feels generally unwell with loss of appetite and is often depressed. According to Starzl they may complain of a localized aching pain over the homograft and in the back—a feature we have not observed. The liver is enlarged. This is most easily demonstrated by scintiscanning which also shows decreased uptake of the isotope throughout the liver.

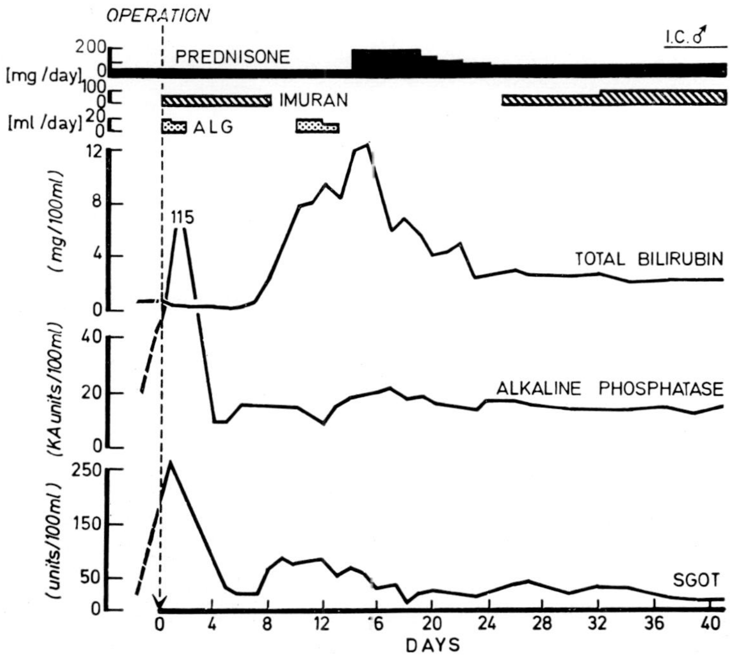

FIG. 1. Illustrating characteristic early episode of jaundice due to rejection in Case IC (from Williams *et al* 1969).

LATE REJECTION

One of our patients developed a relentless cholestatic jaundice which we attributed to chronic rejection. This has also been observed by Starzl in some of his longer survivors. The patient had an early episode of jaundice but was then well during the second month but subsequently there was a progressive rise in serum bilirubin to levels of 30–40 mg/100 ml. during the last month of his life (Fig. 2). The serum transaminase fluctuated

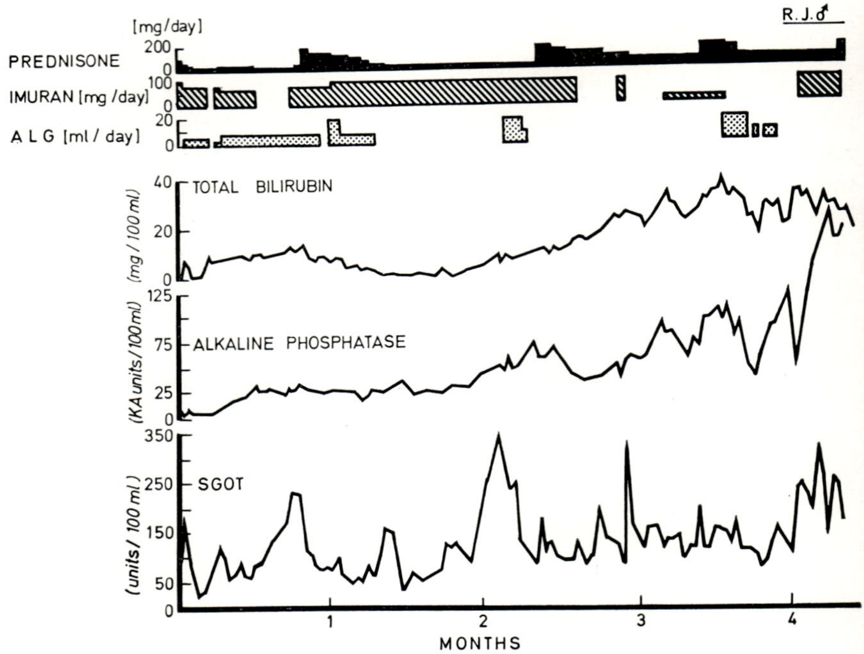

FIG. 2. Liver function tests over a $4\frac{1}{2}$ month period in Case JJ illustrating the relentless cholestatic jaundice of chronic rejection (from Williams *et al* 1969).

around 200 i.u./100 ml, and there was a considerable increase in alkaline phosphatase (up to 170 K.A. u/100 ml). At no time however, did he complain of itching. The initial tissue typing had shown three major incompatabilities and at autopsy at $4\frac{1}{2}$ months there were striking arterial lesions similar to those seen in kidney grafts which have suffered chronic rejection.

OTHER CLINICAL PATTERNS OF REJECTION

Starzl has described an anicteric form of rejection which occurs at about the same time as the early acute episode already described but in which there is some elevation in serum transaminase and alkaline phosphatase but no increase in serum bilirubin and no unequivocal clinical signs, though swelling of the graft can be demonstrated on scintiscanning.

Another variety which Starzl has observed is an indolent rejection in which there is a slow but steady rise in serum bilirubin from the second to third week onwards which reaches a peak at the fourth to seventh week. One of the two patients in which this occurred subsequently improved after the second month, but the other went on to develop avascular areas in the left lobe. By this time the patient was extremely ill and a second transplant was carried out—the first graft when removed showing multiple infarcts.

The different timing and severity of these early rejection episodes may be related to the degree of compatability between donor and recipient though at present this is difficult to prove as will be discussed later. We also have the impression that the initial episode of jaundice is particularly severe when the transplanted liver has sustained considerable ischaemic damage from agonal changes in the donor or a cold ischaemia period of more than 4 h. It is possible also that the intensity with which the immune system of the recipient can react to the graft may have been affected by the previous disease process for example when the recipient had cirrhosis with all its accompanying metabolic and immunological abnormalities. In the rat it has been shown that the presence of obstructive jaundice due to biliary obstruction (induced by ligation of the common bile duct) will significantly delay the rejection of skin grafts done at the same time (Beaudoin & Rabbat 1969).

HYPERACUTE REJECTION

Whether hyperacute rejection similar to that which may occur in kidney transplants when the recipient has lymphocytotoxic antibodies in the serum (due to previous transfusion, pregnancy or other factors) can occur with liver transplantation is at present uncertain.

Such an occurrence would have to be distinguished from the similar effects of severe ischaemic damage. However, Hume and Williams (see Starzl 1969) have described an infant with extrahepatic biliary atresia in whom the conditions for procurement of the donor organ had been excellent and in whom there was no reason to suppose that ischaemic damage to the donor organ had occurred. However, when the child was explored 10 h after completion of transplantation on account of haemorrhage, the surface of the graft was found to be mottled. The left lobe was indurated and a biopsy revealed widespread necrosis. At autopsy 7 days later the liver was almost completely necrotic, although the major vessels were patent. No lymphocytotoxic antibodies could be detected in the serum of the child but eluates of the autopsy liver specimen caused lysis of the cultured renal cells of the original donor.

THE SYNDROME OF SEPTIC INFARCTION

According to Starzl (1969), the three characteristic features of this syndrome are (1) the development of a gram negative septicaemia, (2) a sudden and marked elevation of the serum transaminase indicative of extensive liver cell necrosis (3) large and persistent filling defects on hepatic scintiscanning in which there is no uptake of isotope. It occurred in five of his patients, 2, 24, 25, 52 and 105 days respectively after transplantation. All but one had previously been in good health although they had had occasional spikes of fever for several days or weeks beforehand, thereafter the temperature rose to high levels. Another characteristic feature was hypotension which was often severe. The organisms isolated from a blood culture were similar to those found normally in the intestine.

All five patients were operated on shortly after the diagnosis of septic infarction had been made. One had a formal resection of the major part of the right lobe, the others a debridement procedure carried out through an intercostal approach designed to avoid entry into the chest or abdomen. Patchy, necrotic areas were evident on the surface of the liver and dead tissue of yellow cheesy appearance could be traced into the interior of the liver; frank pus was never found. In only one of these patients was the result satisfactory and after an extensive debridement the defect was filled in slowly by hepatic regeneration as evidenced by serial scintiscanning over a period of 8 months. The others either died shortly afterwards or developed a persistent fistula from which fragments of liver tissue continued to be extruded, the liver at autopsy being shrunken and fibrotic.

Two of our patients developed hepatic infarcts. One (Case EC) a woman of 40, had an orthotopic liver transplant on 2 May 1968 for a carcinoma of the hepatic ducts with complete biliary obstruction. She developed a biliary fistula on the 10th day which persisted despite repeated courses of antibiotics. Prior to the surgery she had also had widespread thrush and leucopenia due to chlorambucil therapy. However, her general condition following transplantation was good and liver function tests returned to normal (Fig. 1, Chapter 25), but in the 10th week she became ill with a high fever and increased jaundice. On exploration the gall bladder was found to be necrosed, and although biliary drainage was re-established she died a few days later. At autopsy a thrombosis of the hepatic artery was found which appeared to have developed at the site of clamping during the surgery. There were numerous infarcts in both right and left lobes and from these and from infarcts in the other organs a variety of organisms and fungi were cultured. In the intervening areas of liver tissue no evidence of rejection could be found.

The second patient was a man aged 51 in whom an orthotopic transplant was carried out on 31 December 1969 for the same diagnosis as the previous patient. Prior to surgery he had a swinging pyrexia up to 103°F and repeated courses of antibiotics had been given. When the liver was sectioned after removal the dilated biliary system was filled with pus and bile. Post-operatively, he did well and liver function returned to normal. On the 5th day the white cell count was increased and on the 12th day bile began to leak from the wound. His condition deteriorated and he became jaundiced and febrile. When re-opened on 16 January 1970 all anastomoses appeared healthy although there was evidence of a bile leak and some infection. The right lobe of the liver was normal but the left lobe contained two large yellow infarcts, which on histological examination showed necrotic tissue but no surrounding cellular infiltration and no demonstrable organisms. Peritoneal drains were inserted and post-operatively the prednisone was reduced rapidly to 10 mg daily, azathioprine being continued in a dose of 100 mg daily. Following this his condition slowly improved although the biliary fistula continued.

Aetiology of hepatic infarction

According to Starzl this syndrome is due to three factors:

1 *Kinking of the hepatic artery.* These five patients that he described were operated on early in his series and at a time when the falciform and other retaining ligaments of the liver were not sutured. Subsequent studies on cadavers in the autopsy room showed that this could lead to displacement and rotation of the liver so that the right hepatic artery became kinked. This would explain why only the right lobe had been affected, and why in four of the patients at autopsy, the right hepatic artery was thrombosed.

2 *Infection.* Following sham abdominal operations in dogs and pigs in which the liver is left exposed an increased number of positive cultures can be obtained from the liver. Following auto-transplantation or orthotopic transplantation the frequency of positive cultures and the development of abscesses is even higher whether or not immunosuppression is given. In man, organisms have direct access to the graft when a cholecyst-duodenostomy or a cholecyst-jejunostomy is performed. Ischaemic damage to the donor organ either before, or during transplantation will also provide suitable areas in which such organisms can multiply.

3 *Rejection.* This, Starzl suggests, is the primary and most important factor in the development of hepatic infarction. Studies in dogs showed that

at the onset of rejection, blood-flow to the liver was reduced and similarly in some patients with an acute early episode of rejection serial scintiscanning showed areas without uptake. However, these were present only temporarily and with control of rejection the scintiscan appearances returned to normal. Failure to recognize the occurrence of rejection in these patients, he suggests, leads to insufficient immunosuppression particularly in the dose of prednisone given. This averaged 1 to 2 mg/kg, whereas since 1968 prednisone has been given in much higher doses (3–4 mg/kg initially) and regional necrosis has not been observed. However, his management has changed in other ways since then. Firstly, the liver is now better fixed which should prevent kinking of the hepatic artery, and secondly, a systematically designed programme of antibiotic cover starting at the time of operation and continuing for 2–6 weeks has been given.

The lack of pus in the infarcts and the absence of organisms in the histological sections of the infarcts in the most recent of our patients suggests however, that infection is not the primary factor although such infarcts may become infected subsequently. The hepatic artery thrombosis may also be a secondary and later event related to infection in the operation area. Neither of our patients had significant rejection as judged biochemically and histologically and indeed the last patient improved when immunosuppression was dramatically reduced. Such infarcts are not seen when hepatic artery blood supply is reduced in other conditions as for instance, following ligation of the hepatic artery for the treatment of secondary hepatic carcinoma. It is also not characteristic of the hepatic lesion of shock in which liver blood flow is considerably reduced. The primary factor we would suggest is either embolization or thrombosis in the interlobular arterial or portal vein radicles. The emboli may come from thrombi forming at sites of operative trauma and the generalized intravascular coagulation present at this time may be a contributing factor. Our approach to management is therefore based on intensification of antibiotic therapy and a reduction of immunosuppressive therapy. Operation is only indicated if biliary drainage becomes compromised with development of biliary obstruction or a major biliary fistula.

REFERENCES

BEAUDOIN J.G. & RABBAT A.G. (1969) Effect of biliary obstruction on skin allograft survival in mice. *Transplantation*, **7**, 576.

STARZL T.E. (1969) *Experience in Hepatic Transplantation.* Philadelphia, London, Toronto: W.B.Saunders.

WILLIAMS R. *et al* (1969) Liver transplantation in man. III. Studies of liver function, histology and immunosuppressive therapy. *Br. med. J.* iii, 12.

CHAPTER 27

Immunosuppressive Therapy

A.L.W.F. Eddleston
I.M. Murray-Lyon and
Roger Williams

CHOICE OF AGENT

The extensive experience now available in the control of rejection of renal transplants suggests that a combination of azathioprine and prednisone is the most consistently effective immunosuppressive regime. It was reasonable to assume, therefore, that this same combination would be satisfactory as the basic immunosuppressive régime in human hepatic transplantation. Starzl, however, using these drugs in his early series of hepatic transplants noted that rejection was poorly controlled and that infection was a serious problem. He has subsequently used antilymphocyte globulin (ALG) and prednisone with only small amounts of azathioprine with more satisfactory results (Starzl 1969). However the exact role that alterations in immunosuppressive therapy have played in the clinical improvement is difficult to analyse. The majority of the earlier cases had poor initial hepatic function which may have interfered with the production of the immunosuppressive metabolites of azathioprine but not the toxic metabolites (see below). In the later cases improvements in surgical technique and organ preservation may have been the most important factors which led to longer survival times. Although it has been claimed that the addition of antilymphocyte globulin significantly improves renal homograft function this has not been a universal finding. There is some evidence that ALG and prednisone may be mutually antagonistic in that they do not prolong the survival of skin allografts in the rat when used in combination (Grogan & Shivers 1969). However, batches of ALG vary greatly in their potency and as there is no generally accepted *in vitro* test of its immunosuppressive activity, data on this subject is difficult to interpret.

In our series we have relied on azathioprine and prednisone as the major immunosuppressive agents and have achieved satisfactory control of rejection without leucopenia. We have found that infections can be overcome provided that the dose of prednisone is kept as low as possible. We have used ALG on relatively few occasions to try to assist in the control of rejection episodes, with variable results.

DOSAGE RÉGIMES

As cadaveric organs must be used for hepatic transplantation it is rarely possible to start immunosuppressive therapy before transplantation and treatment usually begins immediately after the operation. Azathioprine is given in a dose of 50 mg/day to our adult recipients increasing to 75 mg and then 100 mg/day during the first 2 weeks. The oral route of administration is preferred but the drug is usually given intravenously on the first few post-operative days. The dose can be increased to 125 mg/day during the first month if there is no leucopenia and is then usually maintained at this level. Prednisone is first given in a dose of 60 mg/day in divided doses and reduced to 40 mg/day after 3 days. The aim is then to reduce the dose by 5 mg every third day until maintenance levels of 10 to 15 mg/day have been reached. If rejection episodes requiring treatment occur (and this is most difficult to assess since some at least appear to be self limiting) the prednisone dose is increased to 200 mg/day and then reduced by 25 mg every third day until 50 mg/day is being given. Further reduction by 5 mg every third day then follows. In some cases where rejection was not reversed by high doses of prednisone, ALG has been added in doses of 20 ml/day. We have given this intravenously over 4 h in saline, as intramuscular injections are extremely painful and can produce severe local reactions.

Most of Starzl's cases have been young children with biliary atresia and the dose of drugs given has been correspondingly less. The main difference in his régime was a marked reduction in the azathioprine dose in some cases and higher initial doses of prednisone. The average dose of azathioprine he used in the first 3 post-operative weeks in 12 recipients was 1·2 mg/kg/day which is similar to the amount we have used but in some cases the maximum dose of azathioprine which could be used without producing leucopenia was around 0·2 mg/kg/day. This striking intolerance to the drug was apparently not due to the concomitant administration of ALG. The mean prednisone dose in the same period was 3·1 mg/kg/day which is more than three times the average dose which we have used. He described two different approaches to ALG dosage; a low dose scheme using 4 ml/day by intramuscular injection for 10 to 14 days reducing to 4 ml on alternate days, twice a week and finally once a week in the ensuing 4 months (Starzl 1969). The high dosage scheme using double quantities of ALG followed the same pattern initially but thromobyctopenia often developed and the frequency of administration had to be reduced.

IN VITRO DIAGNOSIS OF REJECTION AND THE LEUCOCYTE MIGRATION TEST

Changes in standard liver function tests are non-specific and cannot differentiate between the many causes of jaundice after transplantation. Percutaneous liver biopsies are of great value in this situation but cannot be repeated too often and cannot hope to be predictive. Hepatitis, extra-hepatic obstruction and azathioprine toxicity may all be confused with rejection. There is good evidence of azathioprine hepatotoxicity in man, several case reports have been published, particularly after renal trans-

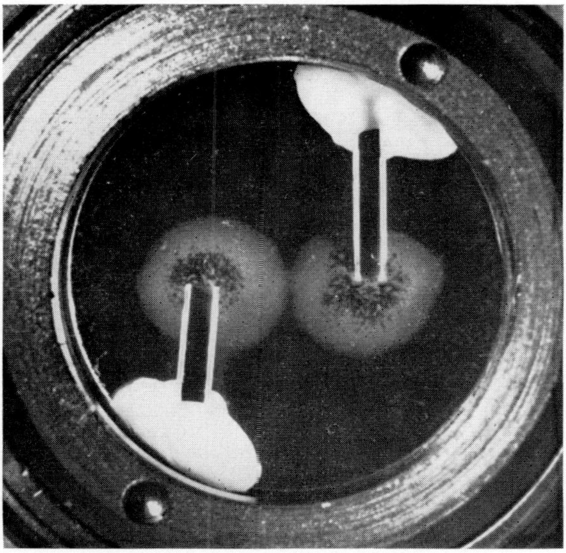

FIG. 1. Showing the migration of peripheral blood leucocytes in tissue culture chambers.

plantation in which azathioprine appeared to cause liver damage which regressed when the drug was stopped or the dose reduced. Such hepatotoxicity is obviously extremely difficult to recognize after hepatic transplantation and from this point of view and because of the dangers of infection the doses of both azathioprine and prednisone must be kept as low as possible. The control of immunosuppressive therapy would therefore be helped by a reliable and specific diagnosis of rejection.

Rejection is mediated initially by sensitized lymphocytes and if these could be detected in the patients peripheral blood, an early and specific diagnosis of rejection might be possible. The leucocyte migration test, studied extensively by Soborg & Bendixen (1967) appears to be an *in vitro* measure of delayed hypersensitivity. We have used this test to follow the changes in cell mediated hypersensitivity after transplantation (Eddleston *et al*; 1969; Smith *et al* 1969). Daily blood samples are taken and the leukocytes placed in capillary tubes mounted in small tissue culture chambers (Fig. 1). The two tubes in each chamber are for duplicate estimations. In the test chamber the medium contains a measured quantity of antigen which is derived either from foetal liver homogenate or from the white cells of the donor from whom the liver was obtained. During incuba-

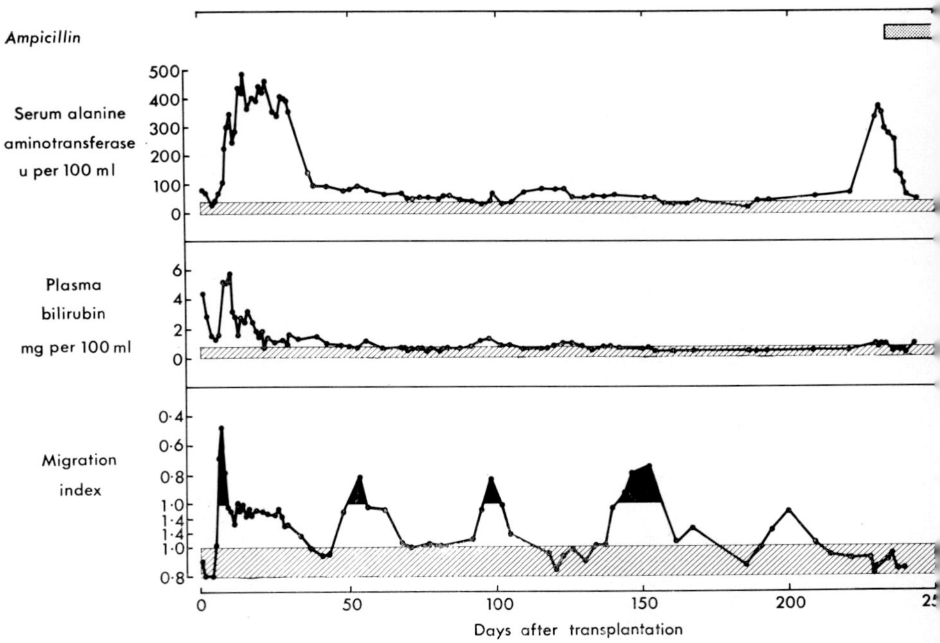

FIG. 2. Illustrating changes in migration index and liver function in patient W.S.—a long-term survivor (from Eddleston *et al* 1971).

tion at 37°C the cells migrate out of the capillary tubes and after 20 h the areas of migration are measured. It has been shown that at any one concentration of antigen, stimulation of migration indicates weak sensitization, and inhibition strong sensitization to that antigen (Soborg 1968).

Figure 2 shows the changes in migration index in relation to liver function in WS—the 44-year-old housewife. On the 8th day after transplantation there was a sharp rise in the serum bilirubin and in the transaminases. Similar changes in liver function at this time in other patients have been associated with histological evidence of rejection on liver biopsy and in this case the deterioration in liver function was preceded by changes in the migration index, with stimulation of migration on the 5th day and marked inhibition on the 7th day. With a short course of an increased prednisone dose the migration index, serum bilirubin and transaminase

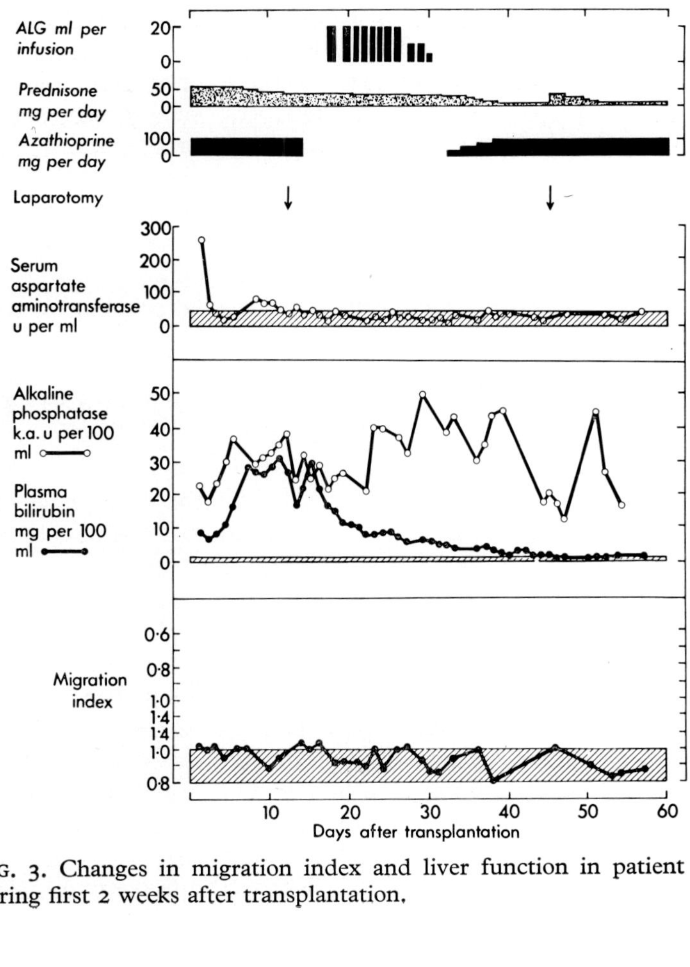

FIG. 3. Changes in migration index and liver function in patient TK during first 2 weeks after transplantation.

returned to normal. She was discharged home on the 30th day and since then there have been three short episodes in which the test has shown inhibition of migration with little if any change in the liver function tests. It is possible that the transplanted organ had become protected from immune attack by the development of some degree of graft adaptation as has been described for renal transplants in dogs (Murray *et al* 1964). The dose of prednisone has been gradually reduced to 10 mg daily and she is also receiving azathioprine 100 mg daily. In the 9th month after transplantation the patient was admitted unwell with an increase in serum transaminase and in serum alkaline phosphatase. There was no change in the migration index and she was treated with ampicillin and rapid clinical and biochemical improvement followed.

Another example of the specificity of the leucocyte migration test in the diagnosis of rejection concerns the immediate post-operative course of patient T.K. (Fig. 3). This patient was given 100 mg/day of azathioprine immediately after the operation. A rise in plasma bilirubin occurred at the end of the 1st week but there was no rise in the serum transaminases and no change in the migration index. Extrahepatic biliary obstruction was suspected clinically but at re-operation the extrahepatic biliary tree appeared patent suggesting that intrahepatic cholestasis was present. The bilirubin levels continued to rise although the migration index remained normal. The azathioprine was discontinued and the plasma bilirubin promptly began to fall. In spite of minimal immunosuppressive therapy provided by small dose of prednisone there was no evidence of rejection.

ASSAY OF SERUM IMMUNOSUPPRESSIVE ACTIVITY

One other *in vitro* test may be of practical help in the management of these patients. Bach *et al* (1969) from Paris have shown that it is possible to assay the immunosuppressive activity attained in the serum of patients on azathioprine. This is done by determining the ability of such serum to inhibit the spontaneous formation of rosettes which occurs when mouse lymphocytes are incubated with sheep red cells at 37°C. Immunosuppressive activity is expressed as a titre—the highest dilution of the serum which will produce at least 25% inhibition of spontaneous rosette formation.

As shown in Table 1 we found a high titre in patient W.S., 1 h after an oral dose of 125 mg at a time when her serum bilirubin was normal. The titre was less in patient G.K., when his serum bilirubin was slightly raised, but it was still within the range found in normal subjects given an equivalent body weight dose of azathioprine (Bach & Dardenne 1969). However,

TABLE 1. Levels of immunosuppressive activity in serum after oral administration of azathioprine to three patients with a liver transplant

	Serum bilirubin (mg/100 ml)	Azathioprine (mg)	Serum immunosuppressive activity 1 h later (titre)
W.S.	0·8	125	1/128
G.K.	3·5	125	1/64
B.P.	12·3	25	1/4
Control serum			1/2–1/4

in patient BP a 3-year-old boy with an auxiliary graft, who had a higher serum bilirubin there was no significant immunosuppressive activity in the serum, the titre being the same as that of control serum. It would appear that the levels of immunosuppressive activity in the serum were related to liver function in these three patients. In one patient S.G. in whom the levels have been estimated daily, 1 h after the oral dose of the drug had been given, there was also a close relationship between liver function and

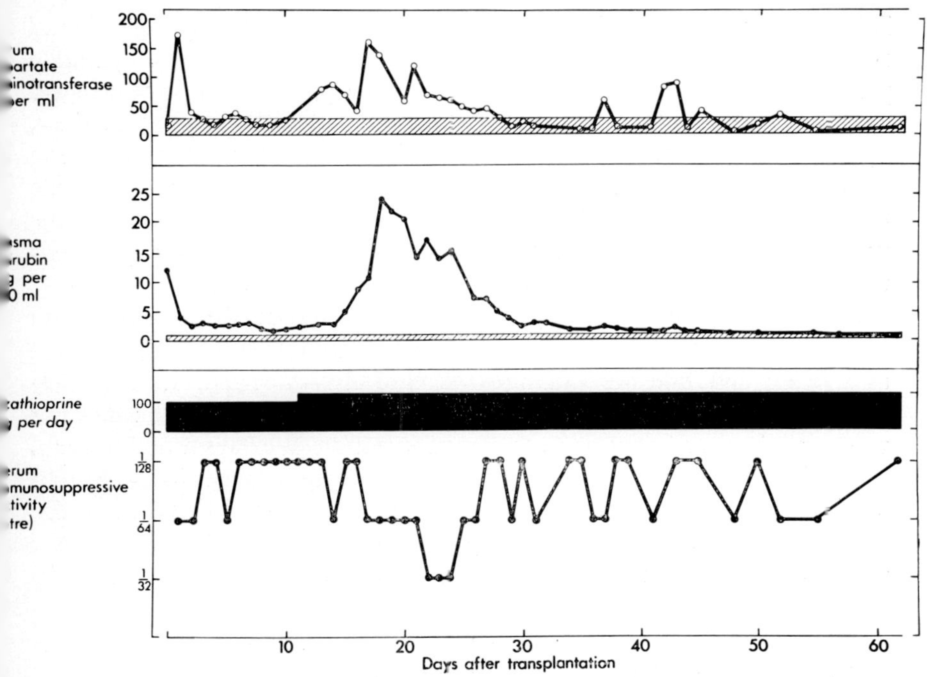

FIG. 4. The correlation between level of immunosuppressive activity in serum due to azathioprine and changes of liver function in Case SG (from Mitchell *et al* (1970)).

immunosuppressive activity in the serum (Fig. 4). An early episode of impaired liver function due to problems with biliary drainage was associated with a moderate fall in serum immunosuppressive activity which was reversed when liver function improved.

Bach & Dardenne (1969) stress that the exact metabolite responsible for the immunosuppressive activity of azathioprine is not known, although its formation is clearly dependent on adequate liver function. There is also some evidence to suggest that the metabolite responsible for the toxic effect of azathioprine upon the marrow is different from that responsible for immunosuppressive activity. Thus we are in a situation where continuation of azathioprine in a patient with impaired liver function due to rejection will expose him to all the hazards of this therapy with none of its benefits. This would be in accord with our own clinical observations and those of Starzl that azathioprine appears to be of little value in either acute or chronic episodes of rejection once they have developed.

INFECTIVE COMPLICATIONS

Infection is a major problem following liver transplantation (Fulginiti *et al* 1968). Of our nine patients who survived the immediate post-operative period six later died of infection, and we have reported the microbiological details of these patients (Murray-Lyon *et al* 1970). Because of debility, cytotoxic therapy or previous surgery some of the patients undergoing operation already have significant infection, and every effort must be made to identify and clear such foci before transplantation proceeds. During the post-operative course careful screening must be continued, for infections tend to become rapidly generalized.

Swabs should be obtained pre-operatively from nose, throat and rectum and mid-stream urine and blood cultures are taken. Other specimens such as sputum and bile are examined as clinically indicated. In the post-operative period the same specimens are cultured at least three times per week even in the absence of overt clinical infection. We have found it useful to tabulate this data in flow charts so that significant changes in the pattern of the flora or its antibiotic sensitivity may be detected early. It is also helpful to examine sera regularly for antibodies against different viruses and to culture fresh urine for cytomegalovirus. Regular chest radiographs should be taken.

Patterns of infection

Patients with carcinoma of the extrahepatic biliary tree, particularly those who have had previous surgery, are liable to have biliary infection prior to transplantation. One of our two patients with carcinoma of the hepatic duct had had a T-tube inserted through the growth at laparotomy 3½ months before transplantation, and a pocket of pus was found in the hilum of the liver at the second operation. Following transplantation this patient had persistant abdominal sepsis which later led to his death. We think that an intensive course of antibiotics effective against gram-negative bacteria (e.g. cephaloridine, kanamycin, gentamicin) should be given before and 2 weeks following transplantation in an attempt to eradicate such infection. Bile should be obtained for culture and sensitivity of the organisms at the time of laparotomy. However, known pre-existing infection is a relative contraindication to liver grafting.

Of the nine patients who had survived the immediate post-operative period at the time of writing four had biliary drainage effected by a choledochodochostomy, a T-tube being left in to support the anastomosis. In three of these patients bile samples regularly contained numerous faecal type organisms usually unaccompanied by inflammatory cells and in none of them was there clinical evidence of cholangitis. Attempts to eradicate these organisms were unsuccessful and often led to colonization with a resistant flora. This use of antibiotics was thought on several occasions to have contributed to the development of serious infection in other sites.

In two of the three patients whose death was due to major abdominal sepsis (Table 2) there was separation of the biliary anastomosis with the development of a biliary fistula. This is a serious complication for it makes eradication of infection virtually impossible.

Biliary drainage by a cholecyst-dochostomy, which preserves the sphincter of Oddi, may protect the patient to some extent from biliary infection although episodes have occurred in two of our patients with this anastomosis.

Septic liver infarction has been discussed already.

Chest infections occurred in eight of our nine patients and were the cause of death in two (Table 2). In one patient fulminating bacterial

TABLE 2. Predisposing factors of the major infections which led to death of six patients

	No. of cases	Predisposing factors
Fungal meningitis	1	Chronic rejection Heavy immunosuppression
Biliary and abdominal sepsis	3	Previous surgery of chemotherapy Biliary fistula
Chest infections	2	Broad spectrum antibiotics Influenza A infection

and fungal pneumonia followed an influenza A virus infection and in the other *Aspergillus fumigatus* pneumonia followed a trivial upper respiratory infection which developed while the patient was at home. Staphylococcal pneumonia developed in four cases and in each case the patient was shown to be a nasal carrier. Pneumonias with gram-positive organisms were rare in Starzl's experience. We have not found any infection with *Pneumocystis carinii*.

Six of the nine patients had bacteriaemia from time to time. Although on occasion these were clinically related to pulmonary and other infection, some were entirely asymptomatic and unattended by pyrexia or leucocytosis.

Oral thrush followed broad spectrum antibiotic therapy in five of our patients and three of these developed *Candida albicans* pneumonia and one systemic candidiasis. The patient who developed *Aspergillus fumigatus* pneumonia had had several prolonged courses of broad spectrum antibiotics in an attempt to clear his bile of organisms. The patient who died at 4½ months with fungal meningitis (Table 2) was the only patient in the series to have developed chronic rejection, and the fungal infection can be regarded as a direct result of the heavy immunosuppression with which he was treated.

Cytomegalovirus complement fixing antibody titres were shown to rise four-fold or more following transplantation in five cases and virus was isolated from the urine in two of these (Table 3). In a further case there was

TABLE 3. Antibody titre to cytomegalovirus serum (the tests were kindly carried out by Dr H.Stern)

Case	Pre-operative	Highest
4*	<8	1024
3	16	64
7	64	128
9*	256	1024
10	16	64
12	64	512

* Also had viruria.

histological evidence of its presence in liver biopsy or lung tissue at autopsy. Five of these patients were considered to have reactivation of latent cytomegalo virus infection because there were significant antibody levels before or immediately following transplantation. Case 4 was a primary infection probably derived from the blood (22 l.) given at operation. Although the cytomegalo virus can cause hepatitis (Toghill *et al* 1967), there was no evidence that these infections caused significant damage to the liver or other organs. Other viruses such as the influenza virus may be important in initiating serious secondary infection.

Treatment

Attention should be paid to minimizing the tendency to infection by keeping immunosuppressive therapy to a minimum. Leucopenia should be particularly avoided. Diabetes mellitus, which was precipitated by corticosteroid therapy in two of our patients, must be carefully controlled.

We have noted that nasal carriers of *Staphylococcus aureus* are particularly liable to develop staphylococcal pulmonary infections. In some cases phage typing has shown organisms of the same type at both sites. Nasal chemoprophlaxis with naseptin may be tried, although there is no proof of its efficacy (Williams *et al* 1966).

Prophylactic antibiotic therapy is now usually considered ineffective in general surgical practice and may, indeed be harmful for it encourages colonization of the body by resistant organisms and fungi (Williams *et al* 1966). We have not used antibiotics prophylactically but in our early cases broad spectrum antibiotics were used freely for minor infections and serious bacterial and fungal infections followed in some of these patients. The use of antibiotics to clear infection prior to transplantation has been mentioned. It is now our practice to use antibiotics sparingly and to rely on narrow spectrum drugs wherever possible guided by the *in vitro* sensitivity tests. If a broad spectrum drug or drug combination is started while the results of cultures are awaited, a change to a narrow spectrum drug is made subsequently. We do not now feel it is necessary or desirable to treat patients with asymptomatic bacteriaemias or colonization of bile obtained from T-tube drainage with antibiotics, although their progress must be carefully watched. In contrast Starzl uses broad spectrum antibiotic therapy for some weeks from the time of operation and frequent changes in the regime are made on the basis of the changing flora in multiple culture sites (Fulginiti *et al* 1968). In some patients pre-operative bowel sterilization has been attempted.

Serious infection in patients after hepatic transplantation can be asymptomatic and in one of our patients a lung abscess was found on a routine chest radiograph. This emphasizes the importance of regular screening for infection so that it is detected and treated early.

REFERENCES

BACH J.F. & DARDENNE M. (1970) The metabolism of axathioprine in renal and hepatic failure. *Proceedings of Nephrology Congress, Stockholm* 1969 (in press).

BACH J.F., DARDENNE M. & FOURNIER C. (1969) *In vitro* evaluation of immunosuppressive drugs. *Nature*, **222**, 989.

EDDLESTON A.L.W.F., WILLIAMS R. & CALNE R.Y. (1969) Cellular immune response during rejection of a liver transplant in man. *Nature, Lond.* **223**, 674.

EDDLESTON A.L.W.F., SMITH M.G.M., MITCHELL C.G. & WILLIAMS R. (1971) Application of the leucocyte migration test to the diagnosis of rejection after liver transplantation (in press).

FULGINITI V.A. *et al* (1968) Infections in recipients of liver homografts. *New Engl. J. Med.* **279**, 619.

GROGAN J.B. & SHIVERS B.J. (1969) Allograft survival after treatment with antilymphocyte serum combined with immunosuppressive drugs. *Surgery*, **66**, 1085.

MURRAY J.E. *et al* (1964) Analysis of mechanism of immunosuppressive drugs in renal homotransplantation. *Ann. Surg.* **160**, 449.

MURRAY-LYON I.M. *et al* (1970) Liver transplantation in man. The significance, patterns and control of infection. *Br. J. Surg.* **57**, 280.

SMITH M.G.M. *et al* (1969) Changes in leucocyte migration after renal transplantation. *Br. Med. J.* iv, 275.

SØBORG M. & BENDIXEN G. (1967) Human lymphocyte migration as a parameter of hypersensitivity. *Acta Med. Scand.* **181**, 247.

SØBORG M. (1968) *In vitro* migration of peripheral human leucocytes in cellular hypersensitivity. *Acta Med. Scand.* **184**, 135.

STARZL T.E. (1969) *Experience in Hepatic Transplantation*. Philadelphia, London, Toronto: W.B.Saunders.

TOGHILL P.J., BAILEY M.E., WILLIAMS R., ZEEGEN R. & BOWN R. (1967) Cytomegalovirus hepatitis in the adult. *Lancet*, i, 1351.

WILLIAMS R.E.O., BLOWERS R., GARROD L.P. & SHOOTER R.A. (1966) *Hospital Infection. Causes and Prevention*, 2nd edition, pp. 106, 174–6. London: Lloyd-Luke.

CHAPTER 28

The Pathology of Liver Transplants

B.M. Herbertson,
P.R. Millard and
I.D. Ansell

I. INTRODUCTION

Following prolonged laboratory studies Starzl in 1963 performed the first human liver transplant (Starzl *et al* 1963) and so initiated the largest series of such operations to date (Starzl & Putnam 1969). Progress has inevitably been slow due to problems of organ procurement and preservation, operative techniques and post-operative management. In this chapter a relatively small amount of our own material is considered and this has been evaluated by comparison with the morphological studies of Porter on Starzl's patients (Starzl & Putnam 1969; Porter 1969b) and with personal experience gained in renal transplantation pathology. The various factors that may affect the morphology of the liver graft are first discussed and then the morphological features of these grafts presented.

II. FACTORS AFFECTING THE LIVER GRAFT

1 Immune rejection

Once some of the technical problems of experimental liver transplantation had been solved it became apparent both in dogs (Starzl *et al* 1965) and in pigs (Calne *et al* 1967) that immune rejection even in the absence of immunosuppression was often more indolent than that of renal allografts. Nevertheless in those dogs not given immunosuppression and in which early rejection episodes occurred Porter (1969a) was able to follow a sequence of events clearly different from those in canine autografts (McBride *et al* 1962; Stuart *et al* 1967) which culminated in the destruction of the graft. Mononuclear cells, principally lymphocytes, but later some plasma cells, appeared around portal veins and later around central veins and in scattered foci throughout the liver lobule. These cells often contained IgG but rarely IgM or components of complement. Electron microscopy demonstrated the migration of these mononuclear cells from the lumen of portal veins and sinusoids, often accompanied by deposits of fibrin in subendothelial spaces of the veins. Within a few days the cellular infiltrate increased and there was progressive destruction of hepatic cells, initially in centrilobular zones and then spreading to periportal regions.

Accompanying these changes there was centrilobular intrahepatic bile stasis and enlargement of Kupffer cells but rarely were arterial lesions observed. Fibrinoid necrosis occurred in less than 25% of all the livers examined. A similar pattern of reaction may occur in pigs (Hunt 1967), rats (Lee & Edgington 1968) and primates (Calne *et al* 1970). However, in pigs immune rejection is generally much less severe and the principal features are a slight increase in fibrous tissue in portal tracts and interlobular septa associated with a slight mononuclear cell infiltrate in these areas. Provided the biliary drainage is adequate (using a choledocho-dochostomy) liver cell necrosis, cholangitis and vascular changes do not occur even after a period of years. Using varying immunosuppressive regimens Starzl *et al* (1965) were able to delay the rejection process in dogs. The effect on morphology in some livers was atrophy of centrilobular liver cells and collapse of the reticulin in these regions with replacement by fibrous tissue and an associated mononuclear cell infiltrate in portal tracts. On occasion some central veins were linked by bands of fibrous tissue and regeneration nodules formed. From these experimental studies it was clear that immune rejection occurred and that its course was unpredictable and its severity less than that of renal allograft rejection. In part these results could be due to chance histocompatibility antigen matches but the work of Calne *et al* (1969) suggests that certainly for pigs other mechanisms are also involved.

Clinical liver transplantation has resulted in similar morphologic observations. Immune rejection in immunosuppressed patients appears to be a low-grade process and in orthotopic grafts severe episodes with resulting fibrinoid necrosis of arteries have not been reported. Also complete cessation of immunosuppression during severe infections has not resulted in acute rejection of the graft and in two patients rapid rejection of a second hepatic allograft did not occur (Starzl & Putnam 1969). Further the immediate rejection seen in presensitized recipients of kidney grafts has not to date been reported. However, severe rejection developing within 7 days of transplantation has been reported in one patient in whom immunosuppressive treatment consisted only of low doses of steroids (Williams 1970).

2 Orthotopic or auxiliary graft

Due to the present lack of adequate artificial supportive measures an individual cannot survive more than a few hours in an anhepatic state. Thus, if the orthotopic position is the site of choice the transplant must function immediately for survival to occur. The complexity and siting of the vascular anastomoses, however, make this technically a very exacting surgical procedure. Theoretically, therefore, the accessory position appears more favourable, leaving the patient's own liver in place so that any remaining function may tide the patient through the immediate post-operative phase and any rejection crises. However, early experience using dogs showed that this unphysiological position was not compatible with normal liver function. Marchioro *et al* (1965) demonstrated in dogs that the auxiliary liver and the animal's own liver appeared to compete with one another, resulting in rapid atrophy of the graft. If, however, the auxiliary liver was provided with an adequate blood supply direct from the small bowel this shrinkage was delayed and function could be expected. Unfortunately in clinical practice further complications associated with the sheer size of the accessory organ, in securely anchoring the graft and in maintaining the patency of the vascular anastomoses have so far mitigated against the theoretical advantages of the auxiliary graft.

3 Ischaemia

The vulnerability of the liver to ischaemia and the morphological and functional consequences are well recognized. Apart from the ischaemia during the transplantation procedure the donor liver may well be relatively ischaemic prior to the death of the donor. By utilizing the preservation techniques discussed in Chapter 3 the surgeon aims to reduce the effects of ischaemia during the transplantation phase. However, despite these measures some biopsies taken from the liver immediately after revascularization show scattered foci of degenerate or necrotic liver cells. Provided well preserved liver cells are also present these appearances are not incompatible with good liver function. On the other hand, biopsy specimens at this time showing widespread liver cell degeneration and liver cell necrosis have generally correlated with a bad prognosis.

After revascularization further ischaemic injury may occur if the blood flow is impaired due to hypotension or vascular obstruction. Thrombosis and kinking of the hepatic artery or its main branches has occurred and results in infarction of liver tissue (Starzl & Putnam 1969). The role of immune rejection and ischaemia in renal transplants is discussed by Retik *et al* (1967). They demonstrated intrarenal arterial spasm with redistribution of blood in canine renal allografts during rejection episodes. It is probable that similar changes occur in arteries within hepatic allografts during rejection episodes resulting in ischaemic injury to the graft. Starzl & Putnam (1969) also suggest that a venous outflow block may occur in acute rejection episodes. Chronic immune rejection in contrast can result in severe intraluminal narrowing of arteries with consequent reduction in blood flow to the tissues and inevitable ischaemia.

4 Regeneration

The substantial regenerative capacity of an animal's own liver has long been recognized and the factors affecting liver cell proliferation extensively studied. Lee & Edgington (1968) have recently shown that similar regeneration can occur in the transplanted liver of the rat and have demonstrated the importance of an adequate blood supply.

Experience following partial hepatectomy in man shows liver cell regeneration with normal morphology can be expected (McDermott 1965). The transplanted liver is inevitably submitted to a wide range of potentially harmful factors including ischaemia, hepatotoxic drugs and immune rejection. Any of these may result in focal or widespread injury to liver cells which will probably be followed by attempts at regeneration with or without alteration in the gross liver structure. Further, regeneration may be modified either by the presence of the cytotoxic drugs used for immunosuppression or by complications at the vascular and/or biliary anastomoses.

5 Infection

The marked susceptibility of patients with liver grafts to severe bacterial, fungal and viral infections was reported by Fulginiti *et al* (1968), and is discussed elsewhere. Starzl & Putnam (1969) suggest that this is associated with a deficiency in the presumed normal 'filtering' effect of the liver following its transplantation. Alternatively, since most liver donors have been maintained on respirators, the source of infection may well be the donor, the infection being transmitted within the transplant. However, whatever the exact mechanism may be any complication of the biliary anastomosis is closely correlated with both systemic and graft infection (Murray-Lyon *et al* 1970). The graft is particularly prone to infection if infarcts are present, resulting in bacterial and fungal abscesses.

The role of virus infection and its effect on morphology of the graft is at present difficult to establish. Cytomegalovirus inclusions have been recognized within cells in hepatic allografts and instances of this virus causing hepatitis in untransplanted patients have been reported (Toghill *et al* 1967). Other virus infections may occur and include serum hepatitis transmitted either by the transplant or via blood. With all types of virus infection, however, the morphological changes are rarely diagnostic and similar features may be produced by a variety of other hepatotoxic agents (Weinbren 1966; Zuckerman 1970).

6 Surgical complications

The complexity of the surgical procedure, whether orthotopic or heterotopic, has been considered elsewhere. Thrombosis and narrowing of the hepatic artery or one of its main branches has been the commonest complication to the vascular anastomoses. This may result either from trauma to the artery during the operation or from kinking. The kinking may be due to too long a segment of artery or to insufficient anchoring of the graft so allowing displacement of the liver and bending of the artery over adjacent structures (Starzl & Putnam 1969). However, provided partial or total obstruction to the arterial flow is not an early post-operative event and collaterals have developed, arterial obstruction may be compatible with long-term survival. The main hepatic artery was occluded by thrombus in a patient dying from carcinomatosis 400 days after transplantation, the liver being largely replaced by tumour but not infarcted and in another patient, alive at that time, stenosis of this artery was demonstrated by arteriography 14 months post-operatively (Starzl & Putnam 1969). Thrombus formation in the main venous and portal vessels is uncommon in orthotopic livers but may occur in auxiliary livers, particularly in children. This probably reflects the difficulty of anastomosing these very small vessels without kinking or twisting occurring post-operatively.

Surgical complications associated with the biliary anastomosis have been common and very often lethal to the patient. They include leakage of bile, complete breakdown of the anastomosis and gangrene of the gall bladder. All of these seem to increase the patient's susceptibility to infection, both systemically and in any infarcts within the graft. Ascending cholangitis may also follow any of these complications and, if chronic, will result in increased portal tract fibrous connective tissue and a variable inflammatory cell infiltrate.

7 Drugs and immunosuppression

The potential variety of morphological consequences of some drugs on the liver are reviewed by Weinbren (1966), and their functional effects by Sherlock (1968). The patient with a liver transplant receives a wide range of drugs some of which may be hepatotoxic. The anaesthetic agents and their potential hepatotoxicity are discussed elsewhere. The methods used for immunosuppression have evolved from those successful in renal transplantation. These include corticosteroids, azathioprine, actinomycin C and antilymphocytic serum. All of these agents are toxic but azathioprine is also hepatotoxic. Stuart *et al* (1967) using normal dogs demonstrated the development of foci of hepatic necrosis associated with a slight localized mononuclear cell infiltrate following the administration of azathioprine. The severity of these lesions was increased with higher doses of the drug. Similarly, lesions occur in the livers of many patients with renal transplants and are associated with hepatic dysfunction (Evans *et al* 1968; Penn *et al* 1969). However, before concluding that these features are due to azathioprine it is important to remember that the morphological picture is not specific to this drug. Similar appearances occur with other hepatotoxic drugs and many forms of virus hepatitis (Zuckerman 1970). Any patient with a liver transplant may be subjected to either of these forms of injury and both may play a role in the pathogenesis of any morphologic changes in the transplanted liver.

8 Nature of original disorder

Liver cell carcinoma, cholangiocarcinoma and biliary atresia have been the commonest reasons for liver transplantation. In contrast portal cirrhosis, primary biliary cirrhosis and viral hepatitis have been the indications in only a minority of cases. In the future this emphasis may well be reversed since preliminary experience suggests that this form of treatment for primary liver tumours may often be palliative. All four of Starzl's long-term survivors given transplants for primary hepatomas developed widespread metastases following operation and in all cases the metastases appeared more anaplastic than the primary growth. None of these patients appeared to have secondary deposits at the time of operation but a careful search at autopsy for metastases in seven short-term survivors revealed unsuspected tumour deposits in one patient (Starzl & Putnam 1969). Similarly in three of six patients with a primary cholangiocarcinoma residual tumour was found at autopsy (Calne & Williams 1970).

The possibility of transmission of viral hepatitis from the recipient to the transplant is self-evident.

III. MORPHOLOGY

A Orthotopic grafts

Of the 15 orthotopic hepatic grafts examined five were from patients who died within 24 h of operation. In the livers of these five patients foci of liver cell necrosis and degeneration associated with congestion were the principal changes. The necrotic foci were often centrilobular and the liver cell damage most probably reflects ischaemic injury. In contrast the livers of the ten longer survivors together showed a wide range of changes. The macroscopic and microscopic appearances of these ten livers are outlined below and some of their features summarized in Table 1.

1 *Macroscopic appearances*

Most livers were firm, deep green to greenish-brown in colour and of approximately normal size and weight. Adhesions, fibrinous or fibrous,

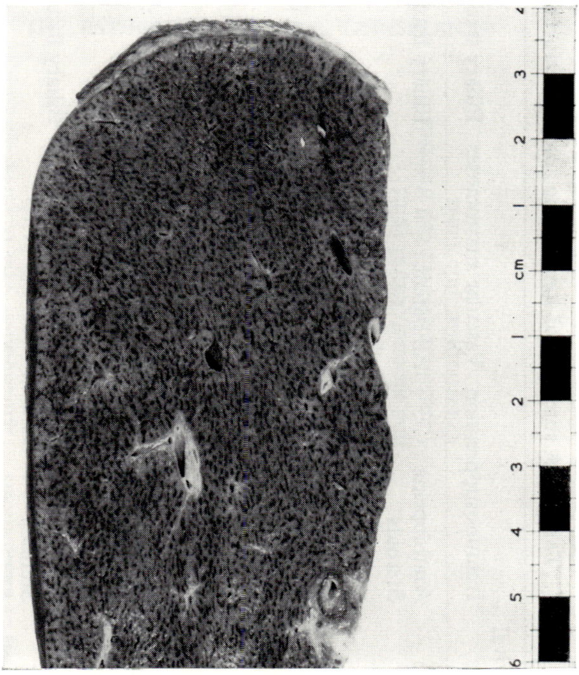

FIG. 1. Liver 22 days after transplantation (Table 1, case 8). Marked centrilobular bile-staining with fibrous adhesions over part of Glisson's capsule. ×0·85.

6	49	Azathioprine Steroids ALG
7	22	Azathioprine Steroids ALG
8	22	Azathioprine
9	7	Azathioprine Steroids
10	7	Steroids

...thotopic liver transplants

	Principal microscopic features
	Centrilobular liver cell necrosis Centrilobular bile stasis Slight increase in portal tract fibrous tissue
	Severe arterial narrowing Moderate fibrous tissue increase in portal tracts and around central veins Centrilobular liver cell necrosis and centrilobular bile stasis
...dder	Large foci of liver cell necrosis with bacterial and fungal infection Ascending cholangitis
	Centrilobular liver cell degeneration Centrilobular bile stasis Slight mononuclear cell infiltrate in portal tracts
	Centrilobular bile stasis Slight mononuclear cell infiltrate in portal tracts

were invariably present on the outer surface binding the liver to surrounding structures. The cut surfaces were deeply bile stained and this was often most prominent in the centres of the lobules (Fig. 1). In some livers there was considerable centrilobular congestion. The liver of one patient (Table 1, case 3) contained bile stained infarcts of variable size in all lobes separated

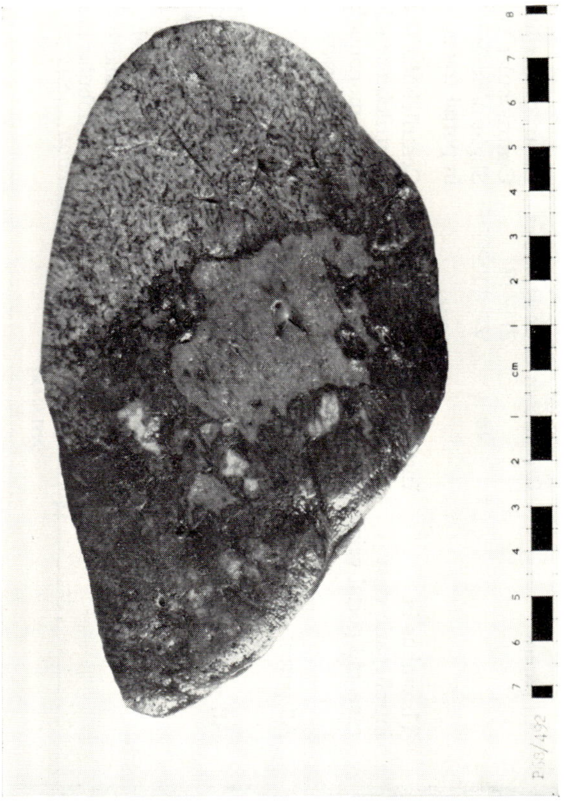

FIG. 2. Liver 78 days after transplantation (Table 1, case 3). Large infarct in centre with congestion of lower two-thirds of the specimen. Thrombus was present in the main hepatic artery. ×0·6.

by large areas of surviving liver tissue (Figs. 2 and 3). Organizing thrombus was present in the main hepatic artery and some of the infarcts were infected. The liver of a patient who survived 336 days (Table 1, case 1) contained two small abscesses but was otherwise unremarkable. Intrahepatic vessels appeared macroscopically normal except in one case (Table 1, case 2). In this liver many intrahepatic arteries were thickened

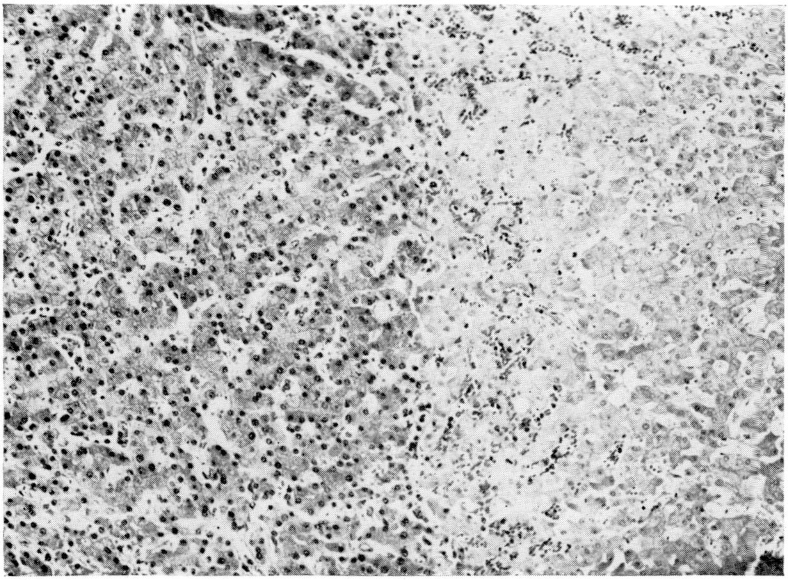

FIG. 3. Liver 78 days after transplantation (Table 1, case 3). Photomicrograph of liver in Fig. 2. Surviving liver tissue adjacent to infarct. No mononuclear cell infiltrate is present in either area. H.E. × 100.

and a bright orange-yellow. The biliary drainage of most livers was defective and a summary of the abnormalities present at autopsy is included in Table 1.

2 *Microscopic appearances*

The principal microscopic changes at autopsy of the ten allografts are shown in Table 1. Similar appearances were also seen in some biopsy specimens. In both types of specimen the changes included a mononuclear cell infiltrate, cholestasis, arterial lesions, an increase in fibrous connective tissue, and degeneration and necrosis of liver cells.

The mononuclear cell infiltrate included lymphocytes, plasma cells and macrophages. Some of these mononuclear cells were pyroninophilic. A few eosinophil polymorphs were also present. The cells were generally confined to portal tracts, occasionally appearing around central veins but rarely spreading into the liver lobules. The infiltrate, particularly in biopsy specimens, was slight and associated with centrilobular cholestasis and centrilobular liver cell degeneration. These appearances were seen at variable times after transplantation but in case 10 (Table 1), a patient

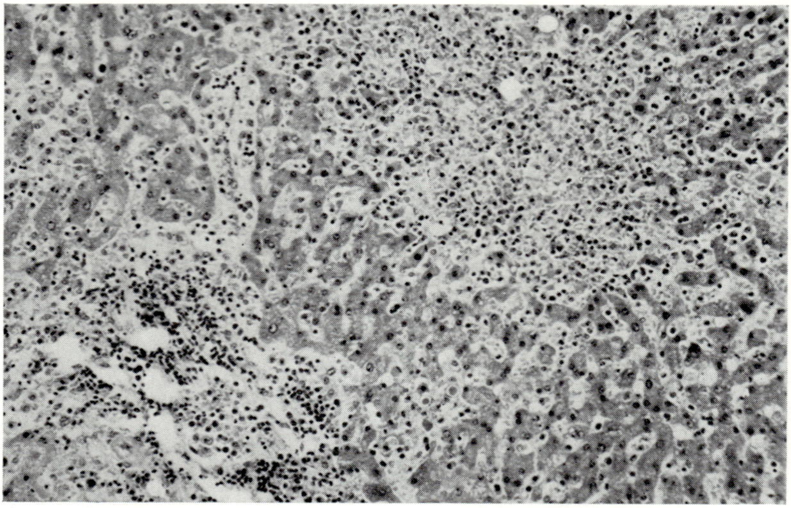

FIG. 4. Liver 7 days after transplantation (Table 1, case 10). Moderate numbers of mononuclear cells in the portal tract with large and small foci of liver cell necrosis in periportal and centrilobular regions. H.E. ×115.

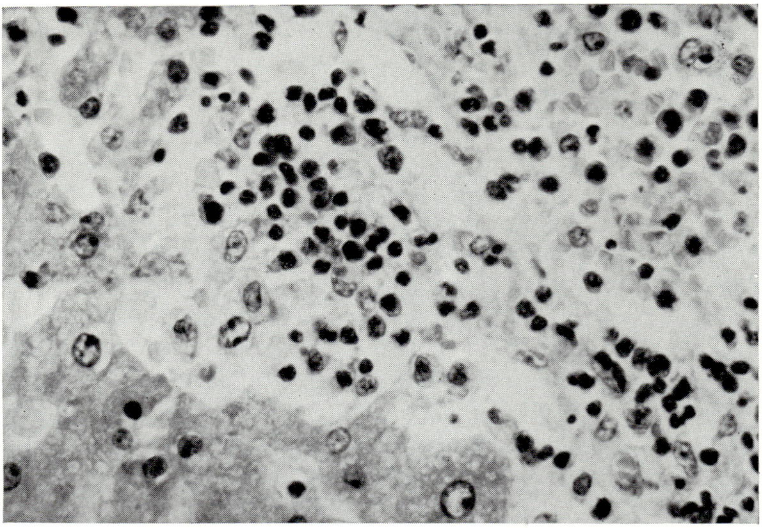

FIG. 5. Liver 7 days after transplantation (Table 1, case 10). Higher power of portal tract of liver in Fig. 4. The cells include large and small mononuclear cells. Many cells were pyroninophilic. H.E. ×450.

receiving only minimal doses of steroids, occurred within 7 days of operation. The cellular infiltrate in this liver was substantial, and associated with wide spread liver cell necrosis (Figs. 4 and 5). The changes in this case are probably due to acute rejection and are similar to those seen in the 10-day graft examined by Porter (1969a), except that no cholestasis occurred in Porter's case. Centrilobular cholestasis is a frequent finding both in autopsy and biopsy specimens. The latter have generally been performed as part of the investigation of persistent jaundice which has often regressed following increased immunosuppression. This observation, even though some of these patients had surgical complications of their biliary tract at the time of biopsy suggests that the cholestasis is at least partly due to immune rejection. The change, in most instances, was confined to the centrilobular regions and bile pigment was also present in liver and Kupffer cells (Figs. 6 and 7).

Rarely, even in biopsy specimens, were all liver cells normal. Generally some centrilobular cells were degenerate and occasionally necrotic. Foci of similar changes in other parts of liver lobules were sometimes observed but in some specimens from longer-term patients atrophy of centrilobular cells was also present. Electron migroscopy of centrilobular cells shows that the mitochondria are enlarged and that the rough endoplasmic reticulum is scanty and dilated. Microvilli are also absent from the sinusoidal borders of cells and several large microbodies were present. Glycogen may or may not be seen (Porter 1969a). Steiner *et al* (1965) record similar changes following other forms of liver cell injury. Pleomorphism of liver cells and increase in the number of cells in mitosis were infrequent findings. Kupffer cells were often enlarged and contained haemosiderin, lipofuscin and bile pigment. Porter (1969a) has made the interesting observation that the donor Kupffer cells were replaced by host cells in three long-term survivors.

Increase in fibrous connective tissue and arterial lesions were conspicuous only in case 2 (Table 1) while increased fibrous tissue alone occurred in case 1 and case 6 (Table 1). A moderate amount of fibrous tissue was seen in portal tracts and around central veins with some spread between the neighbouring liver cells. This tissue was infiltrated by a small number of mononuclear cells and some centrilobular liver cells were degenerate and necrotic. Centrilobular bile stasis was also present. Many small arteries in case 2 (Table 1) were markedly abnormal with their lumens substantially and concentrically narrowed by fat laden cells. Porter (1969a) has shown that these cells include endothelial cells and macrophages. In some of these vessels there were breaks in the internal elastic lamina and on either side of the lamina deposits of IgG and C1q of complement have been reported (Porter 1969a). Other arteries showed similar intimal changes but with loose

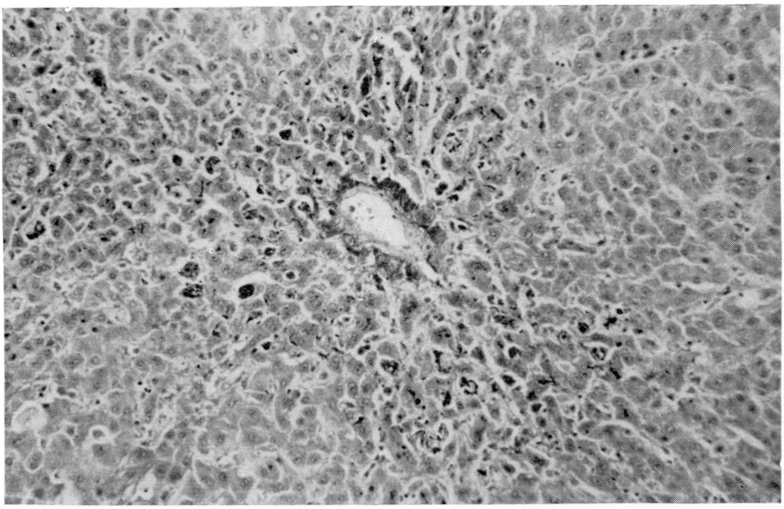

FIG. 6. Liver 141 days after transplantation (Table 1, case 2). Centrilobular vein with bile pigment in surrounding liver cells, Kupffer cells and in bile canaliculi. Slight increase in connective tissue in the wall of the vein. E.P.S. ×115.

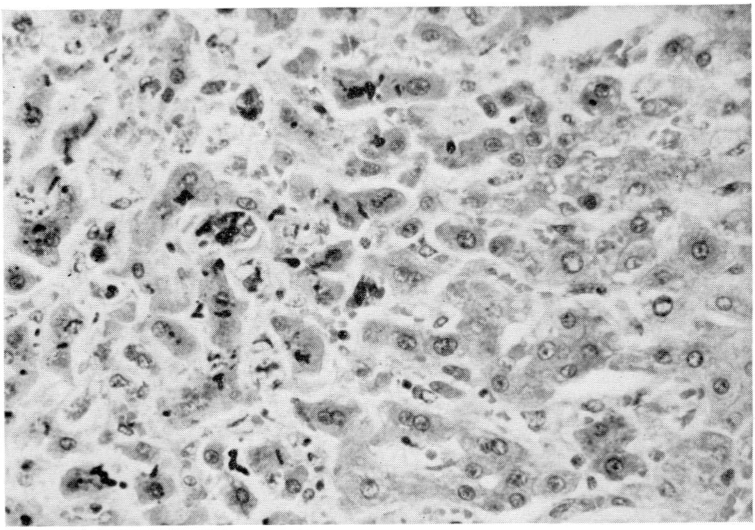

FIG. 7. Liver 141 days after transplantation (Table 1, case 2). Bile pigment in liver and Kupffer cells in the centrilobular region with bile 'thrombi' in some canaliculi. Atrophy of some centrilobular hepatic cells. Some adjacent mid-zonal liver cells are degenerate; others appear normal. H.E. ×275.

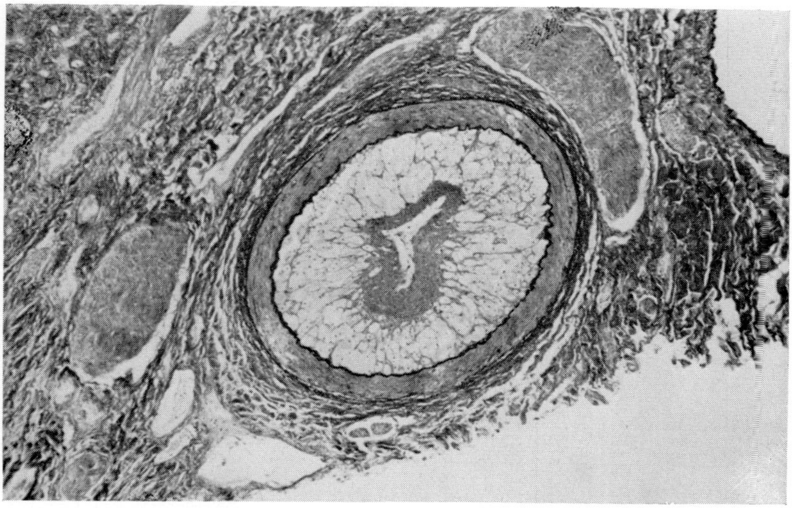

FIG. 8. Artery in liver 141 days after transplantation (Table 1, case 2). Severe narrowing of the lumen of an intrahepatic artery associated with thickening of the intima by fat-laden cells and fibrous connective tissue. Fat-laden cells are also present in parts of the media. The internal elastic lamina is intact. Moderate increase in surrounding connective tissue. E.P.S. ×45.

fibrous tissue separating the fat-laden cells from the lumen (Fig. 8). Alterations in the media often accompanied the intimal changes and included foci of fibrosis and small infiltrates of fat-filled cells. Both the intima and the media of these arteries were slightly infiltrated by mononuclear cells. No changes in portal veins or central veins accompanied these profound arterial appearances. Porter (1969a) reports similar arterial lesions in four cases, the change occurring as early as 68 days after transplantation. These features are seen in human renal transplants and they most probably represent a chronic immune rejection process.

B Auxiliary grafts

Of the four auxiliary livers personally examined only two were from patients surviving the immediate post-operative period. The changes seen in the two short-term survivors are probably entirely due to ischaemia. The principal morphological features of all four livers are summarized in Table 2. Macroscopically, the graft of both longer-term survivors was firm, deeply bile stained and probably swollen. The liver of the 19-day survivor,

TABLE 2. Summary of morphological features in auxiliary hepatic allografts

Case	Immunosuppression	Survival (days)	Vascular anastomoses	Principal morphological features
1	Steroids Azathioprine	34*	Hepatic artery and branches thrombosed at hilum and within liver	Profound loss of liver cells Fibrinoid necrosis and thrombosis of arteries Patchy, slight mononuclear cell infiltrate
2	Steroids Azathioprine	20	All patent	Centrilobular liver cell degeneration Centrilobular bile stasis
3	None	2	Hepatic vein thrombosed	Substantial liver cell necrosis
4	Steroids	1	All patent	Patchy necrosis and degeneration of liver cells Areas of haemorrhage

* Graft removed surgically at 34 days.

who died from pneumonia, showed microscopic features similar to those seen in some orthotopic liver transplants and probably represented an early phase of rejection. The profound liver cell loss and severe vascular changes in the liver removed after 34 days are probably consistent with severe rejection in spite of the presence of only a slight mononuclear cell infiltrate. A severe rejection episode of this type has not been seen in patients with orthotopic livers. This difference is possibly because the patient with an auxiliary liver is able to survive on the remaining function of his own liver so allowing the lesions to progress further than in orthotopic grafts. The features in these two livers are similar to the three auxiliary livers reviewed by Porter (1969b).

IV. CONCLUSIONS

The amount of material presented is small and great caution is needed before forming any firm conclusions. However, the morphological appearances in these grafts are similar to those reported by Porter (1969a) with the difference that in no patient has tumour recurred within the graft or cirrhosis developed. Should cirrhosis frequently complicate liver transplantation this will impose a severe limitation on the procedure. From comparison of the lesions in all of these human liver grafts with those seen in animal liver transplants and human renal allografts, it is apparent that immune rejection occurs. Even so the comparative rarity of arterial fibrinoid necrosis and of chronic obliterative vascular lesions, as well as the absence of immediate rejection, have so far served to distinguish the process from that of human renal allograft rejection. These differences suggest that the process in the liver is less severe, but more experience must be gained in order to evaluate this matter fully. One of the major problems to the patient with a liver transplant is infection. Modifications of the biliary anastomosis have partly contributed towards reducing this complication but the hypothesis that the ability of the transplanted liver to inactivate micro-organisms is inferior to that of the normal liver may be correct (Starzl & Putnam 1969).

REFERENCES

Calne R.Y., Davis D.R., Pena J.R., Balner H., de Vries M., Herbertson B.M., Joysey V.C., Millard P.R., Seaman M.J., Samuel J.R., Stibbe J. & Westbroek D.L. (1970) Hepatic allografts and xenografts in primates. *Lancet*, i, 103.

Calne R.Y., Sells R.A., Pena J.R., Davis D.R., Millard P.R., Herbertson B.M., Binns R.M. & Davis D.A.L. (1969) Induction of immunological tolerance by porcine liver allografts. *Nature, Lond.* **223**, 472.

CALNE R.Y., WHITE H.J.O., YOFFA D.E., BINNS R.M., MAGINN R.R., HERBERTSON B.M., MILLARD P.R., MOLINA V.P. & DAVIS D.R. (1967) Prolonged survival of liver transplants in the pig. *Br. med. J.* iv, 645.

CALNE R.Y. & WILLIAMS R. (1970) Personal communication.

EVANS D.B., MILLARD P.R. & HERBERTSON B.M. (1968) Hepatic dysfunction associated with renal transplantation. *Lancet*, ii, 929.

FULGINITI V.A., SCRIBNER R., GROTH C.G., PUTNAM C.W., BRETTSCHNEIDER L., GILBERT S., PORTER K.A. & STARZL T.E. (1968) Infections in recipients of liver homografts. *New Engl. J. Med.* **279**, 619.

HUNT A.C. (1967) Pathology of Liver Transplantation in the Pig. In *The Liver*, ed. READ A.E., p. 337. London: Butterworth.

LEE S. & EDGINGTON T.S. (1968) Heterotopic liver transplantation utilizing inbred rat strains. *Am. J. Path.* **52**, 649.

MCBRIDE R.A., WHEELER H.B., SMITH L.L., MOORE F.D. & DAMMIN G.J. (1962) Homotransplantation of the canine liver as an orthotopic vascularised graft. Histological and functional correlations during residence in the new host. *Am. J. Path.* **41**, 501.

MCDERMOTT W.V. (1965) Liver and Portal Circulation. In *The Scientific Basis of Surgery*, ed. IRVINE W.I., p. 101. Boston: Little, Brown.

MARCHIORO T.L., PORTER K.A., DICKINSON T.C., FARIS T.D. & STARZL T.E. (1965) Physiologic requirements for auxiliary liver homotransplantation. *Surg. Gynec. Obstet.* **121**, 17.

MURRAY-LYON I.M., EVANS D.B., FOSTER W.D., HOLDEN R.J., RAKE M.O., STERN H., CALNE R.Y. & WILLIAMS R. (1970). Liver transplantation in man: the significance, patterns and control of infection. *Br. J. Surg.* **57**, 280.

PENN I., HAMMOND W., BELL P., MCGUIRE R., HUTT M. & STARZL T.E. (1969) Hepatic Disorders in Renal Homograft Recipients. In *Current Topics in Surgical Research* Vol. I, p. 67.

PORTER K.A. (1969a) Pathology of the Orthotopic Homograft and Heterograft. In *Experience in Hepatic Transplantation*, ed. STARZL T.E. & PUTNAM C.W., p. 408. Philadelphia, London and Toronto: W.B.Saunders.

PORTER K.A. (1969b) Pathology of liver transplantation. *Transplantation Rev.* **2**, 129.

RETIK A.B., HOLLENBERG N.K., ROSEN S.M., MERRILL J.P. & MURRAY J.E. (1967) Cortical ischaemia in renal allograft rejection. *Surg. Gynec. Obstet.* **124**, 989.

SHERLOCK S. (1968) *Diseases of the Liver and Biliary System* 4th edition. Oxford & Edinburgh: Blackwell.

STARZL T.E., MARCHIORO T.L., VON KAULLA K.N., HERMANN G., BRITTAIN R.S. & WADDELL W.R. (1963) Homotransplantation of the liver in humans. *Surg. Gynec. Obstet.* **117**, 659.

STARZL T.E., MARCHIORO T.L., PORTER K.A., TAYLOR P.A., FARIS T.D., HERRMANN T.J., HLAD C.J. & WADDELL W.R. (1965) Factors determining short- and long-term survival after orthotopic liver transplantation in the dog. *Surg.* **58**, 131.

STARZL T.E. & PUTNAM C.W. (1969) *Experience in Hepatic Transplantation.* Philadelphia, London & Toronto: W.B.Saunders.

STEINER J.W., JEZEQUEL A., PHILLIPS M.J., MIYAI K. & ARAKAWA K. (1965) Some Aspects of the Ultrastructural Pathology of the Liver. In *Progress in Liver Diseases*. Volume II, ed. POPPER H. & SCHAFFNER F. London: Heinemann Medical Books.

STUART F.P., TORRES E., HESTER W.J., DAMMIN E.J. & MOORE F.D. (1967) Orthotopic autotransplantation and allotransplantation of the liver: functional and structural patterns in the dog. *Ann. Surg.* **165**, 325.

TOGHILL P.J., BAILEY M.E., WILLIAMS R., ZEEGAN R. & BROWN R. (1967) Cytomegalovirus hepatitis in the adult. *Lancet*, i, 1351.

WEINBREN K. (1966) Diseases of the Liver: the Effects of Hepatotoxic Agents. In *Recent Advances in Pathology* 8th edition, ed. HARRISON C.V., p. 197. London: J. & A.Churchill.

WILLIAMS R. (1970) Transplantation of the liver in man. *Br. med. J.* i, 585

ZUCKERMAN A.J. (1970) *Virus Diseases of the Liver*. London: Butterworths.

ACKNOWLEDGEMENTS

We wish to thank Mr L.Beard, Miss J.Fendick and Mr S.W.Patman for help with the illustrations.

CHAPTER 29

Results of Orthotopic Liver Transplantation

Roger Williams

The overall results when last reviewed (1 January 1971) in our 23 patients who have had an orthotopic transplant are given in Table 1.

Not surprisingly, for an operation of such magnitude carried out in such sick patients, the operative mortality is high. Seven of our 23 patients having an orthotopic transplant died during the operation or within the ensuing 6 days from a variety of technical and other complications. In one of these, a patient early in the series, death was probably due to rejection. This patient had cirrhosis following subacute hepatic necrosis and was not given immunosuppressive therapy because of the supposed risk of activating a presumed earlier infection with the hepatitis virus. Five others did not leave hospital and died between the 3rd and 10th week from infection.

Five patients were discharged home feeling well, fully ambulant and with excellent liver function. Two of these died of infection and one of tumour recurrence after survival periods of 3 to 8 months. One patient who had done extremely well, in the 11th month developed cholangitis and a gram-negative septicaemia from which he died. Three patients are alive at periods of 1 to 4 months since the transplant and another—our longest survivor—is doing extremely well in the 23rd month. Her history is given in more detail later in the chapter.

Analysis of the first 25 cases operated on by Starzl and his group between March 1963 and February 1969 gave a 1-year survival rate of 22%. If the seven patients done before July 1967 are excluded and this seems reasonable since at that time the hazards of ischaemic injury to the donor liver had not been fully realized and all the patients died in the immediate post-operative period, the 1-year survival figure becomes 33%. At the time of writing (1 April 1970) Starzl has six patients alive after an orthotopic transplant, five with biliary atresia, and one with Wilson's Disease. The longest survivor, a boy aged 3 years, at time of transplantation, with biliary atresia, is now in the 25th month after transplantation. Six of his patients have lived a year or more. These are the overall results of the two largest series. Other patients have had orthotopic liver transplants performed at various centres in the USA and in Europe but few details have been reported and none to our knowledge have survived more than 4 months.

RELATION TO TISSUE COMPATABILITY

It is difficult to evaluate the exact relation between tissue typing, the occurrence of rejection and long-term survival following liver transplantation. Many of Starzl's long-term survivors have died of metastases, and his immunosuppressive regime has changed considerably but in his series as a whole there would appear to be little correlation (Starzl 1969). One long-term survivor at 254 days and with normal function had a D match (two or more major mismatches in the Terasaki classification). Another patient in his series who had a Grade A match with complete conformity of all nine antigen groups tested, developed an irreversible rejection within 2 weeks which necessitated re-transplantation, 68 days after the first operation.

As shown in Table 1 one of our patients who survived $4\frac{1}{2}$ months and developed chronic rejection had three major mismatches. The other two, (one who lived 11 months and the other alive and well at 13 months after transplantation and with virtually normal liver function and histology), had a C match with one major mismatch. In a series of patients with

TABLE 1. Overall results in the 23 patients treated by an orthotopic transplantation (analysis on 1 January 1971)

Post operative and early deaths—12	6 died within 6 days 5 died in 3rd to 10th week
Longer survivors including those discharged home—11	6 died in 3rd to 6th month 1 died in 11th month 3 alive in 1st to 4th month 1 alive in 23th month

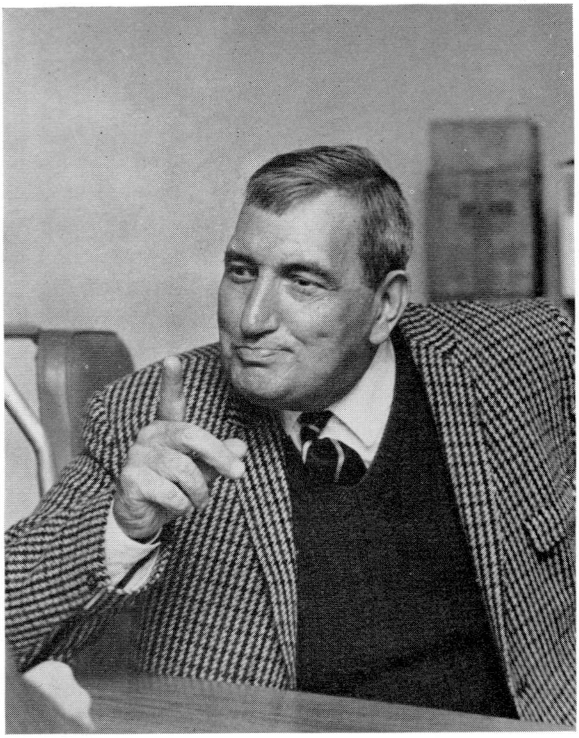

FIG. 1. Patient G.K.

kidney transplants, in whom crossmatching was done with the same antisera, there was a significant correlation between the results of tissue typing and the subsequent clinical status of the patient. Those with two or less major mismatches, like our two long surviving liver transplants, fared significantly better than those with three or more (Batchelor & Joysey 1969).

To achieve a close match it is necessary to have a large pool of recipients and there is no machine like the artificial kidney which will keep patients with advanced liver failure alive, until such times as a donor with the correct tissue type becomes available.

LIVER FUNCTION IN LONG TERM SURVIVORS AND RECURRENCE OF MALIGNANCY

One of our patients (G.K.), the man of 56 who developed chronic hepatic encephalopathy following a portacaval shunt, has already been referred to.

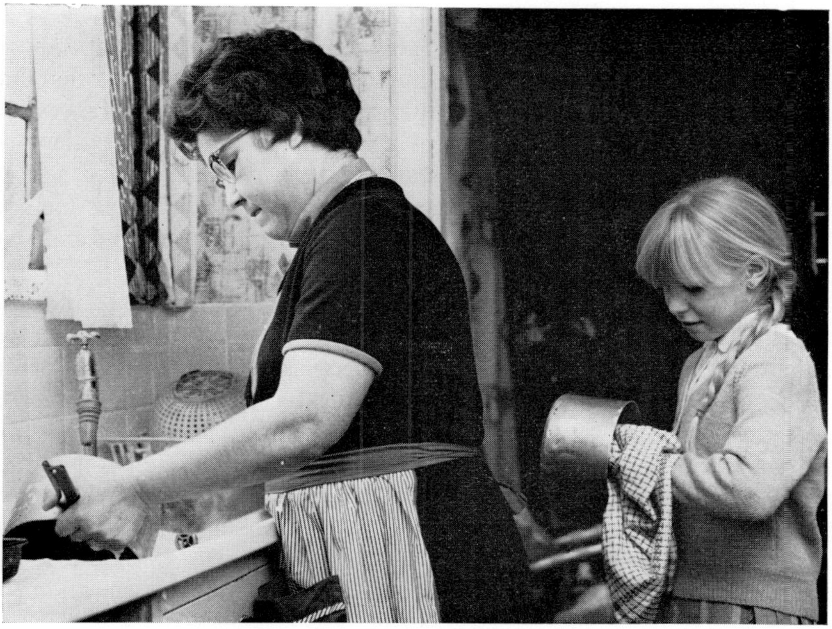

FIG. 2. Patient W.S.

Section of his liver after removal showed multiple nodules of a hepatoma in addition to the underlying cirrhosis. Following transplantation he did well signs of encephalopathy disappearing and he was able to take a normal diet for the first time for 5 years (Fig. 1). He died in the 11th month from a gram-negative septicaemia and at autopsy the liver was virtually normal histologically and there was no sign of recurrence in the graft. The only tumour tissue found was a small nodule in the right adrenal.

The other patient (W.S.), a woman of 44 who had a primary hepatoma, is well 13 months after transplantation. She is able to work as a domestic supervisor and look after her children; do her housework and shopping and

TABLE 2. Tissue typing results (Dr V.Joysey) in three patients surviving more than 3 months

Case	Course	Rejection	Major mismatches	Terasaki grade
J.J.	Died, 4½ months	Chronic	HLA1, HLA7, 4b	D
G.K.	Died, 11 months	Minimal	HLA7	C
W.S.	Alive, 23 months	Minimal	4a, ? HLA5	C

has been away on holiday (Fig. 2). The donor for this patient was a 4-year-old child, the victim of a road accident. The functional capacity of that liver was always adequate even immediately after transplantation and a recent liver biopsy showed virtually normal histological appearances.

The excellent synthetic capacity of the grafts in both these patients is shown by measurements of the albumin synthesis rate carried out in conjunction with Dr A.S.MacFarlane using the ^{14}C carbonate method (Rake *et al* 1970). For G.K. and W.S. the values in g/day, were 29·6 and 17·6 respectively, the normal range being 13·6–24·0.

All five patients in Starzl's series with malignant hepatic disease and who lived long enough to permit meaningful observations after what was thought to be complete excision of the neoplasm developed widespread recurrences. In two of our patients who died soon after the operation microscopic growth was found in remaining lymph nodes. It is possible that immunosuppression could cause a more rapid proliferation of the neoplastic tissue left behind than would otherwise have occurred. Nevertheless the results in our patients G.K. and W.S. show that worthwhile survival can be obtained. As in other types of malignant disease it is the chance of a cure or of worthwhile palliation which is the justification for major surgery.

At the time of writing Starzl has five patients alive after an orthotopic transplant, three with biliary atresia, one with chronic active hepatitis, and one with Wilson's disease. The longest survivor, a boy aged three years at the time of transplantation with biliary atresia, is now in the 31st month after transplantation. Nine of his patients have lived for a year or more.

REFERENCES

BATCHELOR J.R. & JOYSEY V.C. (1969) Influence of HL-A incompatability on cadaveric renal transplantation. *Lancet*, i, 790.

RAKE M.O., WILLIAMS R., FREEMAN T. & MCFARLANE A.S. (1970) Protein synthesis by the liver after transplantation. *Lancet*, ii, 341.

STARZL T.E. (1969) *Experience in Hepatic Transplantation*. Philadelphia, London, Toronto: W.B.Saunders.

Part 4
Heart Transplantation

CHAPTER 30

Cardiac Transplantation

Richard R. Lower

Although experience in the laboratory and with human patients has amply demonstrated that cardiac transplantation is technically and physiologically feasible, prolonged survival of patients has been rarely achieved because of the problems of acute and chronic rejection and the high incidence of infection attendant to the use of immunosuppressants. This chapter reviews the current status of cardiac transplantation and indicates the probable areas of future development. Experience is drawn by the author from operations in over 300 dogs and in five patients. At the time of this writing, 165 cardiac transplants have been performed throughout the world. Twenty-six of the patients are currently surviving for more than 1 year after operation and have served to demonstrate that it is indeed possible by this operation to achieve complete rehabilitation from the terminal stages of certain cardiac diseases which are untreatable by any other available technique.

SELECTION OF THE PATIENT FOR CARDIAC TRANSPLANTATION

No established guidelines exist for the selection of patients for cardiac transplantation. A decision in each case must be based on an assessment of the relative risks of the operation versus continued supportive medical therapy. Physicians and their patients will undoubtedly be influenced not only by the chances for longevity, but also by a consideration of the quality of the patient's existence. Patients who are completely bedridden with intractable congestive failure often will opt for a chance at rehabilitation no matter how slim. Likewise the patient who is in imminent danger of death from an acutely failing myocardium unresponsive to conventional therapy may justifiably take the extreme risk of transplantation—approximately 20–25% chance of survival to 1 year (Haller & Cerruti 1969).

There are at present insufficient data from the small number of transplants to relate ultimate prognosis to the underlying etiology of the patient's heart disease or to associated conditions, e.g. repeated myocardial infarction, cardiomyopathy, myocarditis, hyperlipidemia, diabetes, and pulmonary hypertension. Until significant data are achieved, it does not seem appropriate to consider any condition an absolute contra-indication to cardiac transplantation or to consider any patient 'too sick' for transplantation. In regard to congenital heart disease, it would appear that only two conditions are sufficiently hopeless or without other means of palliation to warrant transplantation, namely the hypoplastic left heart syndrome, and the terminal stages of endocardial fibroelastosis.

Patients with extensive coronary disease make up the largest reservoir of those in terminal heart failure. Yet it is in this group that there is the greatest difficulty in arriving at an accurate prognosis. Newer aggressive surgical approaches to patients with coronary insufficiency, including resection of aneurysms and akinetic areas of myocardium as well as revascularization procedures for ischemic areas, make the indication for transplantation less clear. It is perhaps justifiable in this group to employ transplantation only as a last resort in the dying patient for whom other surgical attempts have been unsuccessful.

SELECTION OF THE DONOR

The concept of brain death has now been quite generally accepted so that when an independent team of neurologists and neurosurgeons conclude that a patient has no spontaneous respirations, no reflexes, and no electroencephalographic evidence of brain activity, death of the patient has in fact occurred, despite the continued maintenance of cardiac activity by artificial ventilation (Alksne 1969). Such a patient is considered a potential cardiac donor if there is no evidence of cardiac disease or injury. The donor invariably requires support of the circulation by continuous intravenous infusion of catecholamines, and closed chest resuscitation is frequently necessary. However, neither of these conditions appears to preclude use of the heart for transplantation. Hearts which have required continuous infusion of catechol amines for several days and sustained repeated arrest have nevertheless recovered well after transplantation. Unsuspected coronary artery disease, congenital lesions or trauma in the donor heart must be excluded insofar as possible.

The problem of size disparity between donor and recipient requires further evaluation. Laboratory experience has shown that transplantation of donor hearts which are between one quarter and one fifth the size of the recipient heart can result in survival of the animal with adequate cardiac function. Acute rejection episodes may, however, be less well tolerated by such small hearts (Thomas *et al* 1970).

Donors and recipients must be compatible by ABO typing, and an attempt is made to minimize histo-incompatibility by prospective typing for HLA antigens (Terasaki *et al* 1969). Because of insufficient data, the relationship between degrees of mismatch with respect to the HLA antigens and the ultimate prognosis of the transplant is unclear. It would seem that with our increasing knowledge of the complexity of the histocompatibility antigens, precise matching is rarely, if ever, achieved. Patients who have had prior blood transfusions, pregnancy or other possible routes of sensitization must be shown *in vitro* to have no preformed antibodies to the lymphocytes of the donor.

Once a compatible donor has been obtained and certified to have complete brain death, every effort must be made to support the circulation of the donor until transplantation can be carried out. When the recipient is readied for cardiopulmonary bypass, the donor is heparinized and the heart is removed by severing the vena cavae, pulmonary veins and the aorta and pulmonary artery a short distance above the valves. The heart is immediately immersed in saline at 8 to 10°C. which results in cold arrest. Laboratory evidence indicates that the heart may be maintained at this temperature up to 4 h with little risk to its recovery after transplantation (Webb & Howard 1957; Lower *et al* 1962; Cleveland & Lower 1967). The donor heart is prepared for implantation by suture ligature of the superior vena cava and by incising the posterior wall of the left atrium between the openings of the pulmonary veins. For convenience the right atrium is not opened further until suture of the left atrium is complete (see below).

THE OPERATION

The patient is prepared as for any open cardiac procedure, using a median sternotomy. Anaesthesia does not differ from the management of other critically ill patients requiring cardiac surgery. Arterial cannulation for cardiopulmonary bypass is via the femoral artery or the ascending aorta. Venous cannulae are placed preferably through pursestring sutures in the lateral aspect of the right atrial wall rather than through peripheral veins. The ascending aorta is clamped and the heart elevated from the pericardial well. The heart is removed by incising the atrial walls and atrial septum leaving a remnant of atrium containing the openings of the cavae and pulmonary veins (Fig. 1) (Lower & Shumway 1960; Lower *et al* 1961b;

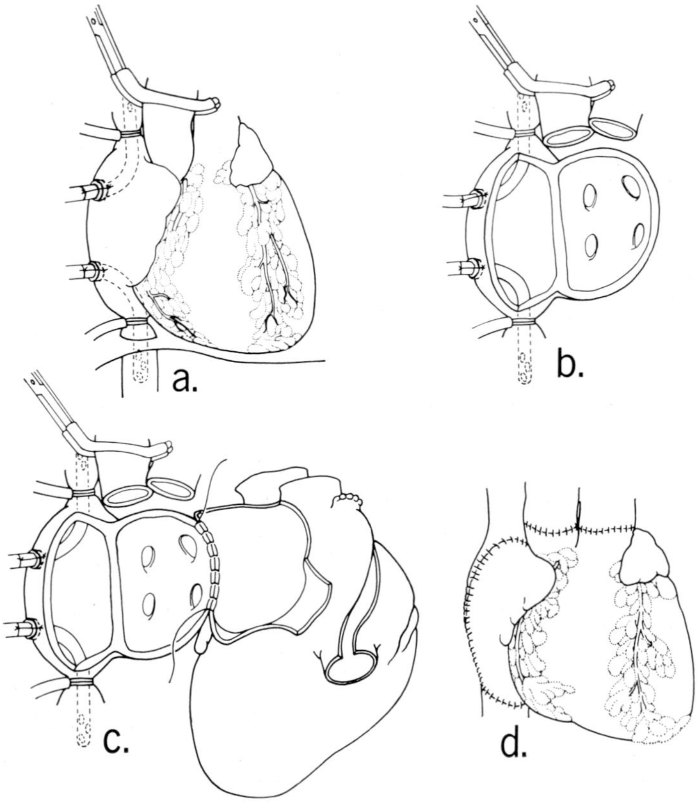

FIG. 1. The operation is performed through a midsternal incision. *A*. Placement of the venous catheters through the wall of the right atrium. *B*. Excision of the recipient heart leaving remnants of both atria and atrial septum. *C*. The left atrium of the donor heart is opened posteriorally and sutured to left atrial remnant of the recipient. The superior vena cava is suture ligated. The right atrium is opened from the inferior cava to base of right atrial appendage and sutured to the right atrial remnant of the recipient. *D*. Implantation of the heart is completed by anastomosis of the pulmonary artery and aorta.

Hardy *et al* 1964; Barnard 1967; Cooley *et al* 1968). The aorta and pulmonary arteries are transected a short distance above the valves. The atrial remnant receives its limited blood supply from bronchial vessels, and thus excessive amounts of residual atrial wall are avoided to insure viability of tissue at the suture line and to minimize the possibility of thrombus formation.

The donor heart is sutured in place by first anastomosing the opened left atrium to the left atrial remnant of the recipient. The suture line is begun in the midpoint of the lateral left atrial wall and carried superiorly and inferiorly as a continuous suture until the free wall and septum are united to the corresponding recipient tissue. The right atrium is then opened from the inferior vena cava to the base of the right atrial appendage. The incision can be carried as far as necessary into the appendage to conform to the size of the recipient's right atrial remnant. A continuous suture is used to join the donor right atrium to the atrial septum and right atrial border of the recipient, thus completing restoration of venous inflow to the heart. The pulmonary artery is joined by continuous suture and lastly anastomosis of the ascending aorta is carried out. During the 45 to 60 min required for suturing, the heart is kept hypothermic by the frequent topical application of cold saline. Prior to the release of the caval tapes and ascending aortic clamp, the ventricles and ascending aorta are carefully aspirated for residual air. Release of the aortic clamp then restores coronary blood flow. In each of our cases, normal cardiac rhythm has resumed either spontaneously or after a single defibrillating shock.

As the patient is weaned from bypass, the right heart has not infrequently shown some dilatation and decrease in contractility. Such evidence of right heart failure may be anticipated when a normal right ventricle is suddenly confronted with an increase in pulmonary vascular resistance. In each instance a good cardiac output has been restored and maintained by an intravenous drip of isoproterenol. It is usually possible to discontinue pharmacological support of the heart within 48 h.

Digitalis and diuretics are continued in the early postoperative period until there is no further evidence of right heart failure and no evidence of rejection. Antibiotics are begun prior to surgery and continued for 24 h after operation; thereafter they are reserved only for the treatment of a specific infection.

THE DIAGNOSIS OF ACUTE REJECTION

The most important aspect of the patient's post-operative management is careful monitoring for the earliest signs of cardiac rejection. Laboratory and clinical experience continues to document that the electrocardiogram is the most specific indicator in the detection of impending cardiac rejection (Figs. 2 and 3) (Lower *et al* 1966; Lower *et al* 1968). Four changes in the electrocardiogram have been convincingly correlated with the onset of an acute rejection crisis, namely a decrease in the voltage, a shift in the frontal plane axis to the right, the appearance of conduction defects such as right bundle branch block, and the appearance of atrial arrhythmias. A decrease in ECG voltage has been the most consistent finding in rejection and its reliability in the early weeks has been increased by the use of a direct myocardial electrode inserted in the right ventricular wall at the time of operation (Fig. 2). The epicardial ECG is less influenced by the accumula-

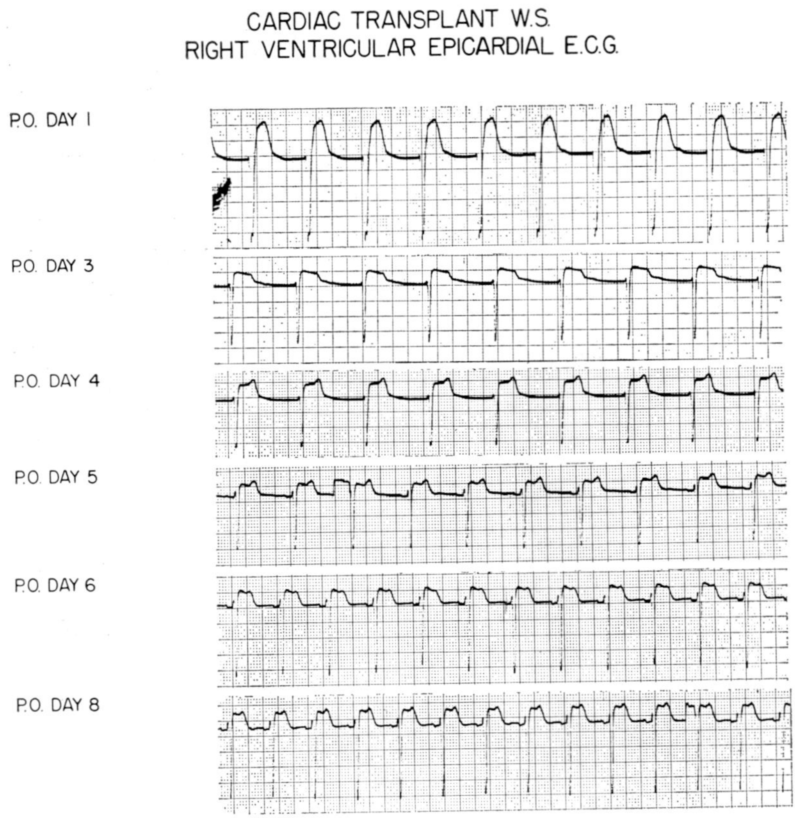

FIG. 2. Epicardial ECG tracings from patient W.S. showing progressive post-operative decrease in voltage. The diagnosis of rejection was further substantiated by the appearance of a pericardial friction rub, gallup rhythm, weight gain and malaise. The patient received a marked increase in steroid therapy and irradiation to the graft on days 5 and 6 with clinical and ECG improvement.

tion of mediastinal fluid or blood clots in the early postoperative period (Sewell *et al* 1969).

Careful daily clinical assessment of the patient is equally important in the detection of right heart failure which appears to be a harbinger of rejection. Weight gain, a right ventricular gallop, and elevation in venous pressure are frequently seen with an early rejection crisis. A friction rub frequently appears but is of less diagnostic value in view of its common occurrence after all types of cardiac surgery. In the later stage of rejection, ventriculr dilatation may result in tricuspid or mitral insufficiency. In order to avoid masking the early appearance of right heart failure as an indicator of rejection, it is suggested that the routine use of digitalis and diuretics be discontinued as soon as paractical in the post-operative course.

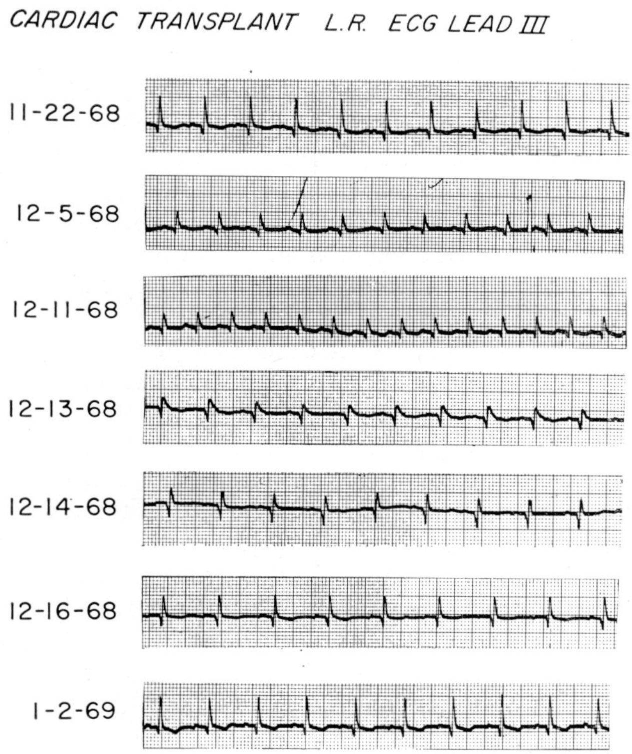

FIG. 3. Post-operative ECG tracings of patient L.R. who received a transplant on 8–24–68. After hospital discharge ECG changes of decreased voltage and right bundle branch block provided the diagnosis of threatened rejection. He was treated with an increase in steroids and irradiation to the graft with improvement in the ECG. Similar episodes were diagnosed and treated at 7 months and at 1 year. He remains alive and well 19 months after operation.

They can of course be reinstituted with the appearance of cardiac dysfunction.

Routine X-ray examinations of the heart have been of little help in the diagnosis of acute rejection. During a rejection crisis, the lung fields may actually exhibit decreased vascularity due to the predominance of right heart failure. There may be little change in the transverse diameter of the heart, but the superior vena cava and right heart chambers may become prominent. Fluoroscopy has frequently demonstrated decreased contractility during the acute rejection episode. The appearance of an infiltrate in the pulmonary parenchyma during the postoperative period is much more likely due to infection or infarction than to cardiac rejection (Weidner *et al* 1969).

Contrary to earlier expectations, the serial determinations of the serum enzymes have not provided a very sensitive indicator of cardiac rejection. A typical rejection episode may occur without a significant rise in the levels of serum enzymes. The isozymes I and II of LDH may increase during a severe rejection crisis and return to normal with the successful use of immunosuppressive therapy, but the increase usually appears later than the diagnostic changes in the electrocardiogram. A rise in the CPK and SGOT is also a late occurrence and probably indicates significant myocardial damage. The LDH isozymes may be of further value in the early detection of azathioprine induced hepatic toxicity by a rise in the level of isozyme V.

The use of ultrasound, ballistocardiography, telemetry and vectorcardiography are currently under study as additional means of monitoring the patient for acute rejection (Schroeder *et al* 1969). It is hoped that eventually an immunologic test will be available to evaluate the adequacy of immunosuppression. The detection of immunofluorescent heart-reactive antibody in the serum may be helpful in the early detection of rejection in some patients (Ellis *et al* 1970). However, the role of antibodies induced by prior myocardial infarctions or by myocardial diseases of other etiology is not clear, and in our experience acute rejection has occurred without a significant rise in the level of antiheart antibody. Tests of lymphocyte or macrophage migration inhibition appear to be a promising approach to the evaluation of the immunologic status of the patient (Smith *et al* 1969).

IMMUNOSUPPRESSIVE THERAPY

Azathioprine remains the basic immunosuppressive drug for the cardiac transplant and is administered in as large a daily dose as tolerated without inducing excessive bone marrow depression or hepatic toxicity. The initial 4 mg/kg dose is tapered to 2 mg/kg or lower with daily monitoring of leukocyte, reticulocyte and platelet counts as well as liver function tests.

Steroid therapy includes 1000 mg of hydrocortisone and 200 mg of prednisone during the operation and the first 12 h after transplantation. The prednisone is tapered to 100 mg by the end of the 1st week and more slowly thereafter. At the time of a suspected rejection crisis, steroid administration is abruptly increased (see below).

Antilymphocyte globulin is initially administered daily in a dose of 10 cc intramuscularly and after 2 weeks the dose is reduced to 5 cc daily. Antilymphocyte globulin has been discontinued whenever a severe adverse reaction is observed.

Pretreatment with ALG and azathioprine would perhaps be beneficial in depressing the patient's initial immunologic response to the graft, but is rarely practical because of the desperate condition of the cardiac patient and the unpredictable availability of cadaver organs. Anticoagulants are not employed routinely, as their role in immunosuppression has not yet been clearly defined. Some surgeons have used anticoagulants prophylactically or during rejection episodes. The risk of anticoagulants as opposed to their theroretical benefits, requires more extensive analysis to establish their proper place.

TREATMENT OF REJECTION CRISES

The primary treatment for an episode of threatened rejection is an abrupt increase in steroid administration (Lower *et al* 1965) usually 1000 mg methylprednisolone intravenously over a 1 to 2 h period and an increase in prednisone orally to 200 mg. The prednisone is then tapered slowly to the prior maintenance does if no further evidence of rejection is noted. In general, earlier rejection crises appear to require more massive doses of steroids than do later episodes of rejection. Because of laboratory evidence showing a beneficial effect of graft irradiation on the rejection process, (Graham *et al* 1969) the patient receives 300 R to the myocardium on each of 2 consecutive days through anterior and posterior ports.

Because of the increased risk of infection during treatment with high doses of steroids, the patient is maintained in strict isolation during rejection crises. Antifungal mouth wash is administered frequently to prevent the oral overgrowth of monilia. As mentioned above, antibiotics are only administered in treatment of specific identifiable bacterial infections. Antacids and bland diet are used liberally to minimize the risk of gastro-intestinal bleeding during the administration of high steroid doses.

Potassium is also given orally to counter the tendency for potassium loss during diuresis or during intensive treatment with steroids. The patient is begun on active exercise as soon as practical to minimize the wasting and osteoporosis which are often secondary to steroid therapy as well as for improvement in patient morale.

PATHOLOGY OF ACUTE REJECTION

Acute rejection of the cardiac transplant resembles the process seen in other homografted organs (Cachera *et al* 1968; Kosek *et al* 1968). The primary target of the immunologic response appears to be the vascular endothelium. Swelling and disruption of the endothelial cells results in

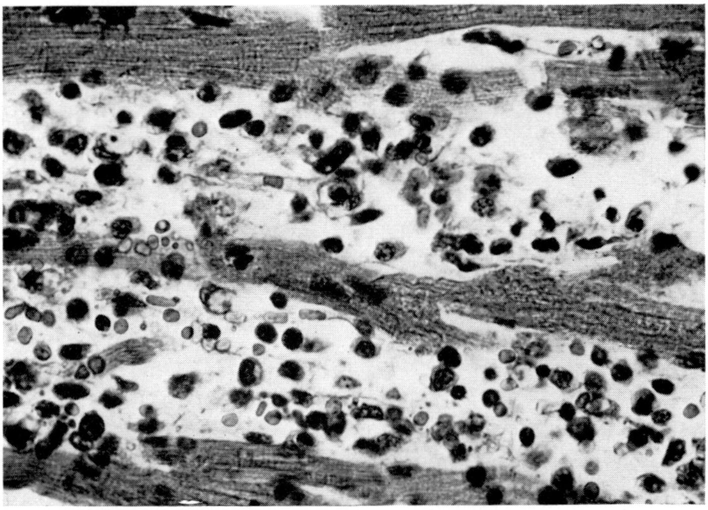

FIG. 4. Photomicrograph of myocardium of patient J.K. who died of acute homograft rejection 7 days after operation. The interstitial spaces show extensive haemorrhage, oedema and infiltration by mononuclear cells.

interstitial oedema and haemorrhage and the concomitant infiltration by the small mononuclear cells termed immunocytes (Fig. 4). The subsequent changes in the myocardial fibers, or myocytes, reflect either anoxic injury as a result of vascular damage or direct immunologic injury from humoral or cellular mechanisms. The electron microscopic changes in the myocytes include swelling of the mitochondria, dilatation of the smooth endoplasmic reticulum, accumulation of lipid droplets and mineral deposits within the mitochondria. Such changes may progress to focal areas of frank necrosis or myocytolysis. In laboratory studies, using serial biopsies, these changes have correlated well with the ECG changes of decreased voltage and the appearance of arrhythmias. Reversal of the early morphologic changes as well as improvement in the ECG has been documented by subsequent biopsies after treatment with high doses of methylprednisolone, and in some cases, after irradiation of the myocardium (Graham *et al* 1969). The irreversible changes of necrosis or myocytolysis persist as residual myocardial scars. Such scarring has been particularly evident in areas of the conduction system, both in laboratory and clinical experience.

The acute rejection process also involves the endothelium of larger coronary vessels with intimal damage and infiltration of the media and perivascular areas by mononuclear cells. Focal degeneration and necrosis of myocytes in the media are also seen in the coronary arteries and may lead to extensive fibrinoid necrosis similar to that seen in polyarteritis nodosa (Kosek *et al* 1969).

Certain modifications of the histologic picture may be seen in human patients with a particularly virulent form of rejection after treatment with massive doses of immuno-suppressants. In one such patient, the gross morphology was typical of acute rejection at 18 days with a markedly haemorrhagic and oedematous myocardium. The microscopic appearance confirmed the presence of vascular injury with extensive interstitial haemorrhage and edema. However, the predominant infiltrating cells present in the myocardium were polymorphonuclear leukocytes. The role of antibody in the clinical course and histopathology of cardiac rejection in some patients has been reviewed elsewhere (Williams *et al* 1969).

CHRONIC REJECTION

The diagnosis and prevention of late failure of the graft due to chronic rejection remains an enigma. The incidence of vascular intimal thickening and occlusion in arterial vessels (Fig. 5) has been high in cases examined beyond 3 months after cardiac transplantation, in man as well as in the dog (Lower & Cleveland 1968; Milam *et al* 1970). Late deaths may be due to ischemic myocardial damage or to arrhythmia. The exact aetiology of the vascular lesions and their relationship to the immune response, thrombosis or atherogenesis awaits further clarification. Whether prolonged anticoagulation or increased immunosuppression can prevent chronic rejection is uncertain; it does appear likely that the vascular lesions can best be avoided by more precise histocompatibility matching between donor and

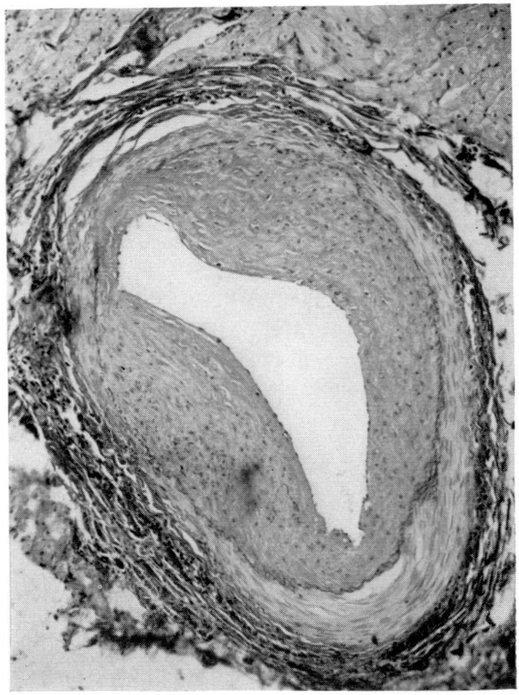

FIG. 5. An epicardial coronary arterial branch from a dog 1 year after homotransplantation of the heart. There is marked thickening of the intimal layer compromising the lumen (from Kosek *et al* (1968) *Lab. Invest.* **19,** 97.

recipient and by the continuous maintenance of immunosuppression for at least 2 years or longer.

A protocol for the long term followup of patients after discharge is difficult to define. The ECG remains the most important means of detecting a rejection episode (Fig. 3) and should probably be performed at least once or twice weekly during the 1st year. Weekly blood counts will aid in the detection of incipient drug toxicity. The appearance of easy fatigability, weight gain or oedema may further alert the physician to the occurrence of a rejection episode.

CARDIAC DENERVATION

The physiologic and metabolic changes resulting from cardiac denervation have been studied in our laboratory and by several other investigators

(Donald & Shepherd 1964; Dong *et al* 1964; Peiss *et al* 1966; Daggett *et al* 1966; Willman *et al* 1968; Lower *et al* 1968). The cardiac autotransplant has been useful in this regard by avoiding the immunologic problems but simulating the homograft in all physiologic respects. It is of particular interest that despite nearly complete depletion of myocardial catecholamines by denervation, post-operative function of human transplanted hearts has been remarkably good even when faced with increased pulmonary vascular resistance. The denervated heart is apparently exquisitely sensitive to alterations in the peripheral secretion of catecholamines (Carleton *et al* 1969) and thus responds appropriately to such forms of stress as exercise and hypoxia (Kontos & Lower 1969).

Reinnervation by sympathetics and parasympathetics has been extensively studied in canine transplants (Dong *et al* 1964; Willman *et al* 1964; Kontos *et al* 1970; Ebert & Sabiston 1970). Responses to nerve stimulation have been seen as early as a few weeks in some animals and confirmed in the majority by 4 months after transplantation. The reappearance of sympathetic fibers within the graft has been documented by fluorescent staining techniques. Nevertheless, biopsies even $2\frac{1}{2}$ years after transplantation have failed to show a return to normal levels of myocardial catecholamines suggesting that reinnervation may never become quantitatively complete. To date evidence of reinnervation in human transplant patients has not been obtained. The exact physiologic significance in terms of risks to patients with cardiac denervation or incomplete reinnervation remains to be clarified.

TRANSPLANTATION OF THE HEART AND LUNGS

Replacement of the heart and both lungs en bloc with a homograft has received scant attention although there are certain patients with extensive damage to both organ systems who could conceivably benefit from such a procedure. The laboratory investigation of this operation has provided data which affirm that despite the extensive denervation of the thoracic viscera, normal ventilation, gas exchange and pulmonary resistance can be maintained, and responses to hypoxia and hypercapnea have been appropriate (Lower *et al* 1961a; Grinnan *et al* 1970). The outstanding problem has been maintaining adequate ventilation for prolonged periods because of the difficulty in controlling rejection in the lungs. Maximum survival in the dog has been 10 days, emphasizing the contrast with heart transplantation alone. Two human attempts have been reported, one an infant who survived for 14 h (Cooley *et al* 1968) and the other an adult male who survived for 8 days (Lillehei 1970). The latter patient died of fulminating rejection and infection, both particularly difficult problems to manage in the lung transplant recipient. It is thus unlikely that this procedure is ready for further clinical trial until animal survival can be vastly improved.

CONCLUSIONS

Although cardiac transplantation has been shown to be eminently feasible on a technical and physiological basis, the rate of survival and complete rehabilitation of the patient will remain unfortunately low until a more specific and less hazardous means is available for controlling the immune response. Until such time, the operation must be reserved for those patients who are desperately ill and for whom no alternative therapy is available. It is now clear that a few such patients can be successfully carried through the transplantation procedure and the postoperative hazards of immunosuppression and can be restored to a full active life.

REFERENCES

Alksne J.F. (1969) Brain death as seen by the neurosurgeon. Presented at the Second World Symposium on Heart Transplantation. Montreal, Canada. 6 June.

Barnard C.N. (1967) A human cardiac transplant. *South African M J.* **41,** 1271.

Cachera J.P., Lacombe M., Buo-Mong-Hung J., Leandri J., Harada S. & DuBost C.L. (1968) Azathioprine et Survie Après Homotransplantation Orthotopique due Coeur Conservé chez le Jeune Chien. In *Advance in Transplantation.* Proceedings of the First International Congress of the Transplantation Society, p. 667. Munksgaard.

Carleton R.A., Heller S.J., Najafi H. & Clark J.G. (1969) Hemodynamic performance of a transplanted human heart. *Circulation,* **40,** 447.

Cleveland R.J. & Lower R.R. (1967) Transplantation of canine cadaver hearts after short-term preservation. *Transplantation,* **5,** 904.

Cooley D.A., Bloodwell R.D., Hallman G.L. & Nora J.J. (1968) Transplantation of the heart. A report of four cases. *J.A.M.A.* **205,** 479.

Cooley D.A., Hallman G.L., Bloodwell R.D., Nora J.J. & Leachman R.D. (1968) Human heart transplantation. *Amer. J. Cardiol.* **22,** 804.

Daggett W.M., Willman V.L., Harada Y., Barner H.B., Cooper T. & Hanlon C.R. (1966) Work capacity and efficiency of the autotransplanted heart. *Surg. Forum,* **17,** 222.

Donald D.E. & Shepherd J.T. (1964) Sustained capacity for exercise in dogs after complete cardiac denervation. *Amer. J. Cardiol.* **14,** 853.

Dong E. Jr., Hurley E.J., Lower R.R. & Shumway N.E. (1964) Performance of the heart 2 years after autotransplantation. *Surgery,* **56,** 270.

EBERT P.A. & SABISTON D.C. (1970) Pharmacologic quantitation of cardiac sympathetic reinnervation. Presented at the 31st Annual Meeting of the Society of University Surgeons. Pittsburgh, Pennsylvania. 13 Feb. To be published in *Surgery*.

ELLIS R.J., LILLEHEI C.W. & ZABRISKE J.B. (1970) Detection of circulating heart-reactive antibody in human heart transplants. *J.A.M.A.* **211,** 1505.

GRAHAM W.H., CHILDS J.W., WEYMOUTH R.J., KOSEK J.C., LIM F. & LOWER R.R. (1969) The reversibility of canine cardiac allograft rejection. *Surg. Forum*, **20,** 145.

GRINNAN G.L., GRAHAM W.H., CHILDS J.W. & LOWER R.R. (1970) Cardiopulmonary homotransplantation. Presented at the 50th Annual Meeting of the American Association for Thoracic Surgery, Washington, D.C., 7 April. To be published in *J. Thor. and Cardiovasc. Surg.*

HALLER J.D. & CERRUTI M.M. (1969) Heart transplantation in man: Compilation of cases. *Amer. J. Cardiol.* **24,** 555.

HARDY J.D., CHAVEZ C.M., KURRUS F.D., NEELY W.A., ERASLAN S., TURNER M.D., FABIAN L.W. & LABECK T.D. (1964) Heart transplantation in man: Developmental studies and report of a case. *J.A.M.A.* **188,** 1132.

KONTOS H.A. & LOWER R.R. (1969) Role of beta-adrenergic receptors in the circulatory response to hypoxia. *Amer. J. Physiol.* **217,** 756.

KONTOS H.A., THAMES M.D. & LOWER R.R. (1970) Responses to electrical and reflex autonomic stimulation in dogs with cardiac transplantation before and after reinnervation. *J. Thoracic and Cardiovasc. Surg.* **59,** 382.

KOSEK J.C., CHARTRAND C., HURLEY E.J. & LOWER R.R. (1969) Arteries in canine homografts: ultrastructure during acute rejection. *Lab. Invest.* **21,** 328.

KOSEK J.C., HURLEY E.J. & LOWER R.R. (1968) Histopathology of orthotopic canine cardiac homografts. *Lab. Invest.* **19,** 97.

LILLEHEI C.W. (1970) As reported in Medical World News, 20 January, p. 21.

LOWER R.R. & CLEVELAND R.J. (1968) The Current Status of Heart Transplantation. In *Advance in Transplantation.* Proceedings of the First International Congress of the Transplantation Society, p. 657. Munksgaard.

LOWER R.R., DONG E. Jr. & GLAZENER F.S. (1966) Electrocardiograms of dogs with heart homografts. *Circulation*, **33,** 455.

LOWER R.R., DONG E. Jr. & SHUMWAY N.E. (1965) Long-term survival of cardiac homografts. *Surgery*, **58,** 100.

LOWER R. R., KONTOS H.A., KOSEK J.C., SEWELL D.H. & GRAHAM W.H. (1968) Experiences in heart transplantation-technique, physiology and rejection. *Amer. J. Cardiol.* **22,** 766.

LOWER R.R., KOSEK J.C., KEMP V.E., GRAHAM W.H., SEWELL D.H. & LIM F. (1969) Rejection of the cardiac transplant. *Amer. J. Cardiol.* **24,** 492.

LOWER R.R. & SHUMWAY N.E. (1960) Studies on orthotopic homotransplantation of the canine heart. *Surg. Forum* **11,** 18.

LOWER R.R., STOFER R.C., HURLEY E.J., DONG E. Jr., COHN R.B. & SHUMWAY N.E. (1962) Successful homotransplantation of the canine heart after anoxic preservation for seven hours. *Amer. J. Surg.* **104,** 302.

LOWER R.R., STOFER R.C., HURLEY E.J. & SHUMWAY N.E. (1961a) Complete homograft replacement of the heart and both lungs. *Surgery*, **50,** 842.

LOWER R.R., STOFER R.C. & SHUMWAY N.E. (1961b) Homovital transplantation of the heart. *J. Thoracic and Cardiovasc. Surg.* **41,** 196.

MILAM J.D., SHIPKEY F.H., LIND C.J. Jr., NORA J.J., LEACHMAN R.D., ROCHELLE D.G., BLOODWELL R.D., HALLMAN G.L. & COOLEY D.A. (1970) Morphologic findings in human cardiac allografts. *Circulation*, **41**, 519.

PEISS C.N., COOPER J., WILLIAM V.L. & RANDALL W.C. (1966) Circulatory responses electrical and reflex activation of the nervous system after cardiac denervation. *Circulation Res.* **19**, 153.

SCHROEDER J.S., POPP R.L., STINSON E.B., DONG E. Jr., SHUMWAY N.E. & HARRISON D.C. (1969) Acute rejection following cardiac transplantation. Phonocardiographic and ultrasound observations. *Circulation*, **40**, 155.

SEWELL D.H., KEMP V.E. & LOWER R.R. (1969) The epicardial ECG in monitoring cardiac homograft rejection. *Circulation*, **39**, Suppl. 1, 21.

SMITH M.G.M., EDDLESTON A.L.W.F., DOMINGUEZ J.A., EVANS D.B., BEWICK M. & WILLIAMS R. (1969) Changes in leukocyte migration after renal transplantation. *Brit. med. J.* iv, 275.

TERASAKI P.I., VON DIEPOW M., DAVIDSON C.J. & MICKEY M.R. (1969) Serotyping for homotransplantation. XXIV. Heart transplantation. *Amer. J. Cardiol.* **24**, 500.

THOMAS K.E., LINEHAN J.D. & LOWER R.R. (1970) Unpublished data.

WEBB W.R. & HOWARD H.S. (1957) Restoration of function of the refrigerated heart. *Surg. Forum* **8**, 303.

WEIDNER W.W., LOWER R.R., KEMP V.E. & VINIK M. (1969) Chest roentgenographic findings in the acute rejection crisis in human cardiac transplants. *Radiology*. **93**, 1267.

WILLIAMS G.M., DEPLANQUE B., GRAHAM W.H. & LOWER R.R. (1969) The participation of antibodies in acute allograft rejection in man. *New Engl. J. Med.* **281**, 1145.

WILLMAN V.L., COOPER T. & HANLON C.R. (1964) Return of neural responses after autotransplantation of the heart. *Amer. J. Physiol.* **207**, 187.

WILLMAN V.L., KAISER G.C., HARADA Y., COOPER T. & HANLON C.R. (1968) Physiological Alterations Following Transplantation of the Heart. In *Advance in Transplantation*. Proceedings of the First International Congress of the Transplantation Society, p. 661. Munksgaard.

Part 5
Lung Transplantation

CHAPTER 31

Lung Transplantation

F. Derom
Ch. R. H. Wildevuur

Although the first lung transplantation was performed by Hardy *et al* 1963, only 24 additional attempts have been made since then (Wildevuur & Benfield 1970). The suggestions and speculations in the following chapters should therefore be accepted with reservation since they must rely upon the limited data available from these cases, which include the experience of the only long term survival in lung transplantation performed by Derom *et al* 1969.

EXPERIMENTAL LUNG TRANSPLANTATION

Experience in lung transplantation has made clear the fact that technical problems are the cause of a large number of graft failures and false conclusions.

The first successful reimplantation of the right lung was carried out in 1951 by Juvenelle *et al* (1951). The experience gained from reimplantation experiments was helpful to define the major technical problems of the pulmonary transplantation, the function ability of the transplanted lung and the problems of pulmonary vascular resistance.

Métras (1950) and Neptune *et al* (1953) described independently a technique which placed the venous anastomosis through the wall of the left atrium. This helped to reduce the problem of pulmonary vein thrombosis and became the standard technique in animals. Continuous suture techniques are usually satisfactory for the vascular anastomosis but they may result under certain conditions to constriction of the circumference of the pulmonary artery and, unless special precautions are taken, may contribute to the high vascular resistance which has been observed in transplanted lungs (Hardy *et al* 1969).

Many investigators reported to have problems with the bronchial anastomosis such as leakage or stenosis. Anastomosis of the bronchus seems both for the investigator and the clinician to be the most challenging technical problem in lung transplantation. Reports about surgical techniques which will avoid these pitfalls are virtually non existent.

No effort is made to restore continuity of the lymphatics, the nerves and the bronchial arteries. Haglin 1970 however believe that the preservation of the bronchial artery supply will prevent complication of the bronchial anastomosis. Most investigators on the other hand believe that the bronchus and its mucosa are able to derive a sufficient blood supply from the pulmonary circulation.

Hardy 1969 found that lymphatic regeneration could be identified by the end of 7 days and that several numbers of lymphatic channels could be seen crossing the bronchial suture line at the end of the 12th day.

The same authors were not able to demonstrate crossing of nerves at the bronchial anastomosis or return of nerve function. Others however, observed a return of the cough and stretch reflexes in the reimplanted lung after 2 to 5 years (Secrist & Trummer 1967). Regeneration of nerves in autotransplantation has however not yet been observed and seems very unlikely to occur.

It has been demonstrated that pulmonary innervation is not essential for sufficient lung function to permit survival in the dog. The respiratory pattern in dogs with denervated lungs is rarely completely normal, although they are able to survive (Faber *et al* 1965). It is generally accepted however that the innervation of the lung in dogs has a more important functional aspect than in man.

There is an immediate decline in lung function following reimplantation. This diminished function however still permits survival of the animal with that lung only if the pulmonary artery anastomosis is distensible (Veith & Richards 1969).

The whole explanation for the immediate decline in function following reimplantation is still open to discussion. Oedema due to handling or ischaemia and hypoxia are possible causes. There is no reliable technique available to protect the lung from ischaemia longer than 2 h (Hardy 1969). Hypothermic perfusion of the lung is considered helpful by some and deleterious by other investigators. Intermittent ventilation of the lung during the ischaemic period seems to improve the function of the transplanted organ. Loss of surfactant is in direct correlation with the ischemia and absence of ventilation of the organ (Yakeishi *et al* 1969). The reduction of function of the transplanted lung lasts about 10 days after which there is a gradual recovery up to almost normal level (Hardy 1969).

Most auto- and homotransplantations of the lung in dogs have been done in the presence of a normal opposite lung. Since this condition is completely different from those which are present in patients undergoing pulmonary transplantation, one should be very careful in the application of experimental conclusions in man. There is a real need for an experimental model similar to restrictive lung disease or a chronic obstructive respiratory disease in man.

Many groups studied lung homotransplantation in order to determine the efficiency of various means of immunosuppression. Although the use of these drugs prolonged host survival for considerable periods up to 2 years (Blumenstock *et al* 1964, 1967), it should be remembered that in all these experiments the animal's own lung contributed for a major part to the ventilatory function. Experiments in homotransplantation, unilateral with exclusion of the contralateral lung, or bilateral lung transplantation should be undertaken in the near future.

I. SUITABLE DONOR

Though a certain number of lungs removed post-mortem after cessation of the cardiac function have been used successfully in human transplantation, there has been a tendency recently to use lungs of donors with brain death and an intact circulation. It is obvious that the use of organs from donors in *coma dépassé* not only simplifies the logistics of the whole procedure, but enables one to study the dying patient more thoroughly and to evaluate his qualities as a potential donor.

It is believed that donors under 50 or 55 years of age, without cardiopulmonary disease, should be accepted. As for other organ transplantations, they should be free of cancer and for the lung it is especially important they also should be free of infection. Prolonged intubation or tracheotomy increases the risk of lung infection. For a donor to be suitable this period should not exceed 48 h.

Although, in the absence of more long-term survivals, it is impossible to make a conclusion about the value of histocompatibility in the cases of lung transplantation, it may be postulated from the experience in kidney transplantation that the intensity of the rejection process will depend on the genetic relationship between donor and recipient. A donor should be compatible with the recipient for ABO and HLA antigens. No strict rules concerning the acceptable numbers of mismatches with the leucocyte antigens will be given here. The critical condition of the recipient may influence the decision of the clinician and the immunologist regarding their choice in selecting the donor. However, it seems to be of importance for the outcome to crossmatch the leucocytes of donor and recipient, and to try to find as good a match as possible.

The size of the donor is also important since the lung has to fit in the hemithorax of the recipient. A slight degree of overexpansion of the transplanted lung seems not to be deleterious, however, one should avoid to compress a large lung in a small thorax which will impair its function.

II. SELECTION AND PRE-OPERATIVE MANAGEMENT OF RECIPIENTS

With one exception, all attempts in lung transplantation have failed within 1 month after surgery. For this reason the only patients whom we feel represent justifiable candidates for lung transplantation are those in very terminal stages of respiratory insufficiency either chronic or acute. Since failure of the transplanted lung to function will usually be fatal, the physician must be exceedingly careful to be sure that the transplantation is the patient's last hope and that no other treatment is available. Very few patients fall in that category since many cases are admitted with a severe respiratory insufficiency to hospital in an almost moribund state but still respond to medical treatment and are able to leave the hospital in reasonable condition for months. The limited success in lung transplantation, the fact that it is extremely difficult to determine when a patient with severe chronic pulmonary insufficiency will die, and the limited number of cases for which it seems justified to propose transplantation as a last chance, are the main reasons why lung transplantation has so seldom been attempted. Careful pulmonary function studies should be performed as completely as possible on the candidate recipient so that as much as possible information can be accumulated before transplantation. The studies should include: right heart catheterization, blood gas studies, Xenon 133 ventilation/perfusion scans and angiocardiography if the condition of the recipient permits.

The most common indications for transplantation in the 25 cases were: respiratory insufficiency (23 cases), of those patients 16 had chronic obstructive pulmonary disease and seven suffered from restrictive lung diseases. Two patients had severe pulmonary hypertension. It seems essential to us to make a distinction between respiratory insufficiency caused by chronic obstructive pulmonary disease and respiratory insufficiency caused by a restrictive lung disease such as silicosis. In considering candidates for a lung transplant it was anticipated that in chronic obstructive diseases such as emphysema, the function of the transplanted lung could be impaired by the patient's own remaining lung. Clinical experiences, as will be discussed later, confirmed this speculation. Patients with restrictive lung disease are better candidates for transplantation, as the remaining lung will not interfere with the function of the transplant. The only long-term survival suffered from severe silicosis. Patients with pulmonary hypertension must be given a transplanted pulmonary vascular bed which is large enough to accept the whole cardiac output. The transplanted lobe in Gago's case (Gago *et al* 1970) was not able to tolerate the whole pulmonary blood flow, the recipient died very quickly of vascular congestion and capillary damage in the transplanted lobe. Doubt has been cast on the ability of one transplanted lung to accept most of the cardiac output but Veith & Richards 1969 have demonstrated experimentally that unilateral canine lung transplants can withstand immediate contralateral pulmonary artery ligation. Derom's case showed that in man, the transplanted lung was also able to handle most of the cardiac output immediately and for a prolonged time. In this case all signs of right heart strain present on the ECG before transplantation disappeared within 24 h after the transplantation was performed. We are therefore convinced that pulmonary hypertension should be considered seriously as an indication for lung transplantation.

The pre-operative management of the patient is restricted. Intermittent periods of artificial ventilation, administration of oxygen, antibiotics and steroids have usually been given with some benefit and their use will be continued. However, very little can be done for the patient, who is not responding to this conservative treatment and is dying from respiratory insufficiency. The hope in those cases is based on a good artificial lung by which the patient can be treated effectively for prolonged periods of time (Landé & Lillehei 1969). Tracheostomy should be avoided since it will increase the susceptibility of the recipient to infection once immunosuppressive drugs are given in the post-transplantation period.

III. THE OPERATION

a Co-ordination

Good planning of the complex procedure of transplanting a lung is essential in order to keep the ischaemia period of the donor lung as short as possible.

The operating teams for the donor and the recipient should co-ordinate their timing very carefully. The anaesthesia of the recipient should start only after the organ to be transplanted appears to be in good condition. It is not possible to be certain however from its appearance that the lung will function well. An absence of immediate good function of the transplanted lung in the post-operative period may lead to the death of the recipient whose lung function has been reduced to a critical level. It has been shown that transplanted lungs rapidly undergo functional derangements during the ischaemic period (Wildevuur 1970). Only 1 to 2 h if ischaemia can be tolerated if there is to be good function in the early post-operative period. Despite intensive investigations in order to try to extend this period with perfusion of various solutions, hypothermia, metabolic inhibitors, etc., no repeatable success has been obtained although sometimes preservation has been prolonged. However, it has been shown that ventilation of the donor lung is of importance (Rangel *et al* 1969). Without ventilation of the donor lung functional derangements will appear even more quickly. Donor lungs have been handled in a variety of ways in clinical transplantation. Neither hypothermia nor perfusion were uniformly used. Some were ventilated, cooled and flushed or perfused. In other cases no efforts at preservation were made. Most of the transplant teams have been able to keep their ischaemia time under 2 h, however adequate function has followed ischaemic times of 2 h and longer.

b **Donor**

It is evident that the use of donors with brain death makes the planning much easier. Whenever possible heparin should be given to the donor before cardiac arrest occurs to avoid intra-vascular clotting in the donor lung. For optimal preservation of the lungs, intermittent ventilation or insufflation should be instituted.

Although it has been suggested (Hardy 1969) to put the donor on cardio-pulmonary by-pass and to cool him simultaneously until the organ has been exposed and removed, it is important to remember that a prolonged period of extra-corporeal circulation is deleterious for the lung and that the absence of left heart decompression may induce lung oedema. The removal of the lung from the donor, should present no difficulties. One should make the stump of the pulmonary artery as long as possible. Most surgeons prefer to divide the pulmonary veins at the atrial level. In the first instant the bronchus should be taken as long as possible permitting intubation to ventilate the lung or to keep it insufflated during the procedure. Before anastomozing the bronchus, it should be cut close to the origin of the upper and lower lobe, to avoid necrosis of the stump.

c Recipient

The recipient lung function in most cases will be limited significantly and problems can be expected at the moment when one of the diseased lungs will be removed in order to make room for the transplant. This may require extra-corporeal circulation, however, the clinical experience has shown that an adequate gaseous exchange can be maintained with artificial respiration, but that acute decompensation of the right ventricle can occur if high vascular resistance exists in the remaining lung. Thus pre-operative evaluation of the haemodynamic status of the patient is important and may indicate the use of extra-corporeal circulation. Since it is not possible to predict with certainty whether or not the patient will withstand temporary occlusion of one pulmonary artery, an extra-corporeal circulation should be ready on a stand-by basis. Prior to lung resection, the pulmonary artery should be temporaly clamped. Since it is easier to connect the patient to the extra-corporeal circuit from the right side, right lung transplantation will be chosen if local conditions are favourable to that side. The recommended sequence of anastomosis is veins or left atrium, artery and bronchus. A generous piece of the patient's own pulmonary artery and veins or atrium will be left attached to the heart, in order to facilitate the anastomosis. Simple continuous suturing is an easy and time saving procedure. The vascular clamps can be removed after termination of the vascular anastomosis, although this can create an important right-left shunt if the transplanted lung is not ventilated at that time. Air may be trapped in the pulmonary veins or the left atrium, this can be aspirated with a syringe. The patient's own bronchus—just as in the donor lung—will be sectioned as close as possible to its division in upper and lower lobe. In this way the innervation of the main bronchus of the recipient will be preserved and this will aid the expectoration of bronchial secretions. To avoid stenosis at the bronchus anastomosis it is recommended that at least half of the anastomotic line should be performed with interrupted sutures.

d Author's technique

In Derom's case the whole transplantation procedure was planned in order to keep the lung ischaemia as short as possible. The donor and the recipient were operated on in two adjacent theatres. The transplantation procedure was started with the thoracotomy of the donor, a patient in *coma dépassé*. The anaesthesia of the recipient began after the right lung of the donor had been found suitable for being transplanted. The right lung has been chosen on the basis of our conviction that surgical technique would be easier on this side. Right thoracotomy also allows easier cannulation for heart-lung by-pass if unavoidable for pneumectomy of the recipient. Temporary clamping of the pulmonary artery demonstrated that the recipient would tolerate removal of his right lung without extracorporeal circulation. Heparine (3 mg/kg body weight) was administered to the donor and the right lung was transplanted with its blood content. The donor lung was neither cooled nor perfused or ventilated. The anastomosis of the pulmonary veins was performed by means of their atrial cuff. The pulmonary artery was anastomozed with a continuous suture. The vascular clamps were removed, permitting perfusion of the lung and reducing ischaemia time to 35 min. The main bronchus, sectioned close to the origin of the upper lobe bronchus, was anastomozed with a continuous posterior suture 000 Tevdek* and interrupted stitches of 0000 Tevdek on the anterior side. The transplanted lung had a normal appearance and consistence: it was very easily inflated on positive pressure ventilation. The whole procedure lasted 3 h and the patient was awake at the end of the operation. In the immediate post-operative period prophylactic artificial ventilation was instituted. The patient was extubated after 13 h: he maintained spontaneous breathing without difficulty.

IV. POSTOPERATIVE CARE

Survival of the recipient will depend mainly upon the function of the transplant. Many lung transplants have shown an adequate lung function during the first days. Every sign of malfunction must be considered for its cause and prophylactic measures have to be taken in order to prevent the occurence of a fatal respiratory insufficiency. Most of them have been discussed above. Post-operative complications such as haemothorax, pneumothorax, atelectasis, accumulation of intra-bronchial secretions must be treated rigorously. The use of mechanical ventilation during the early very critical post-operative period is recommended to promote a satisfactory gaseous exchange source.

a Prevention of infection

Although it is very difficult from the available data to assess the roles which infection or rejection played in causing death in the first post-operative weeks of most transplants, it is of the utmost importance to avoid every known possible cause of infection. An organ undergoing rejection is especially liable to infection. The patient should be completely isolated. Every precaution should be taken to avoid the introduction of additional

* Deknatel, Inc. Queen's Village, N.Y.

bacteria in the patient's airway, ventilator, endotracheal tubes, broncho-scopes, suction catheters etc. The donor lung should be free of infection but the remaining lung of the recipient can form a chronic source of cross infection. Its removal at the moment of transplantation or later may therefore be considered, as will be discussed later. Culture of the bronchial secretions will be repeated at regular intervals in order to recognize the presence of potentially infectious agents as soon as possible. Overdosage of immunosuppressive drugs has to be avoided since these drugs reduce the patient's resistance to infection. Antibiotics should be administrated with great care and prophylactic use of broad spectrum antibiotics may be another source of difficulties. Although infection is a most formidable complication, it has been shown that it is possible to manage a patient with good lung function for nearly 10 months, despite the chronic presence of pseudomonas, Klebsiella, staphylococcae and candida in the sputum (Derom *et al* 1970).

b **Immunosuppression**

The basis of immunosuppressive treatment in these patients is the same as for other organ transplantations. The most commonly used drugs are azathioprine and corticosteroids. Antilymphocyte serum (ALS) may be an important adjuvant in the immunosuppressive treatment although the actual value and indications are not yet clearly established. It has been shown in experimental lung transplantation (Blumenstock *et al* 1969) that ALS can control rejection and ALS has been used in most of the recent clinical cases of lung transplantation. Some patients were given actinomycine C, but its value has not been established. Although one should always be careful to avoid overdosage of immunosuppressive agents with their dangerous toxic side effects, it is important to remember that the lung transplant patient usually has good kidney and liver function and therefore has better drug tolerance than most kidney and liver transplant patients.

The order of drug dosage is as follows:

Azathioprine 2–3 mg/kg body weight.
Prednisolone 35–80 mg.
Actinomycine C 200 γ every 14 days.

Antilymphocyte globulin is given intravenously from the day of operation at the maximum tolerated daily dose. As in kidney transplants, acute lung rejection seems to respond favourably to an increasing dosage of the steroids (Derom *et al* 1970). On the other hand, chronic rejection was not halted by augmentation of the immunosuppressive treatment.

c Complications

Complications encountered in the clinical cases have been various. Since the origin of some of them are related to one of the most essential points in lung transplantation which is the selection of the recipient, we will discuss the complications in detail, namely infection, rejection and malfunction of the transplant. The conclusions and speculations which follow here are based upon the study of the world experience in lung transplantation. The problem of *infection* has already been discussed but it is important to notice that many transplanted patients died of massive pneumonia. Scrupulous criteria for accepting a donor lung might obviate grafting an infected lung. However, cross-infection may result from the recipient's own infected remaining lung and brings up the consideration for contralateral pneumectomy or bilateral lung transplantation. The hazard of the immunosuppressive therapy which reduces the patient's resistance to infection is well known. The search for more selective drugs is of special importance for lung transplantation.

The main problem of *rejection* is the difficulty in differentiating it from infection. The most striking symptoms in Derom's patient who had several acute rejection crises which were treated effectively were: a persistant irritable dry cough, a reticular appearance of the lung on the chest X-ray and decline of lung function. All those features were completely reversible after effective treatment. In several other cases a cloudy appearance of the chest X-ray was interpreted as a possible rejection phase, which later appeared to be probably an infection.

From the practical point of view, when one is in doubt about infection versus rejection, the advice should be: treat them both together since they are likely to co-enact.

Retrospective post-mortem studies have not always determined whether or not rejection had occurred. Infection masked the histological features of rejection.

The malfunction of the transplant can be caused by different factors: As already mentioned a long ischaemia time and a collapsed lung can affect severely the function after transplantation. It has been shown in animal experiments (Wildevuur 1970) that after certain ischaemic periods the immediate post-operative function might be adequate but function will decline in the first post-operative week to critical levels. If the animal survives this period, function may return to normal levels. Malfunction of the transplant may also be due to mechanical factors. In patients with chronic obstructive lung diseases the discrepancy of high expiratory airway resistance in the remaining lung and normal airway resistance of the transplant may result in increasing volume of the remaining emphysematous lung and compression of the transplanted lung. This will lead to disturbance of ventilation and perfusion, the remaining lung receiving most of the ventilation and the transplanted lung most of the perfusion, resulting in a large physiological shunt. Patients with emphysema thus may be poor candidates for unilateral lung transplantation because the high vascular resistance and static compliance of the remaining emphysematous lung predispose it to further hypoperfusion and hyperinflation. This complication has occurred in at least seven of the 16 patients with chronic obstructive lung disease (Wildevuur & Benfield 1970; Stevens *et al* 1970). In three of them it was the direct cause of death. There was no perfusion-ventilation imbalance in the only long-term surviving patient. Radiological studies and lung scanning, showed that this patient's own lung was rigid and non-functional, the haemothorax behaved as after a pneumonectomy. There was a constant opacification of his own remaining lung. Lung scanning demonstrated a complete absence of perfusion in the remaining lung; the total pulmonary blood flow went in the transplanted lung. Inhalation of Xenon showed an uptake of 90% in the transplanted lung. During the whole post-transplant period a gradual shrinkage of the patient's remaining lung was observed and a temporaly asymptomatic pneumothorax on that side also confirmed the functional pneumectomy of the remaining lung. Patients with restrictive lung disease have a high vascular resistance as well as a low compliance in the remaining lung, excluding this lung from function after transplantation. This makes them better candidates for lung transplantation than patients with chronic obstructive disease in which the imbalance of vascular- and airway resistance interferes with the function of the transplant. Another important factor which can impair the function of the transplant is compression of the transplanted lung by implanting too large a lung in a small hemithorax (White *et al* 1966). Functional alteration in the transplanted lung due to ischaemia is difficult to demonstrate and further laboratory investigation is needed. The complications arising from the discrepancy of ventilation and perfusion between the remaining and the transplanted lung can be solved theoretically by performing a bilateral lung transplantation. Although a very major procedure, it seems to us the only possible solution in the treatment of irreversible terminal chronic obstructive lung disease. This procedure will also eliminate the danger of cross infection from the remaining lung in unilateral transplantation. Unilateral transplantation combined with a contralateral pneumectomy may be an alternative. However, from a practical point of view the bilateral lung transplantation will probably be the procedure of choice as a much greater reserve capacity can be obtained with little increase of the operating time and the second lung is likely to be available from the same donor.

V. PATHOLOGY

Flax *et al* 1966 established the histological criteria for rejection of pulmonary tissues in dogs. These microscopic studies revealed that the three main components of rejection were

1 perivascular mononuclear infiltration
2 intra-alveolar oedema and infiltration, peribronchial fibrosis and some thickening of the alveolar walls
3 massive terminal necrosis and haemorrhage.

Up to date information about the clinical lung transplant cases is not yet available. In some patients, the presence of pulmonary infection made the identification of rejection uncertain. Other patients (Wildevuur & Benfield 1970) were thought to have no signs of rejection at the time of death.

One patient died 10 months after transplantation from pneumonia and sepsis due to gram-negative bacteria which developed whilst he was being treated for chronic rejection.

Microscopical studies of this case reveal practically none of the rejection signs quoted above by Flax. There were no vascular changes. The alveolar membrane was normal in the parts without signs of pneumonia. There was only a very limited peribronchial infiltration with mononuclear cell suggesting the possibility of chronic rejection.

VI. LONG TERM RESULTS

Only one patient operated on by one of us (F.D.) survived long enough to demonstrate that lung transplantation is not only possible but that it can be of benefit to the patient.

Analysing the post-operative evolution of that case leads to the following conclusions:

1 The 3 first post-operative weeks were—as in most other cases—the most critical period for the patient: acute rejection, and gram-negative sepsis occurred.
2 One month after transplantation there was a marked improvement of the patient's general condition and pulmonary function which contrasted with his precarious situation before transplantation. With the exception of some minor complications such as herpes, gastric complaints and another crisis of acute rejection, there were no problems until 8½ months after operation. The patient returned home and enjoyed a normal social life.
3 After a traumatic fracture of the femoral shaft, he developed a state of

chronic rejection characterized by dyspnoea, general malaise, lack of appetite and increased expectoration of thick mucus. Various treatments were tried without success, to overcome the rejection. He died from bronchopneumonia. The chest X-ray has been clear until 5 days before his death.

CONCLUSIONS

If one cites the cold statistic that 25 lung transplants have been performed and that only one patient survived longer than 30 days, eventually to succomb to chronic rejection and infection 10 months after operation, the picture is exceedingly discouraging. On the other hand, animal experiments and clinical experience have elucidated various underlying problems that should make it possible to avoid errors in future cases. Choice of donor and preservation of the lung are well defined. The operative tactics and technics are well established. The immunosuppressive treatment allows control of acute rejection in most cases. Despite this, progressive respiratory insufficiency occurred in many patients after transplantation. This indeed was the major problem encountered in the post-operative period. In some cases the recipient's own lung disease led to malfunction of the transplant. It is likely that only patients with restrictive pulmonary disease or pulmonary hypertension can be salvaged by unilateral lung transplantation. Bilateral lung transplantation or unilateral transplantation with contra-lateral pneumectomy should probably be attempted for patients with chronic obstructive lung disease. One patient derived true palliation during his 10-month period of survival following transplantation and it is clear that the transplant not only sustained life as the only functioning lung tissue but also improved the quality of the patient's life significantly and meaningfully.

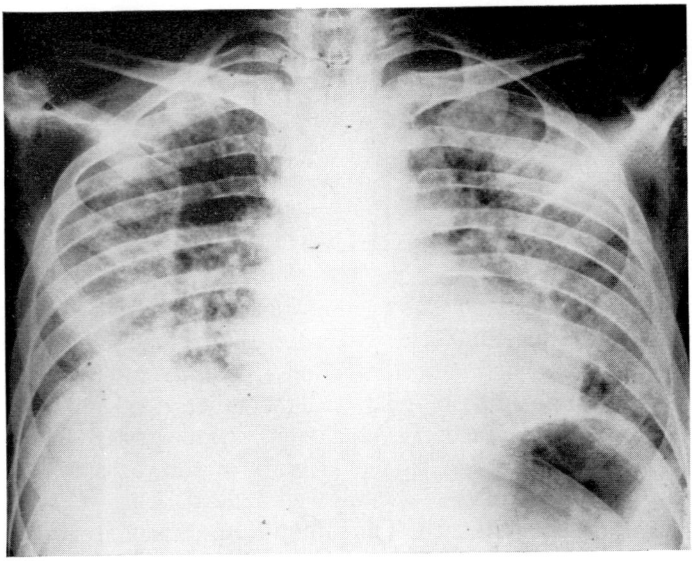

FIG. 1. Chest X-ray of Derom's case $1\frac{1}{2}$ months before transplantation, showing an extensive bilateral silicosis.

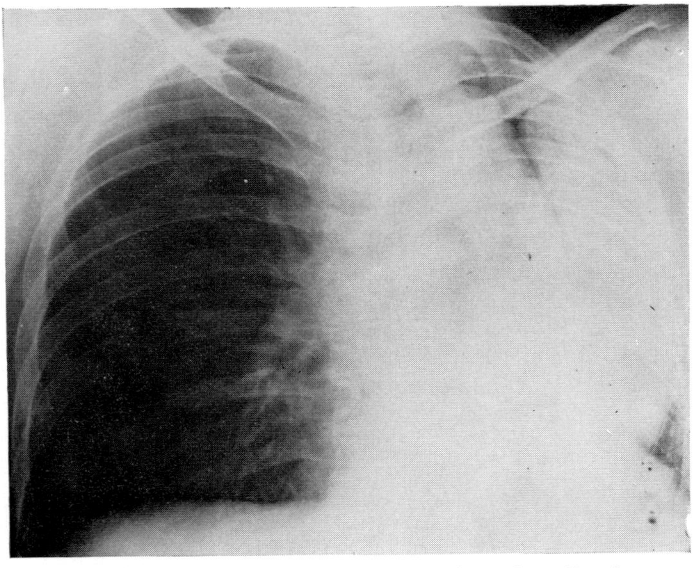

FIG. 2. Chest X-ray 6 months after lung transplantation. Good expansion and ventilation of the right transplanted lung. Retraction of the mediastinal structure to the left with fibrosis atelectasis of the left lung and a small pneumothorax on the left side. This X-ray is typical for all the X-rays which were made after transplantation during the 10 month survival.

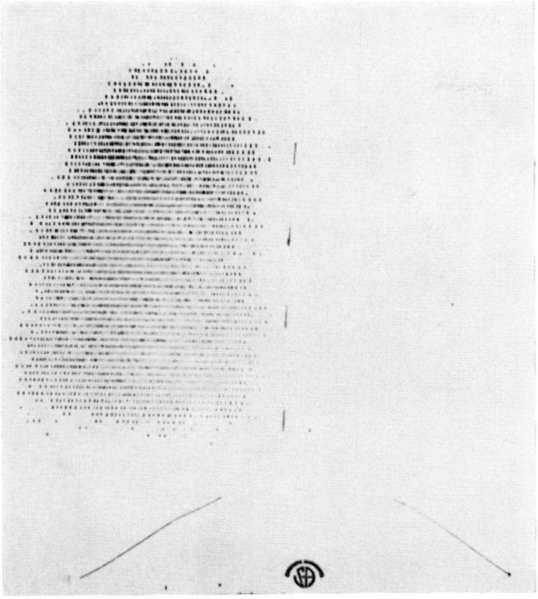

FIG. 3. Lung scanning 4 months after transplantation which shows a complete absence of bloodflow to the left lung.

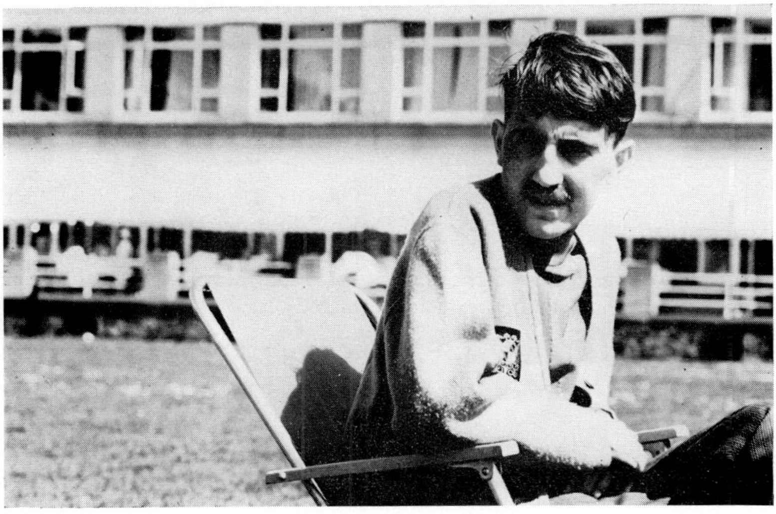

FIG. 4. Picture of the patient 8 months after transplantation.

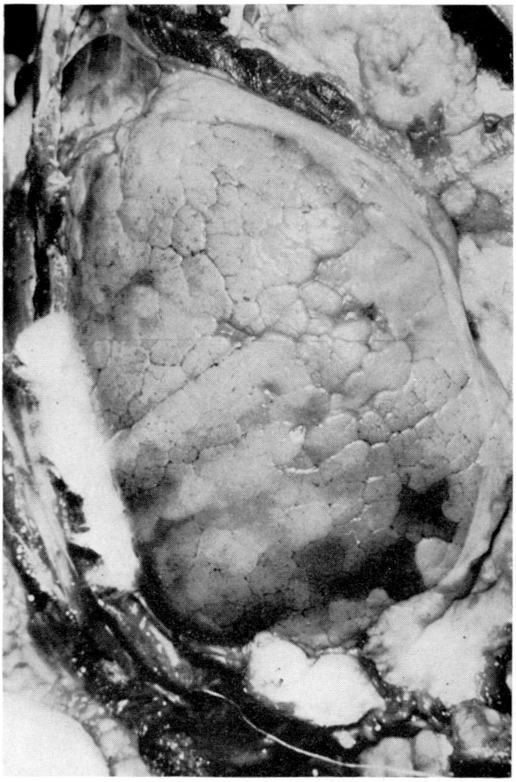

FIG. 5. Close-up of the patient's transplanted lung at autopsy. Macroscopic view of the lung is quite normal. Normal aspect of the visceral surface. An important part of this lung showed bronchopneumonia on further examination.

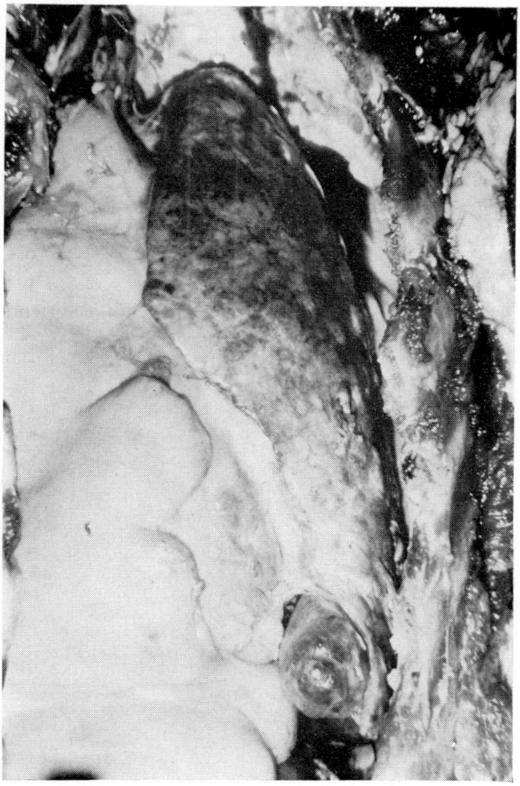

FIG. 6. Patient's own left lung: lung with very firm consistence with coarse nodular surface. This lung had shrunk and showed advanced silicosis with interstitial fibrosis.

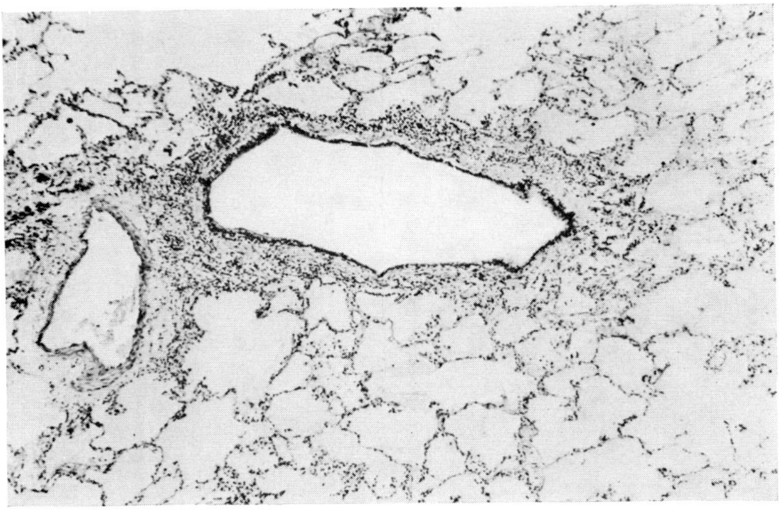

FIG. 7. Microscopic examination: presence of a slight degree of fibrosis and infiltration of plasma cells, lymphocytes and histiocytes in the external bronchial wall. Absence of advanced histologic signs of rejection: no vascular lesions, normal alveolar membrane.

REFERENCES

BLUMENSTOCK D.A., COLLINS J.A. & HECHTMAN H.B. (1964) Lung transplantation in the dog. *Ann. N.Y. Acad. Sci* **120,** 677.

BLUMENSTOCK D.A., GROSJEAN O.V., OTTE H.P. & MULDER M.A. (1967) Experimental allotransplantation of the lung. *J. thorac. cardiovasc. Surg.* **54,** 807.

BLUMENSTOCK D.A., OTTE H.P., GROSJEAN O.B. & MULDER M.A. (1969) Transplantation of the lung. *Transplantation Proceedings,* **I,** 223.

DEROM FR., BARBIER F., RINGOIR S., ROLLY G., VERSIECK J., BERZSENYI G., RAEMDONCK R. & PIRET J. (1969) A case of lung homotransplantation in man. *Tijdschrift voor Geneeskunde,* **25,** 109.

DEROM FR., BARBIER F., RINGOIR S., VERSIECK J., ROLLY G., BERZSENYI G., VERMEIRE P. & VRINTS L. (1970) Ten month survival after lung homotransplantation in man. *J. Thorac. cardiovasc. Surg.*—Submitted for publication.

FABER L.P., PEDREIRA A.L.S., PEVSNER P.H. & BEATTIE E.J. (1965) The immediate and long-term physiologic function of bilateral reimplanted lungs. *J. Thorac. Cardiovasc. Surg.* **50,** 761.

FLAX M.H. & BARNES B.A. (1966) The role of vascular injury in pulmonary allograft rejection. *Transplantation,* **4,** 66.

GAGO O.E. (1970) Personal Communication.

HAGLIN J. (1970) Personal Communicaton—Washington.

HARDY J.D. (1969) Lung Transplantation. In *Organ transplantation today.* Excerpta Medica Foundation, 214.

HARDY J.D., WEBB W.R., DALTON M.L. Jr. & WALKER C.R. Jr. (1963) Lung homotransplantation in man. *J.A.M.A.* **186,** 1065.

HUGGINS C.E. (1959) Reimplantation of lobes on the lung. *Lancet,* i, 59.

JUVENELLE A.A., CITRET C., WILES C.E. Jr. & STEWART J.D. (1951) Pneumectomy with replantation of the lung in the dog for physiologic study. *J. Thorac. Surg.* **21,** 111.

LANDE A.J. & LILLEHEI C.W. (1969) Preclinical evaluation of a practical membrane oxygenator. *Surg. Forum.* **20,** 150.

METRAS H. (1950) Note préliminaire sur la greffe totale du poumon chez le chien. *C. R. Acad. Sci.* **231,** 1176.

NEPTUNE W.B., WELLER R. & BAILEY C.P. (1953) Experimental lung transplantation. *J. Thorac. Surg.* **26,** 275.

RANGEL D.M., STEVENS G.H., YAKEISHI Y., SANCHEZ M. & FONKALSRUD E.W. (1969) Physiologic evaluation of canine lung allografts from cadaver donors. *Surgery,* **66,** 863.

SECRIST W.L. & TRUMMER M.J. (1967) Nerve regeneration following lung reimplantation. *Ann. Thoracic Surg.* **4,** 125.

STEVENS P.M., JOHNSON P.C., BELL R.L., BEALL Jr. A.C. & JENKINS D.E. (1970) Regional perfusion and perfusion after lung transplantation in patients with emphysema. *New Engl. J. Med.* **245,** 282.

VEITH F.J. & RICHARDS K. (1969) Lung transplantation with simultaneous contralateral pulmonary artery ligation. *Surg. Gynec. Obstet.* **129,** 768.

WHITE J.J., TANSER P.H., ANTHONIESEN N.R., WYNANDS J.E., PARS J.A.P., BECKLAKE M.R., MUNRO D.D. & MACLEAN L.D. (1966) Human lung homotransplantation. *Canad. Med. Ass. J.* **94,** 1199.

WILDEVUUR CH.R.H., MEZETTI M. & HOMAN VAN DER HEIDE J.M. (1970) Lung transplantation: problems of lung function. *Les Bronches*, **20**, 144.

WILDEVUUR CH.R.H. & BENFIELD J.R. (1970) A review of 23 human lung transplantations by 20 surgeons a review of 22 cases. *Ann. Thorac. Surg.*, **9**, 489

YAKEISHI Y., NOZAKI M., RANGEL D., STEVENS G. & ADAMS F. (1969) Effect of allotransplantation of the canine lung on pulmonary surfactant. *Surgery, Gynecology, Obstetrics*, **128**, 1264.

Part 6
Other Organs

CHAPTER 32

Transplantation of the Pancreas, Endocrine Organs, Reticulo-Endothelial Elements and Bone

R.A. Sells

I. GLANDULAR GRAFTS IN THE TREATMENT OF HORMONE DEFICIENCY

INTRODUCTION

Other chapters in this book have dealt predominantly with transplantation of organs which are immediately essential to life, for instance, the kidney, liver, heart and the lung. In these cases irreversible and untreatable organ failure present an immediate danger of death, with the exception of renal failure, in which dialysis is available as definitive long-term therapy, or as a preparation for renal transplantation. Failure of the endocrine organs results in a more insidious progression of pathological and biochemical changes, not necessarily fatal in outcome and which can of course be successfully treated in man by replacement therapy using purified hormone preparations derived from mammalian endocrine glands or synthetic preparations. Although advance in endocrinology has thus saved many lives and improved the quality of life in many patients suffering from endocrine deficiencies, certain problems inherent in replacement therapy persist. These problems relate to the control of dosage, immune reactions to heterologous hormone preparations, and the progression of the natural history of the disease despite 'adequate replacement' of the deficient hormone.

If we consider any primary hormonal deficiency state in which life is threatened if the hormone is witheld, then an allograft becomes preferable to injection of heterologous hormone preparations for the following reasons:

1. The regulation of secretions of grafts is effected by normal homeostatic feedback mechanisms. A degree of control is therefore obtainable from a normally functioning graft which should be superior to the relatively crude degree of control achieved in patients receiving injections. Furthermore, injections would not be necessary.
2. Because of this improved control, the quantity of a hormone secreted by a graft would be appropriate to the state of the patients at any particular time. Thus optimal control of hormone dependent reactions would be maintained and long-term effects of dosage mismanagement (for instance, the long-term complications of diabetes, which in certain cases are refractory to insulin) are likely to be avoided. Similarly, acute complications due to overdosage or underdosage should not occur.
3. Although the main physiological active principle secreted by a gland may be known and a purified preparation of it may be obtained suitable for injection into humans, it is known that there are other hormones produced by some glands which do not appear to be essential for the survival, but which almost certainly have a significant effect. The omission of such hormones from a preparation of a purified extract of, say, insulin may cause a response which differs from the total secretions of the gland. One can assume that a normally functioning homograft would supply these additional hormones in correct quantities.
4. It can be assumed that complex hormones secreted by an allograft would be structurally unique to the species from which it arose and therefore similar, if not identical to, the endogenous hormones produced by the recipient. There is no advantage clinically in contemplating graft procedures in the treatment of say hypothyroidism—the existing oral thyroxine preparation is effective, easily administered and is not known to elicit an immune response in the patient. On the other hand, substitution therapy in hypoparathyroidism is attended by an increase in plasma antiparathyroid hormone activity, and subsequent loss of control of calcium metabolism. Immune reaction (and inactivation) would not be expected to occur in the host against homologous hormones originating from an allograft.

These remarks apply to the hypothetical recipient of a graft in whom successful endocrine replacement has been achieved by the graft and in whom no other intercurrent disease exists. At present however, the hazards of immunosuppression in clinical transplantation are such as to contra-indicate transplantation in any patient who is not suffering from an irreversible, lethal or very severely debilitating disorder. Recent encouraging work on the modification of the immune response by biological means suggests that the present dose of immunosuppressive compounds may eventually be reduced or even abandoned. With the attendant reduction in mortality and morbidity transplantation will become a much safer procedure and the use of endocrine allografts will no doubt be considered more seriously in the treatment of endocrine deficiency.

1 The pancreas

Since the discovery of the therapeutic value of insulin in 1922 and the understanding of the nature of diabetes medical treatment with diet, insulinotropic agents or insulin replacement have removed the danger of death from coma in the majority of diabetics, although a hazard of hypoglycaemia faces the insulin dependent diabetic. Furthermore, a disappointing feature of the control of diabetes by insulin is that in a minority of patients the quality of the control of glucose metabolism seems to bear little relationship to the rate of onset and progression of vascular, renal and retinal complications. Thus, in a survey of juvenile onset type diabetes 88% died a premature death due to cardiovascular or renal disease and 100% exhibited fundoscopic changes within 25 years of the onset of the disease. It has been estimated in a large series of juvenile diabetics that the 10-year-old diabetic has a life expectancy of about 30 years (White 1960). This may indicate that the control of insulin dose, which is worked out by the patient himself, or his doctor, on the urinary concentration of sugar, is not accurate enough to ensure stabilization of the blood sugar which in the long term will arrest the progress of complications. Alternatively, it may be that the different types of complications of the disease reflect different abnormalities of tissue chemistry, blood vessels, or hormone action: a study of diabetic neuropathy indicated that nerve damage has occurred in a group of diabetics in whom nephropathy, peripheral vascular disease and retinopathy also have commonly occurred: however, hypercholesterolaemia, coronary artery and myocardial disease form a separate group in whom good control of the diabetes is likely to delay the onset of complications (Pirart 1965). There is evidence that fall-off in control occurs with time. Thirty per cent of juvenile diabetics have good control 15 years after the onset of their disease, yet show a significant incidence of degenerative complications (Lestradet & Billaud 1965).

Early observations on the plasma insulin-like activity in diabetics (using a rat diaphragm bioassay), suggested a reduced reserve of insulin, which became worse with clinical deterioration (Seltzer & Smith 1959). In patients suffering from primary insulin deficiency (the non-obese ketotic type) replacement of insulin by a graft would be expected to enhance control, and it might be hoped that this would have a beneficial effect on the progress of complications. Laboratory investigation of this possibility has not been forthcoming, for as yet no experimental animal which exhibits primary insulin deficiency and diabetes has yet been subjected to long-term pancreatic homografts. Such animals are rare, but diabetes is genetically transmitted, apparently in a manner similar to human diabetes, in the sand rat and in the Chinese hampster, both of which would be useful experimental models for the study of the effect of an allograft on the natural history of diabetes.

The majority of diabetics, however, suffer from a more gradually progressive disease of the obese non-ketotic type, which was thought to result from a defect of peripheral insulin utilization rather than primary insulin deficiency. At least some of these obese diabetics secrete more insulin than non-obese subjects, yet analysis of carbohydrate tolerance and insulin secretory reserve in weight matched patients and controls reveals an overall deficiency of insulin secretory capacity in obese diabetics, resulting in increased insulin requirements (Perley & Kipnis 1966). Despite the fact that such intolerance to carbohydrate may be reversed by careful dieting and weight reduction, a proportion of these patients progress to the stage of insulin dependent diabetes. Whether or not a pancreatic graft would help such patients is not known. If insulin resistance is due to metabolic alterations secondary to the obese state then there is little point in considering such a procedure. If, however, the advent of florid diabetes is due to the vascular and degenerative complications of diabetes within the pancreas, then islet cell grafts with a reducing diet may be a therapeutic and useful measure in this group of patients.

A *The immunological aspects of heterologous insulin injections*

The majority of insulin preparations used in human diabetes are derived from ox or pig pancreas. Preparations of chemically complex hormones from different species can be antigenic, and insulin is no exception, indeed heterologous antibodies can be made to insulin, and anti-insulin serum forms the basis of modern immunochemical insulin assay systems (Yalow & Berson 1959). Furthermore, insulin binding protein has been found in the serum of insulin treated diabetics who had formed antibodies to heterologous insulin (Chao, Karan *et al* 1965). A minority of diabetics develop severe insulin resistance which may lead to refractory coma under conditions of stress, for instance, infection; hyperglycaemic coma and ketosis in a patient with a high level of circulating antibodies may be completely resistant to very large doses of intravenous insulin.

There is some evidence that the therapeutic activity of heterologous insulins are different between species. While this may be explained by specific antibody production and subsequent inactivation, human insulin-binding antibodies certainly seem more avid for ox than pig hormone (Hurn *et al* 1969). Recent investigations have shown that hypoglycaemia may occur in patients on high doses of beef insulin who change to similar doses of porcine insulin, a phenomenon explained by Devlin *et al* (1967) in terms of specific antibody levels. A few insulin dependent patients have been described in whom poor control, due to antibody mediated insulin resistance, was improved by withdrawing the hormone and substituting chlorpropamide; the endogenous hormone was thus able to meet the patient's requirements.

B *Experimental and clinical transplantation of the pancreas*

Several workers have established that pancreatic allografts are technically feasible in dogs, rats, pigs, rabbits and humans. Grafts have been shown to replace adequately essential endocrine secretions in diabetes (experimentally induced by alloxan or pancreatectomy). Dogs have been studied more than other species and the most successful type of graft has been the pancreatico-duodenal transplant. In this preparation the small blood vessels to the gland derived from the pancreatico-duodenal vasculature remain undisturbed and thus thrombotic complications are diminished. Gut-to-gut anastomosis permits the drainage of exocrine secretions. Ligation of the pancreatic duct at the time of transplantation (Largiader *et al* 1968) considerably worsened the result and irradiation to suppress exocrine secretion did not significantly improve dog survival (Merkel *et al* 1968).

Pancreatico-duodenal grafts may be transplanted orthotopically or heterotopically with portal vein drainage to host portal vein (orthotopic) or systemic (ortho and hetertopic) venous channels. The duodenum may be transplanted orthotopically, as a Roux-en-Y loop, as a conduit into the jejunum, or may be brought out to the skin as fistula. The most successful preparation has been the heterotopic graft into the pelvis, devised in the dog and used in humans by Lillehei.

Transplantation of the pancreas alone has been attempted. Burgen has used dog grafts removed from the duodenal arch in which the ducts were ligated at the time of transplantation, and which resulted in graft necrosis, with equivocal evidence of rejection. Reemtsma *et al* (1969) using the dog, and Lillehei *et al* (1969) unsuccessfully in one human case, have transplanted the body and tail of the pancreas heterotopically without drainage of exocrine secretions. In Reemtsma's (1969) experiments improved results were obtained using donors in which the pancreatic duct had been ligated 6 weeks prior to the operation with subsequent atrophy of acinar tissue by the time of transplantation.

In experienced hands experimental pancreatico-duodenal allografts in pancreatectomized dogs have survived many months if immunosuppressive drugs were given to prevent rejection. Most authors agree that pancreatic grafts, perfused or unperfused, will function after a warm ischaemic time of up to 1 hour. Using hyperbaria and hypothermia Idezuki (1969) has preserved dog pancreatico-duodenal grafts for up to 24 hours and has found good immediate function after transplantation. These experimental findings correlated well with his work on *in vitro* estimation of insulin production by the perfused pancreas: grafts stored for more than 24 hours showed *in vitro* inability to secrete insulin in response to a glucose load. Encouraged by these findings Lillehei (1969) has transplanted five patients with insulin dependent juvenile onset diabetes and terminal nephropathy, who received combined renal and pancreatico-duodenal allografts. Two of these patients left hospital with normal function of both grafts. Neither patient had required insulin since transplantation. In one recipient control of the diabetic state had to be re-established post-operatively by insulin therapy during an episode of rejection, while the dose of steroids was raised. Subsequent lowering of immunosuppression caused an improvement in glucose tolerance, and insulin injections were eventually stopped altogether. Lillehei's results suggest also that the pancreas may be less liable to rejections than other organs, a possibility indicated by the fact that his failed cases have succumbed or had their grafts removed for renal rejection rather than for pancreatic rejection.

In experimental animals, pancreatic rejection seems to be a more serious problem than in these human cases. In dogs and rats standard techniques of immunosuppression (prednisone, Imuran, 6-Mercaptopurine, horse-anti-dog lymphocyte serum and irradiation) rarely resulted in prolongation of graft function for further than 40 days. Reemtsma has shown that the rat pancreas appears to be no less prone to rejection than the kidney. There is indirect evidence, however, than the endocrine component of the pancreas may be less antigenic than the exocrine. Certainly de Jode & Howard (1962) described hyperglycaemia as being a terminal phase in graft rejection in the dog: histological examination of the graft frequently revealed extensive pancreatitis, whereas the islet tissues were relatively free of cellular infiltrate. It is interesting that in 'acute allogeneic disease', a type of hyperacute graft-versus-host reaction produced by hyperimmune peritoneal macrophages injected into the peritoneal cavity of mice, a destructive immunological attack occurs on the abdominal organs, including the pancreas, in which the islets of Langerhans appear to remain unscathed, indicating some degree of privilege of endocrine tissue over exocrine in this organ (Weiser *et al* 1965).

C *Biochemical considerations*

All authors since Hédon (1892) have used the blood sugar level as an index of graft activity and latterly other parameters such as amylase, plasma insulin like activity, and plasma lactic dehydrogenase have been used to follow the pancreatic graft function. An interesting and consistent finding following heterotopic pancreatic grafts has been a significantly low fasting blood sugar level, and has been found by Teixeira *et al* (1966) to be associated with higher levels in insulin secretion than normal in response to a glucose load. This is probably due to the drainage of pancreatic venous blood into the systemic, as opposed to the portal circulation. Normally portal venous blood contains a higher insulin like activity than post-hepatic systemic blood, as insulin is altered or inactivated in the liver. Presumably, the diversion of insulin from the liver allows greater peripheral insulin activity and glucose utilization, causing hypoglycaemia. The diversion of pancreatic glucagon away from the liver will also tend to produce hypoglycaemia, although in a different way; glucagon reaching the liver from the portal blood activates phosphorylase, which results in glucagon breakdown and glucose release. It is probable therefore that post-transplant hypoglycaemia results from excessive insulin activity and lack of catabolic glucagon activity, although no experimental evidence is yet available to substantiate this hypothesis.

D *Transplantation of isolated islet tissue*

A byproduct of the search by biochemists for a method of studying islet tissue in diabetic experimental animals has been the technique of 'free' islet transplantation. Utilizing a privileged recipient site (the anterior chamber of the eye) Hultquist & Thorell (1963) using young adult rat minced pancreatic homografts showed histological and biochemical evidence of endocrine graft survival in pancreatectomized recipients, confirming similar histological observations in normal mice of Browning & Resnik (1951) and Coupland (1957). These authors observed that foetal donor material produced more consistently successful results than adult tissue; this may be explained by the fact that foetal pancreatic tissue contains a high proportion of islet cells to acinar tissue (the latter remains undeveloped until birth), and presumably the local release of enzymes and thus subsequent damage to the graft is less from source. House *et al* (1958) showed that similar free pancreatic allografts implanted into the hamster cheek pouch (another 'privileged' site) reversed alloxan induced diabetes in 50% of cases. An intensive study of the histological appearance of free grafts into rat testes by Gonet & Renold (1965) has shown that the surviving cells are predominantly of the β-cell type, stain specifically for insulin and furthermore extraction and assay reveals the presence of the hormone in the graft.

There is little doubt therefore that free transplantation of small pancreatic fragments to immunologically privileged sites in rodents may produce a culture of islet tissue capable of replacing β-cell function after removal or destruction of the host's own pancreas. From histological appearances of the islets in pancreatic canine allografts and acute murine allogeneic disease there is indirect evidence for the hypothesis that islet tissue may be less immunogenic than exocrine tissue (*vide supra*). It might be expected therefore that islet cultures in unprivileged sites would not be rejected as vigorously as the intact vascularized organ allograft. Minced neonatal rat pancreatic allografts have been placed beneath the renal capsule in normal rats (Sells 1969). Subsequent pancreatectomy resulted in a transient hyperglycamia which reverted to normal blood glucose levels after a 3-week period. Rejection was seen in a minority of these grafts, which otherwise looked undistinguishable from islet cultures in privileged situation. The concept of free pancreatic transplantation of the pancreas in diabetics is in some ways a more satisfactory and less heroic alternative to whole pancreas transplantation with its inevitable morbidity due to pancreatitis, immunosuppression and technical hazards. Much more information is needed on the viability and antigenicity of such grafts in various sites and at the moment the latter technique is the only clinically applicable one for transplanting the pancreas.

Lillehei has used combined renal and pancreatic allografts and has thus enabled the inclusion into his clinical transplant programme of the small but significant number of progressive diabetics with end stage renal disease. With the emergence of improved immunosuppression and the exploitation of new types of grafts the groups of diabetics clinically eligible for such grafts will expand.

2 Transplantation of the adrenal, thyroid and parathyroid glands

Introduction

Transplantation of endocrine organs has been an important tool in investigation of endocrine gland function and endocrinology. Indeed the definition of an endocrine gland as one which could exert its effect after excision and revascularization depends on the ability of a graft to function after auto- or homotransplantation. Hormone extraction procedures have enabled successful treatment of endocrine deficiencies to such a degree that clinical endocrine homotransplantation has largely been obviated. Nevertheless, attempts have been made in humans to transplant the adrenal, thyroid and parathyroid glands. The technical problems of reconstituting the blood supply of such small pieces of tissue have encouraged workers to use free transplantation, i.e. fragmentation of tissue and implantation into a suitable site in the recipient. This technique does, however, suffer from several drawbacks. The fact that vascular continuity is not restored rapidly after the removal of the organ from the donor means that a severe degree of ischaemic damage will be incurred by the graft and 'dedifferentiation' is bound to occur. Clearly the extent of recovery of the gland and subsequent function will depend largely on its sensitivity to ischaemia during this early post-transplant period. Thyroid, ovarian and parathyroid tissue all have significantly lower oxygen consumption than adrenal and liver (Brooks & Levy 1968), and this may account for the relative success in terms of survival of thyroid, ovary and parathyroid grafts. In the case of glands where the parenchyma is arranged in a more or less homogenous fashion (e.g. thyroid) one would not expect a major upset of function to occur as a result of dedifferentation; on the other hand a highly complex structure such as the pituitary forms a multiplicity of secreted hormones and has close knit nervous and vascular connections with the hypothalmus; it is doubtful if properly integrated secretory function would ever be achieved by free grafting. The site of transplantation is also important: (the reproductive activity of the ovary could not be expected to occur unless the organ is transplanted to the orthotopic site).

It is well known that adaptation occurs in man and some experimental animals (e.g. the dog) to experimentally induced endocrine deficiencies, for instance, hypoparathyroidism. When investigating the efficacy of allografts in this condition, carefully controlled experiments must be carried out, and functional, as well as histological tests of graft function are mandatory.

Despite these drawbacks most endocrine glands seem capable of surviving in a heterotopic situation and have at least a temporary functional existence. Halstead's law—that endocrine grafts can be successful only when there is an absolute deficiency of their secretions in the host—was originally applied to autografts. It may obtain in allografts, but sufficient experimental evidence is lacking, largely due to the inability of workers to produce long-functioning grafts in deficient recipients.

The adrenal gland

Several authors have reported results of free transplantation of adrenal gland fragments into subcutaneous and muscular sites. Some authors have reported temporary improvement but most have not shown significant graft survival or improvement in the natural history of the disease, as evidenced by biochemical or histological data. One patient reported by Goldseiher & Barishaw (1937) apparently lived for 6 months after intramuscular transplantation of adrenal homograft tissue from a patient with Cushing's syndrome; the recipient suffered from Addison's disease and histologically the transplant at the time of death appeared viable. Woodruff (1952a) reported four patients with Addison's disease treated with intramuscular foetal adrenal allograft tissue and although the patients improved at the time of biopsy no histological evidence of tissue was present. In these and other reports of temporary improvement followed by ultimate failure, few authors have used standard immunosuppressive techniques; the trophic action of ACTH appeared not to have a significant effect on graft survival or function. The success of replacing adrenal hormones by synthetic steroids seems to have excluded the need for clinical adrenal transplantation.

The thyroid

Hypothyroidism is safely, cheaply and conveniently treated by oral thyroid extract or thyroxine. Thyroid transplantation is therefore of more academic than clinical importance. Thyroid tissue is known to survive immune attack if transplanted freely within a diffusion chamber which prevents cellular contact with host immunocytes. However, Brooks *et al* (1960) found that although rejection did not occur, thyroid tissue within a chamber gradually diminished in size and epithelial content, being replaced by fibrous tissue. Because the thyroid is easily transplantable tissue and will 'take' rapidly (being relatively resistant to ischaemia) it has been used successfully as a tool in biochemical research. It was discovered by Woodruff (1952b) that homograft thyroid tissue placed in the anterior chamber of the eye could later be transplanted to another site in the same recipient (for instance, under the skin). The graft would be accepted by the recipient; these experiments led to the concept of graft adaptation. As a research tool, therefore, thyroid grafting has been of some use but clinical transplantation does not seem justifiable.

The parathyroid

Transplantation of the parathyroid gland has been a more popular technique in the treatment of hypoparathyroidism in humans than thyroid transplantation in myxedema. Two basic techniques have been used; transplantation of thyroid and parathyroid using vascular reconstruction, and free transplantation of pieces of parathyroid gland, or cultured fragments, to subcutaneous or intramuscular sites, in some cases within a millipore chamber. In a review of the literature in 1963 Jacob & Dunphy suggested that although considerable clinical experience has been achieved there was little in the follow-up results or histological data to suggest that the grafts had significantly altered the natural history of hypoparathyroidism in humans, and that some of the supposedly successful grafts have been implemented at a time when adaption of the recipient to his disease would be likely to occur. Although many cases of clinical improvement have been known there appears not to be sufficient evidence to judge the efficacy of this measure.

3 The ovary

The clinical applications of ovarian transplantation are probably limited to Turner's syndrome and young castrated females. When improved methods of immunosuppression eventually make endocrine transplantation a safer procedure then no doubt there will be a sudden demand for orthotopic vascularized allotransplantation of the ovary in the treatment of sterility; the ethical question of whether artificial genetic transference by transplantation of functioning oöcytes is acceptable or unacceptable is outside the scope of this book. Despite the limited application of ovarian grafting the subject has received much attention from experimental immunologists. There was an early hypothesis that endocrine grafts, in particular the ovary, provide an antigenic stimulus which only ellicits a partial immunological response. It was suggested that this might be due to the presence of fewer histocompatability antigens. Certainly ovarian allograft tissue is just as effective as skin in eliciting transplantation immunity yet it has been shown that transplanting mouse ovary together with skin across a weak histocompatability barrier resulted in indefinite prolongation of the skin graft survival in comparison to solitary skin graft controls.

On the assumption that ovarian tissue was capable of adapting to the host, Sturgis & Castellanos (1958), have used a biological type of diffusion chamber by wrapping ovarian grafts within corneal tissue in an attempt to prevent cellular contact between host immune cells and the graft. In the rabbit this technique has been exploited by Shaffer & Hulka (1969) to investigate the extended survival of ovarian tissue in the mammal. Ovarian tissue remained viable within the corneal capsule for periods up to 30 weeks, despite repeated challenges of donor skin. If the grafts were shelled out of their capsule and replaced in the original donor after 6 weeks no rejection was seen, indicating that an alteration in antigenic constitution was not the mechanism of survival. Rejection time for other allografts were the same as controls, indicating that the hosts were not immunologically tolerant. It has been suggested that the less antigenic cells within the capsule have been passively selected for survival, the more antigenic cells having been deleted, although enhancing antibody cannot be excluded as a possible cause of the graft protection.

Autotransplantation of the ovary in the ewe by means of vascular reconstruction (Golding *et al* 1966) has been followed by normal cyclical progesterone secretion, although oöcyte production in ovarian transplantation appears to be impaired even in the orthotopic situation. Orthotopic allotransplantation of the ovary in the pig leads to rejection at about 1 week (Harrison 1969). Review of the literature on clinical allografting reveals that no surviving allograft has yet been carried out. Although several authors have demonstrated reversal of endocrine abnormalities in Turner's syndrome for periods of up to 6 months, these experiences have been followed uniformly by graft atrophy and fibrosis and return of endocrine abnormality.

The treatment of gastrointestinal deficiency by bowel homografts

Transplantation of the small bowel has been carried out in the investigation of malabsorption and the effect of denervation and deprivation of bowel lymphatics in this condition. Auto- and allotransplantation of short segments of bowel to the neck in the dog has been performed (Lillehei *et al* 1967; Hardy *et al* 1970). Study of 15 cm long autografts has shown that after revascularization severe diarrhoea and malabsorption may occur with recovery after 1 to 2 weeks; orthotopic autografts of larger segments of bowel have been demonstrated to develop a lymphatic supply within 2 to 3 weeks of transplantation. Glucose and arabinose absorption and gut motility remain unimpaired after the first week of transplantation. Allografts in the unsuppressed dog, however, are normally rejected within a week, preceded by rapid fall off in glucose absorption associated with oedema and cyanosis of the gut stoma. Histologically, rejection of bowel is characterized by the destruction of surface epithelium, absence of mucin secreting cells, dilatation of the central lacteals and marked perivascular round cells infiltration. Hardy *et al* (1970) have shown that with a combination of antilymphocyte serum, prednisone and Imuran, bowel allografting in the dog may enjoy a functional prolongation of survival of 21 to 54 days (mean 38 days).

Transplantation of large segments of the small bowel have produced a distinctly different effect on the host. Lillehei *et al* (1959) described death of dogs after transplantation of the small bowel with what appeared to be a normal allograft. Non-survival was ascribed to graft-versus-host reaction. This was presumably a consequence of transplanting a large population of lymphocytes normally resident in Peyer's patches which migrated out of the graft and attacked the host tissue.

Intestinal transplantation in man

There are few conditions in man which would justify an attempt at transplantation of the bowel, but in widespread mesenteric infarction, it is tempting to improve the debilitating diarrhoea and malabsorption which results from extensive resection of bowel by inserting an allograft. Such a patient presented at Minnesota in 1967 and was gravely ill with massive infarction of her bowel from the ligament of Treitz to the rectum. After bowel resection a total small bowel allograft was inserted but the patient died soon after the operation from thromboembolism (Lillehei *et al* 1967).

It seems likely that problems would have been encountered with graft-versus-host reaction in such a situation, although the tissue typing data are not known. Theoretically, it would be possible to irradiate the graft during a period of preservation prior to transplantation in an attempt to diminish the immune properties of the gut lymphocytes. Unfortunately, the sensitivity of gut epithelium to X-rays makes this procedure impracticable. Perfusion of the mesenteric vessels with a lymphotoxic agent might be expected to impair donor lymphocyte reactivity. From observations on the survival of the duodenum in pancreatico-duodenal allografts, where a duodenal stoma allowed serial biopsy of the mucosa, it appears that small bowel in humans may survive for long periods of time with conventional immunosuppression (Lillehei 1967). Given adequate technical facilities it seems that this particular type of graft may be practical in the future in the treatment of deficiency states following extensive bowel resection.

II. RETICULO-ENDOTHELIAL GRAFTS

Transplanting cellular elements of the reticulo-endothelial system poses special problems: the transfer of other organs between individuals calls forth predictable and, to a greater or lesser extent, suppressible reactivity against the graft on the part of the host. The grafted tissue of the kidney, lung, heart, or even liver has not been known to modify the recipient except in those effects which may appear secondary to graft failure or over activity. Reticulo-endothelial grafts, however, will contain cells normally capable of the full range of immune reactivity and their transfer to a foreign environment will cause graft reactivity to appear against the hosts tissues. The host naturally will exhibit the usual reactivity to the grafted tissue, and so bidirectional cellular attack occurs within the host. In modified recipients the outcome of this contest depends on several factors as will be seen from the following account: to put it simply, the grafted cells may be rejected, and die, in which case the host's condition remains unchanged, or the graft-versus-host reaction may overwhelm the recipient, producing a well known syndrome (termed in the irradiated experimental mammalian recipient 'secondary disease') which usually leads to death. When the condition of the recipient is one of immune deficiency then as the host reactivity is attenuated or absent the transplantation situation is more simple, as rejection is operating on one direction only (against the host). However it will be seen that the possible indications for such transplantation procedures will not remain confined to these comparatively rare disorders of reticulo-endothelial aplasia.

1 Biological considerations

Historical review

The early progress of reticulo-endothelial grafting was helped by optimistic claims of enthusiastic haematologists and others who used bone-marrow grafts in the treatment of diseases such as leukaemia and anaemia. The more hopeful claims of the early workers were not justified; initially living cells were not administered parenterally to the recipients, so it is fairly certain that no long term cures were achieved by marrow repopulation. Without properly controlled trials it is difficult to assess accurately the effect of a new therapeutic measure on the natural history of a disease, particularly one so capricious in its behaviour as leukaemia. The earliest attempts in this disease were made by Brown-Sequard & d'Arsonaval in 1891, who administered bone marrow orally. Other authors administered extracts of marrow or dead cells by mouth in the treatment of anaemia, and in 1938 an isolated case of agranulocytosis was reported, treated successfully with marrow extracts; Leake & Leake (1923) infused red marrow and spleen intravenously for secondary anaemia. It is of course possible that such procedures fortuitously resulted in the patient receiving a much needed dose of the appropriate mineral or hormone, a possibility which still cannot be discounted, but it seems inconceivable that a cure by grafting could occur without the infusion of live donor cells capable of leading a separate existence in the host. This was substantiated in 1949 by Osgood who reported probably the first case of successful bone marrow grafting for aplastic anaemia. It is difficult to prove however that remission of a disease is due to the permanent persistence of grafted allogeneic cells without cytological tests for their identification, which have only recently been developed; the possibility of spontaneous remission of the disease with disappearance of the grafted cells must always remain a realistic alternative to complete success of the transplant.

It became apparent that orthotopic placement of the graft within the marrow cavity is not necessary, and it was subsequently discovered by Gregusova & Hupka (1961) that in experimental animals intravenously infused appogeneic marrow cells settle in the lungs where they may reside for about 24 h before passing back into the systemic circulation to colonize the splenic and bone marrow parenchyma.

Modification of the recipient prior to grafting

Early attention was directed to reducing the reactivity of the host to allogeneic cells. Radiation and, less successfully, radiomimetic drugs were used in preparing the host for the graft, and although the irradiated rodent and the cancerous patient receiving X-ray therapy were somewhat similar immunologically in relation to a marrow graft, difficulties were encountered in the experimental model in achieving the correct sub-lethal dose and distinguishing the effect of irradiation from those of graft-versus-host reaction. Uphoff & Law (1957) were able to separate the effect of immune attack from those due to radiation by performing marrow transplants reciprocally between F_1 hybrids of H2 incompatible inbred mouse strains, and parental strain mice: parental strain grafts caused secondary disease in hybrid recipients, but hybrid donor cells did not behave similarly in parental strain recipients. Syngeneic grafts into irradiated recipients also failed to cause secondary disease. The syndrome therefore appeared to be due to graft versus host activity on the part of grafted cells.

Autologous spleen or marrow may restore normal physiological parameters in irradiated animals. Jacobson *et al* (1950) showed that shielding the spleen during radiation in mice protected the animal from the subsequent anaemia seen in the unshielded animal, a protection also afforded by intravenous intraperitoneal injection of syngeneic or allogeneic marrow (Congdon 1962). Furthermore, excision of the shielded spleen 1 hour after irradiation did not abolish this protective effect: the explanation for this could be that (a) the spleen provides a reservoir of unmodified cells which pass into the circulation to repopulate the marrow, or (b) a humoral factor produced by the spleen exerts a protective or even trophic effect upon otherwise critically irradiated erthyopoietic cells. But it has been shown beyond doubt (Lindsley *et al* 1955; Ford *et al* 1956) that cellular transfer is responsible for recovery rather than humoral factors.

The choice of graft

In rodents the cell which most efficiently repopulates the irradiated marrow recipient is probably the small lymphocyte—it has been shown that the restorative capacity is proportional to the number of lymphocytes transfused. In primates, lymphocyte-rich grafts produced a high incidence of severe graft-versus-host disease, and Van Bekkum (1968) has used a method of centrifugation of marrow cells on a discontinuous bovine albumen gradient whereby harmless donor marrow cells capable of restoring host marrow activity (thought to be stem cells) may be separated from mature immunocytes. Such selective allogeneic grafts have produced 100% 90-day survival in irradiated mice, and this technique shows promise in immunosuppressed primates. It has indeed been successfully used in a human recipient of a marrow graft (*vide infra*).

The genetic source of the graft is important if long-term chimerism is being attempted; isogeneic material, rarely available in humans, will produce neither graft-versus-host or rejection reaction, and thus constitutes the ideal type of graft. In allogeneic grafting the graft/host relationship may vary widely within acceptable limits of genetic difference, and allogeneic grafting across weak histocompatability barriers have produced long-term chimeras, whereas extreme dissimilarities preclude transplantation. It has been found that the dose of cells required to produce a successful 'take' is proportional to the genetic difference between donor and host (Yamada & Wakeyama 1961). In human allografts a marrow dose about 0·5% of the total normal marrow mass is thought to be adequate. In man the choice of the best donor/recipient relationship may be made by carrying leukocyte antigen typing, assessing lymphocyte reactivity in a mixed culture (in both directions) and by testing the reactions of donor and recipient leukocytes in the dermis of an irradiated hamster (Mathé 1968).

Graft-versus-host reaction could theoretically be overcome in disparate donor/recipient relationships by employing tolerant or potentially tolerant graft sources. Classical tolerance has already been referred to in the context of non-identical cattle twin chimeras and tolerance induction has been described in foetal rodents by artificial exposure to antigen during the adaptive phase of lymphoreticular development. This concept allows two possible manoeuvres: (1) the use of marrow from donors made artificially tolerant of recipient cells by injection during the adaptive period, (2) the use of marrow cells derived from donors near the end of the adaptive period.

In either case specific tolerance might be expected to occur, with consequent lack of secondary disease; the problem would only be solved in one direction, however, as 'host-versus-graft' rejection would not be influenced by this sort of selection. Duplan & Monier (1961) found that this method produced success only in certain strain combinations and that rejection of the graft occurred after recovery of the irradiated host bone marrow.

The use of pooled cells from multiple donors has been suggested by Mathé *et al* (1968). The rationale being that the more disparate cells are rejected before the onset of secondary disease, and the suitable compatible cells repopulate the marrow. It is unlikely, however, that such an approach would be superior to that of chosing the best donor/recipient relationship prior to grafting by tissue-typing and testing mutual reactivity in mixed lymphocyte culture.

Prior treatment of donor marrow with cytotoxic agents has not been successful, as the efficacy of the graft is depressed as well as the anti-host reactivity. Cosgrave *et al* (1958) showed a diminution of secondary disease in irradiated F_1 hybrid mice injected with parental spleen cells after prior incubation with recipient strain liver, suggesting some modifying action of liver tissue on the reactivity of lymphocytes, a topic discussed elsewhere. However, it is not clear whether this is a non specific effect of liver tissue or whether incubation *per se* will also alter reactivity.

Treatment of the recipient after grafting

In primates treatment of recipients following a marrow allograft with Amethopterin and cyclophosphamide has improved survival and diminished graft-versus-host activity (van Bekkum 1968). Antilymphocyte serum also appears effective in diminishing secondary disease. An interesting method of producing selective proliferation of one moiety of bone marrow has been exploited by Congdon (1969). The post-irradiation anaemia found in mice may be averted by subjecting the grafted animals to chronic hypoxia ('hypoxic caging'); under these conditions selective erythropoietic proliferation occurs which dominates leukopoiesis, with consequent reduction in the incidence of secondary disease. Although this method is not applicable clinically, the use of trophic hormones, e.g. erthropoietin, may lead to a useful physiological method of suppressing graft activity against the host.

2 **Possible clinical indications for reticuloendothelial grafting procedures, and results**

From the point of view of the transplantation immunologist, immune deficiency syndromes fall into three main groups:

1. stem cell deficiency
2. thymic deficiency
3. erythroid, myeloid and platelet marrow deficiency
4. haemophilia.

A brief account follows of the main features of these conditions and the outcome of attempts made to cure them by transplantation.

1. *Stem cell deficiency*

A deficiency characterized by combined loss of cellular and humoral immune mechanisms is the disease known as Swiss agamma-globulinaemia. Typically gamma-globulin is undetectable in the serum, there is lymphopenia and inability to mount a delayed hypersensitivity response (e.g. reject a skin allograft). It may be that this arises from a defect of stem cell development with consequent lack of plasma cells and lymphocytes. The disease is fatal in infancy, the cause of death being infection which the patient has little power to resist. Thymus grafting (1 mm fragments of foetal thymus placed in the rectus muscle) has not been successful in restoring cellular immunity, as evidenced by lack of serum IGG response and continued inability to reject allograft tissue. However, bone marrow transplantation has been effective in these respects, although patient survival is difficult to achieve because of the poor initial state of the recipient and the consequent unusual susceptibility to graft-versus-host disease. Two cases illustrate the application of this technique.

Rosen *et al* (1966) described the case of a negro boy with Swiss disease who, after unsuccessful thymic grafting, received a graft of unmodified maternal marrow. A rise in peripheral lymphocyte count was noted, with a concommitant return of delayed hypersensitivity response. Unfortunately, the child died of pulmonary sepsis which was present before the graft took place. There was not convincing evidence of graft-versus-host disease at autopsy. A 5-month-old male child with a similar disease was treated by de Koning *et al* (1969) with a combination of foetal thymus tissue graft taken from a 15-week abortus, and a bone marrow infusion from the patient's sister. The leucocyte antigen profile was identical in brother and sister and mutual cellular reactivity, measured *in vitro* by mixed lymphocyte culture, was nil. Although these tests suggested very little likelihood of severe graft-versus-host activity, the marrow was treated by centrifugation on a discontinuous albumen gradient and fraction 2 was infused (this fraction contained the least reactive population of stem cells as seen in the rhesus monkey model of van Bekkum). The child was nursed in sterile conditions and apart from a mild exanthema during the 3rd and 4th weeks after treatment, has remained well, having shown a return to normal of cellular immune reactivity and normal serum immunoglobulin levels. The exanthema was thought to represent a mild graft-versus-host response.

The success of this case emphasizes the importance of proper genetic selection of donor and recipient. The authors make the point that siblings, not necessarily twins, are likely to be good donor/recipient pairs because the HLA antigens being governed by one genetic locus, siblings will have a one in four chance of receiving the same HLA antigens from each parent.

It also seems likely from this case that prior treatment of the marrow graft by eliminating reactive immunocytes lessens the chances of graft-versus-host disease.

2. *Thymus deficiency*

A type of cellular immune deficiency with *normal* antibody synthetic mechanisms is found in association with thymic aplasia, congenital hypoparathyroidism and abnormalities of the great vessels (Di George's syndrome). This combination of deficiency arises from failure of development of third and fourth ventral branchial arch derivatives. The immune status of these rare children is exactly that of the neonatally thymectomized mammal: they cannot reject skin allografts nor mount delayed hypersensitivity reactions to chemical antigens or tuberculin. Lymphocytes are present in peripheral blood, but do not undergo blast formation on exposure to foreign antigen or phytohaemagglutinins. By contrast, serum immunoglobulin levels are normal, and humoral antibody responses may be elicited to antigen. Transplantation of fragments of foetal thymus to the rectus sheath has resulted in dramatic restoration of cellular immune competence (August *et al* 1968; Cleveland *et al* 1968) with rapid improvement in clinical condition. The behaviour of this type of graft is particularly interesting in that the return of cellular responsiveness was extremely rapid (within 48 hours of the graft), and that in one male child who received a female thymus graft the reactive lymphocytes were of host antigen type. Furthermore graft-versus-host disease was not found to be a problem. This provides good evidence of an inductive role for the thymus graft rather than the establishment of a chimeric state by thymus derived cells. There is a good deal of scepticism regarding the possibility of early activity of free thymus grafts (Dempster 1969) but this field of therapy is very promising in the treatment of this and other forms of thymic aplasia, as well as being of great interest to cellular immunologists.

3 *Deficiency of the erythroid, myeloid, and platelet series of bone marrow cells*

The principle benefit of bone marrow grafts in this category of diseases has been claimed in the treatment of thrombocytopenia accompanying aplastic anaemia although a very small number of truly successful grafts appear to have been carried out. One such case was described by Calarusso *et al* in 1962—an adult female suffering from iatrogenic thrombocytopenia purpura secondary to bismuth and arsenic therapy. She received numerous blood transfusions and was eventually treated by multiple intramedullary unmodified marrow infusions from her husband. Her improvement and prolonged survival suggest the development of true chimerism. With strict selection of donors by tissue typing and *in vitro* assessment of graft reactivity no doubt marrow grafting in aplastic anaemia and thrombocytopenia will become feasible.

Another theoretical use for marrow grafting is in the repopulation of marrow in patients with fatal reticulosis following ablative sub-lethal doses of whole body irradiation. The main objection to this type of treatment lies in the fact that if the radiation dose is kept below the level which would cause fatal gastrointestinal and cutaneous complications, a truly ablative dose to the tumour will not be attained. This means that although the population of malignant tumour cells is drastically reduced, resurgence of tumour activity seems inevitable; exposure of the patient to the dangers and miseries of severe radiation and grafting do not seem justifiable at present. Mathé *et al* (1968) described allogeneic bone marrow grafting in 24 non-irradiated leukaemic patients, 17 of whom exhibited successful 'takes', 13 of these succumbed to secondary disease.

The severity of this syndrome was however attentuated by using cortisone during marrow infusion and amethopterin and cyclophosphamide in the post-transplantation phase, which confirmed the observations made by van Bekkum on the treatment of secondary disease using these drugs in rhesus monkeys. Pegg, in his comprehensive review (1966) of this subject noted a high incidence of fatal secondary disease and a low proportion (about 10%) of recipients who appeared to have derived any benefit from marrow grafts.

4 *Haemophilia (factor VIII deficiency)*

The treatment of haemophilia consists of transfusion of antihaemophilic factor (AHF) either in the form of whole plasma or in the more convenient cryo- or glycine precipitated concentrate. In either case the half life of AHF in the haemophiliac is 8–12 h, so long term prophylactic therapy to prevent spontaneous haemorrhage is currently impracticable. It has been shown by *ex-vivo* perfusion in the dog, pig and man that the spleen, amongst other organs (in particular the liver) produces AHF. A successful splenic allograft might therefore appear to be a hopeful therapeutic measure in such patients. Experimenters in this field were fortunate in the availability of a colony of dogs in which factor VIII deficiency (analogous to human haemophilia) occurs spontaneously, which could therefore be used as the recipients of normal spleens for the evaluation of this procedure. Several authors have reported improvement in clotting ability following ortho- and hetertopic splenic allografting procedures (Webster *et al* 1967; Norman *et al* 1968; Sise *et al* 1968), and prolongation of graft survival with Imuran

(Marchioro *et al* 1964). Graft-versus-host reaction is a surprisingly not conspicuous feature in these observations. The clinical use of splenic transplantation has been reported by Marchioro *et al* (1964). Five patients received grafts, four suffered from widespread tumour growth (in whom it was hoped that the immunological properties of the grafted splenic cells would cause remission of the cancer), and one patient had hypo-gammaglobulinaemia. No successes were achieved. Hathaway *et al* (1969) from the same centre described a severe haemophilic boy who received a splenic graft from his father. The spleen was placed heterotopically in the iliac fossa and the recipient received Imuran and antilymphocyte serum. Tissue typing revealed one major antigen detectable in the donor and absent in the recipient. AHF levels rose from 0% and persisted at 30% for 110 h, when the patient became shocked. Exploration of the graft showed a laceration of its surface and haemorrhage from this necessitated its removal. The cause of this complication was not apparent.

Despite early disappointments, reticuloendothelial grafts are being used in wider contexts of haematological and immune disorders. Although the safety of the recipient is still definitely at risk from graft-versus-host disease, an improved understanding of the mechanisms involved will no doubt produce better results in future. Crucial to this improvement seem to be the selection of ideal donor/recipient matches, selective marrow grafting and more specific chemotherapy in the early post-operative phase. Developments in this field will be watched with great interest by those concerned with transplantation biology.

III. BONE GRAFTS

A very large amount of literature has accumulated on the subject of foreign bone grafts, and descriptions range from the efficacy of allogeneic bone chips to whole limb and joint replacement. The following account outlines some of the pathological and clinical features of bone grafting but makes no attempt at a comprehensive survey. The fascinating surgical technique of whole limb autotransplantation (replacement) is not described here and the reader is referred to an authorative monograph by J.S.Horn on this subject (1969).

Surgical techniques for bone grafting have now been available for more than half a century, yet it was only recently with the development of interest in transplantation biology that an objective comparison of autologous and homologous bone graft has been felt necessary by orthopaedic surgeons. The results of current series suggest that the early optimism which led to homologous and heterologous tissue grafts should be tempered with caution; lack of detail concerning technique, type of graft and clinical and radiological outcome make comparison of autologous and homologous bone graft very difficult.

1 Bone autografts

The behaviour of autotransplanted bone has been fully studied (for summary see Burwell 1969), in humans and experimental animals, and the pathological sequence of events seems to be as follows. Free bone grafts, being temporarily deprived of a blood supply, undergo partial necrosis, but the surviving cellular elements soon show mitosis and proliferation, the endosteal cells being more active than the periosteal in this regard (Reynolds & Oliver 1950). Revascularization occurs from host tissue in 1 to 3 weeks (Deleu & Trueta 1965). Bigger fragments of bone largely die at this stage and are slowly revascularized from both ends by vessels entering the medulla. However, smaller fragments form the site of new bone formation after vascularization, and there is evidence that osteogenesis occurs from the grafted bone as well as from the surrounding tissues. The endosteal tissue in autogenous bone is found to be more productive of new bone than periosteal tissue, and for this reason cancellous chip autografts are more satisfactory in the clinical treatment of bony defects. It is probable that as the endosteal surface of cancellous bone is much greater in area than in cortical bone, osteogenic induction is greater, the bone is more rapidly vascularized, and more rapidly remodelled (Abbott *et al* 1947). Following osteogenesis, cortico-medullary differentiation, remodelling and growth follow the pattern seen in a united fracture.

Several factors are known to determine the success of autografts, the most important being the size of grafted fragments, the source of the bone, the vascularity of the bed, and the age of the patient. It appears that the ideal autogenous bone graft is in a young child consisting of cancellous bone chips transplanted into the marrow and covered with well vascularized muscle. Boiled or frozen autografts are not as successful since their contribution to bone formation is nil and the graft acts as a rather weak dead strut which is slowly removed and replaced by host bone. It appears also that mechanical compression is a stimulus to graft survival: heterotopic non weight-bearing autogenous bone fragments waste away without forming organized bone (Howlem 1952).

2 Bone allografts

Bone, like other tissues, contains in its cells histocompatibility antigens representative of the donor in type, and is therefore antigenic when transplanted. The mineral in bone is not antigenic, and does not therefore excite an immune response; deproteinizing bone may however diminish antigenicity. After free grafting of allogeneic bone chips an inflammatory response is seen between 6 and 12 days characterized by round cell, plasma cell and macrophage infiltration and eventual impairment of the blood supply due to thrombosis and depressed vascularization. The allogeneic bone cells die and therefore osteogenesis is impaired. The mineral bone remains, and after 1 month induced bone growth in the surround host tissue takes place. Remodelling is slow and consists of destruction of the donor tissue and creeping substitution by new bone (accretion). Allotransplantation of bone into a recipient previously sensitized to donor skin results in early signs of acute rejection. Despite initial immune damage, after as long an interval as 1 year, dog allografts have been observed to form a satisfactory bridge in a major skeletal defect of long bone (Herndon 1960).

3 Clinical use of bone allografts

Bone autografts are ideal for reconstituting small defects encountered in orthopaedic practice, but in some cases stored allograft bone would be more convenient and safe, for instance, in extensive spinal fusion for scoliosis in children, filling of bone cysts, treatment of delayed fractures and replacing extensive bone loss following radical surgery for cancer or trauma. The primary disadvantages are the rejection process and the fact that stored grafts are dead and cannot contribute to bone formation. However, the ability of even dead allograft bone to induce osteogenesis in surrounding tissue has produced a measure of clinical success. As pointed out earlier, the objective assessment of success or failure in bone allografts is difficult, due to variability in technique and other factors. Some authors have indeed favoured allograft bone rather than autogenous bone (Sicard & Binet 1950), though the general consensus of opinion points to the reverse being true. An attempt to compare the fate of fresh autografts and frozen irradiated homologous bone transplants was made by Bosworth *et al* (1953) using a standard technique for both types of graft in the Hibbs spinal fusion operation for tuberculosis. Based on radiological assessment 13·3% of the autografts and 32·7% of stored allografts were judged to have failed, an observation broadly confirmed by McElroy in 1963. The method of storage undoubtedly influences the fate of allogeneic bone: the most satisfactory graft appears to be frozen bone chips, and the least satisfactory methiolate preserved bone.

Massive frozen bone allografts implanted after radical resections for tumour have been variously reported and some degree of functional success has been achieved, despite varying amounts of bone absorption and cartilage necrosis (Ottolenghi 1966). Eighty-two per cent success was claimed by

Merle d'Aubigné *et al* (1966) and a similar figure is quoted by Afanassieff in a review of the Russian literature (1967). No immunosuppression was given in these patients, and though functional survival may have been achieved, it is doubtful whether many of these cases constituted success from the biological point of view.

In summary, bone autografts are ideal and stored bone allografts freely transplanted into bony defects may give acceptable results. It is possible that with attention to donor/recipient matching and immune suppression, in conjunction with improved storage methods to keep bone tissue alive, that bone allografts of limited size will approach autografts in efficiency, safety and long term survival.

REFERENCES

ABBOTT L.C., SCHOTTSTAEDT E.R., SAUNDERS J.B. & DEC. BOST F.C. (1947) The evaluation of cortical and cancellous bone as grafting material. A clinical and experimental study. *J. Bone Jt. Surg.* **29,** 381.

AFANASSIEF A. (1967) Les reconstructions articulaires partielles ou totales par homogreffes. *La Presse Medicale,* **75,** 669.

AUGUST C.S., ROSEN F.S., FILLER R.M., JANEWAY C.A., MANKOWSKI B. & KAY H.E.M. (1968) Implantation of a foetal thymus restoring immunologic competence in a patient with thymic aplasia (Di George's syndrome). *Lancet,* ii, 1210.

BOSWORTH D.M., WRIGHT H.A., FIELDING J.W. & GOODRICH E.R. (1953) A study in the use of bank bone for spine fusion in tuberculosis. *J. Bone Jt. Surg.* **35A,** 329.

BROOKS J.R., HILL G.J., II, SCOVILLE A. DE, PRIARIO J., CROCKER D. & SELENKOW H.A. (1960) A study of the survival and function of homografted thyroid tissue in membrane filter chambers in the rat. *Endocrinology,* **66,** 392.

BROOKS J.R. & LEVY J. (1968) Endocrine Transplantation. In *Human Transplantation,* ed. DAUSSET J. & RAPAPORT F.T., p. 271.

BROWNING H. & RESNIK P. (1951) Homologous and heterologous transplantation of pancreatic tissue in normal and diabetic mice. *Yale J. Biol. & Med.* **24,** 141.

BURWELL G. (1969) The Fate of Bone Grafts. In *Recent Advances in Orthopaedics,* Ed. APLEY A.G., p. 115.

CALARUSSO A., BILE G. & DE BIASI R. (1962) Erythrocyte antigenic constitution and seroimmunological data in a woman subjected ten years before to repeated transplants of bone marrow. *Rif. med.* **76,** 101.

CASTELLANOS H., STURGIS S.H. (1958) Ovarian homografts: Survival with millipore filter chambers in the monkey. *Obst. & Gynec. (N.Y.),* **12,** 603.

CHAO P.Y., KARAN J.H. & GRODSKY G.M. (1965) Insulin I-131 binding in serum from normal and diabetic subjects by ultracentrifugation and gel filtration. *Diabetes,* **14,** 27.

CLEVELAND W.W., FOGEL B.J., BROW W.T. & KAY H.E.M. (1968) Foetal thymic transplant in a case of Di George's syndrome. *Lancet,* ii, 1211.

CONGDON C.C., UPHOFF D. & LORENZ E. (1962) 'Modification of acute irradiation injury in mice and guinea pigs by injection of bone-marrow: A histological study. *J. Nat. Cancer Inst.* **13,** 73.

CONGDON C.C. (1968) Secondary Disease in Radiation Chimeras. In *Bone Marrow Conservation, Culture and Transplantation.* International Atomic Energy Authority, Vienna (1969), p. 21.

COUPLAND R.E. (1957) Growth of pancreatic islet tissue in the anterior chamber of the eye. *Nature, Lond.* **179,** 51.

DE JODE R.L. & HOWARD J.M. (1962) Studies in pancreatico-duodenal transplantation. *Surg. Gynec. & Obst.* **114,** 553.

DE KONING J., VAN BEKKUM D.W., DICKE K.A., DOOREN L.J., VAN ROOD J.J., RADL J. (1969) Transplantation of bone marrow cells and fetal thymus in an infant with lymphopenic immunological deficiency. *Lancet,* **1,** 1223.

DELEU J. & TRUETA J. (1965) Vascularisation of bone grafts in the anterior chamber of the eye. *J. Bone Jt. Surg.* **47B,** 319.

DEMPSTER W.J. (1969) Transplantation and the thymus. *Lancet,* i, 468.

DEVLIN J.G., BRIEN T. & STEPHENSON N. (1967) Relation between antibody and insulin dose. *Brit. med. J.* i, 542.

DUPLAN J.F. & MONIER R. (1961) Evolution of radio chimeras as a function of the bone-marrow or foetal liver origin of the grafted haemopoietic cells. *Cr. Soc. Biol. (Paris),* **155,** 712.

FORD C.E., HAMERTON J.L., BARNES D.W.H. & LOUTIT J.F. (1956) Cytological identification of radiation chimeras. *Nature, Lond.* **177,** 452.

GODING J.R., MCCRACKEN J.A. & BAIRD D.T. (1967) The study of ovarian function in the ewe by means of a vascular autotransplantation technique. *J. Endocr.* **39,** 37.

GOLDZEIHER M.A. & BARISHAW S.B. (1937) Transplantation of adrenal tissue in Addison's disease. *Endocrinology,* **21,** 394.

GONET A. & RENOLD A.E. (1965) Homografting of fetal rat pancreas. *Diabetologia,* **1,** 91.

GRAINGER G.A., WEISTER R.S. & HOLMES B. (1965) The pathogenesis of acute allogeneic disease in mice studied by parabiosis. *Transplantation,* **3,** 524.

GREGUSOVA V. & HUPKA S. (1961) On the distribution of ^{51}Cr-labelled bone marrow cells in irradiated rats. *Neoplasma (Bratisl),* **8,** 577.

HARDY M.A., QUINT J. & STATE D. (1970) The effect of antilymphocyte serum and other immunosuppressive agents on canine jejunal allografts. *Ann Surg.* **171,** 51.

HARRISON F.A. (1969) Personal communication.

HATHAWAY W.E., MULL M.M., GITHENS J.H., GROTH C.G., MARCHIORO T.L. & STARZL T.E. (1969) Attempted spleen transplantation in classical hemophilia. *Transplantation,* **7,** 73.

HÉDON M.E. (1892) Greffe sous-cutanée du Pancreas-son importance dans l'étude due diabéte pancreatique. *Archive de Physiologie Normale et Pathologique.* 5° *series* IV.

HERNDON C.H. (1960) Principles of bone graft surgery—different methods of operative procedure and indications for each. *American Academy of Orthopaedic Surgeons (Instructional Course Lecture),* **17,** 149.

HORN J.S. (1969) The Reattachment of Severed Extremities. In *Recent Advances in Orthopaedics,* ed. APLEY A.G. London: J. & A.Churchill, p. 49.

HONG R., KAY H.E.M., COOPER M.D., MENWISSEN H., ALLAN M.J.G. & GOOD R.A. (1969) Immunological restitution in lymphopenic immunological deficiency syndrome. *Lancet*, i, 503.

HOUSE E.L., BURTON C., COOPER H., ANDERSON E. (1958) The implantation of neonatal pancreas in the cheek pouch of the alloxan diabetic hamster. *Endocrinology*, **63**, 389.

HULTQUIST G.T. & THORELL J. (1963) Isolering av pankreas övävnad genom transplantation. *Nordisk Medicin*, **69**, 247.

HURN B.A.L., FARRANT P.C., YOUNG B.A. & GRAHAME A. (1969) Insulin binding antibody and hormone dosage in non-resistant diabetes. *Postgraduate Medical Journal supplement on Diabetes*, 819.

IDEZUKI Y., GOETZ F.C. & MERKEL F.K. (1968) Experiences with pancreaticoduodenal allotransplantation. *Rev. Francaise Etud. Clin. Biol.* **13**, 996.

IDEZUKI Y., GOETZ F.C. & MERKEL F.K. (1968) Experiences with pancreatico duodenal allotransplantation. *Rev. Franc. Etud. Clin. Biol.* **13**, 996.

JACOB S.W. & DUNPHY J.E. (1963) 'Successful' parathyroid transplantation. A review of the literature. *Amer. J. Surg.* **105**, 196.

JACOBSON L.O., SIMMONS E.L., MARKS E.K., ROBSON M.J., BETHARD W.F. & GASTRON E.E. (1950) The role of the spleen in radiation injury and recovery. *J. Lab. clin. med.* **35**, 746.

LARGIADER F., HEGGLIN J., JAKOB A., MEILI H.U. (1968) Erhaltens exokrine Funktion als Voraussetzung für den Erfolg der Pankreastransplantation. *Helvetica Chirugica Acta.* **1**, 2321.

LEAKE C.D. & LEAKE B.W. (1923) The erythropoietic action of red bone marrow and splenic extracts. *J. Pharmacol. exp. Ther.* **22**, 75.

LESTRADET H. & BILLAUD L. (1968) Degenerative complications after 15 years infantile diabetes. *La Presse Medicale*, **76**, 303.

LILLEHEI R.C., GOOT B. & MILLER F.A. (1959) The physiological response of the dog small bowel to ischaemia, including prolonged *in vitro* preservation of the bowel with successful replacement and survival. *Ann. Surg.* **150**, 543.

LILLEHEI R.C., MANAX W.G. & LYONS G.W. (1966) Transplantation of gastrointestinal organs including small intestine and stomach. *Gastroenterology*, **51**, 936.

LILLEHEI R.C., IDEZUKI Y., FEEMSTER J.A. DIETZMAN R.H., KELLY W.D., MERKEL F.K., GOETZ F.C., LYONS G.W., MANAX W.G. (1967) Transplantation of stomach, intestine and pancreas: experimental and clinical observations. *Surgery*, **62**, 721.

LINDSLEY D.L., ODELL T.I. & TAUSCHE F.G. (1955) Implantation of functional erythropoietic elements following total body irradiation. *Proc. Soc. exp. Biol. (N.Y.)*, **90**, 512.

MACELROY D.K. (1963) Failure of bank bone. *J. Bone Jt. Surg.* **45A**, 1555.

MARCHIORO T.L., FUDENBERG H., ROWLANDS D.T., RIFKIND D., WADDELL W.R. & STARZL T.E. (1964) Splenic Homotransplantation. *Ann. N.Y. Acad. Sci.* **120**, 626.

MATHÉ G., SCHWARTZENBERG L.,AMIEL J.L., SCHNEIDER M.,CATTAM A. & SCHLUMBERGER J.R. (1968) Effects and Complications of Bone Marrow Transplantation in Man, In *Bone Marrow Conservation, Culture and Transplantation* Moscow, July 1968. International Atomic Energy Agency, Vienna 1969, p. 47.

MERLE D'AUBIGNÉ R., MËARY R. & THOMINE J.M. (1966) La resection dans le traitment des tumeurs des os. *Rev. Chir. Orthop.* **52**, 305.

MERKEL F.K., KELLY W.D., GOETZ F.C. & MANEY J. (1968) Irradiated heterotopic segmental canine pancreatic allografts. *Surgery*, **63**, 2291.

MINKOWSKY J. (1892) Weitere Mitteilung über den Diabetes mellitus nach Exstirpation des Pankreas. *Berl. klin. Wchnschr.* **29**, 90.

NORMAN J.C., COVELLI V.H. & SISE H.S. (1968a) Transplantation of the spleen. Experimental cure of hemophilia. *Surgery* **64**, 1.

OTTOLENGHI C.E. (1966) Massive osteoarticular bone grafts. *J. Bone Jt. Surg.* **48B**, 646.

PEGG D.E. (1966) Bone Marrow Transplantation, p. 96. London: Lloyd-Luke.

PERLEY M. & KIPNIS D.M. (1966) Plasma insulin response to glucose and tolbutamide of normal weight and obese diabetic and non-diabetic subjects. *Diabetes*, **15**, 867.

PIRART J. (1965) Diabetic neuropathy: A metabolic or a vascular disease? *Diabetes*, **14**, 1.

QUINT J., HARDY M.A. & STATE D. (1968) Effect of ALS on absorptive function and survival of dog intestinal allografts. *Surg. Forum*, **19**, 184.

REEMSTMA K., GIRALDO N., DEPP D.A. & EICHWALD E.J. (1968) Islet-cell transplantation. *Ann. Surg.* **168**, 436.

REYNOLDS F.C. & OLIVER D.R. (1950) Experimental evaluation of homogenous bone grafts. *J. Bone Jt. Surg.* **32A**, 283.

ROSEN F.S., GOTOFF S.P., CRAIG J.M., RITCHIE J. & JANEWAY C.A. (1966) Further observations on Swiss agammaglobulinaemia—the effect of syngeneic marrow cells. *New Engl. J. Med.* **274**, 18.

SELLS R.A. (1969) Pancreatic Ileus Transplantation. Presented to the meeting of the Surgical Research Society, The Society of University Surgeons and the European Society for Experimental Surgery in London, July 1969.

SELTZER H.S. & SMITH W.L. (1959) Plasma insulin activity after glucose: Index of insulinogenic reserve in normal and diabetic man. *Diabetes*, **8**, 417.

SHAFFER C.F. & HULKA J.F. (1969) Ovarian graft-host interactions in corneal encapsulated homografts. *Americal Journal of Obst. & Gynec.* **103**, 78.

SICARD A. & BINET J-P. (1950) La conservation des transplants osseux et leur emploi en chirurgie. *Presse Medicale*, **58**, 433.

SISE H.S., COVELLI V.H. & NORMAN J.C. (1968) *Splenic Transplantation for Haemophilia.* Read before 49th Annual session of the American College of Physicians, in association with the Royal College of Physicians, London: Boston, April, 1968.

SNELL G.D. (1970) Immunologic enhancement. *Surg. Gynec. & Obst.* **130**, 1109.

STURGIS S.H. & CASTELLANOS H. (1958) Ovarian homografts *Obstet. & Gynec.* **12**, 603.

TEIXEIRA E., SHARKEY E., COLWELL J. & BERGAN J.J. (1966) Insulin and glucose levels following pancreas allografting. *Surgical Forum*, **17**, 205.

UPHOFF D.E. & LAW L.W. (1957) Histocompatibility genes and irradiation protection by bone marrow inoculation in mice. *Radiat. Res.* **7**, 456.

VAN BEKKUM D.W. (1968) Prevention Control of Secondary Disease Following Allogeneic Bone Marrow Transplantation. In *Bone Marrow Conservation, Culture and Transplantation.* International Atomic Energy Agency, Vienna, 35, 1969.

WEBSTER W.P., PENICK G.D., PEACOCK E.E. & BRINKLAW K.M. (1967) Allotransplantation of the spleen in haemophilia. *N. Carolina Med. J.* **28**, 505.

WEISER R.S., GRANGER G.A., BROWN W., BAKER P., JUTILA J. & HOLMES B. (1965) Production of acute allogeneic disease in mice. *Transplantation*, **3**, 10.

WHITE P. (1960) Childhood diabetes, its course and influence on the second and third generations. *Diabetes*, **9**, 345.

WOODRUFF M.F.A. (1952a) Surgical replacement therapy. *Postgrad. med. J.* **28**, 534.

WOODRUFF M.F.A. (1952b) Transplantation of homologous tissue and its surgical applications. Hunterian Lecture. *Ann. Royal Coll. Surgeons England*, **11**, 173 (September).

YALOW R.S. & BERSON S.A. (1959) Assay of plasma insulin of human subjects by immunological methods. *Nature, Lond.* **184**, 1648.

YAMADA K. & WAKAYAMA E. (1961) Studies on some immunologic aspects of bone marrow transplantation. *Acta haemat. J.* **24**, 702.

Part 7
Ethics, the Law and the Future

CHAPTER 33

Ethics, the Law and the Future

R.Y. Calne

ETHICS AND THE LAW

The publicity that followed the first cardiac allograft in man highlighted many ethical aspects of organ grafting, yet the main result has been confusion rather than an understanding of the problems. The immense emotional excitement concerning heart grafting was eagerly exploited by the mass media and unfortunately also by some medical men. Initial unwarranted optimism and adulation were followed by bitter criticism. In particular, since the operation can be performed by any competent cardiac surgeon, the prestige of the individual and institution appeared to influence some centres in deciding to pursue heart grafting even in the absence of any previous interest or research background in the subject. Some of those who did not share in the apparent glory were particularly vindictive in their criticism and did not hesitate to denounce all transplantation in press and on the radio and television. Some of the emotive phrases such as vulture 'human vivisector' have had a disastrous influence on all organ transplantation and undermined the public's confidence in the medical profession. If some surgeons have lacked seriousness and sufficient responsibility in their approach to transplantation, their misdemeanours are trivial compared with the prejudiced and ignorant vituperation of some of the critics, whose efforts have resulted in needless deaths of many young people awaiting kidney transplantation.

The plight of those in need of organ grafting is the main ethical problem, and it has received remarkably little attention. A community that can afford vast expenditure in arms designed to destroy, can certainly cover the relatively minor financial burden required to treat the sick by organ grafting—moreover a successful organ graft is of fiscal benefit to the state, restoring an individual to work and costing often little more, and sometimes even less than conventional palliative hospital care, with a tragic fatal end. To argue that the money could be better spent in preventative medicine or under-developed countries is irrelevant. Suffering from disease is not confined to poor communities. Valuable treatment, expensive in its development, will become increasingly less costly as techniques improve and then the benefits will be available to all.

It is a very sad indictment of the community in the United Kingdom that only 10% of young people with terminal renal disease are receiving treatment in the form of transplantation and dialysis. More than 2000 are dying each year without help. The Government Department of Health is spending large sums in setting up transplantation and dialysis centres, but these cannot operate adequately when donor organs do not become available. Yet there are more than enough deaths from accidents, cerebral tumour and haemorrhage to provide all the kidneys required. The failure is a result of two main difficulties which are inter-related, namely co-operation with the profession and public understanding and confidence.

There must be few people in a civilized community, who would prefer their organs to be burned or buried after death, rather than that they should save another's life. There are, however, three points of worry—

1 Can there be assurance that the best medical care will be utilized in their terminal illness with no thought of sparing therapeutic effort to facilitate organ donation?

2 Will irreversible death have occurred *beyond any doubt whatsoever* before organ removal commences?

3 If organs are used for grafting can the privacy of the bereaved relatives be respected by the mass media?

These points will now be considered further.

1 On this first matter, experience would suggest that reassurance is fully justified. The usual result of the possibility of organ grafting being raised, is for the medical and nursing staff looking after the sick patient to redouble their efforts to try and treat him. The only fear is that these efforts can be over-enthusiastic in cases with irreversible brain damage, who may be kept 'alive' artificially. This results in the tragic situation of caring for a perfused but slowly decomposing corpse.

2 A consideration of death, irreversible and beyond doubt is more complicated although it should be made clear that the diagnosis of death in most cases presents no difficulty. The patient is usually known to be suffering from a fatal disease. Deterioration occurs and eventually the heart stops beating and breathing ceases. If this situation persists for more than 5 min in an individual at normal body temperature, then death can be diagnosed with complete confidence. Stories of people awaking in the mortuary or a coffin have been a haunting fear to some who have asked for an artery to be incised to make sure that they are dead. At least this danger of premature burial is eliminated by being an organ donor! In the context of proposed organ removal, great care in diagnosing death is usually taken by several doctors. In the extremely unlikely event of a mistake being made, the error would be revealed and rectified by the first touch of the knife.

There are cases, often especially suitable as organ donors, where the diagnosis of death is less straightforward. These are patients who have suffered cardiac arrest or brain damage sufficient to abolish spontaneous respiration and in whom the circulation and/or pulmonary ventilation have been maintained by artificial means. The only satisfactory management of such cases is for resuscitation to be continued until brain death is apparent beyond any doubt. Thus whilst there is still any difficulty in being sure no effort is spared in trying to save the patient. Once however irreversible brain death is established, pursuance of resuscitative efforts can do no good, in fact the reverse is true. The patient will not benefit and his relatives will suffer or, even worse, become indifferent, when they realize that the perfused tissues they visit have no relationship to the person they once loved.

If all the following features are present then the brain must be dead beyond doubt:

1 Fixed wide dilated pupils.
2 Absent cerebral reflexes.
3 Absence of spontaneous respiration in the presence of adequate CO_2 drive.
4 Absent cerebral circulation demonstrated by carotid and/or vertebral angiography and/or brain scanning.
5 A persistently flat EEG.
6 Cessation of the retinal circulation with red cell sludging on ophthalmoscopic examination.

It is usually not necessary to perform the special tests to decide to cease resuscitation, but they can be valuable where there is difficulty, for example, in cases of barbiturate poisoning or in patients who are hypothermic. The consideration so far has had *absolutely nothing* to do with transplantation.

The decision to abandon resuscitation is related *solely* to the case of the afflicted patient, once made however, the transplantation team should be informed as soon as possible so they can prepare the instruments, operating theatre and personnel. As soon as the donor is dead the quicker the organs are cooled and removed the more likely are they to function well after grafting.

A powerful argument has been advanced and is gaining increasing acceptance in America and the continent of Europe, to permit organ removal from patients with established brain death—*coma depassé*—whilst ventilation of the lungs is continued and the circulation is intact. This allows the surgeon to remove the organs unhurriedly whilst they are perfused with oxygenated blood and undoubtedly improves the transplantation results. There are many doctors, however, particularly in the United Kingdom who find this procedure of organ removal from patients with *coma depassé* unacceptable. They argue that no matter what precautions are taken, there is still the possibility of diagnosing brain death erroneously. If however resuscitation is abandoned and the organs are not removed until the circulation has ceased, then the brain must be dead from ischaemia and the irreversibility of the process will have been demonstrated. Following this conventional diagnosis of death, livers have been transplanted successfully. Since the liver is the most sensitive organ to ischaemic damage, with the exception of the brain itself, conventional diagnosis of death is compatible with all types of organ transplantation and has the immensely reassuring feature of *revealed* irreversibility of death that provides the public and the profession with adequate safeguards. It must be admitted, nevertheless, that the practical advantages of removing organs from 'living corpses' will produce better results.* The chances of making a mistake in the diagnosis of *coma depassé* must be infinitesimal, if the assessment is undertaken by experienced neurologists or neurosurgeons. There can however be an irrational uneasiness in the minds of many that should not be disregarded. Reassurance is only certain when brain death is *revealed*. Thus few would object of organ removal from a decapitated body, an anencephalic monster or an individual whose whole brain has been visibly extruded after an accident, even though in each of these instances the heart were still beating and providing an adequate circulation and the lungs were ventilated mechanically. These 'living corpses' would be surely acceptable organ donors on ethical grounds. In other cases where death of the brain is established by means other than visible absence of the brain, a difference of opinion will doubtless persist amongst members of the

* Which type of donor has been used is often not specified in comparisons of organ transplantation results from different centres—a serious omission, since *coma depassé* cases from the point of view of ischaemic damage are 'live' unrelated donors.

profession and the laity, as to whether organ removal whilst there is a good circulation is or is not justifiable. To wait for circulatory arrest after cessation of resuscitation can induce misgivings in none and is compatible with good organ grafting results. The merits are obvious.

It is very sad that the charitable donation of organs after death cannot remain private. The callous disregard of the feelings of bereaved relatives by the mass media has been scarcely credible. Photographs have been published with personal information quite unrelated to the operation. In the United Kingdom where complaints have been made that this information has been obtained and published contrary to the expressed wishes of the relatives, the Press Council, one of whose functions is meant to be to protect the public from such abuses, has twice rejected the complaints on the grounds that publishing the material was in the general 'public interest'. The result, as could be anticipated, has been a reluctance on the part of bereaved relations to give permission for organ removal from the deceased next of kin, specifically because of the fear of publicity, which the doctors cannot prevent and the Press Council has condoned. How little sympathy have those responsible for the young patients suffering from kidney disease, who have died needlessly and for their tragically bereaved relatives.

THE LAW

In most countries, legislation relating to the disposal of dead bodies has not been framed to facilitate organ grafting. In some states, such as the United Kingdom, the law is confused on several important matters that have not so far been tested. It is unlikely that there will be sufficient organs for grafting until it is regarded as routine practice by the public and the profession for organs to be removed from all suitable cadaver donors. Then no doubt the mass media would lose interest and organ removal from corpses would be no more newsworthy than a coroner's autopsy—which is compulsory by law and is seldom objected to by individuals or public opinion and is not a subject of detailed ghoulish discussion.

In the United Kingdom, unless the donor in his lifetime had clearly expressed his wish to be an organ donor after death, it is necessary to obtain permission from the relatives. Moreover, if the case is under the jurisdiction of the coroner, his consent must also be obtained. Frequently, relatives and/or the coroner cannot be contacted in the short time available before irreversible ischaemic damage will have occurred to the organs required. Thus many organs are wasted when, in fact, it later transpires that both the patient in his lifetime and his relatives would have wished them to be used. Doctors looking after dying patients often refuse to inform the transplantation team for fear that the request to the relatives will cause them further unnecessary distress. This can be true—especially in cases of sudden unexpected death, but the reverse is by no means rare. A not unusual reply is—'I am glad you asked doctor because I am sure he would have wished it and then perhaps some good may come from our personal tragedy'.

In Sweden, Denmark, France, Italy and Israel permission from the relatives is not required. This is probably the only form of legislation that will permit satisfactory development of organ grafting. Contracting into a scheme of voluntary donation would never produce sufficient response, although it would be helpful.

A reasonable legislative framework could be constructed on the following lines.

1 *The individual's wishes should be respected* so that any who did not want their organs used for grafting would register an objection on behalf of themselves and/or their children. Suitable machinery would be set up to record and retrieve this information. This should present no serious problems of computerization. It would be necessary for the names of objectors to be determined by a hospital at any time—day or night. As an added precaution, objectors could carry a card on their person stating their wishes. It should be possible to specify organs with regard to permission and also for an individual to change his mind at any time. Those feeling strongly that they wished to be organ donors could 'contract in' under the same scheme.

2 *If active objection had not been made—permission would be assumed.* After death—established by traditional criteria—namely cessation of the circulation and spontaneous respiration, organs could be removed. Permission from the relatives would not be necessary, but if they were available they would certainly be consulted as to the deceased's wishes and should the relatives object, their feelings would be respected, since this would be the only humane action.

3 If it was felt desirable to remove organs whilst the circulation continued after *coma depassé* had been diagnosed, permission of the relatives after full explantation would be necessary even in cases where the patient had 'contracted in' as a donor. In such cases signatures from two consultants experienced in neurology and/or neurosurgery should testify brain death.

4 The potential donor in his lifetime should not be interfered with in any way not specifically directed towards his own treatment for purposes of transplantation except for removal of a few ml of blood for tissue typing. He should not be moved to another hospital to facilitate organ removal unless he had specifically requested that this were done.

5 Doctors *not* concerned with the transplantation operation should care for the donor, decide if and when to abandon resuscitation, if resuscitative measures had been taken and diagnose death.

6 In cases coming under the jurisdiction of the coroner, arrangements with the coroner and/or his pathologist, should allow organ removal to proceed, this forming part of the coroner's autopsy examination. The surgeon removing the organs would report in detail to the coroner any relevant findings. In certain specified cases, which would be infrequent, where organ removal might interfere with establishing the cause of death, the coroner's pathologist should partake in the operation.

7 Publicizing the names of donors by the mass media would be unlawful even if the relatives wished it. Any complaint of an irregularity occurring would be reported to the coroner, who would then hold a public inquest.

This framework of proposed legislation would probably be acceptable to the public of most civilized communities provided accurate information was fully available. No matter what laws are devised, eventually doctors have to make decisions based on their knowledge and experience and the only real safeguard is the trust of the public in the integrity of the medical profession. Such trust is an essential feature of all clinical practice. Operative or medical treatment given for any illness implies a bond of trust between the patient and his doctor that the treatment is necessary. Moreover it will be undertaken by the doctor conscientiously to the best of his ability. The same confidence is necessary in all aspects of transplantation surgery relating both to the donor and the recipient.

Live donors

The ethical factors have been considered in Chapter 10. It was suggested that with an adult close blood relative medically suitable and of a good tissue match with the recipient, if failure to donate a kidney would lead to a genuine feeling of deprivation, then to proceed is justified. The law in the United Kingdom does not provide for organ donation from live volunteers, which technically constitutes an assault. It is, however, most unlikely that this could ever be successfully upheld in court.

The recipient

Provided fatal disease of a vital organ has failed to respond to conventional treatment—if there are no obvious contra-indications and an organ graft would seem to be a feasible form of treatment, then it is surely correct to bring this possibility to the patient's attention. In most cases, however, the patient will have already requested an organ transplant. It is important that the current situation is carefully explained to the patient, including the attendent risks. If after careful consideration the patient and his relatives wish to proceed then this is the correct course. A similar argument is used to decide whether or not to perform all major risky surgery. If death is 100% certain in a few weeks without treatment, and organ grafting has only a 5% chance of restoring the patient to a normal life for a year, then the patient should be given that chance if he wishes. Fortunately, as has been described in early chapters, the chances are much better than 5% with most organ grafts.

THE FUTURE

Transplantation is already an established and valuable therapeutic procedure for kidney disease and has helped a number of patients dying from liver and heart diseases. There can be no doubt that the results will continue to improve and more organs will be successfully transplanted.

If the confidence of the public is restored so that new legislation can be introduced to help provide more organs, many young people now dying could be restored to a happy and healthy existence. Advances in tissue typing, logistics of organ distribution and preservation can be anticipated. If, as seems likely, safer and more specific immunosuppression is developed then clinical organ transplantation will be able to help an increasing number of people and will constitute a most valuable part of surgery.

Index